Tropical Medicine
Lecture Notes

This title is also available as an e-book.
For more details, please see
www.wiley.com/buy/9780470658536
or scan this QR code:

Tropical Medicine
Lecture Notes

Edited by

Nick Beeching

Senior Lecturer in Infectious Diseases
Liverpool School of Tropical Medicine
Liverpool, UK

Geoff Gill

Emeritus Professor of International Medicine
Liverpool School of Tropical Medicine
Liverpool, UK

Seventh Edition

WILEY Blackwell

This edition first published 2014 © 2014 by John Wiley & Sons, Ltd
Previous editions: 1981, 1985, 1990, 1995, 2004, 2009

Registered office: John Wiley & Sons, Ltd, The Atrium, Southern Gate, Chichester, West Sussex,
PO19 8SQ, UK

Editorial offices: 9600 Garsington Road, Oxford, OX4 2DQ, UK
The Atrium, Southern Gate, Chichester, West Sussex, PO19 8SQ, UK
111 River Street, Hoboken, NJ 07030-5774, USA

For details of our global editorial offices, for customer services and for information about how
to apply for permission to reuse the copyright material in this book please see our website at
www.wiley.com/wiley-blackwell

Library of Congress Cataloging-in-Publication Data
Lecture notes. Tropical medicine. – Seventh edition / edited by Nick Beeching, Geoff Gill.
    p. ; cm.
  Tropical medicine
  Includes bibliographical references and index.
    ISBN 978-0-470-65853-6 (pbk.) – ISBN 978-1-118-73452-0 – ISBN 978-1-118-73453-7 –
ISBN 978-1-118-73454-4 (eMobi) – ISBN 978-1-118-73455-1 (ePdf) – ISBN 978-1-118-73456-8 (ePub)
  I. Beeching, N., editor of compilation.   II. Gill, Geoffrey V., editor of compilation.   III. Title:
Tropical medicine.
  [DNLM: 1. Tropical Medicine. WC 680]
  RC961
  616.9'883–dc23
                                                                    2013024789

A catalogue record for this book is available from the British Library.

Wiley also publishes its books in a variety of electronic formats. Some content that appears in print
may not be available in electronic books.

Cover image: iStock: world map © Pavel Khorenyan; mosquito © James Benet
Cover design by Grounded Design

Set in 8.5/11pt Utopia Std by Aptara® Inc., New Delhi, India

Printed in the UK

Contents

Contributors, vii

Preface, ix

List of abbreviations, x

New drug names, xiii

How to use your textbook, xiv

About the companion website, xvii

Part 1   A general approach to syndromes/symptom complexes, 1

1   Gastrointestinal presentations, 3

2   Respiratory presentations, 11

3   Neurological presentations, 16

4   Febrile presentations, 24

5   Dermatological presentations, 29

6   The patient with anaemia, 33

7   A syndromic approach to sexually transmitted infections, 38

8   Splenomegaly in the tropics, 47

Part 2   Major tropical infections, 51

9   Malaria, 53

10   Visceral leishmaniasis, 70

11   Cutaneous leishmaniasis, 77

12   Tuberculosis, 82

13   HIV infection and disease in the tropics, 96

14   Onchocerciasis, filariasis and loiasis, 126

15   African trypanosomiasis, 141

16   South American trypanosomiasis (Chagas' disease), 148

17   Schistosomiasis, 151

18   Leprosy, 163

Part 3   Other tropical diseases, 175

19   Amoebiasis, 177

20   Bacillary dysentery, 183

21   Cholera, 186

22   Giardiasis and other intestinal protozoal infections, 190

23   Intestinal cestode infections (tapeworms) including cysticercosis, 195

24   Soil-transmitted helminths, 199

25   Viral hepatitis, 205

26   Liver and intestinal flukes, 214

27   Hydatid disease, 218

28   Pneumonia, 222

29   Lung flukes, 229

30   Tropical pulmonary eosinophilia, 231

31   Pyogenic meningitis, 233

32   Cryptococcal meningitis, 241

33   Encephalitis, 243

34   Acute flaccid paralysis, 248

35   Spastic paralysis, 251

36   Rabies, 254

37   Tetanus, 259

38   Brucellosis, 262

39   Typhoid and paratyphoid fevers, 267

40   Arboviruses, 273

41   Viral haemorrhagic fevers, 276

42   Dengue and yellow fever, 283

43   Relapsing fevers, 289

44   Rickettsial infections, 292

45   Leptospirosis, 294

46   Melioidosis, 297

47   Tropical ulcer, 299

48   Buruli ulcer, 301

49   Myiasis, 305

50 Cutaneous larva migrans, 307

51 Scabies and lice, 309

52 Strongyloidiasis, 311

53 Guinea worm infection
    (dracunculiasis), 315

54 Histoplasmosis, 317

55 Other fungal infections, 319

56 Haemoglobinopathies and red cell
    enzymopathies, 321

57 Haematinic deficiencies, 326

58 Bites and stings, 330

59 Non-communicable diseases, 334

60 Refugee health, 351

61 Syndromes of malnutrition, 358

62 Eye disease in the tropics, 364

63 Neglected tropical diseases, 372

Index, 381

Contributors

Imelda Bates Professor, Liverpool School of Tropical Medicine, Pembroke Place, Liverpool L3 5QA; Honorary Consultant Haematologist, Royal Liverpool University Hospital, Prescot Street, Liverpool L7 8XP
Chapters 6, 8, 56, 57

Mike Beadsworth Honorary Lecturer, Liverpool School of Tropical Medicine, Pembroke Place, Liverpool L3 5QA; Consultant Physician, Tropical & Infectious Disease Unit, Royal Liverpool University Hospital, Prescot Street, Liverpool L7 8XP
Chapters 1, 4

Nick Beeching Senior Lecturer, Liverpool School of Tropical Medicine, Pembroke Place, Liverpool L3 5QA; Clinical Director, Tropical & Infectious Disease Unit, Royal Liverpool University Hospital, Prescot Street, Liverpool L7 8XP
Chapters 1, 5, 18, 25, 27, 29, 30, 31, 38, 41, 53

David Bell Consultant in Infectious Diseases, Brownlee Centre, Gartnavel General Hospital, Great Western Road, Glasgow G12 0YN
Chapter 9

Tom Blanchard Honorary Fellow, Liverpool School of Tropical Medicine, Pembroke Place, Liverpool L3 5QA; Honorary Senior Lecturer, Institute of Translational Medicine, University of Manchester, Oxford Road, Manchester M13 9P; Consultant in Infectious Diseases & Tropical Medicine, North Manchester General Hospital, Delaunays Road, Manchester M8 5RB
Chapter 4

Martin Dedicoat Consultant in Infectious Diseases, Heart of England Foundation Trust, Bordesley Green East, Birmingham B9 5SS
Chapter 13

Tom Doherty Consultant Physician, The Hospital for Tropical Diseases, Tottenham Court Road, London W1T 7DN
Chapter 61

Neil French Professor, Institute of Infection and Global Health, University of Liverpool, West Derby Street, Liverpool L69 7BE; Honorary Consultant Physician, Tropical & Infectious Disease Unit, Royal Liverpool University Hospital, Prescot Street, Liverpool L7 8XP
Chapters 2, 28

Geoff Gill Emeritus Professor, Liverpool School of Tropical Medicine, Pembroke Place, Liverpool L3 5QA; Consultant Physician, Aintree University Hospital, Lower Lane, Liverpool L9 7AL
Chapters 44, 47, 49, 50, 51, 52, 54, 59

Stephen Gordon Professor, Liverpool School of Tropical Medicine, Pembroke Place, Liverpool L3 5QA; Honorary Consultant Physician, Royal Liverpool University Hospital, Prescot Street, Liverpool L7 8XP and Aintree University Hospital, Lower Lane, Liverpool L9 7AL
Chapters 2, 28, 30

Malcolm Kerr-Muir Honorary Lecturer, Liverpool School of Tropical Medicine, Pembroke Place, Liverpool L3 5QA; Consultant Ophthalmologist, Cambridge University Hospitals Trust, Addenbrooke's Hospital, Hills Road, Cambridge CB2 0QQ
Chapter 62

Rachel Kneen Consultant Paediatric Neurologist, Alder Hey Children's Foundation NHS Trust, Eaton Road, Liverpool L12 2AP; Honorary Senior Clinical Lecturer, Institute of Infection and Global Health, University of Liverpool, West Derby Street, Liverpool L69 7BE
Chapters 3, 33, 34

David Lalloo Professor and Dean, Faculty of Clinical Sciences and International Public Health, Liverpool School of Tropical Medicine, Pembroke Place, Liverpool L3 5QA; Honorary Consultant Physician, Tropical & Infectious Disease Unit, Royal Liverpool University Hospital, Prescot Street, Liverpool L7 8XP
Chapters 9, 15, 16, 32, 37, 46, 55, 58

Diana Lockwood Professor, London School of Hygiene & Tropical Medicine, Keppel Street, London WC1E 7HT; Consultant Physician and Leprologist, The Hospital for Tropical Diseases, Tottenham Court Road, London W1T 7DN
Chapter 18

Alastair Miller Honorary Fellow, Liverpool School of Tropical Medicine, Pembroke Place, Liverpool L3 5QA; Honorary Senior Lecturer, Institute of Infection and Global Health, University of Liverpool, West Derby Street, Liverpool L69 7BE; Consultant Physician, Tropical & Infectious Disease Unit, Royal Liverpool University Hospital, Prescot Street, Liverpool L7 8XP
Chapter 45

David Molyneux Emeritus Professor, Centre for Neglected Tropical Diseases, Liverpool School of Tropical Medicine, Pembroke Place, Liverpool L3 5QA
Chapter 63

Kevin Mortimer Senior Lecturer, Liverpool School of Tropical Medicine, Pembroke Place, Liverpool L3 5QA; Honorary Consultant in Respiratory Medicine, Aintree University Hospital, Lower Lane, Liverpool L9 7AL
Chapter 59

Tim O'Dempsey Senior Lecturer, Liverpool School of Tropical Medicine, Pembroke Place, Liverpool L3 5QA; Honorary Consultant Physician, Tropical & Infectious Disease Unit, Royal Liverpool University Hospital, Prescot Street, Liverpool L7 8XP
Chapters 10, 11, 14, 19, 20, 22, 23, 24, 26, 27, 43, 48, 60

Chris Parry Honorary Research Fellow, Liverpool School of Tropical Medicine, Pembroke Place, Liverpool L3 5QA
Chapter 39

Paul Shears Consultant Microbiologist, Microbiology Department, Wirral University Teaching Hospital NHS Foundation Trust, Wirral CH63 4JY
Chapter 21

Rebecca Sinfield General Practitioner; Associate Tutor of Clinical Education, Faculty of Education, Edge Hill University, St Helens Road, Ormskirk L39 4QP
Chapter 61

Tom Solomon Professor of Neurological Sciences and Head, Institute of Infection and Global Health, University of Liverpool, West Derby Street, Liverpool L69 7BE; Honorary Consultant Physician, The Walton Centre NHS Foundation Trust, Lower Lane, Liverpool L9 7JL
Chapters 3, 33, 34, 35, 36, 40, 41, 42

Bertie Squire Professor, Liverpool School of Tropical Medicine, Pembroke Place, Liverpool L35QA; Honorary Consultant Physician, Tropical & Infectious Disease Unit, Royal Liverpool University Hospital, Prescot Street, Liverpool L7 8XP
Chapter 12, 17

Russell Stothard Professor, Liverpool School of Tropical Medicine, Pembroke Place, Liverpool L3 5QA
Chapter 17

Miriam Taegtmeyer Senior Lecturer, Liverpool School of Tropical Medicine, Pembroke Place, Liverpool L3 SQA; Honorary Consultant Physician, Tropical & Infectious Disease Unit, Royal Liverpool University Hospital, Prescot Street, Liverpool L7 8XP
Chapters 7, 13

Jecko Thachil Consultant Haematologist, Manchester Royal Infirmary, Oxford Road, Manchester M13 9WL
Chapters 6, 8, 56, 57

Ralf Weigel Lecturer, Liverpool School of Tropical Medicine, Pembroke Place, Liverpool L3 5QA; Honorary Consultant Paediatrician, Alder Hey Children's NHS Foundation Trust, Eaton Road, Liverpool, L12 2AP
Chapter 13

Maureen Wilkinson Consultant Psychiatrist, Cheshire and Wirral Partnership NHS Foundation Trust, Countess of Chester Health Park, Chester CH2 1BQ
Chapter 59

Preface

It is now over 30 years since the first edition of *Lecture Notes in Tropical Medicine* appeared (1981). This was entirely conceived and written by Dr Dion Bell, Reader and Honorary Consultant Physician at the Liverpool School of Tropical Medicine. The book rapidly became very popular both in the United Kingdom and the tropics. Dion was one of the greatest tropical clinicians and teachers of his time; and he wrote *Lecture Notes* in a practical, authoritative and entertaining style. Two more editions followed over the next few years, again entirely self-written, and the book became a classic of its type, and required reading for doctors taking the DTM&H (Diploma in Tropical Medicine and Hygiene) diploma at either the Liverpool or London tropical schools.

By the time of the 4th edition in 1994, the spectrum of tropical disease had expanded considerably (particularly with the emergence of HIV/AIDS), and in view of this other authors from the Liverpool School became involved to cover specific topics. After this edition, Dion retired and later sadly died. It has been a privilege for us to take over editorship of this important project. In the 5th edition, we continued and expanded the principle of multi-authorship, but ensured that all writers had practical experience of their topics, and that they were either staff or associated teachers or examiners of the Liverpool School of Tropical Medicine. For this edition we also introduced syndromic chapters on subjects such as fever, splenomegaly, skin disease etc. New chapters were also added on emerging problems such as refugee health and non-communicable diseases (NCDs).

In the 6th edition, a chapter on nutritional syndromes was added, and a mental health section was added to the NCD chapter. The layout of the book changed, with a move to colour text and incorporation of clinical images throughout the chapters instead of being placed on separate colour plates in the centre of the book. In the current 7th edition, all chapters have been updated, particularly important with rapidly evolving topics such as malaria, tuberculosis and HIV/AIDS. New chapters on tropical ophthalmology and neglected tropical diseases (NTDs) have been added, and we welcome on board the authors of these chapters – respectively Malcolm Kerr-Muir and David Molyneux. We have tried to retain the emphasis on practical issues of importance at the bedside and in the clinic. Two exciting developments for this edition are that an electronic version will be available, and also that a set of online multiple-choice questions (MCQs) for each chapter have been written with explanatory answers. For this project we are very grateful to Dr Dom Colbert. We believe that both these innovations will greatly enhance the availability and educational experience of the book. A final change for the 7th edition is that though the editorial team remains the same as in the last two editions (Geoff Gill and Nick Beeching), the lead editor role has moved from Geoff Gill to Nick Beeching.

Finally, as well as continuing the style and philosophy of the book, we have continued the financial arrangements with the publishers begun by Dion Bell in 1981. No author or editor has ever accepted payment, and all royalties are given directly to a fund held at the Liverpool School of Tropical Medicine. This is used to award bursaries to Liverpool medical students undertaking elective periods in tropical countries.

We hope that this new edition is useful to both students and practitioners of medicine in the tropics. As always, we welcome any comments and criticisms.

Nick Beeching
Geoff Gill

List of abbreviations

3TC	Lamivudine		BMI	body mass index
AAFB	acid- and alcohol-fast bacilli		BP	blood pressure
Ab	antibody		b.p.m.	beats per minute
ABC	abacavir		BT	borderline tuberculoid leprosy
ACE	angiotensin-converting enzyme		cAMP	cyclic adenosine monophosphate
ACPR	adequate clinical and parasitological response		cART	combination antiretroviral therapy
ACR	adequate clinical response		CATT	card agglutination test for trypanosomes
ACT	artemisinin combination therapy		CBT	cognitive behaviour therapy
ADLA	acute dermatolymphangioadenitis		CCA	circulating cathodic antigen
AFB	acid-fast bacilli		CCHF	Crimean–Congo haemorrhagic fever
AFL	acute filarial lymphangitis		CD4	CD4 positive T lymphocyte (formerly T-helper cell)
Ag	antigen			
AgB	antigen B		CDC	Centers for Disease Control and Prevention (USA).
AHI	acute HIV infection			
AIDP	acute inflammatory demyelinating polyneuropathy		ComDT	Community directed treatment with ivermectin
			CFT	complement fixation test
AIDS	acquired immune deficiency syndrome		CHE	complex humanitarian emergency
ALA	amoebic liver abscess		CHK	chikungunya virus
ALB	albendazole		CIATT	card indirect agglutination test for trypanosomes
AMAN	acute motor axonal neuropathy			
AmB	amphotericin B		CL	cutaneous leishmaniasis
APOC	African Programme for Onchocerciasis Control		CM	cryptococcal meningitis
			CMI	cell-mediated immunity
AQ	Amodiaquine		CMR	crude mortality rate
ARB	angiotensin receptor blocker		CMV	cytomegalovirus
ARC	AIDS-related complex		CNS	central nervous system
ARDS	acute respiratory distress syndrome		COPD	chronic obstructive pulmonary disease
ARI	annual risk of infection		CQ	chloroquine
ART	antiretroviral therapy		CRP	C-reactive protein
ARV	antiretroviral drug		CSF	cerebrospinal fluid
AST	aspartate transaminase		CT	computerized tomography
ATB	antibiotic		CTC	community based therapeutic care
AVPU	Alert, responds to Voice, to Pain, or Unresponsive		CTF	Colorado tick fever
			CVP	central venous pressure
AZT	zidovudine		CXR	chest x-ray
BB	borderline leprosy		DALY	disability adjusted life year
BCG	bacille Calmette–Guérin		DART	Development of Anti-Retroviral Therapy
b.d.	twice daily		DAT	direct agglutination test
BI	bacterial index		d4T	stavudine
BL	borderline lepromatous leprosy			

DCL	diffuse cutaneous leishmaniasis
ddI	didanosine
DD5	double diffusion test for arc 5
DEN	dengue virus
DDS	4,4-diaminodiphenylsulphone
DDT	dichlorodiphenyl-trichloroethane
DEC	diethylcarbamazine citrate
DF	dengue fever
DHF	dengue haemorrhagic fever
DHFR	dihydrofolate reductase
DHPS	dihydropteroate synthetase
DIC	disseminated intravascular coagulation
DKA	diabetic ketoacidosis
DOT	directly observed therapy
DOTS	directly observed short course therapy
DSS	dengue shock syndrome
DTH	delayed-type hypersensitivity
DTM&H	diploma in tropical medicine and hygiene
DTP	diptheria, tetanus and pertussis
EBV	Epstein–Barr virus
ECG	electrocardiogram
EEE	eastern equine encephalitis
EEG	electroencephalography
EFV	efavirenz
EHEC	enterohaemorrhagic
EIA	enzyme immunoassay
EITB	enzyme-linked immunoelectrotransfer blot
ELISA	enzyme-linked immunoabsorbent assay
EMF	endomyocardial fibrosis
ENL	erythema nodosum leprosum
EPI	extended programme of immunization
ERCP	endoscopic retrograde cholangiopancreatography
ESR	erythrocyte sedimentation rate
ETF	early treatment failure
EFV	Efavirenz
FAR	fever–arthralgia–rash
FAST	fast agglutination-screening test
FBC	full blood count
FCPD	fibrocalculous pancreatic diabetes
FES	fasciola excretory–secretory
FEV1	forced expiratory volume in 1 second
FGM	female genital mutilation
FGT	formol gel test
FTC	emtricitabine
FUO	fever of unknown origin
FVC	forced vital capacity
G6PD	glucose-6-phosphate dehydrogenase
GABA	γ-aminobutyric acid
GAELF	Global Alliance for the Elimination of Lymphatic Filariasis
GAVI	Global Alliance for Vaccines and Immunization
GBS	Guillain-Barré syndrome
GCS	Glasgow coma score
GDP	gross domestic product
GPELF	Global Programme to Eliminate Lymphatic Filariasis
GSK	GlaxoSmithKline
GTT	glucose tolerance test
HAV	hepatitis A virus
HbA	adult haemoglobin
HbF	foetal haemoglobin
HbS	sickle haemoglobin
HBeAg	hepatitis B 'e' antigen
HBIg	hepatitis B immunoglobulin
HBsAg	hepatitis B surface antigen
HBV	hepatitis B virus
HCC	hepatocellular carcinoma
HCV	hepatitis C virus
HDCV	human diploid cell vaccine
HDV	hepatitis D virus
HEV	hepatitis E virus
HFRS	haemorrhagic fever with renal syndrome
Hib	*Haemophilus influenzae* type b
HIV	human immunodeficiency virus
HLA	human leucocyte antigen
HNK	hyperosmolar non-ketotic coma
HPV	human papilloma virus
HRP-2	histidine-rich protein 2
HSV2	herpes simplex virus type 2
HTLV-1	human T lymphotrophic virus type 1
HUS	haemolytic uraemic syndrome
ICT	immunochromatographic card test
IDP	internally displaced person
IFAT	indirect fluorescent antibody test
IFN	interferon
Ig	immunoglobulin
IGRA	interferon gamma release assays

IL	interleukin	MRI	magnetic resonance imaging
i.m.	intramuscular	MSF	Médecins sans frontières
IMAI	Integrated Management of Adult Illness strategy	MTB	*Mycobacterium tuberculosis*
		MTCT	mother to child transmission
IMCI	Integrated Management of Childhood Illness strategy	MUAC	mid-upper arm circumference
		MVE	Murray Valley encephalitis
INR	international normalized ratio	NAAT	automated nucleic acid amplification tests
IPT	intermittent presumptive therapy	NCD	non-communicable disease
IRD	immune reconstitution disease	NGO	non-governmental organizations
IRIS	immune reconstitution inflammatory syndrome	NK	natural killer
IRS	indoor residual spraying	NNN	Novy, MacNeal and Nicolle's medium
ITNs	insecticide-treated bednets	NNRTI	non-nucleoside reverse transcriptase inhibitor
i.v.	intravenous	NRTI	nucleoside reverse transcriptase inhibitor
IVDU	intravenous drug use	NSAID	non-steroidal anti-inflammatory drug
IVF	intravenous fluids	NTDs	neglected tropical diseases
IVM	ivermectin	NTS	non-typhi *Salmonella*
JEV	Japanese encephalitis virus	NVP	nevirapine
JHR	Jarisch–Herxheimer reaction	OCP	Onchocerciasis Control Programme
KS	Kaposi's sarcoma	OCR	Oculocephalic (doll's eye) reflex
LACV	La Crosse virus	OEPA	Onchocerciasis Elimination Program for the Americas
LBRF	louse-borne relapsing fever		
LDH	lactate dehydrogenase	OLM	ocular larva migrans
LED	light emitting diode	ONN	o'nyong nyong virus
LF	lymphatic filariasis	ORS	oral rehydration solution
LL	lepromatous leprosy	ORT	oral rehydration therapy
LP	lumbar puncture	OTF	outpatient treatment facility
LR	leishmaniasis recidivans	OTP	outpatient therapeutic programme
LRTI	lower respiratory tract infection	OVR	Oculovestibular reflex
LTF	late treatment failure	PAIR	Puncture, Aspiration, Injection, Reaspiration
MAEC	minianion exchange column technique	PAS	periodic acid–Schiff
MAT	microscopic agglutination test	PCECV	purified primary chick embryo cell vaccine
MCH	mean corpuscular haemoglobin	PCP	*Pneumocystis jirovecii* (formerly *P carinii*) pneumonia
MCHC	mean corpuscular haemoglobin concentration		
MCL	mucocutaneous leishmaniasis	PCR	polymerase chain reaction
MCV	mean corpuscular volume	PCV	packed cell volume
MDA	mass drug administration	PDEV	purified duck embryo vaccine
MDR	multidrug resistant	PE	pre-erythrocytic
MDT	multidrug therapy	PEG	pegylated
Mf/mL	microfilariae per millilitre	PI	protease inhibitors
MHCT	microhaematocrit	PID	pelvic inflammatory disease
ML	mucosal leishmaniasis	PF	peak flow
MMDM	malnutrition-modulated diabetes mellitus	PGL	persistent generalized lymphadenopathy
MOTT	mycobacteria other than tuberculosis	PHC	primary health clinic
MRDM	malnutrition-related diabetes mellitus	PITC	provider-initiated testing and counselling

PKDL	post-kala-azar dermal leishmaniasis
pLDH	Plasmodium lactate dehydrogenase
PML	progressive multifocal leucoencephalopathy
PMTCT	prevention of mother to child transmission
PPD	purified protein derivatives
PRR	parasite reduction ratio
PTSD	post-traumatic stress disorder
PUO	pyrexia of unknown origin
PVCV	purified vero cell vaccine
PVRV	purified Vero cell vaccine
QBC	quantitative buffy coat
q.d.s.	four times a day
QTc	corrected QT interval (electrocardiographic)
RAPLOA	rapid assessment procedures for loiasis
RBM	Roll Back Malaria
RDT	rapid diagnostic test
ReSoMal	rehydration solution for the malnourished
RIG	rabies immune globulin
r.p.m.	revolutions per minute
RR	respiratory rate
RRV	Ross River virus
RTA	road traffic accident
RUTF	ready to use therapeutic food
RVF	Rift Valley fever
SACD	subacute combined degeneration of the spinal cord
SAFE	surgery–antibiotics–facial cleanliness
SAM	severe acute malnutrition
SAT	standard agglutination test
SbV	Pentavalent antimonials
SFP	selective feeding programme
SLE	systemic lupus erythematosus
SLE	St Louis encephalitis
SMB	suckling mouse brain
SP	sulfadoxine-pyrimethamine
STD	sexually transmitted disease
STI	sexually transmitted infection
TB	tuberculosis
TBE	tick-borne encephalitis
TBRF	tick-borne relapsing fever
TCBS	thiosulphate citrate bile salt sucrose
TDF	tenofovir
t.d.s.	three times daily

TFC	therapeutic feeding centre
TIF	thiomersal, iodine and formol
TNF	tumour necrosis factor
TPE	tropical pulmonary eosinophilia
TT	tuberculoid leprosy
U&E	urea and electrolytes
UFM	under-fives mortality
UN	United Nations
UNICEF	United Nations Children's Fund
UTI	urinary tract infection
VCT	voluntary counselling and testing
VEE	Venezuelan equine encephalitis
VHF	viral haemorrhagic fever
VIMTO	vascular, infectious, metabolic, tumours trauma and toxins, other
VL	visceral leishmaniasis
VLM	visceral larva migrans
W/H	weight-for-height index
WBC	white blood cell count
WBCT20	20-min whole blood clotting test
WHO	World Health Organization
WNV	West Nile virus
XDR	extremely drug resistant
YF	yellow fever
ZDV	Zidovudine
ZN	Ziehl–Neelsen

New drug names

New	Old
aciclovir	acyclovir
amoxicillin	amoxycillin
anthelmintic	antihelminthic
beclometasone	beclomethasone
chlorphenamine	chlorphenyramine
hydroxycarbamide	hydroxyuria
lidocaine	lignocaine
nonoxinol '9'	non-oxynol 9
phenobarbital	phenobarbitone
sulfamethoxazole	sulphamethoxazole
tiabendazole	thiabendazole
thioacetazone	thiacetazone

How to use your textbook

Features contained within your textbook

Every chapter ends with a summary of key points for quick revision.

 SUMMARY

- The main features of respiratory disease are breathlessness, cough and chest pain.
- Together with the duration of symptoms and presence of fever, important additional points in the history are use of tobacco, exposure to domestic smoke or other air pollutants, and features suggestive of HIV.
- A raised respiratory rate may be caused by systemic illness rather than a primary respiratory problem.
- In resource-poor settings, chest X-rays should be reserved to clarify complex diagnostic problems and not be used to confirm obvious clinical signs.
- Asthma and tobacco-related lung disease and cancer are increasing in the tropics.

Your textbook is full of photographs, illustrations and tables.

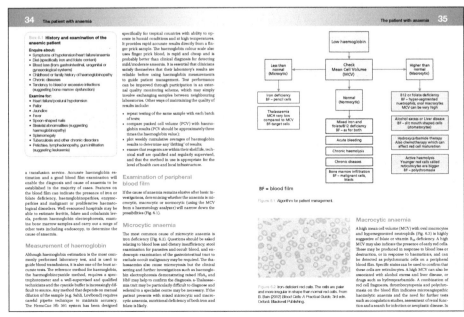

The anytime, anywhere textbook

Wiley E-Text

Your book is also available to purchase as a **Wiley E-Text: Powered by VitalSource** version – a digital, interactive version of this book which you own as soon as you download it.

Your **Wiley E-Text** allows you to:

Search: Save time by finding terms and topics instantly in your book, your notes, even your whole library (once you've downloaded more textbooks)

Note and Highlight: Colour code, highlight and make digital notes right in the text so you can find them quickly and easily

Organize: Keep books, notes and class materials organized in folders inside the application

Share: Exchange notes and highlights with friends, classmates and study groups

Upgrade: Your textbook can be transferred when you need to change or upgrade computers

Link: Link directly from the page of your interactive textbook to all of the material contained on the companion website

The **Wiley E-Text** version will also allow you to copy and paste any photograph or illustration into assignments, presentations and your own notes.

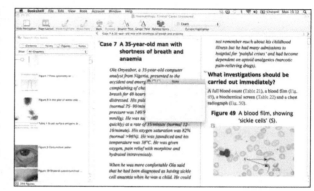

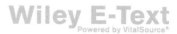

To access your Wiley E-Text:

- Visit **www.vitalsource.com/software/bookshelf/downloads** to download the Bookshelf application to your computer, laptop or mobile device.
- Open the Bookshelf application on your computer and register for an account.
- Follow the registration process.

The VitalSource Bookshelf can now be used to view your Wiley E-Text on iOS, Android and Kindle Fire!

- **For iOS:** Visit the app store to download the VitalSource Bookshelf: **http://bit.ly/17ib3XS**
- **For Android:** Visit the Google Play Market to download the VitalSource Bookshelf: **http://bit.ly/ZMEGvo**
- **For Kindle Fire, Kindle Fire 2 or Kindle Fire HD:** Simply install the VitalSource Bookshelf onto your Fire (see how at **http://bit.ly/11BVFn9**). You can now sign in with the email address and password you used when you created your VitalSource Bookshelf Account.

Full Wiley E-Text support for mobile devices is available at: **http://support.vitalsource.com**

CourseSmart

CourseSmart gives you instant access (via computer or mobile device) to this Wiley-Blackwell e-book and its extra electronic functionality, at 40% off the recommended retail print price. See all the benefits at: **www.coursesmart.com/students**

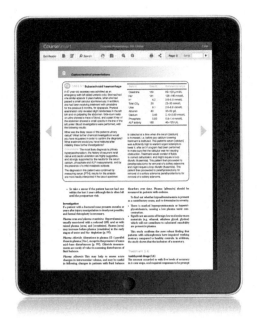

Instructors . . . receive your own digital desk copies!

CourseSmart also offers instructors an immediate, efficient, and environmentally-friendly way to review this book for your course.

For more information visit **www.coursesmart.com/instructors**.

With CourseSmart, you can create lecture notes quickly with copy and paste, and share pages and notes with your students. Access your **CourseSmart** digital book from your computer or mobile device instantly for evaluation, class preparation, and as a teaching tool in the classroom.

Simply sign in at **http://instructors.coursesmart.com/bookshelf** to download your Bookshelf and get started. To request your desk copy, hit 'Request Online Copy' on your search results or book product page.

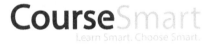

We hope you enjoy using your new book. Good luck with your studies!

About the companion website

Don't forget to visit the companion website for this book:

 www.lecturenoteseries.com/tropicalmed

There you will find valuable material designed to enhance your learning, including:
- Interactive multiple-choice questions (written by Dom Colbert)
- Revision summaries in PDF and PowerPoint format
- All the figures from the book in PowerPoint format

Part 1

A general approach to syndromes/ symptom complexes

Gastrointestinal presentations

Nick Beeching and Mike Beadsworth
Liverpool School of Tropical Medicine

The most important gastrointestinal presentation in the tropics is diarrhoea, and the majority of this chapter is devoted to this problem. However, other presentations of gastrointestinal disease are discussed first.

Dysphagia/odynophagia

Significant recent-onset dysphagia should always raise the possibility of oesophageal carcinoma. This malignancy is particularly common in certain parts of the tropics, e.g. some areas of Central and East Africa. Oesophageal candidiasis (HIV-related) is also a common cause of tropical dysphagia, together with ulceration due to herpes simplex and cytomegalovirus infections in patients with HIV. In South America, the mega-oesophagus of Chagas' disease should be considered. Finally, achalasia, peptic strictures, corrosive chemical ingestion and foreign bodies (fish bones especially in some areas) may also be important causes of impaired swallowing.

Haematemesis

In all areas of the world, an upper gastrointestinal haemorrhage can be caused by peptic ulceration, gastritis, oesophagitis, and gastric or oesophageal carcinoma. Gastritis, gastric erosions and gastric ulcers may be drug-related, e.g. corticosteroids and non-steroidal anti-inflammatory drugs (NSAIDs). *Helicobacter pylori* is recognized globally as a major cause of gastric and duodenal inflammation and/or ulceration. Oesophageal varices may be a particularly common cause of haematemesis in many tropical areas – at least 25% of all cases in some series. The underlying liver disease can be the late result of alcohol abuse, chronic viral hepatitis, or schistosomal hepatic fibrosis. Liver disease related to metabolic syndromes is becoming a global probem.

Abdominal pain

In 'Western' populations, severe abdominal pain can result from appendicitis, mesenteric adenitis, perforated peptic ulcers, biliary colic, cholecystitis and intestinal obstruction (commonly because of adhesions or malignancy). The irritable bowel syndrome and variants are common and in some cases may be triggered by infections, particularly by organisms that cause invasive colitits. This list is far from exhaustive, but serves to demonstrate that the spectrum of causes in the tropics is much wider. The following 'exotic' causes of acute severe abdominal pain may need to be considered.

- Abdominal tuberculosis
- Amoebic colitis (including perforation)
- Amoebic liver abscess (which may rupture)
- Ectopic ascariasis (e.g. biliary and/or pancreatic obstruction)
- Hydatid cyst rupture
- Hyperinfection syndrome of strongyloidiasis
- Intestinal obstruction caused by *Ascaris lumbricoides*
- Sickle cell crisis

Tropical Medicine Lecture Notes, Seventh edition. Edited by Nick Beeching and Geoff Gill. © 2014 John Wiley & Sons, Ltd. Published 2014 by John Wiley & Sons, Ltd.

- Splenic rupture
- Typhoid (including typhoid perforation)

Malabsorption

Malabsorption can be a feature of infection with *Giardia lamblia, Strongyloides stercoralis*, intestinal tuberculosis (TB) infection, as well as AIDS. Perhaps the most common cause, however, is the temporary lactase-deficient situation that may occur after any significant acute infective diarrhoeal illness. Milk and milk products may need to be avoided, although yoghurt is usually tolerated, because of its high bacterial lactase content.

Tropical sprue

A particularly well-described form of tropical malabsorption is 'tropical sprue'. This occurs predominantly in India and South East Asia, as well as the Caribbean and Central America. Patients develop non-bloody diarrhoea (sometimes steatorrhoea) often with abdominal bloating and significant weight loss. There may be a history of initial acute diarrhoeal illness, which is thought to be the precipitant (although the exact mechanism is unknown). As well as biochemical features of malabsorption, duodenal biopsy typically shows partial villous atrophy. The illness can be prolonged and debilitating. Traditional treatment with tetracycline (for associated bacterial small bowel overgrowth) and folic acid is often highly effective.

Diarrhoea

Diarrhoeal illness is one of the most important causes of morbidity and mortality in the tropics, causing over 6 million deaths per year. It is the fifth most common communicable cause of death worldwide and is clearly linked with poor hygiene and contamination of water and food. A wide variety of viral, bacterial and parasitic pathogens have been implicated in the pathogenesis of diarrhoea but it is impossible and unnecessary to test for all of these in individual cases. Systematic review of epidemiological, clinical and host factors usually enables a sensible working aetiological diagnosis to be established. The working diagnosis can be used to decide whether specific investigation should be performed, or to direct empirical antimicrobial therapy in the minority of cases in which it is required. The mainstay of management of diarrhoeal illness is the assessment and maintenance of appropriate fluid and electrolyte balance, irrespective of the aetiology, as well as the introduction of control measures in an epidemic setting to prevent further cases.

Pathophysiology and definitions

Diarrhoea may be thought of as 'water malabsorption' with excessive secretion of ions, usually Na+ and Cl-, followed by the release of large volumes of water from the small intestine causing diarrhoea. Of the 9 litres of fluid which enter the intestine each 24 hours, approximately 2 litres are ingested and the rest is made up of salivary, gastric, pancreatic, biliary and intestinal secretions. Most is absorbed in the small intestine, with around 1.5 litres entering the large bowel. Of this, 1.3 litres is absorbed, leaving a final stool volume of approximately 200 ml. The colonic functional reserve is 5–6 litres, so a significant insult or dysfunction is required within the small intestine to cause clinical diarrhoea. Diarrhoea can be classified according to aetiology, pathogenesis and clinical presentation, and each system has merits and problems. For example, definitions using abnormal stool consistency or frequency may be helpful for clinical assessment, but are not always helpful in determining the aetiology. A simple classification for bedside use separates non-inflammatory (secretory) diarrhoea from inflammatory/invasive disease.

History

It is essential to establish that both the doctor and the patient are talking about the same thing, especially if interpreters are being used to take the clinical history. A useful working definition of diarrhoea is the passage of three or more loose or watery bowel motions in 24·h. The distinction between soft or loose diarrhoea is more difficult, but bowel motions can be described as diarrhoeal when they assume the shape of the collecting container. This definition works with acute diarrhoeal illness but is less satisfactory with chronic diarrhoeal illness related to malabsorption, in which bulky sticky soft bowel motions are abnormal but may not be fluid enough to move around in the container. Key features in the history are the presence or absence of visible blood in the stool (dysentery), the presence and degree of abdominal pain, the presence of tenesmus and the presence of fever. The duration of illness is important – chronic diarrhoea is the passage of three or more loose or watery stools a day for 28 days or more.

In the historical assessment of fluid balance, the volume and frequency of faecal loss should be estimated, together with the frequency and approximate volume of any vomiting. The amount of fluid intake should be checked, as should the frequency of urinary output during the last 24 h.

The epidemiological setting is important. Illness in close family contacts should be ascertained, and enquiry made about whether the patient has attended any functions or eaten unusual foods in the preceding 48–72 h. If so, have any other guests had similar illness? Point source outbreaks can be caused by toxin-mediated food poisoning, in which case vomiting is often a predominant feature and incubation periods are usually shorter than 24 h. This may be difficult to distinguish from outbreaks of norovirus infection, in which vomiting is a predominant feature and contacts are readily infected. Unusual systemic pathogens (e.g. anthrax of the gut) or non-infectious poisoning caused by adulterated or contaminated food products must always be considered. Bacterial pathogens causing small or large bowel diarrhoea usually have intermediate incubation periods of 12–72 h. More detailed food histories are not otherwise very helpful, except in the case of expatriates who have unwisely overindulged in very spicy foods ('tasting the chilli twice'), or who have recently arrived in the tropics (traveller's diarrhoea). Diarrhoea developing in patients who are already hospitalized suggests a nosocomial or antibiotic-associated cause, while outbreaks of diarrhoeal illness in a refugee or camp setting imply specific infections such as shigellosis or cholera (see Fig. 1.1).

Other illness

Diarrhoea can be a prominent feature of many systemic illnesses, including malaria, pneumonia and enteric fever, especially in children, and evaluation of the patient should exclude these as potential causes. Surgical and other intra-abdominal conditions may mimic gastroenteritis, as can inflammatory bowel disease. In older or immobile patients, constipation with overflow diarrhoea must be excluded. Alcohol and drugs frequently cause diarrhoea with or without nausea and vomiting (see Table 1.1).

Table 1.1 **Non-infectious causes of diarrhoea**

Exogenous
Alcohol
Drugs
  Antibiotics
  Antihypertensive drugs: beta-blockers, calcium channel antagonists, methyldopa
  Antiretroviral therapy
  Biguanides
  Cardiac glycosides
  H_2 receptor antagonists
  Non-steroidal anti-inflammatory drugs
  Laxatives: all classes cause diarrhoea, apart from those that bulk-form
Traditional and complementary therapies

Endocrine
Addison's disease
Carcinoid syndrome
Diabetes mellitus
Thyroid disease
Tumours, e.g. MEN syndrome, gastrinoma, VIPoma

Enteropathy
Bacterial overgrowth
HIV enteropathy and malabsorption
Pancreatic insufficiency

Small bowel disease
Coeliac disease
Intestinal lymphangectasia
Surgery
Tropical sprue
Whipple's disease

Colonic
Inflammatory bowel disease
Ischaemic colitis
Microscopic colitis
Radiation coitis/enterocolitis
Surgery

Malignancy
Colorectal adenocarcinoma
Kaposi's sarcoma
Lymphoma

Motility disorders
Faecal incontinence
Chronic constipation
Irritable bowel syndrome

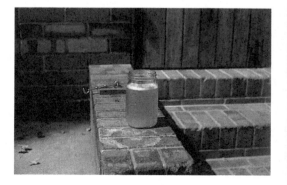

Figure 1.1 Though it looks like urine, this is the 'ricewater' stool from a patient with cholera.

Host factors

Conditions that cause hypochlorhydria (e.g. gastric surgery, H_2 antagonists and proton pump inhibitors) reduce the gastric acid barrier to many bacterial pathogens, so a smaller infective dose is required. Patients with established cardiovascular or renal disease are less likely to tolerate dehydration, as are those on diuretics and patients with poorly controlled diabetes. Preexisting large bowel problems such as inflammatory bowel disease predispose to complications of dysenteric infections such as toxic megacolon, signs of which may be partly masked by concurrent steroid therapy. Bowel tumours can produce diarrhoea with or without blood or weight loss. Small bowel problems, including lymphoma, can cause prolonged diarrhoea. Immunosuppression of the patient, particularly by HIV, predisposes to increased invasiveness (local and systemic) of bacterial pathogens such as non-typhoidal *Salmonella*, increased recurrence of such pathogens, and chronic diarrhoea caused by a variety of protozoa.

Examination

General examination must include assessment of the state of hydration. This is more difficult to quantify clinically in adults than in children but key features are summarized in Table 1.2. Measurement of any postural drop in blood pressure is particularly useful. Rectal examination should be performed, except in obvious cases of cholera for example, and is particularly important in older patients who are more likely to have non-infectious bowel problems. Systemic causes of diarrhoea and signs of immunosuppression (e.g. zoster scars and oral candidiasis) should be sought.

Clinical syndromes of diarrhoea

Apart from acute toxin-mediated food poisoning, diarrhoeal illness can be broadly classified into small bowel secretory diarrhoea, small bowel malabsorption and large bowel inflammatory diarrhoea. Each of these groups may be acute or chronic, and there is considerable overlap (Table 1.3).

Small bowel secretory diarrhoea is exemplified by cholera and non-invasive *Escherichia coli* infections, in which toxins specifically promote secretion of water and electrolytes into the bowel lumen and inhibit their reabsorption. Such secretion can be competitively overcome by a steady intake of balanced electrolyte solutions containing adequate amounts of glucose, but not too much to produce an osmotic diarrhoea. This is the scientific basis for the success of oral rehydration therapy, in which the correct quantities of salts and glucose are added to sterile water for rehydration.

Table 1.2 Clinical classification of severity of dehydration in adults

	Mild	Moderate	Severe
Subjective			
General state	Alert, active, up and about	Weak, lethargic, able to sit and walk	Dull, inactive, unable to sit or walk
Ability to perform daily activities	Able to perform daily activities without difficulty	Able to perform daily activities with some difficulty, e.g. stays away from work, needs support	Unable to perform daily activities, stays in bed or needs hospitalization
Thirst	Not increased	Increased thirst	Feels very thirsty
Objective			
Pulse	Normal	Tachycardia	Tachycardia
Blood pressure	Normal	Normal or decrease, 10–20 mmHg systolic	Decrease > 20 mmHg systolic
Postural hypotension	No	Yes or no	Yes
Jugular venous pressure	Normal	Normal or slightly flat	Flat
Dry mucosa (mouth, tongue)	No	Slight	Severe
Skin turgor	Good	Fair	Poor
Sunken eye balls	No	Minimal	Sunken
Body weight loss	< 5%	5–10%	> 10%

Table 1.3 Clinical features of inflammatory and non-inflammatory diarrhoea

Non-inflammatory	Inflammatory
Symptoms	
Nausea, vomiting; abdominal pain and fever not major features	Abdominal pain, tenesmus, fever
Stool	
Voluminous, watery	Frequent, small volume; blood-stained, pus cells present, mucus
Site	
Proximal small intestine	Distal ileum, colon
Mechanism	
Osmotic or secretory	Invasion of enterocytes leading to mucosal cell death and inflammatory response
Faecal leucocytes	
Absent	Present

Malabsorption is a common complication of infectious diarrhoea in the tropics, as many races have relatively low disaccharidase activity in the small bowel enterocytes. Disruption of 'normal' bowel activity readily leads to failure to break down sugars and a moderately prolonged lactose intolerance. This is particularly common after infections that cause flattening of the small bowel mucosa (such as giardiasis and cryptosporidiosis). Large bowel diarrhoea is usually caused by direct invasion of the bowel by pathogens such as *Entamoeba histolytica,* bacteria such as *Campylobacter* species, or *Clostridium difficile* after antibiotic therapy. Other parasites such as *Schistosoma mansoni* can also cause prolonged large bowel diarrhoea. In heavy *Trichuris trichiura* infections, oedema of the rectal mucosa together with continued efforts to defaecate resulting from tenesmus can lead to rectal prolapse. A summary of the major pathogens in inflammatory and non-inflammatory diarrhoea is shown in Table 1.4.

Investigations

A useful algorithmic approach to individual patient diagnosis and management is summarized in Figure 1.2. In most tropical settings, microbiological investigation proves impossible or very limited. Microscopy of faeces for leucocytes, suggestive of invasive pathogens in the large bowel, is commonly advocated but is of questionable time-effectiveness compared with macroscopic inspection of faeces

Table 1.4 Pathogens in inflammatory and non-inflammatory diarrhoea

Non-inflammatory	Inflammatory
	Viruses
Rotavirus	Nil
Adenovirus 40/41	
Astrovirus	
Norovirus (Norwalk agent)	
Calicivirus	
Small round structureless virus	
Coronavirus	
Torovirus	
Bredavirus	
Picobirnavirus	
	Bacteria
Enterotoxigenic *E. coli* (ETEC)	Enteroinvasive *Escherichia coli* (EIEC)
Enteropathogenic *E. coli* (EPEC)	Enterohaemorrhagic *E. coli* (EHEC), e.g. 0157
Vibrio cholerae	Enteroaggregative *E. coli* (EAggEC)
Vibrio parahaemolyticus	*Aeromonas hydrophila*
Campylobacter spp.	*Campylobacter* spp.
Salmonella spp.	*Salmonella* spp.
Plesiomonas shigelloides	*Shigella* spp.
Bacillus cereus	*Yersinia enterocolitica*
Clostridium perfringens	*Clostridium difficile*
	Protozoa
Cryptosporidium spp.	*Entamoeba histolytica*
Giardia lamblia	*Balantidium coli*
Cyclospora cayetanensis	
Cystoisospora belli	
Microsporidia (e.g. *Enterocytozoon bieneusi*)	
	Helminths
Strongyloides stercoralis	*Schistosoma* spp.

for blood (and smell) when resources are limited. However, cholera vibrios may be observed with their characteristic 'shooting star' motility even without dark ground facilities, and this is very useful when culture is not available. Investigations for faecal parasites should be limited to specific settings (e.g. chronic diarrhoea complicating HIV), and are almost never indicated in nosocomial diarrhoea. Fresh stool

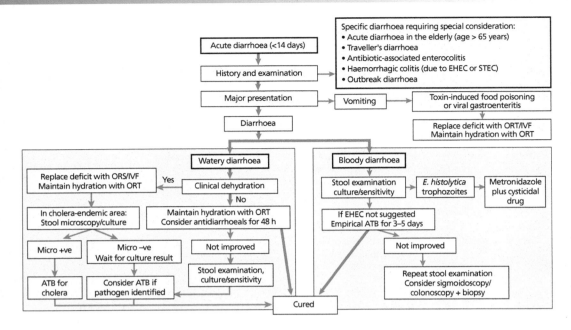

Figure 1.2 Algorithm for the management of diarrhoea in adults. (Adapted from Manatsathit *et al. (2002)* with permission.) Stool examination and culture depends on local availability, affordability and practice. In suspected cholera, dark field microscopy is ideal (or, if not available, a search for 'shooting star' bacteria on light microscopy will do). In epidemic situations, a clinical diagnosis is sufficient. When antibiotics are used, the choice either depends on culture and sensitivity results, or local experience. If available, ciprofloxacin is a good choice, except in Asia where resistant campylobacter responds better to azithromycin. ATB, antibiotic; EHEC, enterohaemorrhagic *Escherichia coli;* IVF, intravenous fluids; ORT, oral rehydration therapy.

microscopy for active trophozoites should only be requested when amoebic dysentery is truly suspected. Blanket requests for faecal microscopy for 'ova, cysts and parasites' on all patients are a waste of time in most settings. Such requesting patterns overload laboratories, demoralize their staff and lead to reports of questionable quality with little effect on clinical management decisions.

In an outbreak setting, full microbiological identification of the pathogen and assessment of the antimicrobial resistance patterns is very helpful, and should be pursued even if outside assistance is required. In sporadic cases, detailed microbiological tests may be inappropriate, but clinicians need to be aware of the local antibiotic sensitivities of organisms such as *Shigella, Salmonella* and *Campylobacter* if they are to use empirical antimicrobial therapy in a responsible and effective manner. Other investigations, such as serum electrolytes, peripheral white cell count and blood cultures, are performed in a hospital setting but again may not be available routinely.

Management

Detailed management of individual pathogens is beyond the scope of this brief chapter. The key is the correction of fluid and electrolyte imbalance. Severely dehydrated patients need rapid intravenous replacement of fluid loss, preferably using normal saline or a physiologically balanced electrolyte solution such as Hartmann's or Ringer's lactate (see also Chapter 21: Cholera, p. 187). Large volumes of dextrose solution can be dangerous. Intravenous fluid can be supplemented and rapidly replaced by oral rehydration, which is more successful if small volumes of fluid are taken steadily rather than large volumes at a time. Specific World Health Organization (WHO) oral rehydration solution is ideal, but the water in which it is dissolved must be clean and safe to drink – preferably by prior boiling and cooling. Alternative oral rehydration therapy mixtures can also be used for adults and food, including milk products, is usually reintroduced as early as possible after initial resuscitation of children. Fluid balance should be carefully monitored and a cholera bed is useful for less mobile patients with profuse diarrhoea. The fluid faeces can then be collected through a hole in the middle of the bed directly into a measuring bucket. If a large-bore disposable Foley's urinary catheter is available, this can be inserted into the rectum when diarhoea is profuse and watery (e.g. in cholera), removing the need for frequent evacuation, and allowing accurate measurement of faecal losses by volume.

Laxatives should be stopped, as should other drugs and traditional/complementary therapies that may cause diarrhoea. Antidiarrhoeal agents such as codeine or loperamide should be avoided in patients with acute invasive or large bowel disease, and should not be used in young children. Antiemetics should be used sparingly and again avoided in young children. Zinc supplementation is beneficial for children, but the roles of probiotics and use of lactose free feeds are less clear. Empirical or specific antimicrobial treatment should be reserved for specific situations such as proven amoebiasis, prolonged severe infection in a vulnerable host, or in outbreak settings, e.g. cholera or shigellosis. Chronic diarrhoea presents a different challenge and patients with HIV-related diarrhoea often progress through successive therapeutic trials of co-trimoxazole, metronidazole, fluoroquinolones, albendazole or nitazoxanide. Such patients may need 'hospital at home' support including provision of adequate antidiarrhoeal medications (Chapter 13).

In a refugee camp outbreak setting, logistical support must be requested at an early stage for detailed epidemiological investigation, triage and treatment facilities; as well as provision of an adequate water supply, rehydration solutions and latrines (Chapter 60).

> - In addition to gastrointestinal infection, diarrhoea may be prominent in many systemic infections including pneumonia, sepsis and malaria.
> - Most patients with gastroenteritis can be managed using simple algorithms that include assessment of the degree of dehydration to determine the amount and speed of administration of balanced oral rehydration solution.
> - Chronic diarrhoea is likely to be associated with underlying bowel or pancreatic disease or immunosuppression, especially due to HIV.

 Visit www.lecturenoteseries.com/tropicalmed to test yourself on this chapter using interactive MCQs.

FURTHER READING

Al-Abri SA, Beeching NJ, Nye FJ (2005) Traveller's diarrhoea. *Lancet Infectious Diseases* **5**: 349–60. [Overview of aetiology, epidemiology, management and prevention of this common problem for travelers.]

Elliott EJ (2007) Acute gastroenteritis in children. *BMJ* **334**: 35–40. [Concise evidence based review, very practical and useful.]

Hart CA (2003) Introduction to acute infective diarrhoea. In GC Cook, A Zumla (eds), *Manson's Tropical Diseases*, 21st edn. London: Elsevier Science, pp. 907–13. [Good overview with references of both adult and paediatric diarrhoea causes and effects.]

Manatsathit S, DuPont H, Farthing M *et al.* (2002) Guideline for the management of acute diarrhoea in adults. *J Gastroenterol Hepatol* **17** (Suppl): S54–S71. [Superb working party report produced by acknowledged experts from Thailand, India and Africa as well as 'Western' authorities. Detailed definitions, practical approaches and many references.]

Navaneethan U, Giannella RA (2008) Mechanisms of infectious diarrhea. *Nat Clin Pract Gastroenterol Hepatol* **5**(11): 637–47. doi: 10.1038/ncpgasthep1264. Epub 2008 Sep 23. [Recent review.]

Thomas PD *et al.* (2003) Guidelines for the investigation of chronic diarrhoea, 2nd edn. *Gut* **52**: 1–15. [British guidelines for assessment of both infectious and non-infectious causes of chronic diarrhoea.]

SUMMARY

- Oesophageal varices are an important cause of haematemesis in the tropics, related to infections such as schistosomiasis and chronic viral hepatitis together with rising prevalences of both alcohol abuse and non-alcoholic fatty liver disease.
- Diarrhoeal illness remains a leading cause of infection-related mortality worldwide, especially in children aged less than 5 years.
- The aetiology of diarrhoeal illness can be predicted from its duration, the presence or absence of systemic features or of blood in faeces, and knowledge of local pathogen prevalence.

World Health Organization (2005) Diarrhoea – assessment and management of diarrhoea in children in tropical settings. In *Handbook IMCI Integrated Management of Childhood Illness*. Geneva: WHO, ch. 8, pp. 25–31. [Summary of WHO guidelines for use at clinic level. Full manual and other IMCI and nutrition-related resources freely downloadable from WHO Child and adolescent health development website http://www.who.int/child_adolescent_health/topics/en/]

World Health Organization (2005) *The Treatment of Diarrhoea. A Manual for Physicians and Other Senior Health Workers*. 4th edn. Geneva: WHO. [Comprehensive review with algorithms for assessment and management of children and adolescents in particular, appropriate for resource poor settings.]

World Health Organization (2006) *Implementing the New Recommendations on the Clinical Management of Diarrhoea. Guidelines for Policy Makers and Programme Managers*. Geneva: WHO. [Summary of recommendations for use of the 2003 low osmolarity ORS mixture and zinc supplementation, plus programme guidance.]

2

Respiratory presentations

Stephen Gordon[1] and Neil French[2]
[1]Liverpool School of Tropical Medicine; [2]University of Liverpool

Disorders of the respiratory tract are among the most important cause of ill health in human populations around the world. The normal physiological functioning of the respiratory tract exposes it to prolonged and intimate contact with the external environment, leading to a steady exposure to airborne pollutants and pathogens with disease-causing potential.

Infectious diseases dominate acute respiratory illness in the tropics in all age groups; acute viral and bacterial infections in childhood, and tuberculosis and bacterial pneumonia in adults. The enormous global burden of respiratory impairment due to chronic obstructive pulmonary disease (COPD) has recently been described and shown to be worst in Africa and Asia where the disease is mainly caused by exposure to tobacco smoke in men and indoor air pollution from cooking with biomass fuel in women. Global concern regarding the health effects of tobacco smoke has now resulted in important international treaties to limit tobacco products and smoking bans effective in public places have had a positive impact both in developed (Scotland) and tropical countries (Kenya).

Assessment

History

The predominant symptoms of respiratory illness are breathlessness, cough and chest pain. Symptom duration and the concurrence of fever are useful descriminators – common presentations in adults and children are summarized in (Table 2.1).

Breathlessness

Shortness of breath should be characterized by duration, progression and whether it is constant or intermittent. Orthopnoea (breathlessness on lying flat) suggests a cardiac cause or a structural abnormality of the thoracic cage. Nocturnal dyspnoea is a feature of asthma and obstructive airways disease.

The effort required to precipitate breathlessness provides a good gauge of the level of respiratory impairment. Breathless at rest or inability of a young child to feed indicate severe restriction. Shortness of breath in an adult should be quantified in terms of tasks completed or failed, or distance walked.

Cough

Cough is both a reflex (from any organ supplied by the vagus nerve) and a conscious act, therefore discriminating between causes of cough can be difficult. Cough may be productive or non-productive but a **productive** cough is often evidence of pulmonary infection and investigation for tuberculosis should be prompted by any persistent cough.

The quantity of sputum produced may provide diagnostic information about chronic obstructive pulmonary disease or bronchiectasis. The expectoration of mucopurulent material is an indicator of neutrophil activity and infection.

Haemoptysis is often an indicator of serious underlying pathology, but it is important to establish that blood is being coughed and not coming from the upper airway, throat or upper gastrointestinal tract. Tuberculosis, bronchiectasis and neoplasia are primary concerns.

Extreme paroxysms of coughing in a child, particularly in association with the characteristic whoop,

Tropical Medicine Lecture Notes, Seventh edition. Edited by Nick Beeching and Geoff Gill. © 2014 John Wiley & Sons, Ltd. Published 2014 by John Wiley & Sons, Ltd.

Table 2.1 **Shortness of breath in adults and children**

Sudden (hours)	Acute (days)	Chronic (weeks, months)
Adults		
Pneumothorax	Pneumonia	Tuberculosis
Pulmonary embolus	Bronchitis	COPD
Asthma	Lung abscess	Kaposi's sarcoma
	Acute left ventricular failure	Lung cancer
	Allergic alveolitis	Heart failure
	Pulmonary eosinophilia	Silicosis / asbestosis
Children		
Pneumothorax	Pneumonia	Tuberculosis
Inhaled foreign body	Bronchitis	Heart failure
Asthma		

indicates a diagnosis of whooping cough. A 'barking' cough with inspiratory stridor is the hallmark of laryngotracheobronchitis – croup.

Chest pain

Complaints of chest pain should be assessed for their association with breathing and coughing. Pain derived from the pleura will be noticeable on breathing and is localized. Tracheal pain has a tearing or burning quality and is felt retrosternally, particularly on coughing.

Respiratory history

In addition to the presenting symptoms it is important to enquire about:

- **tobacco smoking** (quantify in pack years);
- **occupation**: identify occupationally-related symptoms and exposures including asbestos, inhaled proteins and fumes;
- risk factors for **HIV** infection and contact with **tuberculosis** cases, particularly in children failing to thrive.

Non-respiratory illness

Non-respiratory illness may present with predominantly respiratory symptoms – most commonly anaemia or heart failure presenting with dyspnoea. Breathlessness is a feature of metabolic acidosis which may be caused by diabetic ketoacidosis, poisoning, severe sepsis or renal failure. Alteration of breathing pattern and breathlessness can occur with neurological injury, during the early stages of tetanus and botulism and following envenomation.

Examination in respiratory cases

A respiratory examination is used to test hypotheses generated by the history. The signs elicited are rarely diagnostic in isolation.

The general condition of an individual provides clues to a diagnosis. In particular, cachexia, or failure to thrive in a young child, will indicate malnutrition or chronic underlying illness. Oral thrush, skin rashes and old herpes zoster scars are highly indicative of HIV infection, heightening the possibility of pneumococcal pneumonia or tuberculosis.

Tachypnoea (rapid breathing) can be a feature of any respiratory illness. In the context of an acute presentation, rates in adults above 30/min suggest severe disease particularly in association with systolic blood pressure below 90 mmHg and/or tachycardia pulse greater than 120. The criteria for tachypnoea in childhood are very different from adults. It is diagnosed only if the respiratory rate is over 60/min before the age of 2 months, over 50/min from 2–12 months, over 40/min from 1–5 years and over 30/min (as for adults) above the age of 5 years.

Cyanosis should be looked for in the oral mucosa but is always a difficult sign. Pulse oximetry is now affordable in most settings and provides accurate information to guide the use of supplemental oxygen.

Altered consciousness and confusion usually indicate severe acute disease and can necessitate specific management to protect the airway. Meningism can be found with severe pneumonia, with or without pneumococcal meningitis.

Percussion of the chest will identify a large pleural effusion (dull note). Lobar consolidation is common in pneumonia or tuberculosis and can be diagnosed on the basis of bronchial breathing. Many patients present with non-specific signs or scanty chest signs. In these cases, a suggestive history should lead to further investigation as a normal chest examination does not exclude significant pathology.

Investigation of respiratory disease

Chest X-ray

Limited resources must be carefully rationed in order to optimally investigate respiratory patients in the tropics. In particular, a chest X-ray should be used to extend the examination in difficult cases and not simply to confirm diagnoses made confidently on auscultation. Patients with severe acute respiratory illness or those who fail to respond to therapy including smear-negative cases of chronic cough are the ones most frequently requiring a chest X-ray. A normal chest X-ray does not exclude infection, particularly in HIV-infected adults.

Sputum/respiratory secretions

Sputum examination is essential in the investigation of suspected TB (see Chapter 12: Tuberculosis) and is of value in cases of chronic disease when Gram staining defines dominant bacteria. Occasionally, an unstained wet preparation of sputum examined under low power may be useful for identifying strongyloidiasis, paragonimiasis or fungal elements. Cytology for malignant cells can also be performed on sputum but requires a skilled pathologist. Other sputum include direct immunofluorescence for viruses and *Pneumocystis jirovecii*, urinary antigen detection for pneumococci (Gram stain described in Chapter 12) and molecular techniques for several organisms in sputum including tuberculosis, but these methods are not yet resource-efficient in developing countries.

When sputum cannot be produced, placing the patient in a head-down position or simple chest physiotherapy (drumming) for 2–3 minutes will help. Lung aspiration increases the diagnostic yield in young children with lung consolidation. A needle and syringe primed with 1 mL normal saline or sterile water is passed into the consolidated tissue through the thoracic wall and aspirated. The aspirated material can be smeared onto slides for examination and injected into liquid culture media. In young children when sputum is difficult to collect, early morning gastric washings yield swallowed sputum for the investigation of possible tuberculosis (mycobacteria are gastric acid resistant).

Blood cultures

Blood cultures are a valuable investigation in febrile patients. Recovery of a pathogen allows confident treatment and is frequently the investigation by which an unusual cause of pneumonia is established, e.g. *Salmonella typhi, Cryptococcus spp, Burkholderia pseudomallei* (melioidosis), *Rhodococcus equi.*

Pleural fluid

Sampling of pleural fluid is simple to perform and should be considered for most effusions as the management of simple effusion and empyema are different. Fluid is aspirated by use of a needle and syringe, avoiding the neurovascular bundle at the inferior margin of each rib. Occasionally, this fails because pleural fluid is loculated, has formed a thick empyema or the chest examination findings result from chronic pleural scarring. Pleural fluid should be defined as transudate (protein below 30 g/dl) or exudate and exudates subjected to pH, amylase, microscopy and culture. Inflammatory cells and pH<7.2 suggest empyema.

Lung function testing

Chronic lung disease cannot be precisely defined without spirometry. Lung function can now be measured using handheld technology and stored on a laptop computer. Asthma prevalence is increasing and COPD is recognized as a significant burden of chronic disease in Africa, so the provision of spirometry is increasing.

Common presentations

In general, respiratory presentations in the general medical clinic tend to fall into a small number of syndromes.

Acute breathlessness and fever in the small child

Lower respiratory tract infection (LRTI) is a leading killer of children. Consequently, early assessment and management of this syndrome is a core component of the Integrated Management of Childhood Illness (IMCI) strategy promoted by the World Health

Organization (WHO). Vaccination against pneumococcal and *Haemophilus influenzae* infections are also global priorities.

Simple assessment at the primary care level using features of rapid breathing and subcostal recession (chest indrawing) of a child with fever and cough is used to distinguish children with a LRTI who require antibiotics and possible hospital admission, from those with an upper respiratory tract infection (Fig. 28.1). Early initiation of therapy is essential for a good outcome.

Although many LRTIs are initiated by viral infections (amongst which respiratory syncitial virus, parainfluenza, adenovirus and measles are important), super-added bacterial infections with *Streptococcus pneumoniae* and *Haemophilus influenzae* type b are common. The presentation of tuberculosis in infants is often occult.

Acute breathlessness, cough and fever in adults

Acute bacterial pneumonia is the principal diagnostic consideration and the diagnosis and management of this is covered in Chapter 28. Non-infectious causes become more prevalent in older adults.

Chronic cough and malaise

Many chronic respiratory problems present this way. It is important to exclude or confirm tuberculosis, which represents a serious public health threat but is readily treatable (Chapter 12). A small number of conditions are specific to the tropics and may need to be considered under the right epidemiological circumstances: paragonimiasis in South East Asia and restricted areas of West Africa (Chapter 29); endemic mycoses in South and Central America (Chapter 54); and pulmonary complications of schistosomiasis in endemic regions (Chapter 17). The incidence of tobacco smoking associated lung cancer is increasing in developing countries.

Breathlessness and wheeze

Asthma is an increasingly important problem in the tropics, particularly in urban centres. The expiratory wheeze or whistling associated with lower airways obstruction must be differentiated from inspiratory phase stridor, which indicates upper airway obstruction. The presence of paroxysmal or diurnal cough, breathlessness and wheeze preferably supported by variation in peak flow measurements reliably indicates airways obstruction. An important differential

diagnosis of asthma is tropical pulmonary eosinophilia (Chapter 30).

Pleural effusion

Symptoms associated with pleural effusions can be of short or long duration, depending on the nature of the underlying problems, but large effusions are straightforward to find on examination. Pleural fluid should be sampled as described above. In HIV endemic regions, TB is the most common cause of pleural effusion. Parapneumonic effusions, empyema or tuberculous effusions should be suggested by the history. Malignant effusions must be considered when an infective aetiology is not readily apparent. Effusions may indicate extrapulmonary or systemic problems (Table 2.2).

Respiratory disease and HIV

Respiratory problems head the list of conditions leading to hospital admission of HIV-infected adults (Table 2.3). Bacterial (particularly pneumococcal) pneumonia is strongly associated with HIV infection. It has a similar predictive value for HIV infection in adults to herpes zoster – around 90% in eastern and southern Africa. HIV infection is the principal factor driving the tuberculosis epidemic in Africa, where the prevalence of HIV coinfection varies between 50 and 70% in patients with TB. HIV testing should be considered in all cases of pneumonia and tuberculosis.

Table 2.2 Causes of pleural effusion

Common	Infrequent	Rare
Tuberculosis (primary and post-primary)	Neoplasia – Lung carcinoma – Kaposi's sarcoma – Burkitt's lymphoma – Mesothelioma	Thoracic duct damage
Para-pneumonic	Constrictive pericarditis	Pancreatitis
Empyema – pneumococcal – staphylococcal – mixed and anaerobic		Haemorrhagic fever
Heart failure		Filariasis
		Hypothyroidism

Table 2.3 Respiratory problems complicating HIV infection

Problems complicating HIV infection	
Common	Infrequent
Bacterial pneumonia	*Pneumocystis jirovecii* pneumonia*
Tuberculosis	*Rhodococcus equi* infection
Acute bronchitis	Nocardiasis
Sinusitis	Lymphoid interstitial pneumonitis[†]
Bronchiectasis	Lymphoma
Pulmonary cryptococcosis	Pulmonary hypertension
Pulmonary Kaposi's sarcoma	Penicillinosis[‡] Melioidosis[‡] Invasive mycoses[§]

*Common in children under 1 year old.
[†]Common in children.
[‡]South East Asia.
[§]South and Central America.

Cough is a frequently reported symptom in individuals with advanced immunosuppression and chronically ill AIDS patients frequently present with intractable breathlessness. These cases are difficult to manage as pulmonary Kaposi's sarcoma, sputum-negative TB, bacterial pneumonia, pulmonary cryptococcosis and fungal pneumonia can all potentially be present at one time – each of these diagnoses is hard to make and treatment unlikely to be successful. Careful consideration must be made about when symptom-directed palliative care is the most appropriate strategy.

 SUMMARY

- The main features of respiratory disease are breathlessness, cough and chest pain.
- Together with the duration of symptoms and presence of fever, important additional points in the history are use of tobacco, exposure to domestic smoke or other air pollutants, and features suggestive of HIV.
- A raised respiratory rate may be caused by systemic illness rather than a primary respiratory problem.
- In resource-poor settings, chest X-rays should be reserved to clarify complex diagnostic problems and not be used to confirm obvious clinical signs.
- Asthma and tobacco-related lung disease and cancer are increasing in the tropics.

 Visit **www.lecturenoteseries.com/tropicalmed** to test yourself on this chapter using interactive MCQs.

FURTHER READING

Ait-Khaled N, Odhiambo J, Pearce N, *et al.* (2007) Prevalence of symptoms of asthma, rhinitis and eczema in 13- to 14-year-old children in Africa: the International Study of Asthma and Allergies in Childhood Phase III. *Allergy* **62**: 247–58.

Buist AS, McBurnie MA, Vollmer WM, *et al.* (2007) International variation in the prevalence of COPD (the BOLD Study): a population-based prevalence study. *Lancet* **370**: 741–50.

Ezzati M, Kammen D (2002) Indoor air pollution from biomass combustion and acute respiratory infections in Kenya: an exposure-response study. *Lancet* **358**: 619–24.

http://www.fctc.org The website of the Framework Convention Alliance, and NGO supporting the actions of the Framework Convention for Tobacco Control.

3

Neurological presentations

Tom Solomon[1] and Rachel Kneen[2]
[1]University of Liverpool; [2]Alder Hey Children's Foundation NHS Trust

Neurological presentations are more common in the tropics than in the developed industrial world. Infectious diseases make a major contribution, but non-infectious causes are also important (Table 3.1). A complex mixture of socioeconomic and environmental factors contribute to the increased incidence.

Reasons for increased incidence of neurological disorders in the tropics

- Non-infectious neurological disorders – trauma is more common in the tropics, especially road traffic accidents. Patterns of vascular disease are catching up with those in the developed world, but the usage of drugs to control them lags behind.
- Infectious neurological diseases – the climate supports transmission of insect-borne pathogens (malaria, trypanosomiasis, arthropod-borne viruses). Environmental factors include the close proximity of homes to zoonotic infections. Vaccine-preventable diseases are more common (e.g. measles, tetanus, diphtheria, polio). There is also unregulated use of over-the-counter antibiotics, leading to the partial pretreatment of central nervous system (CNS) infections, which hampers diagnosis and therapy, and promotes the development of antibiotic resistance.

- Poverty, overcrowding, poor sanitation and lack of education about disease risk factors and prevention are important. These may lead, for example, to cysticercosis and typhoid.
- Immunosuppression, particularly as a result of HIV, allows many other infections such as cryptococcal and tuberculous meningitis. Many patients with HIV have no access to combination antiretroviral therapy (cART).

Neurological syndromes

Neurological diseases – particularly infections – can present with a range of syndromes.

- *Encephalopathy* – a reduced level of consciousness from any cause (infectious, metabolic, vascular, traumatic).
- *Meningism* – clinical signs of meningeal irritation (headache, neck stiffness, Kernig's sign; see below).
- *Paralysis* – weakness of one or more limb, respiratory or bulbar muscles, which may be a result of damaged upper motor neurones, lower motor neurones, peripheral nerves, or muscles.
- *Chronic neurological presentations* – insidious presentation over weeks or months, often with changes in personality, behaviour or other psychiatric illness. Fever may not be prominent, even with an infectious cause (Table 3.2).
- *Headache* – may be the only symptom (e.g. in cryptococcal meningitis).
- *Other focal neurological signs* – including hemispheric signs, brainstem signs, seizures and movement disorders.

Tropical Medicine Lecture Notes, Seventh edition. Edited by Nick Beeching and Geoff Gill. © 2014 John Wiley & Sons, Ltd. Published 2014 by John Wiley & Sons, Ltd.

Table 3.1 **Causes of neurological disease (mnemonic = VIMTO)**

Vascular
Hypertension/hypotension
Ischaemia/infarct
Subarachnoid/subdural/extradural/intracerebral
  haemorrhage

Infectious
Direct effect on CNS
Bacteria
Meningococcus, streptococci, *Haemophilus
  influenzae*, tuberculosis, leprosy, *Mycoplasma
  pneumoniae,* listeria, *E. coli* (neonates),
  Mycobacterium tuberculosis

Viruses
Arboviruses, herpes viruses, enteroviruses, rabies,
  paramyxoviruses (measles, mumps), influenza and
  parainfluenza viruses, adenoviruses, Nipah virus

Parasites
 Protozoans
   African trypanosomiasis (*Trypanosoma gambiense*
     and *T. rhodesiense*)
   amoebiasis (*Entamoeba histolytica)*
   malaria *(Plasmodium falciparum)*
   toxoplasmosis (*Toxoplasma gondii)*
 Trematodes (flukes)
   paragonimiasis
   schistosomiasis (especially *Schistosoma japonicum*)
 Cestodes (tapeworms)
   cysticercosis (*Taenia solium*)
   hydatidosis (*Echinococcus granulosus*)
 Nematodes (roundworms)
   ascariasis (*Ascaris lumbricoides*)
   gnathostomiasis (*Gnathostoma spinigerum*)
   parastrongyliasis (*Parastrongylus cantonensis*)
   trichinosis (*Trichinella spiralis*)

Spirochaetes
 Leptospirosis (*Leptospira* species)
 Louse-borne/epidemic relapsing fever (*B. recurrentis*)
 Lyme disease (*Borrelia burgdorferi*)
 Neurosyphilis (*Treponema pallidum*)
 Tick-borne/endemic relapsing fever (*B. duttonii*)

Rickettsiae
 Endemic/murine/flea-borne typhus (*R. typhi/
   R. mooseri*)
 Epidemic/louse-borne typhus (*Rickettsia
   prowazekii*)
 Rocky Mountain spotted fever (*R. rickettsii*)
 Scrub typhus (*O. tsutsugamushi*)

Fungi
 Aspergillosis
 Blastomycosis
 Candidiasis
 Coccidioidomycosis
 Cryptococcosis
 Histoplasmosis
 Nocardiasis*
 Paracoccidiomycosis

Prion
Creutzfeldt-Jakob disease (sporadic, new-variant,
  iatrogenic)
Indirect effect of infection
Immune-mediated post-infectious inflammatory (GBS,
  acute disseminated encephalomyelitis, transverse
  myelitis)
Toxin-mediated infectious diseases (tetanus,
  diphtheria, shigellosis)

Metabolic
Addison's disease
Diabetic ketoacidosis
Hepatic encephalopathy
Hypoglycaemia
Hyponatraemia
Hypothyroidism/hyperthyroidism
Mitochondrial encephalopathies, e.g. Leigh syndrome
Uraemia

Tumours/trauma/toxins
Alcohol
Drugs (medical, recreational, traditional)
Pesticides
Poisons

Other
Degenerative
Epilepsy (non-convulsive status epilepticus)
Hydrocephalus
Hypertensive encephalopathy
Inflammatory (e.g. multiple sclerosis)
Limbic encephalitis (autoimmune or paraneoplastic)
Nutritional
Psychiatric disease (psychogenic)
Vasculitis

Abbreviations: CNS, central nervous system; GBS, Guillain–
Barré syndrome.
**Nocardia* are actinomycete bacteria which are grouped with
fungi because of their morphology and behaviour.

Pathological processes

These neurological syndromes are explained by a range of pathological processes.

- *Encephalitis* – inflammation of the brain substance, usually in response to viral infection, but also in response to other pathogens.
- *Meningitis* – inflammation of the meningeal membranes covering the brain, in response to bacterial, viral or fungal infection.
- *Myelitis* – inflammation of the spinal cord. This may occur across the whole cord (causing transverse myelitis, which is often post-infectious) or be confined to the anterior horn cells).
- *Neuropathy* – damage to peripheral nerves, e.g. diphtheria, Guillain–Barré syndrome, leprosy, rabies, vitamin deficiencies, unwanted effects of antiretroviral therapy (ART).

Table 3.2 Causes of chronic neurological presentations in the tropics

Infectious	Other
Bacterial abscesses	Chronic subdural haemorrhages
Cryptococcal meningitis and other fungi	Dementia
HIV encephalopathy	Drugs
Neurosyphilis	Lead, other heavy metal poisoning
Partially treated bacterial meningitis	Toxins
Sleeping sickness (*Trypanosoma rhodesiense*, *T. gambiense*)	Tumours
Subacute sclerosing panencephalitis	Vitamin deficiencies
Toxoplasma gondii and other parasitic space-occupying lesions	
Tuberculous meningitis	

- *Mononeuritis multiplex* – damage to at least two individual nerves. Can be caused by HIV, leprosy, Lyme disease, hepatitis A.
- *Polyradiculopathy* – inflammation of the nerve roots, often presents as a cauda equina syndrome. May occur in HIV infection caused by CMV, syphilis, and HSV2.
- *Space-occupying lesions* (Table 3.3) – these cause pathology in the brain or spinal cord directly (by interrupting neuronal pathways) and indirectly

Table 3.3 Causes of central nervous system space-occupying lesions in the tropics

Bacterial abscesses

Fungi
    Aspergillosis, blastomycosis, nocardiasis

Haemorrhage

HIV-related – toxoplasmosis, primary CNS lymphoma, tuberculomata

Tuberculomata

Tumours and metastases

Parasites
    Cestodes (cysticercosis, hydatidosis)
    Nematodes (ascariasis)
    Protozoa (toxoplasmosis, amoebiasis)
    Trematodes (paragonimiasis, schistosomiasis)

(by causing localized swelling, raised intracranial pressure and brainstem herniation syndromes). Typically, they present with focal signs or a chronic insidious deterioration.

Rapid assessment of patient with coma in the tropics

1 **Stabilize the patient**, and treat any immediately life-threatening conditions.
   - Airways.
   - Breathing – give oxygen; intubate if breathing is inadequate or gag reflex impaired.
   - Circulation – establish venous access.
     - Obtain blood for immediate bedside blood glucose test (hypoglycaemia?).
     - Malaria film (look for parasites and pigment of partially treated malaria).
     - Full blood count, urea and elecrolytes, blood cultures, arterial blood gases.
   - Disability.
     - Give intravenous (i.v.) glucose (e.g. 10% glucose 50 mL in adults, 5 mL/kg in children), irrespective of blood glucose.
     - Give adults 100 mg thiamine i.v., especially if alcohol abuse is suspected.
     - Immobilize cervical spinal cord if neck trauma is suspected.
   - Rapidly assess AVPU scale (Alert, responds to Voice, to Pain, or Unresponsive).
     - If patient responds to pain or is unresponsive, examine the pupils, eye movements, respiratory pattern, tone and posture for signs of cerebral herniation (see below).
     - If herniation is suspected start treatment for this.
   - If purpuric rash is present give penicillin or chloramphenicol (or third generation cephalosporin) for presumed meningococcal meningitis (after taking blood cultures).
   - Look for and treat generalized seizures, focal seizures and subtle motor seizures (mouth or finger twitching, or tonic eye deviation).
2 **Take a history,** while preliminary assessment and resuscitation proceeds. This is the single most useful tool in determining the cause of coma. In particular:
   - Duration of onset of coma.
     - Rapid onset (minutes–hours) suggests a vascular cause, especially brainstem cerebrovascular

accidents or subarachnoid haemorrhage. If preceded by hemispheric signs, then consider intracerebral haemorrhage. Coma caused by some infections (e.g. malaria, encephalitis) can also develop rapidly, especially when precipitated by convulsions.

- Intermediate onset (hours–days) suggests diffuse encephalopathy (metabolic or, if febrile, infectious).
- Prolonged onset (days–weeks) suggests tumours, abscess or chronic subdural haematoma (see Table 3.2).
- Any drugs?
- Any trauma?
- Important past medical history (e.g. hypertension)?
- Family history (e.g. tuberculosis)?
- Known epidemic area (e.g. viral encephalitis)?

3 **Perform a rapid general medical examination,** and in particular:

- Check pockets for drugs.
- Note temperature (febrile or hypothermia) and blood pressure (hypo- or hypertensive).
- Examine for signs of trauma (check ears and nose for blood or cerebrospinal fluid (CSF) leak).
- Smell the breath for alcohol or ketones (diabetes?).
- Examine the skin for:
  - rash (meningococcal rash, dengue or other haemorrhagic fever, typhus, relapsing fever);
  - needle marks of drug abuse;
  - recent tick bite or eschar (tick-borne encephalitis, tick paralysis, tick-borne typhus or relapsing fever);
  - chancre, with or without circinate rash (trypanosomiasis, especially *Trypanosoma rhodesiense*);
  - healed dog bite (rabies);
  - snake bite.
- Examine for lymphadenopathy (e.g. Winterbottom's sign of posterior cervical lymphadenopathy in African trypanosomiasis).
- Examine the fundi for papilloedema (longstanding raised intracranial pressure) or signs of hypertension.

4 **Determine the coma score** to allow subsequent changes to be accurately monitored. The scale in Box 3.1 is for adults and children over 5 years of age and in Box 3.2 for young children. Simpler still is to use the AVPU score as in 1 above.

5 **Neurological examination.** A detailed description of the neurological examination is beyond the scope of this chapter. For most practical purposes

---

Box 3.1 Modified Glasgow coma scale for adults and children over 5 years

Best motor response
6 Obeys command
5 Localizes supraorbital pain
4 Withdraws from pain on nail bed
3 Abnormal flexion response
2 Abnormal extension response
1 None

Best verbal response
5 Oriented
4 Confused
3 Inappropriate words
2 Incomprehensible sounds
1 None

Eye opening
4 Spontaneous
3 To voice
2 Pain
1 None

Total score is the sum of best score in each of the three categories (maximum score 15). 'Unrousable coma' reflects a score <9

---

the ability to recognize the following four clinical patterns (and combinations of them) will allow appropriate classification and subsequent investigation and treatment.

- *Meningism* – with or without encephalopathy.
- *Diffuse encephalopathies* – usually metabolic or infectious.

Box 3.2 Blantyre coma scale for young children

Best motor response
2 Localizes painful stimulus
1 Withdraws limb from pain
0 Non-specific or absent response

Best verbal response
2 Appropriate cry
1 Moan or inappropriate cry
0 None

Eye movements
1 Directed (e.g. follows mother's face)
0 Not directed

Total score is sum of best score in each of three categories (maximum score 5). 'Unrousable coma' reflects score <2

- *Supratentorial focal damage* (above the cerebellar tentorium) – usually manifests as hemispheric signs.
- *Damage in the diencephalon or brainstem* (midbrain, pons or medulla) – may indicate a syndrome of cerebral herniation through the tentorial hiatus or the foramen magnum (Fig. 3.1). The importance of these syndromes is being increasingly recognized in non-traumatic coma (particularly that caused by infections). Although the level of brainstem damage is given in brackets below (and in Fig. 3.1), recognizing the presence or absence of brainstem signs, and in particular early signs of reversible damage, is usually more important than determining their exact localization.

Assessment of the following five points allows most patients to be classified.

1 **Check for neck stiffness** (if no trauma), and Kernig's sign (extension of knee when hip is already flexed causes pain).
2 **Examine pupil reaction to light** (Fig. 3.1). A normal reaction (constriction) is seen in a diffuse encephalopathy. A unilateral large pupil is seen in herniation of the uncus of the temporal lobe. The pupils are reactive (small or mid-sized) in the diencephalic syndrome. Unreactive pupils occur in brainstem lesions (mid-sized in midbrain or pontine lesions; large in medullary lesions). Pinpoint pupils occur following opiate or organophosphate overdose, or in isolated pontine lesion. Other drugs can cause large unreactive pupils.

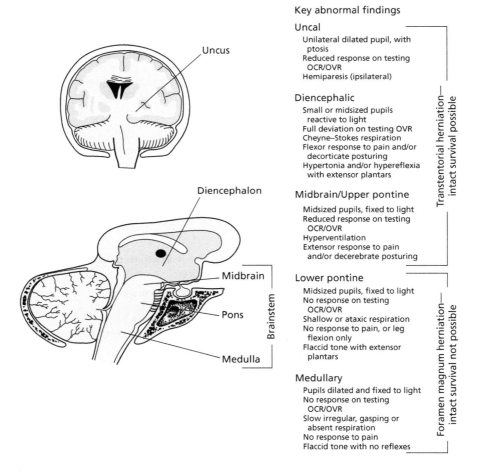

Key abnormal findings

Uncal
Unilateral dilated pupil, with ptosis
Reduced response on testing OCR/OVR
Hemiparesis (ipsilateral)

Diencephalic
Small or midsized pupils reactive to light
Full deviation on testing OVR
Cheyne–Stokes respiration
Flexor response to pain and/or decorticate posturing
Hypertonia and/or hyperreflexia with extensor plantars

Midbrain/Upper pontine
Midsized pupils, fixed to light
Reduced response on testing OCR/OVR
Hyperventilation
Extensor response to pain and/or decerebrate posturing

Lower pontine
Midsized pupils, fixed to light
No response on testing OCR/OVR
Shallow or ataxic respiration
No response to pain, or leg flexion only
Flaccid tone with extensor plantars

Medullary
Pupils dilated and fixed to light
No response on testing OCR/OVR
Slow irregular, gasping or absent respiration
No response to pain
Flaccid tone with no reflexes

Transtentorial herniation—intact survival possible

Foramen magnum herniation—intact survival not possible

Uncus

Diencephalon

Midbrain

Pons

Medulla

Brainstem

Figure 3.1 Sagittal section of brain showing anatomy and key abnormal findings of midline herniation syndromes, and (above) coronal section showing herniation of the uncus of the temporal lobe – this compresses the ipsilateral third nerve (to cause a palsy of CNIII), and the contralateral cerebral peduncle (to cause an ipsilateral hemiparesis).

3 **Assess eye movements** (holding eyelids open if necessary).
- *Spontaneous eye movements* – eyes spontaneously roving or eyes following indicates the brainstem is intact (a diencephalic syndrome or a diffuse encephalopathy).
- *Oculocephalic (doll's eye) reflex* (OCR) – when rotating the head, the eyes normally deviate away from the direction of rotation. A normal response indicates that the brainstem is intact (diffuse encephalopathy). Reduced or absent responses occur in uncal herniation, brainstem damage or, rarely, deep metabolic coma.
- *Oculovestibular reflex* (OVR) – caloric response to water should be tested if the result of the oculocephalic reflex is unclear. Check that the eardrum is not perforated, then irrigate by injecting 20 mL ice-cold water. Nystagmus is the normal response and indicates 'psychogenic coma'. Both eyes deviate towards the irrigated ear in coma with the brainstem intact. A reduced or absent response indicates an uncal syndrome or a damaged brainstem.
4 **Assess breathing pattern.** A normal pattern occurs in diffuse encephalopathy. Cheyne–Stokes breathing and hyperventilation occur in reversible herniation syndromes. Shallow, ataxic or apnoeic respiration occurs in more severe syndromes (Fig. 3.1). Hyperventilation also occurs in acidosis or may be caused by aspiration pneumonia, which is common in coma.
5 **Assess response to pain** by applying painful stimulus to the supraorbital ridge and nail bed of each limb.
- *Hemiparesis* – most often indicates supratentorial hemispheric focal pathology (other signs include asymmetry of tone and focal seizures), but also occurs in uncal herniation.
- *'Decorticate posturing'* – flexion of arms with extension of legs, indicating damage in the diencephalon, and *'decerebrate posturing'* (extension of arms and legs caused by midbrain/upper pontine damage) may both be reversible. No response, or leg flexion only, are more severe.

Symmetrical posturing (decorticate or decerebrate) and hemiparetic focal signs are also occasionally seen in metabolic encephalopathies (e.g. hypoglycaemia; hepatic, uraemic or hypoxic coma; sedative drugs), cerebal malaria, and intra- or postictally. Other pointers to metabolic disease include asterixis, tremor and myoclonus preceding the onset of coma.

Classification and further investigation of patients with coma

At this stage, if the history, general examination and preliminary investigation have not made one diagnosis extremely likely, most comatose patients will fall into one of three categories, based on the presence or absence of meningism, supratentorial and brainstem signs.

1 **Coma only** (no hemispheric signs, brainstem signs or meningism – 'sleeping beauties').
- If patient is febrile (or has a history of fever), suspect CNS infection (especially cerebral malaria) or metabolic coma plus secondary aspiration pneumonia.
- If afebrile, coma is likely to be metabolic (hypoglycaemia, drugs, alcohol, diabetic ketoacidosis, toxins), psychogenic (test caloric response to water – causes nystagmus), or, occasionally, resulting from subarachnoid haemorrhage or other cerebrovascular accident.
2 **Coma with meningism,** but no focal signs.
- If febrile, CNS infection (especially bacterial meningitis) is likely.
- If afebrile, subarachnoid haemorrhage is likely.
3 **Coma with focal signs** (with or without meningism). Decide if the signs are 'hemispheric signs', 'brainstem signs', or both.
- *Hemispheric signs only.* If febrile, consider CNS infection (especially encephalitis, bacterial meningitis, abscess, etc.). If afebrile, consider space-occupying lesion (Table 3.3), cerebrovascular accident or trauma.
- *Brainstem signs only* may be caused by either focal pathology within the brainstem (e.g. encephalitis) especially if markedly asymmetrical signs, or by herniation of the brainstem (through the foramen magnum) secondary to a diffuse process (e.g. diabetic ketoacidosis, or late bacterial meningitis) causing raised intracranial pressure.
- *Hemispheric and brainstem signs* may be a result of either a supratentorial lesion causing hemispheric signs and sufficient swelling to precipitate brainstem herniation (e.g. cerebral bleed, abscess) or patchy focal pathology in the hemispheres and brainstem (e.g. toxoplasmosis, viral encephalitis).

Indications and contraindications for lumbar puncture in suspected CNS infections (Table 3.4)

For many years lumbar puncture was performed in all patients with suspected CNS infections, in both the tropics and Western industrialized nations. It has gone out of fashion in the latter, following concerns that it was being performed on patients with contraindications, and may have precipitated herniation.

In patients with a contraindication, treatment should be started and then a lumbar puncture reconsidered later. In many tropical settings in Africa and Asia, where CNS infections are very common, lumbar puncture is still considered an essential investigation. Here the benefits of accurate diagnosis and

Table 3.4 Guidelines for lumbar puncture in patients with suspected central nervous system (CNS) infections

All patients with suspected CNS infection should have a lumbar puncture, except those with the following contraindications:
- Deteriorating level of consciousness, or deep coma (responsive only to pain, GCS < 8)
- Focal neurological signs present:
  Absent 'doll's eye' movements
  Decerebrate or decorticate posturing
  Hemiparesis/monoparesis (in patients with coma)
  Papilloedema
  Unequal, dilated or poorly responsive pupils
- Hypertension and relative bradycardia
- Obtunded state with poor peripheral perfusion or hypotension
- Within 30 min of a short convulsive seizure
- Following a prolonged convulsive seizure or tonic seizure

Abbreviation: GCS, Glasgow coma score.

Table 3.5 Cerebrospinal fluid (CSF) findings in central nervous system infections.

	Acute bacterial meningitis	Viral meningo-encephalitis	Tuberculous meningitis	Fungal	Normal
Opening pressure	Increased	Normal/increased	Increased	Increased	10–20 cm*
Colour	Cloudy	'Gin' clear	Cloudy/yellow	Clear/cloudy	Clear
Cells/mm³	High–very high	Normal–high	Slightly increased	Normal–high	
	1000–50 000	0–1000	25–500	0–1000	<5
Differential	Neutrophils	Lymphocytes	Lymphocytes	Lymphocytes	Lymphocytes
CSF: plasma glucose ratio	Low	Normal	Low–very low (e.g. <30%)	Normal–low	66%
Protein (g/L)	High >1	Normal–high 0.5–1	High–very high 1–5	Normal–high 0.2–5.0	<0.5

Normal values
*Normal CSF opening pressure is <20 cm water for adults, <10 cm for children below age 8.
A normal CSF glucose is usually quoted to be 66% that of the plasma glucose, but in many tropical settings a cut-off of 40% is found to be more useful.
A bloody tap will falsely elevate the CSF white cell count and protein. To correct for a bloody tap, subtract 1 white cell for every 700 red blood cells/mm³ in the CSF, and 0.1 g/dL of protein for every 1000 red blood cells.

Some important exceptions
In patients with acute bacterial meningitis that has been partially pretreated with antibiotics (or patients <1 year old) the CSF cell count may not be very high and may be mostly lymphocytes.
In viral CNS infections, an early lumbar puncture may give predominantly neutrophils, or there may be no cells in early or late lumbar punctures.
Tuberculous meningitis may have predominant CSF polymorphs early on.
Listeriosis can give a similar CSF picture to tuberculous meningitis, but the history is shorter.
CSF findings in bacterial abscesses range from near normal to purulent, depending on location of the abscess and whether there is associated meningitis or rupture.
An India ink test, and if negative a cryptococcal antigen test, should be performed on the CSF of all patients in whom cryptococcosis is possible.

appropriate treatment may outweigh the theoretical risk of herniation, and even patients with relative contraindications often receive lumbar punctures with no apparent harm.

Cerebrospinal fluid findings in CNS infections

Although most patients with CNS infections will have findings that are straightforward to interpret, there may be considerable overlap (Table 3.5). Ideally, the decision about starting antibiotics should await the result of the lumbar puncture (if it is available quickly). However, antibiotics should be started immediately for patients with a typical meningococcal rash, because of the speed with which meningococcal septicaemia can become fatal. In such patients, if it is certain that the rash is meningococcal it has been argued that the lumbar puncture is not necessary, because the diagnosis is already made, though others advocate always doing a lumbar puncture.

 FURTHER READING

Kelly CA, Upex A, Bateman DN (2004) Comparison of consciousness level assessment in the poisoned patient using the alert/verbal/painful/unresponsive scale and the Glasgow Coma Scale. *Ann of Emerg Med* **44**: 108–13. [Validation of AVPU score.]

Kirkham FJ (2001) Non-traumatic coma in children. *Arch Dis Child* **85**: 303–12. [An excellent review of pathophysiology and management.]

Kneen R, Solomon T, Appleton RA (2001) The role of lumbar punctures in CNS infections. *Arch Dis Child* **87**: 181–3. [Detailed discussion of the use of lumbar puncture.]

 SUMMARY

- Presentations with neurological features are more common in the tropics due to more frequent head trauma as well as a variety of infections including malaria, tuberculosis, bacterial meningitis and viruses causing viral encephalitis.

- Assessment of patients with neurological presentations should include search for systemic diseases as well as determination of the level of consciousness and the presence of focal upper or lower neurological signs.

- The level of consciousness should be graded using simple scoring systems such as modified Glasgow Coma score or the AVPU score, both to determine immediate severity and to follow progress.

- Clinicians should have a high index of suspicion for meningitis, which merits immediate empirical antibiotic therapy if essential investigations such as lumbar puncture cannot be performed urgently.

Visit **www.lecturenoteseries.com/tropicalmed** **to test yourself on this chapter using interactive MCQs.**

4

Febrile presentations

Mike Beadsworth[1] and Tom Blanchard[2]
[1]Liverpool School of Tropical Medicine; [2]North Manchester General Hospital

Pathogenesis and symptomatic treatment of fever

Fever (pyrexia) is the most common physiological response to infection, however non-infective causes including malignancy, autoimmune, drugs and others must always be considered. Resetting of thermoregulation in the hypothalamus, mediated by prostaglandins, is caused by activation of cytokines, including IL-1, tumour necrosis factor and interferon-alpha. Antipyretics in common use act by inhibition of pyrogenic prostaglandin production: these are either non-steroidal anti-inflammatory drugs or paracetamol (acetaminophen). Although antipyretics are widely used and have beneficial properties in terms of analgesic effects and reducing discomfort, they do not improve mortality. Paracetamol is the antipyretic of choice because it is free of side-effects at normal dosage and, unlike aspirin, it is not associated with Reye's syndrome in children.

Clinical approach to the patient with fever

History

A comprehensive history is key to determining aetiology of fever, and should include: when did the fever begin, where and what exposures may have taken place? A sexual history is also vital. Incubation periods of infection may be calculated allowing a differential diagnoses list to be developed. Where the patient is located allows further development of this list (e.g. is it a malarious area?) Finally, exposure to risk factors such as insect bites, abrasions and bites should also be queried, to help determine the causes. For example, water and soil contact may herald leptospirosis in regions where it is present, and contact with rivers and freshwater lakes in Africa suggest schistosomiasis (Katayama fever).

Important symptoms are headache, photophobia, cough, sputum, pleurisy, localized pain, diarrhoea (especially if bloody) and urinary symptoms. Coryza and upper respiratory symptoms generally suggest a viral illness. Prior treatment with antibiotics may make diagnosis difficult. Recent travel (within 3 weeks) to high-risk countries should always raise the possibility of viral haemorrhagic fever. The pattern of fever is rarely helpful in making a diagnosis in practice. Older children will give a history in the same way as adults. For infants and babies, enquiry should be made about feeding, weight gain (often charted), general activity and the health of the parents.

Examination

A temperature >38.0 °C is clinically significant. If there is a convincing history of fever but no significant pyrexia on presentation, and the patient does not require admission to hospital, a self-recorded temperature chart can be helpful. A pulse rate >100 or <60 or systolic blood pressure <100 mmHg in an adult suggests the patient is seriously ill and needs urgent physiological support and empirical treatment. Conscious level, orientation and neck stiffness need to be assessed.

Spontaneous haemorrhage suggests a viral haemorrhagic fever. A full clinical examination should be undertaken. The eyes should be inspected for anaemia, jaundice, conjunctival injection (mea-

Tropical Medicine Lecture Notes, Seventh edition. Edited by Nick Beeching and Geoff Gill. © 2014 John Wiley & Sons, Ltd. Published 2014 by John Wiley & Sons, Ltd.

sles and leptospirosis) and the fundi examined if lumbar puncture is likely to be needed or if endocarditis is possible. Psychosis may be a manifestation of typhoid. The mouth should be examined for candidiasis (HIV infection), Koplik's spots (measles) and pharyngitis. The tympanic membranes of all young children should be inspected, but only in adults if there are relevant symptoms. Cervical and axillary lymphadenopathy should be sought (pharyngitis, HIV, cytomegalovirus [CMV], Epstein–Barr virus [EBV], tuberculosis, lymphoma, toxoplasmosis, syphilis) and also occipital lymphadenopathy (rubella, trypanosomiasis). The skin should be carefully inspected for rash (viral exanthems, non-blanching meningococcal petechiae), an eschar (tick-borne rickettsial infection) or anaesthetic patches with pigmentary change (leprosy). Severe skin and soft tissue infections (usually streptococcal or staphylococcal) are common causes of fever.

The chest and heart require examination for signs of consolidation (pneumonia often fails to give respiratory symptoms), pleural or pericardial effusion (tuberculosis, HIV, empyema) and heart murmurs (bacterial endocarditis, rheumatic heart disease). In infants and babies a raised respiratory rate may be the only evidence of pneumonia. Abdominal tenderness and peritonism should be sought (appendicitis, peritonitis, pelvic inflammatory disease). Localized right lower intercostal tenderness suggests amoebic liver abscess. Hepatomegaly (malaria, tuberculosis, hepatitis, schistosomiasis, hepatoma, amoebic liver abscess) and splenomegaly (malaria, typhoid, leishmaniasis, HIV, infectious mononucleosis, lymphoma and leukaemia, portal hypertension, brucellosis, disseminated tuberculosis) are important signs. Demonstrable ascites requires a diagnostic tap Any detectable joint effusion should also be tapped. Urinalysis should, of course, be part of the examination.

Initial investigation

Laboratory tests that are useful to discriminate those who require further investigation and treatment from those who require symptomatic management only, are malaria films and full blood count. A malaria film should always be performed if there has been a visit to a malarious area and there is fever or symptoms suggestive of fever, irrespective of the patient's presentation. It is useful triage to arrange a malaria film as soon as a febrile patient presents, even before seeing a doctor. Where facilities are available, measurement of urea and electrolytes (renal failure in sepsis syndromes, shock, severe malaria, leptospirosis, haemolytic uraemic syndrome; hyponatraemia

in tuberculosis), liver function tests (viral hepatitis) and C-reactive protein (CRP) are helpful. If the CRP is <10mg/L, significant underlying pathology is much less likely. The ESR is simple to perform and may be helpful as a non-specific marker of inflammation (bearing in mind that the ESR may be raised in the elderly and in the general population in the tropics). It is good practice to save a specimen of acute serum. A chest X-ray should be performed if no obvious cause of fever is present. Appropriate bacterial cultures are important and, where available, should always be performed prior to starting antibiotic treatment. These include: blood cultures, especially if typhoid or paratyphoid is possible; urine culture, where symptoms or urinalysis suggest urinary tract infection; and stool microscopy and culture, if bloody diarrhoea is present. At least two sets (aerobic and anaerobic on each occasion) of blood cultures should be taken: these do not have to coincide with spikes of fever, but should be taken from different sites and as little as 10–20 minutes apart if antibiotic treatment is urgent. If bacterial endocarditis is suspected then at least three sets of blood cultures should be taken, preferably spaced over several hours. Sputum culture is generally not helpful, except for tuberculosis, and is often unavailable in resource-poor settings. Sputum microscopy for acid-fast bacilli should be available in most settings, and is important if pulmonary tuberculosis is suspected (chronic cough, weight loss, night sweats). Lumbar puncture is necessary if symptoms and signs suggest meningitis. In well-resourced settings there is massive overuse of CT scanning prior to lumbar puncture: CT scan is only indicated if there are recent onset seizures, focal neurology, significantly depressed Glasgow Coma Score (<8), papilloedema, or immunosuppression (e.g. by HIV) is likely. Unnecessary CT scans are a waste of money, cause significant delays in lumbar puncture, impair bacteriological diagnosis and appropriate treatment. Infants and babies may give no specific clues of meningitis, so lumbar puncture should be performed if they are significantly unwell with no other identifiable cause of fever and a negative malaria film. An adult patient who has severe headache but no meningism, and in whom HIV is known or suspected, requires lumbar puncture in order to exclude cryptococcal meningitis. Usually, evidence of raised intracranial pressure is a contraindication to lumbar puncture, but it has a therapeutic role in cryptococcal meningitis provided that space occupying lesions such as cerebral toxoplasmosis have been excluded. Genital swabs for microscopy and culture should be taken if sexually transmitted infection is suspected; syphilis serology is also relevant, especially with a rash extending to the palms and soles. Viral tests are usually restricted to serology, generally for HIV and hepatitis B, in resource-poor settings.

Acute fevers with a negative malarial blood film

The white blood cell count (WBC) divides this group into two, as shown in Box 4.1.

Box 4.1 Acute fevers with a negative malarial blood film

Polymorphonuclear leucocytosis?

Yes	No
Pyogenic infection	Viral infections
Leptospiral infection	Typhoid
Relapsing fevers	Rickettsial
Amoebic liver abscess	infections
Gout	

Treatment of common causes of fever lasting <2 weeks

It is important to remember that in general in at least 50% of adults and older children with genuine fever, no cause will be identified and the fever will resolve spontaneously in a few days. These patients come to no harm from their presumed infection, and the important thing is to keep diagnostic procedures and therapeutic intervention to a minimum. In young children and babies many infections are viral, and if the cause is not immediately apparent, it may become so in a few days. Such infections require symptomatic treatment only, with the exception of suspected measles which requires high-dose vitamin A supplements (see Chapter 62: Eye disease, p. 364). In adults, even when there is likely to be an underlying cause for infection, it is preferable to delay anti-infective treatment until the diagnosis is established, and certainly cultures should always be taken first where possible. In children with neutrophilia who appear unwell there may be a case for giving antibiotics. There are instances where empirical treatment should be started immediately, but treatment has to be guided by the diagnostic and therapeutic options available. For example, it is bad practice blindly to give treatment for malaria unless there are no diagnostic facilities whatsoever. Semi-immune people in endemic areas may have a few detectable malaria parasites circulating harmlessly, with their fever caused by something entirely different. Malaria does not cause a raised neutrophil count, but thrombocytopenia is very common and requires no intervention unless very low with spontaneous bleeding. Empirical treatment should be started immediately for meningitis if the patient is ill (with appropriate symptoms and signs) or if there is going to be a delay in obtaining the results of lumbar puncture. In practice, this usually means treatment with chloramphenicol or a third generation cephalosporin is preferred. Similarly, a patient with severe sepsis requires empirical antibiotics immediately after blood cultures have been taken. Follow local or national guidelines for antimicrobial prescribing.

Rickettsial infection is often a clinical diagnosis; the patient should be treated with a tetracycline once investigations have been performed to exclude malaria and typhoid. Dengue fever should be suspected if there is general body pain and severe retro-orbital headache with generalized blanching erythema and a negative malaria film. Treatment is supportive only, and the diagnosis is only established retrospectively when serology is available. The fever should not last longer than 2 weeks and classically has a saddleback pattern. Treatment for pneumonia should be started on clinical grounds, although chest X-ray is certainly helpful. A low threshold for treating severe pharyngitis with penicillin V is reasonable in the tropics, partly because post-streptococcal complications are seen much more frequently, and because the rare but severe Lemierre's syndrome has increased in frequency as antibiotic treatment for sore throat has become unfashionable.

Common non-infectious causes of fever

Autoimmune and connective tissue disorders

- Familial Mediterranean fever
- Giant cell arteritis
- Polyarteritis nodosa
- Polymyositis/dermatomyositis
- Rheumatoid arthritis

- Still's disease
- Systemic lupus erythematosus
- Wegener's granulomatosis

Malignancy

- Lymphoproliferative disorders
- Myeloproliferative disorders
- Renal and hepatic malignancy

Other

- Drug fevers and adverse reactions (including erythema multiforme etc.)
- Factitious fever
- Inflammatory bowel disease
- Thyrotoxicosis

Common causes of fever lasting >2 weeks

The following list contains the most common causes of prolonged fever, simply subdivided according to the most usual white blood cell (WBC) picture.

1 **Chronic fever with neutrophilia:**
  - amoebic liver abscess
  - cholangitis
  - deep sepsis
  - erythema nodosum leprosum
  - relapsing fever
2 **Chronic fever with eosinophilia:**
  - acute lymphangitic exacerbations of *Wuchereria bancrofti* and *Brugia malayi* infections
  - gross visceral larva migrans caused by *Toxocara canis*
  - invasive (toxaemic) *Schistosoma mansoni* and *S. japonicum* infections
  - invasive *Fasciola hepatica* infection
3 **Chronic fever with neutropenia:**
  - brucellosis
  - disseminated tuberculosis
  - malaria
  - visceral leishmaniasis
4 **Chronic fever with normal WBC:**
  - brucellosis
  - chronic meningococcal septicaemia
  - HIV-related (see below)
  - endocarditis
  - localized tuberculosis
  - secondary syphilis

- systemic lupus erythematosus
- toxoplasmosis
- trypanosomiasis
5 **Chronic fever with a variable WBC picture:**
  - drug reactions
  - lymphomas
  - tumours

Omitted from the list are those conditions where the localizing signs are apparent. Fever in association with HIV is covered in Chapter 13.

Common clinical problems with febrile patients

Managing a febrile patient with no localizing symptoms or signs and little or no laboratory or radiological back-up is a common problem. If the patient is unwell, empirical treatment has to be given. In a malarious area, the first line should be antimalarials, and a significant fall in fever would be expected after 2–3 days.

If there is no response, then the next pathogen of importance is typhoid. It used to be standard practice to treat with chloramphenicol, but resistance is widespread so ciprofloxacin or a third generation cephalosporin is to be preferred if available. Typhoid fever should respond to appropriate treatment in 4–5 days, but it can take 7–10 days if there is low-grade ciprofloxacin resistance. If there is still no response, empirical antituberculous therapy may be indicated, although regimens containing rifampicin will treat other infections as well as tuberculosis.

Another difficult scenario is a fever (>38.3 °C on at least two occasions) which has lasted >4 weeks and has not resolved after at least 3 days of inpatient investigation, i.e. pyrexia/fever of unknown origin (PUO or FUO). Such patients should be clinically assessed at regular intervals in case new signs or symptoms come to light. There is very little information regarding underlying causes of PUO in the tropics. When PUO in the developed world is investigated, then infection accounts for about one-third of cases (mainly intra-abdominal abscess, tuberculosis, infective endocarditis and complications of HIV infection), neoplasia for 20% (especially lymphoma and occasionally renal cell carcinoma), autoimmune disorders for 10% (e.g. adult Still's disease, temporal arteritis, Wegener's granulomatosis, systemic lupus erythematosus and polyarteritis nodosa), miscellaneous causes for 15% (e.g. drug fever, non-infective granulomatous disorders, haematomas, e.g. subdural), and cause is unknown in 25%. Travel and exposure history, symptoms and signs should guide investigation and laboratory results. If available, an ultrasound is non-invasive and helpful for demonstrating hepatic disease (e.g. tumour, abscess, schistosomiasis, fascioliasis), splenomegaly, ascites and renal tract disorders. A computerized tomography (CT) scan of the thorax, abdomen and pelvis is relatively non-invasive and has a high diagnostic yield for abscesses, tumours and lymphadenopathy, but is not widely available in the tropics. Other potentially useful investigations include lymph node biopsy (if enlarged), bone marrow aspirate, trephine and culture, and liver biopsy. In the tropics, tuberculosis, osteomyelitis, dental sepsis, hepatoma and SLE appear to be more common than in adults with PUO in Europe. There is very little written about PUO affecting babies and children in the tropics, but it is safe to say that infections secondary to HIV-induced immunosuppression are increasing in importance, and neoplasia is less common than in adults.

PUO in HIV-infected adults in the tropics presents a different spectrum of disease, and is usually associated with a CD4 count $<200 \times 10^6/L$ (Chapter 13). PUO has become less common since the advent of combination antiretroviral therapy (cART), but the causes of PUO remain essentially unchanged. A series of patients investigated in Brazil found (in descending order) tuberculosis, *Pneumocystis jirovecii*, *Mycobacterium avium* complex, non-Hodgkin's lymphoma, cryptococcal meningitis, sinusitis, salmonellosis, histoplasmosis, neurosyphilis and cystoisosporiaisis. A similar investigation in Thailand found tuberculosis, *Cryptococcus neoformans*, *Pneumocystis jirovecii*, *Toxoplasma gondii* and salmonella bacteraemia. Up to 25% of HIV-infected patients with PUO will have two or more opportunistic infections simultaneously. PUO is associated with a high mortality in HIV infection, so it is unwise to wait the statutory 4 weeks before investigating thoroughly. Traditionally infectious disease physicians have waited to obtain a clear response to treatment of opportunistic infection before initiating cART, because of the complexity of interactions and interpreting the side effects of all the drugs involved, with the added difficulty of recognizing immune reconstitution inflammatory syndrome. There is accumulating evidence that better outcomes are obtained if cART is started earlier rather than later, an important point because most of the HIV-infected patients who present with PUO will have low CD4 counts and will not have started antiretrovirals (see Chapter 13).

Finally, there are many exotic and uncommon infective causes of fever. Some, like trypanosomiasis, *Borrelia recurrentis* and babesiosis will show up unexpectedly on examination of the blood film. Others have to be thought of and deliberately sought, such as bartonellosis, *Borrelia burgdorferi* and Q fever.

 SUMMARY

- Fever is the most common physiological response to infection but may also be caused by non-infectious illness.
- The likely causes can be predicted from careful history and examination of the patient, coupled with knowledge of local pathogens causing fever of short duration (less than two weeks) or longer duration.
- The diagnosis can usually be clarified further by simple tests such as the total and differential peripheral white cell count and malaria films.
- In resource poor settings, detailed investigation should be reserved for patients whose fever does not settle spontaneously or as a result of treatment based on a local algorithmic approach.
- Fever in patients with HIV may be multifactorial and/or due to a wider range of pathogens than in the immunocompetent.

 Visit www.lecturenoteseries.com/tropicalmed **to test yourself on this chapter using interactive MCQs.**

📖 FURTHER READING

Fletcher TE, Bleeker-Rovers CP, Beeching NJ (2013) Fever. *Medicine* 41(2): 70–6. 10.1016/j.mpmed.2012.11.002. [Review of fever syndromes in different settings and algorithm for managing PUO.]

Surviving sepsis campaign website http://www.survivingsepsis.org/Pages/default.aspx [Recent guidelines and pointers to improving recognition and management of sepsis. These can be adapted for different tropical settings.]

5

Dermatological presentations

Nick Beeching
Liverpool School of Tropical Medicine

Skin disease is ubiquitous among the poor of underdeveloped countries. Bacterial infections, often secondary to insect bites or scabies, are particularly likely in childhood and superficial fungal infections, especially pityriasis versicolor, are present in many adults. Several of the major tropical diseases also have skin manifestations and it is essential that the clinician should not miss the diagnosis of leprosy.

Whenever possible take a systematic history to include details of any travel, contact with insects or sensitizing agents, use of drugs or skin applications, similar rashes in family or contacts and the evolution of the skin problem. Examine the entire skin surface together with the scalp and mucous membranes in a good light, and note the character and distribution of all skin lesions, distinguishing the original lesions from modifications caused by scratching or secondary infection. Don't panic – non-dermatologists can reach a sensible differential diagnosis by describing the rash in terms of its distribution and characteristics:

Distribution of lesions

- Solitary or multiple (few or many)
- Discrete or coalescent
- Symmetry
- Distribution
  - Centripetal (limbs)
  - Centrifugal (trunk)
- Face
- Mucous membranes (mouth, nose, conjunctivae, genitalia)
- Palms and soles

Characteristics

- Dolor (pain)
- Rubor (redness/heat)
- Tumor (swelling)
- If redness is present, does it blanch on pressure (vasodilatation)?
- Is it itchy?

Very few conditions commonly affect the palms of the hands and soles of the feet:

- Syphilis, yaws
- Drugs including arsenicals
- Erythema multiforme including Stevens-Johnson syndrome
- Rickettsiae
- Enteroviruses
- Parvovirus
- Psoriasis group (pustular prosiasis etc)
- Monkeypox (and formerly smallpox), whereas involvement rare in chickenpox

Skin ulcers

Trauma and insect bites account for many acute skin ulcers but these usually heal quickly. All the causes of chronic ulceration seen in temperate climates (including diabetic ulcers, venous and arterial ulcers), are seen but their frequency is less in most young tropical populations. Some of the more important causes of chronic ulcers are given in Table 5.1.

Tropical Medicine Lecture Notes, Seventh edition. Edited by Nick Beeching and Geoff Gill. © 2014 John Wiley & Sons, Ltd. Published 2014 by John Wiley & Sons, Ltd.

Table 5.1 **Chronic ulcers**

Type of ulcer	Main characteristics	How diagnosis is established
Tropical ulcer	Painful; rapid onset, usually lower leg	Heals on non-specific regimen
Buruli ulcer	Extensive; mainly painless; very deep undermined edges	Finding acid-fast bacilli in edge of ulcer
Cutaneous leishmaniasis	Single or multiple; often with infiltrated edges; not undermined	Amastigotes in edges of lesions. Culture or PCR
Desert sore, veld sore (cutaneous diphtheria)	Usually single, painful onset with vesicle; adherent slough, undermined, paralysis from toxin	Culture, as well as the clinical combination of ulcer with neurological deficit
Tertiary syphilis (gumma)	Chronic, usually painless ulcers on extremity	Serological tests for syphilis Spirochaetes cannot be found
Tuberculous ulcer	Frank ulcers often follow subcutaneous TB; there may be adjacent cold abscess or evidence of TB elsewhere	Microscopy for AAFB. Culture
Sickle cell disease in adults	Rare in Africa where few adults with the disease survive. Ulcers often symmetrical on lower legs	Patient obviously anaemic and sickling test positive
Dracunculiasis (guinea worm)	The pearly prolapsed uterus is seen early	By identifying the worm, or larvae expelled after exposure to water
Trophic ulcer of leprosy	Painless; may be deeply penetrating on the sole	Associated evidence of nerve damage: thick nerves, loss of sensation
Diabetic ulcer	In the tropics usually neuropathic. On soles of feet over bony prominences. Usually painless	Evidence of neuropathy. Known or newly diagnosed diabetes
Malignant ulcer	Squamous cell carcinoma	Biopsy and histology
Mycoses (subcutaneous or deep)	Usually ulcerates within a preformed granulomatous nodule. May have proximal sporotrichoid spread	Biopsy, culture and histology Microscopy for hyphae and spores

Abbreviations: AAFB, acid- and alcohol-fast bacilli; PCR, polymerase chain reaction; TB, tuberculosis.

Skin itching

A very wide range of dermatological conditions and health problems may cause itching but in the tropics the most common causes include the following.

- *Scabies* – typical distribution (rarely affects head and neck), but burrows are often masked by secondary infection.
- *Norwegian scabies* – atypical with massive exfoliation which is highly infectious; associated with HIV, HTLV-1.
- *Insect bites* – papular urticaria on exposed surfaces.
- *Superficial fungal infection* – examine scrapings for hyphae after clearing in 10% potassium hydroxide.
- *Eczema* – often a personal or family history of allergy or recent exposure to drugs or topical sensitizer.

- *Onchocerciasis* – geographical distribution, examine for nodules and take skin snips.
- *Metabolic disorders* – e.g. chronic uraemia.

Creeping eruptions

- Larva migrans from dog hookworms form a slowly extending, persistent, itching track most often on the foot or lower leg. Multiple infections cause severe itching.
- Track-like lesions from the larvae of some species of *Paragonimus*, *Gnathostoma spinigerum* or from some fly larvae are less common.
- Larva currens is the name given to rapidly moving tracks caused by migrating *Strongyloides stercoralis* larvae. These urticaria-like tracks are found between the neck and the knees and last for hours or a day or two only.

Papules

- Milia
- Molluscum contagiosum (umbilicated)
- Onchocerciasis
- HIV-related
- Scabies
- Insect bites
- Acne
- Cercarial dermatitis
- Tungiasis (typically in feet)

Skin nodules

- Furuncle
- Furuncular myiasis
- Leprosy. The nodules are frequently over the ears, eyebrows and face. The diagnosis is readily confirmed by slit skin smears for acid-fast bacilli
- Erythema nodosum resulting from leprosy is sometimes widespread. Tuberculosis, streptococcal infection and sarcoidosis are other causes
- Leishmaniasis. Single or multiple nodules may take months to ulcerate; they are predominantly on exposed surfaces but spread along lymphatics occurs. Diffuse cutaneous leishmaniasis and nodular post-kala-azar dermal leishmaniasis can resemble nodular leprosy
- Kaposi's sarcoma. Chiefly affecting limbs of older persons in endemic areas, but any skin surface and mucosae often with lymph node enlargement in AIDS
- Fungal infections including chromoblastomycosis, sporotrichosis, *Histoplasma duboisii* and *H. capsulatum, Paracoccidioides brasiliensis, Penicillium marneffei*. Some are particularly common as secondary infections in the immunosuppressed
- Subcutaneous nodules are a feature of onchocerciasis
- Cysticercosis
- Juxta-articular nodules are found in late yaws

Remember also 'non-tropical' causes such as rheumatoid nodules, gouty tophi and neurofibromata.

Changes in pigmentation

Hypopigmented macules

- Post-inflammation and scarring
- Pityriasis versicolor. 'Raindrop' patches over trunk with slight scaling

- Leprosy. Loss of sensation, enlarged nerves. Hair loss
- Onchocerciasis. Patches chiefly over shins; nodules and positive skin snips
- Yaws. Mainly affects palms and soles; positive syphilis serology
- Vitiligo. Usually white and well-demarcated, sometimes hyperpigmented borders; symmetrical; association with autoimmune disease
- Post-kala-azar dermal leishmaniasis

Hyperpigmentation

- Pellagra. Affects sun-exposed skin
- Pregnancy
- Chronic arsenic poisoning. Slatey-grey colour of trunk with small areas of normal skin. Hyperkeratosis of palms and soles
- Addison's disease. Look for pigment in oral mucosa
- Hypertrophic lichen planus. Warty patches typically involving calves, forearms and lower back
- Kaposi's sarcoma
- Fixed drug eruptions. Especially after sulfa-containing drugs. Associated with systemic upset
- Rickettsial eschar – black. Often hidden in hair-line or in underwear areas
- Cutaneous anthrax – evolving black lesion, clues are oedema but relative lack of pain

Urticaria

Acute urticaria may follow jellyfish stings or other envenomation, contact with plants, arthropods or drugs such as penicillin. The diagnosis of the cause of chronic urticaria can be very difficult because such a wide variety of both internal and external causes may be responsible. Some common causes acquired in the tropics are as follows.

- Papular urticaria from insect bites
- Katayama syndrome in schistosomiasis. Follows freshwater exposure by weeks to months and associated with cough, wheeze and marked eosinophilia
- Intestinal helminths including roundworms and hookworms and migrating larvae of *Strongyloides stercoralis*
- Filarial infection
- Drugs
- Food additives

Vesicles and bullae

The main differential diagnosis of vesicular lesions includes chickenpox and herpes zoster (often HIV associated), localized or disseminated herpes simplex and poxviruses. Larger fluid-filled blisters may result from a variety of causes; some of the more common ones in the tropics include the following.

- Bullous impetigo
- Insect bites/contact, usually multiple
- Sunburn
- Burns and scalds
- Drug eruptions
- Snake bite and other causes of envenoming
- Larva migrans
- Pemphigus including Brazilian pemphigus foliaceous
- Porphyria associated with sun exposure

Petechial rashes

- Meningococcal septicaemia
- Dengue and dengue haemorrhagic fever
- Rickettsial infections. May involve palms, look for eschars and lymphadenopathy
- Viral haemorrhagic fevers including Lassa, Ebola and Crimean–Congo
- Vasculitis including Henoch–Schönlein purpura
- Disseminated intravascular coagulation
- Infective endocarditis
- Drug rashes

 Visit www.lecturenoteseries.com/tropicalmed to test yourself on this chapter using interactive MCQs.

 SUMMARY

- Skin disease is very common in the tropics in all age groups.
- A sensible working diagnosis can be achieved by describing the rash in textbook terms, which narrows down the differential diagnosis.
- The differential diagnosis must be interpreted in the context of geography and any other illness that the patient may have.
- Presence of itch always suggest scabies, which rarely affects the head and neck.
- Any atypical skin lesion, pale or anaesthetic patch should prompt careful search for other features of leprosy such as nerve thickening.

📖 **FURTHER READING**

Caumes E, Carriere J, Guermonprez G, *et al.* (1995) Dermatoses associated with travel to tropical countries: a prospective study of the diagnosis and management of 269 patients presenting to a tropical disease unit. *Clin Infect Dis* **20**: 542–8. [A description of travellers with dermatological conditions acquired abroad.]

Hay R, Bendeck SE, Chen S, *et al.* (2006) Skin diseases. In DT Jamison *et al.*, *Disease Control Priorities in Developing Countries,* Chapter 37, pp. 707–21. World Bank. http://publications.worldbank.org/index.php?main_page=product_info&cPath=0&products_id=21135.

Naafs B (2004) The skin. In EPO Parry, R Godfrey, D Mabey, GV Gill (eds), *Principles of Medicine in Africa*, 3rd edn. Cambridge University Press, pp. 1264–1305.

Naafs B (2009) Rural dermatology in the tropics. *Clin Dermatol* **27**: 252–70. [A useful review of dermatological disease in the rural tropics, including a section on tropical ulcer.]

6

The patient with anaemia

Jecko Thachil[1] and Imelda Bates[2]
[1]Manchester Royal Infirmary; [2]Liverpool School of Tropical Medicine

Anaemia is the most common medical condition worldwide, but it is not a diagnosis in itself. Whenever possible, the underlying cause should be determined and alleviated to prevent recurrence. It is important to have knowledge of the local causes of ill health as this can help to prioritize investigations and treatment, especially when diagnostic resources are limited. Where schistosomiasis is common this may be a frequent local cause of anaemia, whereas amongst rural farming communities it may be chronic hookworm infestation. In poorer countries the aetiology of anaemia is often multifactorial and exacerbated by poor nutrition and high levels of infections and infestations.

Causes of anaemia

The aetiology of severe anaemia in developing countries is complex as it is usually the end result of several interdependent factors. In some studies 'anaemia' has been assumed to be due to iron deficiency and this imprecision has further complicated understanding about the factors that cause anaemia.

Infections are probably the commonest cause of anaemia in the tropics:

- In malaria-endemic areas of Africa, there is a clear correlation between anaemia and malaria.
- Severe anaemia is also seen in individuals affected by HIV. This is especially the case if there is coexisting tuberculosis infection.
- Bacterial infections can be a common cause of anaemia in children by causing increased bleeding and underproduction due to cytokine-induced bone marrow suppression.

- Hookworm infestation is a common cause even in very young children (e.g. those less than 2 years old in Malawi). Surprisingly, hookworm infections are more common in HIV-negative than HIV-positive adults.
- Vitamin A deficiency has been noted in approximately one-third of anaemic patients possibly related to its antibacterial protective effect.

Haematinic deficiency as a cause of anaemia in the tropics is discussed separately.

Clinical diagnosis of anaemia

Examination of the degree of pallor of tongue, nails and conjunctivae can provide a reasonable indication of anaemia when it is severe but is not helpful for detecting mild/moderate anaemia. Clinical examination alone is 66% sensitive and 68% specific for haemoglobin levels of 50–80 g/L in Malawian children and 82% sensitive and 65% specific for haemoglobin levels of less than 70 g/L in pregnant women in Kenya. A laboratory test to estimate haemoglobin levels is therefore necessary to detect and guide treatment of mild/moderate anaemia and to prevent the development of severe anaemia. A good clinical history and examination are essential in determining the cause of anaemia (Box 6.1).

Laboratory investigations

At smaller hospitals, the laboratory may provide tests such as haemoglobin, blood film examination and malaria slide microscopy. It may also offer

Tropical Medicine Lecture Notes, Seventh edition. Edited by Nick Beeching and Geoff Gill. © 2014 John Wiley & Sons, Ltd. Published 2014 by John Wiley & Sons, Ltd.

has been designed specifically for tropical countries with ability to operate in humid conditions and at high temperatures. It provides rapid accurate results directly from a finger prick sample. The haemoglobin colour scale also uses finger prick blood, is rapid and cheap and is probably better than clinical diagnosis for detecting mild/moderate anaemia. It is essential that clinicians satisfy themselves that their laboratory's results are reliable before using haemoglobin measurements to guide patient management. Test performance can be improved through participation in an external quality monitoring scheme, which may simply involve exchanging samples between neighbouring laboratories. Other ways of maintaining the quality of results include:

- repeat testing of the same sample with each batch of tests;
- compare packed cell volume (PCV) with haemoglobin results (PCV should be approximately three times the haemoglobin value);
- plot weekly cumulative averages of haemoglobin results to determine any 'drifting' of results;
- ensure that reagents are within their shelf life, technical staff are qualified and regularly supervised, and that the method in use is appropriate for the level of health care and local infrastructure.

a transfusion service. Accurate haemoglobin estimation and a good blood film examination will enable the diagnosis and cause of anaemia to be established in the majority of cases. Features on the blood film can indicate the presence of iron or folate deficiency, haemoglobinopathies, enzymopathies and malignant or proliferative haematological disorders. Well-resourced hospitals may be able to estimate ferritin, folate and cobalamin levels, perform haemoglobin electrophoresis, examine bone marrow samples and carry out a range of other tests including endoscopy, to determine the cause of anaemia.

Measurement of haemoglobin

Although haemoglobin estimation is the most commonly performed laboratory test, and is used to guide blood transfusions, in practice, it is also one of the least accurate tests. The reference method for haemoglobin, the haemoglobincyanide method, requires a spectrophotometer and well-supervised and qualified technicians and the cyanide buffer is increasingly difficult to source. Any method that depends on manual dilution of the sample (e.g. Sahli, Lovibond) requires careful pipette technique to maintain accuracy. The HemoCue Hb 301 system

Examination of peripheral blood film

If the cause of anaemia remains elusive after basic investigations, determining whether the anaemia is microcytic, macrocytic or normocytic (using the MCV from a haematology analyzer) will narrow down the possibilities (Fig. 6.1).

Microcytic anaemia

The most common cause of microcytic anaemia is iron deficiency (Fig. 6.2). Questions should be asked relating to blood loss and dietary insufficiency; stool examination for parasites and occult blood, and endoscopic examination of the gastrointestinal tract to exclude occult malignancy may be required. The thalassaemias also cause microcytosis but the clinical setting and further investigations such as haemoglobin electrophoresis demonstrating raised HbA_2 and HbF may help to confirm the diagnosis. α-thalassaemia trait may be particularly difficult to diagnose and referral to a specialist centre may be necessary. If the patient presents with mixed microcytic and macrocytic anaemia, nutritional deficiency of both iron and folate is likely.

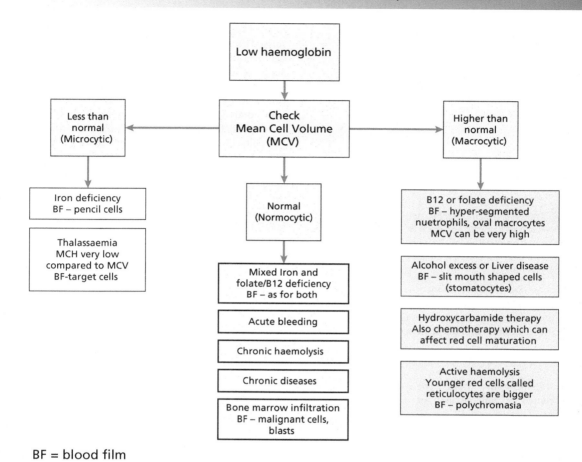

```
                    ┌─────────────────┐
                    │ Low haemoglobin │
                    └─────────────────┘
```

Low haemoglobin

Less than normal (Microcytic) ← Check Mean Cell Volume (MCV) → Higher than normal (Macrocytic)

Normal (Normocytic)

Less than normal (Microcytic):

Iron deficiency
BF – pencil cells

Thalassaemia
MCH very low compared to MCV
BF-target cells

Normal (Normocytic):

Mixed Iron and folate/B12 deficiency
BF – as for both

Acute bleeding

Chronic haemolysis

Chronic diseases

Bone marrow infiltration
BF – malignant cells, blasts

Higher than normal (Macrocytic):

B12 or folate deficiency
BF – hyper-segmented nuetrophils, oval macrocytes
MCV can be very high

Alcohol excess or Liver disease
BF – slit mouth shaped cells (stomatocytes)

Hydroxycarbamide therapy
Also chemotherapy which can affect red cell maturation

Active haemolysis
Younger red cells called reticulocytes are bigger
BF – polychromasia

BF = blood film

Figure 6.1 Algorithm for patient management.

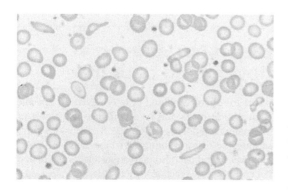

Figure 6.2 Iron-deficient red cells. The cells are paler and more irregular in shape than normal red cells. From B. Bain (2002) *Blood Cells: A Practical Guide*, 3rd edn. Oxford: Blackwell Publishing.

Macrocytic anaemia

A high mean cell volume (MCV) with oval macrocytes and hypersegmented neutrophils (Fig. 6.3) is highly suggestive of folate or vitamin B_{12} deficiency. A high MCV may also indicate the presence of early red cells. These may be produced in response to blood loss or destruction, or in response to haematinics, and can be detected as polychromatic cells on a peripheral blood film. Specific stains can be used to confirm that these cells are reticulocytes. A high MCV can also be associated with alcohol excess and liver disease, or drugs such as hydroxycarbamide. A combination of red cell fragments, thrombocytopenia and polychromasia on the blood film indicates microangiopathic haemolytic anaemia and the need for further tests such as coagulation studies, assessment of renal function and a search for infection or neoplastic disease. In

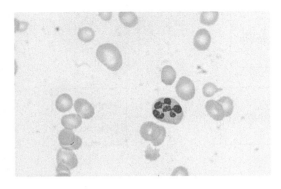

Figure 6.3 Oval macrocytes and hypersegmented neutrophils in folate deficiency. B. Bain (2002) *Blood Cells: A Practical Guide*, 3rd edn. Oxford: Blackwell Publishing.

conditions of altered bone marrow function (myelodysplastic syndromes) which is usually seen in older individuals, macrocytic anaemia may be noted since the maturation process of the red cells is affected.

Normocytic anaemia

Normochromic normocytic anaemia is usually caused by inflammation or an underlying chronic non-haematological disease. Investigations should include screening for renal disease, infections, autoimmune diseases and neoplasia. In the presence of anaemia, a lack of polychromasia and reticulocytes suggests failure of erythropoiesis due to true or functional lack of haematinics, or bone marrow suppression. A combination of fever, anaemia and thrombocytopenia may indicate acute leukaemia and a blood film should be examined urgently for the presence of blasts. Examination of the bone marrow may be helpful to detect aplastic anaemia, infiltrations, infections (e.g. tuberculosis) or myelodysplastic syndrome. Bone marrow examination is not always necessary for the diagnosis of leukaemia as immunophenotyping can be performed on the abnormal peripheral blood by specialist laboratories.

Management of anaemia in the absence of a laboratory

At health centres without laboratory facilities the management of anaemia will by guided by knowledge of the locally prevalent diseases. Good clinical skills are essential to elicit relevant information and

to detect possible causes. Mild anaemia is likely to be missed if haemoglobin cannot be measured (for management of anaemia see Box 6.2). Recent evidence suggests that the traditional approach of treating anaemia presumptively with iron and folic acid may not be be appropriate in all circumstances. Although iron administration may help some children who have iron deficiency, it has been linked to increased mortality in children in malarious areas. In Africa folate supplementation has not been shown to have a dramatic effect on haemoglobin levels and there is a suggestion that folic acid might reduce the efficacy of anti-folate malarial treatment. Because anaemia can be caused my multiple factors health consultations should be used as an opportunity to detect and treat both the anaemia and any underlying conditions.

> **Box 6.2 Suggested management of anaemia if no laboratory tests are available**
>
> - Give iron, folate and antihelmintics and monitor response (clinically detectable improvement should occur within 4 weeks and the haemoglobin should rise at rate of 5–10 g/L each week).
> - Continue iron for at least 3 months after normal haemoglobin is achieved.
> - If acute life-threatening haemolysis is suspected (anaemia with jaundice and dark urine) and there is no obvious cause or underlying infection, a trial of folate and prednisolone 0.5–1 mg/kg (1–2 weeks) may be worthwhile until transfer to a higher level facility can be arranged.
> - If still no response, refer to specialist centre.

Blood transfusion in developing countries

Blood transfusions should only be given for specific clinical indications and in accordance with local or international guidelines (Box 6.3). Transfusions carry serious risks of transmitting infections such as HIV and hepatitis B, and can also be responsible for acute and delayed immune reactions. These risks are increased if the laboratory does not have rigorous quality-checking processes. Critical blood shortages are not uncommon in resource-poor countries so it is imperative to retain all potential blood donors; all blood donors should be unpaid. Repeat donations should be encouraged as repeat donors have the lowest risk of transmitting

> **Box 6.3 Prescribing blood: a checklist for clinicians**
>
> Always ask yourself the following questions before prescribing blood or blood products for a patient.
>
> 1 What improvement in the patient's clinical condition am I aiming to achieve?
> 2 Can I minimize blood loss to reduce this patient's need for transfusion?
> 3 Are there any other treatments I should give before making the decision to transfuse, such as intravenous replacement fluids or oxygen?
> 4 What are the specific clinical or laboratory indications for transfusion in this patient?
> 5 What are the risks of transmitting HIV, hepatitis, syphilis or other infectious agents through the blood products that are available for this patient?
> 6 Do the benefits of transfusion outweigh the risks for this particular patient?
> 7 What other options are there if no blood is available in time?
> 8 Will a trained person monitor this patient and respond immediately if any acute transfusion reactions occur?
> 9 Have I recorded my decision and reasons for transfusion on the patient's chart and the blood request form?
>
> Finally, if in doubt, ask yourself the following question:
> If this blood was for myself or my child, would I accept the transfusion in these circumstances?

infections. Patients with severe anaemia, usually children or obstetric emergencies, need blood transfusion rapidly as an emergency life-saving measure. Before prescribing blood transfusions, clinicians need to carefully balance the risks and benefits. Transfusions should only be used as a last resort and clinicians should satisfy themselves that all other options, such as intravenous fluids and haematinics, have been explored.

 SUMMARY

- Anaemia is the most common medical condition globally, but is not in itself a diagnosis, and needs investigation and evaluation.
- Malaria and hookworm infection account for a large proportion of anaemia in the tropics.
- Laboratory support is vital. Even simple classification into microcytic, macrocytic and normocytic anaemia is diagnostically and therapeutically helpful.
- In the absence of laboratory support, it may be reasonable to give empirical iron, folic acid and anthelmintics; and observe the response.

 Visit www.lecturenoteseries.com/tropicalmed to test yourself on this chapter using interactive MCQs.

 FURTHER READING

Cheesbrough M (2006) *District Laboratory Practice in Tropical Countries*. Vol. 2. Cambridge, UK: Tropical Health Technology, 2nd edn. [Widely recognized as a leading standard laboratory manual for developing countries. Clearly written and well illustrated with basic explanations of rationale and principles of tests.]

Critchley J, Bates I (2005) Haemoglobin colour scale for anaemia diagnosis where there is no laboratory: a systematic review. *International Journal of Epidemiology* **34**: 1425–34. [Review of techniques used for anaemia diagnosis where there is no laboratory with focus on haemoglobin colour scale.]

van Hensbroek MB, Jonker F, Bates I (2011) Severe acquired anaemia in Africa: new concepts. *Br J Haematol* Jun 28 doi: 10.1111/j.1365-2141.2011.08761.x. [Epub ahead of print]. [Review of the aetioapthogensis, diagnosis and management of severe anaemia in Africa.]

World Health Organization (1999) *The Clinical Use of Blood*. Geneva: WHO/BTS/99.2. [Provides prescribers of blood with information to assist them to make appropriate decisions about the use of blood and to avoid unnecessary transfusions. A pocket handbook is available to accompany this publication.]

7

A syndromic approach to sexually transmitted infections

Miriam Taegtmeyer
Liverpool School of Tropical Medicine

The global prevalence of chronic viral sexually transmitted infections (STIs) is likely to be over a billion. In some populations, almost every adult has either active or latent infection with viruses such as genital herpes virus, genital human papilloma virus (HPV), hepatitis B or HIV. In addition, the World Health Organization (WHO) estimated the incidence of curable bacterial STIs such as gonorrhoea, chlamydia and syphilis was 340 million annually in 2005. In view of this it is hardly surprising that the management of individuals with STIs and the consequences thereof constitutes a significant proportion of the outpatient workload in high-prevalence settings.

The need for a public health approach

From early on in the HIV epidemic it was clear that STIs have a role in the spread of HIV. Individuals with recurrent presentations of genital ulcer or discharge were shown to be at a higher risk of acquiring HIV. In addition, HIV-infected individuals with an ulcer or discharge were found to have higher rates of viral shedding of HIV and therefore to be more infectious to partners. Because rates of shedding revert to lower levels after treatment, the appropriate management

of STIs reduces the risk of HIV transmission. It makes sense therefore to include STI management as an HIV prevention strategy. Currently, however, the public health benefits of this approach have not been realized on a large scale.

Syndromic management

In 1991, the WHO developed a system of syndromic management for STIs. The aim was effective management of STIs in resource-poor countries with high prevalence rates of STIs. The emphasis was on an integrated approach at primary health care centres, with no requirement for specialist clinics, highly trained personnel or laboratory facilities. Syndromic management is based on the identification of consistent groups of symptoms and easily recognized signs (syndromes) (Table 7.1). A patient with an STI syndrome presents to a health facility for care and the practitioner has merely to tell the difference between a genital ulcer and a discharge. Once identified, a step-by-step flowchart guides the practitioner. A single course of treatment is provided at the first clinic visit, which deals with the majority of the organisms responsible for producing each syndrome in a given area.

Tropical Medicine Lecture Notes, Seventh edition. Edited by Nick Beeching and Geoff Gill. © 2014 John Wiley & Sons, Ltd. Published 2014 by John Wiley & Sons, Ltd.

Table 7.1 **Some common syndromes and their aetiologies**

Syndrome	Infectious causes	Aetiological agent*	Non-infectious causes
Urethral discharge	Gonococcal urethritis Non-gonococcal (NSU)	***Neisseria gonorrhoeae*** No aetiology (25%) ***Chlamydia trachomatis*** ***(most of the rest)*** *Ureaplasma urealyticum* *Trichomonas vaginalis* *Candida albicans*	Physiological Trauma
	Intra-urethral ulcers or warts	Herpes simplex HPV	
Vaginal discharge	Vaginal infections	*C. albicans* *Gardnerella vaginalis* *T. vaginalis*	Physiological, trauma, retained products, tampons
	Cervical infections	***C. trachomatis*** ***N. gonorrhoeae*** Herpes simplex HPV *Treponema pallidum*	Carcinoma of cervix (linked with HPV infection)
Genital ulcer			
Multiple and painful	Herpetic Chancroid Scabies	Herpes simplex *Haemophilus ducreyi* *Sarcoptes scabiei*	Behçet's disease Stevens–Johnson syndrome
Single and painful	TB Superinfection of painless ulcers	*Mycobacterium tuberculosis* ***Staphylococcus aureus***	Carcinoma
Multiple and painless	Secondary syphilis	*T. pallidum*	
Single and painless	Primary syphilis LGV	*T. pallidum* *C. trachomatis* *(LGV strains)*	
	Granuloma inguinale	*Klebsiella granulomatis*	
Bubo			
Genital ulcer visible	Chancroid	*H. ducreyi*	
No genital ulcer visible	LGV	*C. trachomatis*	
Non-sexually transmitted infections	Plague Filariasis Infections of the lower limb		

Abbreviations: HPV, human papilloma virus; LGV, lymphogranuloma venereum; NSU, non-specific urethritis; TB, tuberculosis.
*Bold italic indicates infections targeted by syndromic management.

Local adaptations

Local data on aetiology and bacterial sensitivity patterns are taken into consideration when designing a flowchart for the syndromic management of STIs. For example, penicillin resistance amongst *Neisseria gonorrhoeae* is on the increase globally. In some countries as much as 50% of gonorrhoea cases are resistant to penicillin. This represents a major threat to the cheap and effective treatment of urethral and cervical discharge syndromes. Moreover, as in the treatment of pneumococcal disease, penicillin resistance is associated with resistance to multiple antibiotics including macrolides. The inevitable consequence has been therapeutic failures and higher priced therapies such as ciprofloxacin being included in syndromic management.

The successful implementation of syndromic management programmes requires that the appropriate drugs be accessible, available and affordable. Unfortunately, many of the antibiotics used for the treatment of STIs in the West (such as quinolones) are too expensive for STI control programmes or individuals to afford in resource-poor countries. The choice of drugs in most countries is therefore often a compromise between what is affordable and what is therapeutically required. Drugs are generally dispensed at health centre level where other more urgent conditions may put demands on supplies originally intended for STI treatment only. Ensuring that the supply of STI drugs is used for the treatment of STIs and guarding it against drug theft are additional challenges on a strained system.

Each country therefore has a slightly different flowchart validated in its own setting according to local prevalence and incidence rates of STIs. This chapter contains simplified versions of the WHO flowcharts in use that manage the following common clinical situations:

- urethral discharge syndrome in men (Fig. 7.1);
- vaginal discharge (Fig. 7.2);
- lower abdominal pain in women (Fig. 7.3);
- genital ulcer disease (Fig. 7.4).

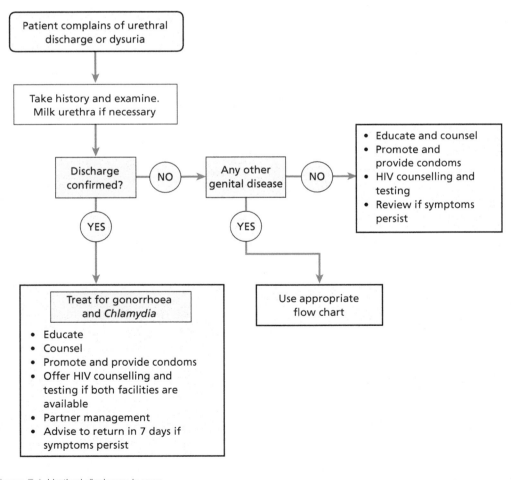

Figure 7.1 Urethral discharge in men.

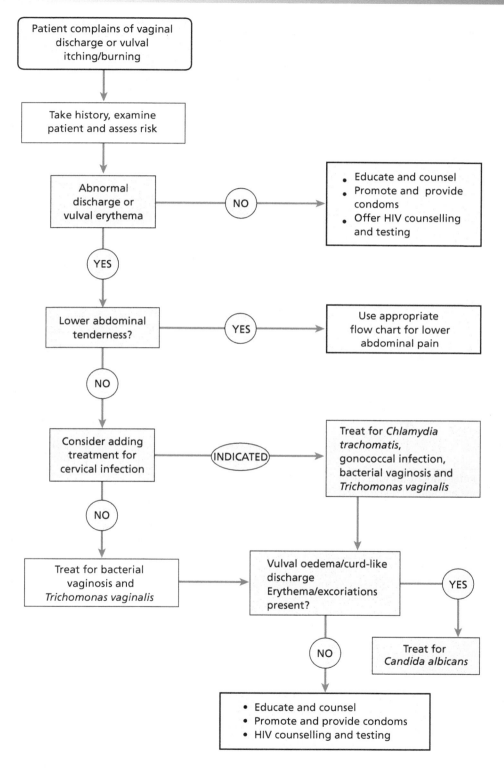

Figure 7.2 Vaginal discharge.

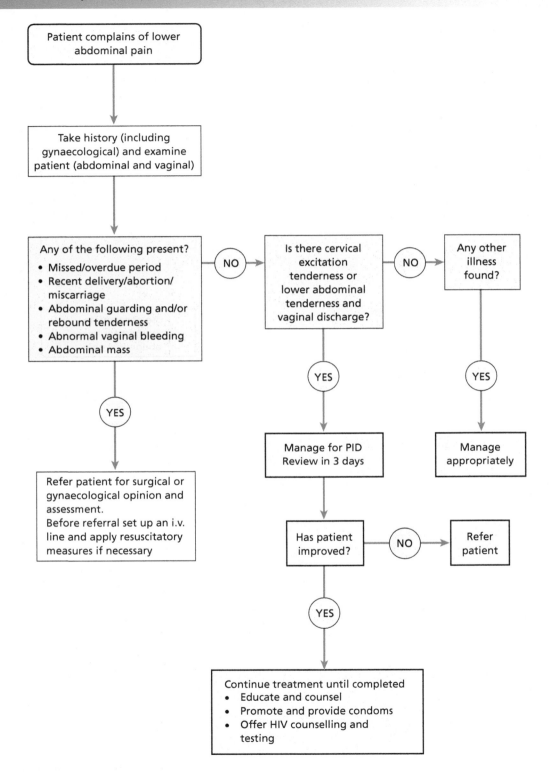

Figure 7.3 Lower abdominal pain in women.

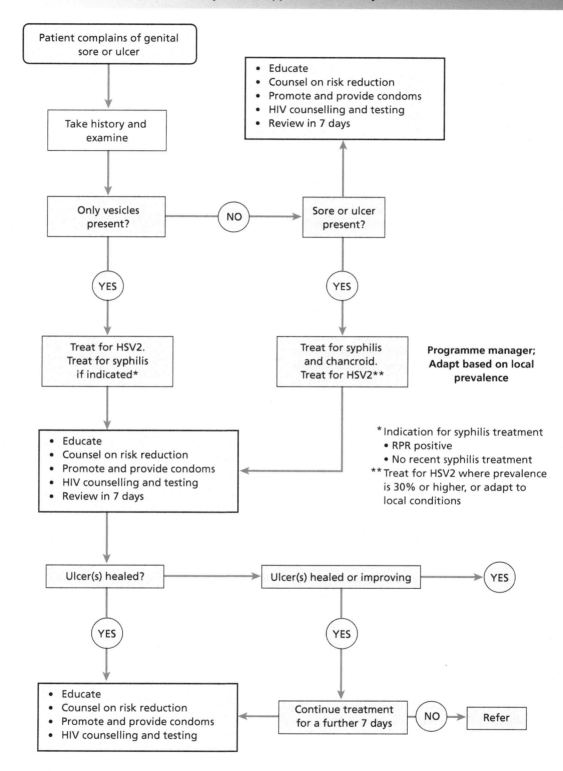

Figure 7.4 Genital ulcer disease.

How to use the flowcharts

1 Symptoms determine which flowchart to select. Patients should be specifically asked about the onset of symptoms and whether the condition is associated with pain.
2 Signs indicate the likelihood of pathology. Patients must be examined for the presence of ulcers, in males the urethra milked for discharge and in females a bimanual examination should be performed. Speculum examination of the cervix should be performed if available as a cervix that bleeds easily when touched or a mucopurulent discharge from the cervix are indications that treatment for cervical infection should be added.
3 Investigations are limited in many settings. If a microscope is available, a Gram stain provides a sensitive indicator of gonococcal infection in urethral discharge. A wet mount from the vaginal specimen will reveal *Candida albicans, Trichomonas vaginalis* and clue cells of bacterial vaginosis. However, investigation with microscopy does not improve the sensitivity and specificity of the flowcharts for lower abdominal pain and vaginal discharge in women. To identify women at greater risk of cervical infection, questions have been added about partners' symptoms, sex work and whether the woman feels she has been exposed to an STI. Laboratory-assisted diagnosis is rarely helpful in genital ulcer disease as mixed infections are common.
4 Management should be guided by the local guidelines. Alternatives are recommended on the locally produced flowcharts for patients with allergies. Special circumstances such as pregnancy are also covered. In general, quinolones are recommended to treat gonorrhoea and tetracyclines to cover chlamydial infection. Concurrent therapy for chlamydia and gonorrhoea should be given to all patients with gonorrhoea, as dual infection is common. While the treatment of choice for syphilis remains intramuscular benzylpenicillin, the penicillins and tetracyclines have no place in the treatment of chancroid owing to widespread resistance in all geographical areas. To cover chancroid a quinolone or macrolide must be added.
5 Some patients fail to respond to treatment. The likeliest causes are reinfection from partner, poor compliance or drug resistance. In the case of persistent urethral discharge, *Trichomonas vaginalis* should be considered before referral, as there are high prevalence rates in some geographical settings. In the case of genital ulcer disease, if symptoms persist after adequate treatment of the index case and partner, the patient should be referred to rule out other causes, including chronic viral STIs, coinfection with HIV, carcinoma or a non-sexually transmitted disease. Where prevalence rates of HIV infection are high, a large number of genital ulcers are likely to be brought about by atypical herpes simplex virus infection.

The nine elements of case management and the 'five C's' of syndromic management

Regardless of whether the diagnosis is presumptive or aetiological, correct case management of STI includes nine elements: history; physical examination; diagnosis; early and effective treatment; advice on sexual behaviour; promotion and provision of condoms; partner notification and treatment; case reporting and, if necessary, clinical follow-up. One of the greatest barriers to the successful implementation of syndromic management has been the attitude of health care workers. Training on the use of flowcharts therefore always includes training on basic counselling skills. This is the first 'C'. Emphasis in training is also put on Confidentiality, Contact tracing, Compliance and Condoms.

Advantages of syndromic management

The syndromic approach to STI management is simple and problem-orientated and can be integrated into existing health facilities without requiring specialist clinics, doctors or nurses. It allows for rapid diagnosis and treatment of the individual at the first visit, thus saving resources for the client and the provider and improving surveillance. Flowcharts developed for the treatment of urethral discharge in men are robust and well validated in numerous settings. Cases of genital ulcer disease resulting from chancroid and syphilis have dropped dramatically in Nairobi, Kenya as a result of intensive syndromic management in high-risk cohorts. Studies of a population-wide approach to syndromic management in Mwanza, Tanzania showed a 42% reduction in rural HIV incidence rates in those receiving access to syndromic management of STIs. However, reduction of HIV incidence was not demonstrated in a study conducted in neighbouring Rakai district in Uganda where a similar cohort was enrolled in a mass STI treatment campaign. A closer analysis of the two data sets reveals different baseline HIV and gonococcal prevalence rates as well as different risk behaviour levels. Syndromic management may therefore be most likely to influence HIV incidence in areas with high levels of risk behaviour and low prevalence of HIV.

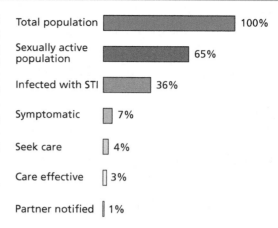

Total population	100%
Sexually active population	65%
Infected with STI	36%
Symptomatic	7%
Seek care	4%
Care effective	3%
Partner notified	1%

Figure 7.5 Operational model of treatment-seeking

Disadvantages of syndromic management

The focus on syndromic management has public health limitations. The main disadvantage is that the uninfected are not targeted and therefore asymptomatic infections are not detected and there is no provision for screening. In addition, there is insufficient emphasis on partner notification and a lost opportunity to promote condom use and provide information on STIs. The approach relies entirely on the self-presentation of those who perceive themselves to have symptoms. In the majority of settings the flowcharts have a low sensitivity and specificity for cervical gonococcal and chlamydial infections in symptomatic women. This frequently leads to overtreatment of the individual and possible increased rates of antibiotic resistance. A lack of consideration of the differential diagnoses is commonplace.

The design of STI control programmes in the tropics has been much enhanced by the widespread use of the syndromic management approach. However, programmes need to combine the simple management of syndromes with interventions that target the general population, promote condoms and educate on other prevention methods. Levels of appropriate health-seeking behaviour are low (Fig. 7.5). Work in the community and with health care workers themselves is therefore needed to challenge stigma, gender roles and myths surrounding STIs. Partner notification and treatment are essential to interrupt the chain of transmission and prevent reinfection and programmes should be accompanied by access to other services such as counselling and testing. Efforts to improve partner notification should be voluntary and ensure the confidentiality of patients and their partners, as fear of rejection and of domestic violence are very real concerns that underlie poor rates of partner notification in many programmes. Good STI

management challenges traditional views of medicine as clinicians work closely with public health specialists and all sectors of the community for it to be a success.

HIV testing in STI clinics

infection with HIV should be excluded as part of routine practice in STI management. WHO guidance on provider-initiated HIV testing and counselling (PITC) recommends that an HIV test is performed on every STI patient and repeated in those who previously tested negative with each new attendance. Rapid HIV antibody testing can be conducted by trained personnel in STI clinics, who should also consider repeat testing of individuals at risk of acute HIV infection (seroconversion) and who require repeat testing at the end of the window period. Knowledge of HIV status allows appropriate referral to HIV treatment and care as well as risk reduction counselling and behaviour change (see Chapter 13). To maximize uptake STI clinics should operate an 'opt-out' policy on HIV testing.

 SUMMARY

- The incidence of curable sexually transmitted infections (STI) is extremely high in the tropics and this facilitates HIV transmission.
- The increasing prevalence of antimicrobial resistance threatens this success.

- Syndromic management of STI has been successfully implemented for over 20 years, using simple flowcharts to guide management of conditions such as urethral discharge syndrome in men, vaginal discharge, lower abdominal pain in women and genital ulcer disease.

- Management flowcharts should be modified to take into account local pathogen prevalence and antibiotic resistance profiles and the availability of drugs.

- The nine elements of correct case management include adequate: history; physical examination; diagnosis; early and effective treatment; advice on sexual behaviour; promotion and provision of condoms; partner notification and treatment; case reporting and, if necessary, clinical follow-up.

- The 5 'C's that underpin this are adequate training of staff in Counselling skills, and ensuring Confidentiality, Contact tracing, Compliance and Condoms.

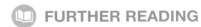 **Visit** www.lecturenoteseries.com/tropicalmed to test yourself on this chapter using interactive MCQs.

FURTHER READING

Dallabetta G, Laga M, Lamptey P, *et al.* (2001) *Control of Sexually Transmitted Diseases: A Handbook for the Design and Management of Programmes.* Arlington: AIDSCAP/Family Health International. [This manual was developed primarily for programme managers in resource-poor settings.]

Mabey D, Ndowa F, Latif A (2010) What have we learned from sexually transmitted infection research in sub-Saharan Africa? *Sex Transm Infect* **86**(7): 488–92. doi: 10.1136/sti.2009.041632. [Summarizes high quality studies in Africa that have provided important information to the benefit of STI control programmes worldwide.]

Mayaud P, Ndowa F, Richens J, Mabey D (2004) Sexually transmitted infections. In EPO Parry, R Godfrey, D Mabey, GV Gill (eds), *Principles of Medicine in Africa*, 3rd edn. Cambridge: Cambridge University Press, pp. 241–83. [A detailed and exhaustive chapter on the modern approach to tropical STDs.]

Ng BE, Butler LM, Horvath T, Rutherford GW (2011) Population-based biomedical sexually transmitted infection control interventions for reducing HIV infection. *Cochrane Database Syst Rev* **16**(3): CD001220. doi: 10.1002/14651858.CD001220.pub3. [Review – evaluates the evidence for STI as an HIV prevention method and shows no strong evidence confirming this hypothesis.]

Wisdom A (1992) *A Colour Atlas of Sexually Transmitted Disease.* London: ELBS edition. [Available at low cost and still popular after all these years.]

www.who.int/Reproductive_health [Useful source for the latest guidelines for the management of sexually transmitted infections with several flowcharts that can be downloaded.]

8

Splenomegaly in the tropics

Jecko Thachil[1] and Imelda Bates[2]

[1]Manchester Royal Infirmary; [2]Liverpool School of Tropical Medicine

Enlarged spleens are common in tropical practice. The disorders that cause splenomegaly in temperate regions are also present in the tropics but, in addition, other factors such as infections and parasitic infestations can contribute to splenomegaly. The spleen responds to infections by augmenting its major physiological functions of phagocytosis and antibody production. The subsequent splenic enlargement is particularly common in children living in areas of high malaria transmission, where the population rates of splenomegaly are used as an indicator of malaria transmission intensity. This 'spleen rate' may reach 100% in children and then decline to less than 10% in adults as they acquire clinical malarial immunity. In areas with stable endemic malaria, adults' spleens are about twice as large as those in non-malarious areas.

Reasons for enlarged spleens

Spleens can enlarge:

- in response to a need for excess physiological activity (e.g. phagocytosis of abnormal red cells as in haemoglobinopathies; antibody production to combat infection);
- because of a structural abnormality (e.g. portal hypertension; infiltration by malignant cells).

The degree to which the spleen enlarges depends on the underlying cause (Box 8.1) but in most cases the spleen size rarely exceeds 10 cm when measured from the left costal margin to the spleen tip. Acutely enlarged spleens are often tender and soft on examination, and are associated with a higher risk of rupture than chronically enlarged spleens which tend to be firmer and more fibrous. Conditions in which the spleen may be moderately (<10 cm) enlarged include chronic haemolysis (e.g. recurrent malaria, haemoglobinopathies, spherocytosis), portal hypertension and haematological malignancies such as chronic lymphocytic leukaemia, lymphomas, acute leukaemias and myeloproliferative disorders.

Massive tropical splenomegaly

The most common causes of massive splenomegaly in the tropics are hyperreactive malarial splenomegaly (formerly called tropical splenomegaly syndrome), lymphomas, schistosomiasis, visceral leishmaniasis, haemoglobinopathies, chronic myeloid leukaemia, myelofibrosis and miscellaneous disorders such as splenic cysts, tumours and lipid storage diseases (Fig. 8.1). Although massive splenomegaly has been reported to be common in many tropical African countries there are few data available on prevalence. Published rates in Africa vary from 1–2% in Nigeria to 0.4–1.2% in the Gambia. The highest prevalence of massive splenomegaly is in Papua New Guinea where up to 80% of some ethnic groups are affected by hyperreactive malarial splenomegaly. The diagnosis and management of most of the conditions associated with massive splenomegaly are discussed in other chapters.

Tropical Medicine Lecture Notes, Seventh edition. Edited by Nick Beeching and Geoff Gill. © 2014 John Wiley & Sons, Ltd. Published 2014 by John Wiley & Sons, Ltd.

Diagnostic clues in a patient with an enlarged spleen

1 Blood count
   – A high white cell count – infections, chronic myeloid leukaemia
   – A high platelet count – acute infections, myeloproliferative disorders
   – A high red cell count – myeloproliferative disorders
   – Low platelet count – malaria, liver disease, associated bone marrow infiltration
   – Low haemoglobin – malaria, liver disease, myelofibrosis, storage diseases
2 Clinical lymphadenopathy
   – Lymphomas (chronic and non-tender)
   – Tuberculosis (chronic)
   – HIV (chronic)
   – Viral infections (acute and tender)
3 Blood film
   – Malaria
   – Haemoglobinopathies
   – Leishmaniasis
   – Leukaemias
4 Bone marrow examination
   – Lymphomas
   – Myeloproliferative diseases
   – Leukaemias
   – Tuberculosis
   – Storage diseases

Hyperreactive malarial splenomegaly

Hyperreactive malarial splenomegaly is caused by an abnormal response to repeated malaria infections which results in overproduction of immunoglobulin M (IgM). The consequent immune complexes are removed by the spleen, which can enlarge to huge proportions (Fig. 8.2). Malaria parasites are rarely found in patients with hyperreactive splenomegaly. The disorder is more common in women and predominantly affects those aged between 20 and 40 years. Patients are surprisingly asymptomatic but eventually develop symptoms of anaemia, malaise and abdominal discomfort. Pregnant women with hyperreactive malarial splenomegaly can experience sudden episodes of haemolysis which may be life-threatening. A mild reduction in platelets and white cells secondary to hypersplenism is common in hyperreactive malarial splenomegaly. Almost all patients have anaemia and hepatomegaly and there may be increased susceptibility to bacterial infections. Interestingly a study from Ghana showed that relatives of patients with hyperreactive splenomegaly are more likely to have splenomegaly.

Criteria for a diagnosis of hyperreactive splenomegaly include splenomegaly over 10 cm from the left costal margin and a sustained reduction in spleen size of at least 40% on antimalarial treatment. Differentiation from splenic involvement by

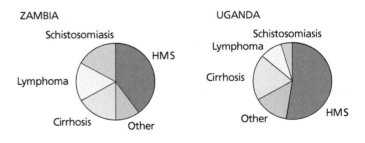

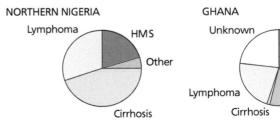

Figure 8.1 Causes of massive splenomegaly from various African countries. HMS: hyperreactive malarial splenomegaly.

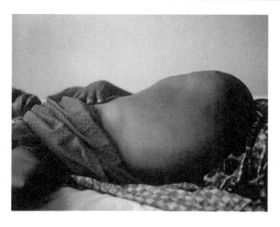

Figure 8.2 Patient with massive splenomegaly.

lymphoma may be difficult without molecular techniques but a diagnosis of hyperreactive malarial splenomegaly is more likely if the patient is under 40 years of age and has a peripheral blood lymphocyte count of less than $10 \times 10^9/L$. There is some evidence to suggest that hyperreactive splenomegaly may occasionally transform into B cell-lymphoma, possibly as a result of B-cell proliferation from repeated exposure to malaria.

In some patients the splenomegaly may resolve spontaneously, whereas in others life-long treatment may be necessary to prevent recurrence of the splenomegaly. Proguanil 100 mg/day is the drug of choice as it is safe for continued use over many years. Treatment usually results in resolution of the haematological abnormalities and the spleen slowly shrinks although it may never become impalpable.

Splenectomy in the tropics

The indications for splenectomy in tropical practice are similar to those in temperate regions but the balance between risk and benefit may be altered by, for example, the lack of blood products and intensive peri-operative care in poorer countries. Elective splenectomy for patients with enlarged spleens in Uganda had an early post-operative mortality of 4.8% and the risks of splenectomy include the following:

- Larger spleens make the procedure technically difficult.
- Hypersplenism leads to reduced platelet counts with increased risk of peri-operative bleeding, exacerbated by shortages of blood supplies and unavailability of platelet transfusions.
- Increased susceptibility to bacterial infections, especially encapsulated organisms. Septicaemia with these organisms can be associated with disseminated intravascular coagulation, which has a mortality of 50–80% in established cases. Lifelong antibiotic prophylaxis and vaccination for *Haemophilus influenza* type B, *Neisseria meningitidis* and *Streptococcus pneumoniae* should be given if available.
- Very few data are available about the risk of malaria infection post-splenectomy. It is likely that the risk is less than in non-immunes if the individual acquired malarial immunity at an early age and has been a long-term resident in a malarious area.
- To reduce the risk of post-splenectomy infections, a partial rather than total splenectomy could be performed, leaving a portion of spleen with arterial structures *in situ*.
- An increased incidence of pulmonary hypertension and both arterial and venous thromboembolism have been observed in individuals who have undergone splenectomy possibly due to alterations in lipid metabolism, platelet hyperreactivity, haemolysis and the lack of protective effect of the spleen itself.

 SUMMARY

- Splenomegaly is common in the tropics, and has a wide differential diagnosis.
- Recurrent malaria, leishmaniasis, haemoglobinopathies, schistosomiasis, leukaemias and lymphomas are important causes.
- Hyperreactive malarial splenomegaly is due to recurrent malarial attacks and is immune complex mediated. The spleen size can be very large.

 Visit **www.lecturenoteseries.com/tropicalmed** **to test yourself on this chapter using interactive MCQs.**

📖 FURTHER READING

Bates I (1991) Hyperreactive malarial splenomegaly in pregnancy. *Trop Doct* **21**: 101–3.
Bates I, Bedu-Addo G, Rutherford TR, Bevan DH (1997) Circulating villous lymphocytes--a link between hyperreactive malarial splenomegaly and splenic lymphoma. *Trans R Soc Trop Med Hyg* **91**: 171–4.

Bedu Addo G, Bates I (2002) Causes of massive tropical splenomegaly in Ghana. *Lancet* **360**: 449–54. [Review of causes of massive splenomegaly in tropical, malaria-endemic country determined using current technology.]

Doherty T, Mabey D (2004) The spleen. In EPO Parry, R Godfrey, D Mabey, GV Gill (eds), *Principles of Medicine in Africa*, 3rd edn. Cambidge: Cambridge University Press, pp. 1026–9.

Part 2

Major tropical infections

Malaria

David Bell[1] and David Lalloo[2]
[1]Gartnavel General Hospital; [2]Liverpool School of Tropical Medicine

Malaria is the most important tropical parasitic infection and one of the world's leading causes of death and morbidity. Around three billion people live in one of the 106 countries endemic for malaria. In 2010, there were an estimated 216 million episodes of malaria and around 655 000 deaths, of which 91% were in Africa. It is estimated that 86% of malaria deaths worldwide were in children less than five years old.

There are over 120 species of the protozoan genus *Plasmodium,* but only 4 species commonly cause human disease: *P. falciparum, P. vivax, P. ovale* and *P. malariae.* Other plasmodia were thought only to infect animals, but *P. knowlesi,* which usually infects monkeys in South East Asia, has recently been recognized to cause human disease.

Malaria epidemiology

The geographical distributions of the species vary. *P. vivax* has the widest geographical range, but predominates in the Indian subcontinent, Mexico, Central America and China. Vivax accounts for over half of all malaria infections outside Africa and approximately 10% of those in Africa. *P. ovale* is found mainly in West Africa and *P. malariae* has a patchy distribution throughout tropical and temperate regions. *P. falciparum,* found throughout the tropics, is responsible for the vast majority of deaths. In Africa, falciparum is the cause of over 75% of malaria infections (Fig. 9.1).

The incidence of episodes of illness and death and the intensity of transmission are closely related. More intense transmission is associated with the development of protective malaria-specific immunity, so that severe disease is less common with increasing age.

Intensity of transmission in a community can be estimated in a number of ways:

- the parasite rate: the prevalence of blood stage infections;
- the spleen rate: the proportion of individuals with a palpable spleen;
- the Entomological Inoculation rate: the number of infected bites per year.

Based on these measures, the terms hypoendemic, mesoendemic, hyperendemic and holoendemic are used to describe the intensity of transmission, increasing from low to high respectively. Hypoendemic regions have little transmission while in holoendemic areas, transmission is perennial and a high degree of immunity is established. The terms low, moderate and high transmission areas are also used interchangeably. Stable malaria transmission describes countries with high transmission and with little change in the intensity year on year, though there may be seasonal fluctuations. Unstable malaria transmission occurs in communities with little transmission. A change in environmental conditions, e.g. prolonged rains, may lead to an explosion in mosquito populations and epidemics of malaria in a population with little or no immunity.

Life-cycle

Malaria infection occurs at the time of biting by the female *Anopheles* mosquito (Fig. 9.2). The infecting agents, the sporozoites, are inoculated in the saliva of the mosquito and circulate in the blood to the liver where they invade hepatocytes. Sporozoites disappear from the blood within hours. Within the hepatocytes there is a period of asexual replication, termed

Tropical Medicine Lecture Notes, Seventh edition. Edited by Nick Beeching and Geoff Gill. © 2014 John Wiley & Sons, Ltd. Published 2014 by John Wiley & Sons, Ltd.

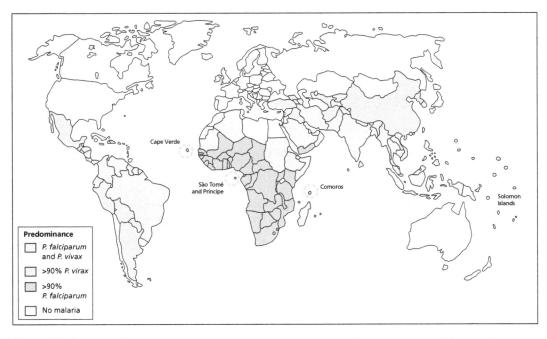

Figure 9.1 Countries affected by malaria, showing relative predominance of falciparum or vivax infections. *Source*: Adapted from RGA Feacham *et al.* (2010) *Lancet* **376**: 1566–78.

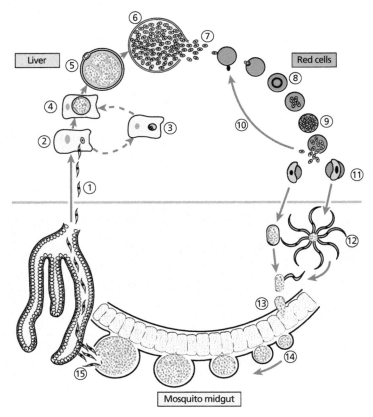

Figure 9.2 Malaria life-cycle. 1, Sporozoites, injected through the skin by female anopheline mosquito; 2, sporozoites infect hepatocytes; 3, some sporozoites develop into 'hypnozoites' (*Plasmodium vivax* and *P. ovale* only); 4, liver-stage parasite develops; 5–6, tissue schizogony; 7, merozoites are released into the circulation; 8, ring-stage trophozoites in red cells; 9, erythrocytic schizogony; 10, merozoites invade other red cells; 11, some parasites develop into female (macro-) or male (micro-) gametocytes, taken up by mosquito; 12, mature macrogametocyte and exflagellating microgametes; 13, ookinete penetrates gut wall; 14, development of oocyst; 15, sporozoites penetrate salivary glands.

'exo-erythrocytic' schizogony leading to the development of cyst-like structures called pre-erythrocytic schizonts, which contain thousands of merozoites. On maturation, these schizonts rupture, liberating the merozoites into the blood stream. Merozoites attach to and invade circulating red blood cells using a variety of cell surface receptors and disappear from the blood within minutes. The time from the mosquito bite to the appearance of circulating infected red blood cells varies between species; for *P. falciparum*, it is 7–30 days, usually ten days.

Several rounds of asexual replication then take place within the infected red cells, termed 'erythrocytic' schizogony, with the parasites deriving nutrition from haemoglobin in the red cell. As the parasites mature, they change from merozoites (very early ring forms) to trophozoites (mature rings) and to schizonts. Schizogony occurs in the circulating blood in *P. vivax*, *P. ovale*, *P. malariae* and *P. knowlesi* infections and schizonts are commonly seen in the peripheral blood films from patients infected with these species. In contrast, *P. falciparum* schizonts are rarely visible in blood films. Mature falciparum trophozoites express receptors on the red cell surface, which bind or cytoadhere the infected cells to other red cells and to endothelial cells lining capillaries in microvascular beds in the brain (Fig. 9.3), gut, spleen and other organs. In falciparum malaria, schizogony occurs in these deep capillary beds. The sequestration of large numbers of mature parasites in deep tissues prevents the removal of circulating parasitized red cells by the spleen. This is a unique feature of falciparum and together with its rapid replication potential, results in the severe pathology associated with *P. falciparum* infection.

After approximately 48 or 72 hours, depending on the infecting species, the erythrocytic schizonts rupture, releasing 12–24 merozoites per red cell (to infect more red cells) and other parasite antigens. It is at this point that clinical symptoms first occur. Some of the merozoites entering red cells do not develop into schizonts but differentiate into male or female gametocytes, the stage of the parasite which is infectious to biting mosquitoes; gametocytes are not pathogenic to humans. Falciparum gametocytes appear in the peripheral blood around ten days after the peak in numbers of asexual ring forms. In other malaria species, gametocytes appear earlier, around the same time as the peak in asexual forms. Haploid male and female gametocytes are ingested by the female mosquito during a blood meal and sexual reproduction occurs within the mosquito gut leading to the formation of a diploid zygote. In a polyclonal infection, male and female gametocytes are present from different parasite strains and during zygote formation, genetic mixing between different strains occurs. This is important in the origin and spread of drug resistance.

Zygotes develop into motile ookinetes which migrate from the mosquito gut lumen into the gut wall where they develop further into oocysts. Sporozoites develop inside oocysts and are released into the body cavity after oocyst rupture, migrating thereafter to the salivary glands. At the next blood meal, these sporozoites are inoculated by the biting mosquito causing human infection. The duration of the life-cycle within the mosquito is approximately ten days. Rarely, malaria infection may be transmitted between persons by other means, including blood transfusion, accidental inoculation or needle-sharing, or across the placenta.

P. vivax and *P. ovale* have an additional stage in their life-cycles called 'hypnozoites'. These dormant forms develop in the liver from sporozoites. Months or years after the initial infection, these may resume replication, develop into pre-erythrocytic schizonts and cause a further blood stage infection. This 'relapse' in clinical symptoms occurs despite successful treatment of the primary infection. Late recurrence of infection can also occur in *P. malariae* due to recrudescence of dormant red cell stages.

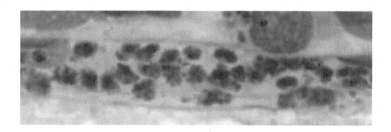

Figure 9.3 Brain smear in fatal malaria. A cerebral venule is packed with late-stage *P. falciparum* parasites (late trophozoites and schizonts). As a result of such sequestration in various deep tissues, these stages of *P. falciparum* are not usually seen in the peripheral blood. (Photo courtesy of D Milner. Oil immersion, × 1000, reversed Field's stain.)

Malaria immunity and other determinants of disease severity

Asymptomatic infection occurs when an individual is able to tolerate the presence of parasitaemia without exhibiting symptoms. This is common in adults and older children who grow up in areas of high malaria transmission. Asymptomatic infection is not always clinically insignificant; it may lead to anaemia and infected individuals are infectious to mosquitoes and a significant reservoir of infection. This immune tolerance, known as premunition, is due to the development of malaria-specific partial immunity following repeated falciparum infections, usually with a limited number of locally prevalent isolates. In order to maintain this immunity, frequent re-exposure to infection is required. If re-exposure does not occur, the immunity wanes over a period of a few years. In high transmission areas, for example much of sub-Saharan Africa, this immunity is built up during early childhood and comes at a great cost, with malarial morbidity and mortality concentrated in young children. In contrast, travellers and people living in countries with low-intensity or sporadic malaria transmission develop little immunity, and malaria infection causes symptomatic disease in all age groups.

Several host genetic factors are also important determinants of disease severity. The best documented of these is the protection afforded against severe falciparum malaria by the heterozygous state for haemoglobin S (genotype AS). The sickle trait prevents the development of high parasitaemia, probably partly as a result of the parasitized red cells sickling in the circulation and being removed by the spleen before they can develop into schizonts. However, malaria infection in patients with sickle-cell anaemia (genotype SS) is usually of severe consequence. Protection against severe falciparum is also conferred by alpha and beta thalassaemia traits. *P. vivax* is unable to infect red cells lacking the Duffy blood-group antigen. This is believed to account for the natural resistance of some populations of sub-Saharan African origin (who lack the Duffy antigen) to infection with this parasite.

HIV (human immunodeficiency virus) and malaria coexist at high intensity in many countries. The immunosuppressive effect of HIV results in a higher incidence of episodes of symptomatic malaria and an increased likelihood of developing severe disease. These risks rise as the HIV induced immunosuppression increases. There is also some evidence to suggest that HIV-infected adults are at greater risk of malaria treatment failure. Acute episodes of malaria are associated with transient increases in plasma HIV viral load, a factor that may be important in enhancing mother-to-child and person to person transmission of HIV.

Clinical features

The consequences of malaria infection are classified into two clinical syndromes, uncomplicated malaria and severe malaria; the latter is usually associated with *P. falciparum* infection. The clinical features of uncomplicated malaria are non-specific and common to each of the malaria species and to many other infections. There are no recognized symptoms associated with the liver stage of malaria infection; symptoms occur during the blood stage of infection and include fever, malaise, headache, myalgia and minor gastrointestinal symptoms. Anaemia occurs due to haemolysis of red cells and also to bone marrow suppression. Splenomegaly is common in acute malaria and may persist after repeated attacks and lead to secondary hypersplenism. Fever is related to the release of pyrogens from the rupture of red cells and is usually irregular. The patterns of regular periodic fever gave rise to the traditional names for the different types of malaria; tertian malaria (*P. falciparum, P. vivax* and *P. ovale*) with fever every third day (i.e. every 48 hours) and quartan malaria (*P. malariae*) with fever every fourth day (every 72 hours). However, these patterns are rarely seen unless illness has continued untreated for a week or more. *P. knowlesi* causes daily fever cycles.

Although severe and fatal disease is also described with *P. vivax* and *P. knowlesi* infections, the vast majority of acute malaria associated deaths each year are a result of *P. falciparum* infection. Nevertheless, there is increasing recognition that background morbidity and mortality due to *P. vivax* may be substantial in endemic settings.

The processes of cytoadherance and sequestration make *P. falciparum* much more pathogenic than the other species. The precise mechanisms by which sequestration leads to the life-threatening complications like cerebral malaria are not known, although several hypotheses are proposed (Fig. 9.3). These include mechanical obstruction of the microvasculature causing local ischaemia and alterations in capillary permeability and the blood–brain-barrier leading to oedema and the release of pro-inflammatory cytokines detrimental to surrounding tissue.

Approximately 1–2% of uncomplicated falciparum infections progress to severe and life-threatening malaria, characterized by the development of organ or tissue complications. Severe malaria has a mortality rate of between 10–20% depending on the setting. Prompt effective treatment reduces the risk of progression to severe disease. The major clinical features of severe malaria are shown in Table 9.1. In children growing up in areas of high malaria endemicity, cerebral malaria, severe anaemia and respiratory distress/acidosis predominate whilst in adults (who are usually non-immune), the most common features are cerebral malaria, renal failure, acidosis and ARDS. In non-immune children, severe anaemia is less prominent. One or several of these features may be present in an individual, the prognosis worsening with the number of complications

Specific features of severe disease

- *Cerebral malaria* is a diffuse disturbance of cerebral function, characterized by altered consciousness that persists despite correction of metabolic defects (hypoglycaemia or acidosis), severe anaemia and seizures and no other explanation for the coma can be found. It is commonly accompanied by convulsions, flaccidity of limbs, or by any combination of hypertonicity, posturing and opisthotonos. Convulsions range from grand-mal episodes to minor repetitive muscle movements. With effective treatment most children with cerebral malaria will recover with a minority (5–10%) left

with a neurological deficit, such as hemiparesis, cerebellar ataxia or epilepsy. In many cases these will resolve over a period of months, but some are permanent. We do not know how many individuals may suffer more subtle impairment (e.g. of memory or intelligence) after cerebral malaria. Recently, a characteristic retinopathy has been observed in children and adults with cerebral malaria. The changes consist of areas of retinal whitening, best seen immediately around the fovea (but always sparing the fovea itself), and orange or white discoloration of retinal vessels and capillaries in scattered parts of the retina. These features are sufficiently distinctive to be diagnostically helpful. Most children with cerebral malaria also have white-centred retinal haemorrhages, and about 10% have some degree of papilloedema, neither of these being distinctive of malaria (Fig. 9.4).

- *Severe anaemia* (haemoglobin less than 50 g/L) is most common in children in endemic areas with intense transmission and may be related to repeated malaria infections.
- *Acidosis* occurs due to tissue hypoxia resulting from parasite sequestration, anaemia, hypovolaemia and seizure activity. In children, it is strongly associated with respiratory distress which may partly be a compensatory physiological response.
- *Hypoglycaemia* occurs due to impaired hepatic gluconeogenesis, glucose consumption by the parasites themselves and the effects of quinine stimulating pancreatic insulin secretion. Blood glucose should be regularly checked in severe malaria.

Table 9.1 Major features of severe or complicated malaria

Major features of severe or complicated malaria	
Children	**Adults**
Impaired consciousness or seizures	Impaired consciousness or seizures
Respiratory distress or acidosis (pH < 7.3)	Renal impairment (oliguria < 0.4 ml/kg bodyweight per hour or creatinine > 265 mmol)
Hypoglycaemia (< 2.2 mmol/l)	Acidosis (pH < 7.3)
Haemoglobin < 50 g/dL (packed cell volume < 15%)	Hypoglycaemia (< 2.2 mmol/l)
Prostration	Pulmonary oedema or acute respiratory distress syndrome (ARDS)
Hyperparasitaemia (threshold depends upon endemicity – increased risk from > 2.5% red blood cells parasitized in low endemic areas)	Haemoglobin < 50 g/L
	Spontaneous bleeding/disseminated intravascular coagulation
	Shock (algid malaria) BP < 90/60 mmHg
	Intravascular haemolysis and haemoglobinuria (without G6PD deficiency) 'Blackwater fever'

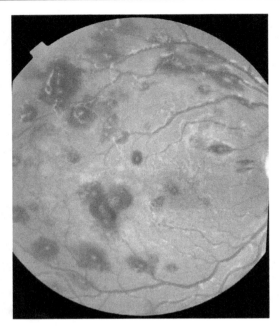

Figure 9.4 Fundus of a child with cerebral malaria showing malarial retinopathy. The edge of the optic disc is on the extreme right. In addition to many white–centred haemorrhages, there are multiple patches of retinal whitening which are most evident temporal to the macula (left-hand side of the photo). Retinal whitening is due to focal areas of retinal ischaemia. (Photo courtesy of Nick Beare.)

Other malaria complications

Malarial nephrosis is an occasional complication of *P. malariae* infection in children. Antigen–antibody complex binds to the glomerular basement membrane causing an intractable nephrotic syndrome which is not responsive to corticosteroids nor eradication of the malaria. Hyperreactive malarial splenomegaly (formerly known as Tropical Splenomegaly syndrome) is a marked splenomegaly in *P. falciparum* infection due to infiltration of the hepatic sinusoids with lymphocytes, with or without features of secondary hypersplenism. This condition usually resolves within a few months if the patient is given continuous effective chemoprophylaxis (see Chapter 8).

Malaria in pregnancy

Malaria during pregnancy is a risk factor for the development of severe disease in both non-immune and semi-immune women, especially primigravida.

It is also a risk factor for foetal growth retardation, low birth weight and infantile death. Anaemia is a common consequence, and many women enter labour with a low haemoglobin concentration, making peripartum blood loss more dangerous. In endemic areas, it is common to find malaria parasites in umbilical venous blood; it is less common to find them in the neonate's peripheral blood, and these usually disappear within the first few days of life. Illness brought about by congenital infection is rare in endemic areas due to transfer of protective maternal IgG to the newborn, but may develop in infants born to non-immune mothers.

Malaria diagnosis

The diagnosis of malaria is usually made by examining a peripheral blood slide for the presence of parasites or by the detection of parasite antigens in a drop of blood applied to a test-strip or rapid diagnostic test (RDT). A thin film consisting of a monolayer of red cells is used for speciation and determination of parasitaemia (Fig. 9.5), while a thick film of haemolysed red cells about 10–20 deep is most sensitive for determining if malaria infection is present (Fig. 9.6). Malaria microscopy is time consuming and requires training and equipment but, in skilled hands, is still the most sensitive method of detecting infection. RDTs (Fig. 9.7) may detect antigens present in

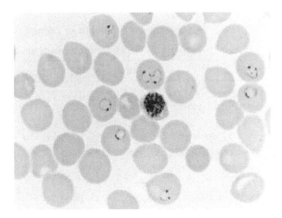

Figure 9.5 Thin blood film showing substantial *P. falciparum* parasitaemia, with double chromatin dot ring forms (like headphones) and two parasites in one red cell, both typical features of falciparum. Unusually, a schizont is present in the centre red cell, indicating severe infection (Leishman stain).

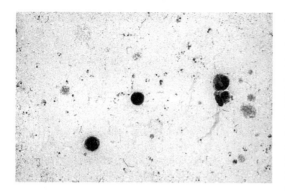

Figure 9.6 Thick blood film showing moderate *P. falciparum* infection. The red cells have been lysed, leaving white cells and numerous falciparum ring forms on an amorphous background (Field's stain).

all Plasmodium species, e.g. lactate dehydrogenase (pLDH) and aldolase, or antigens specific to one species only, e.g. histidine-rich protein 2 (HRP-2) which is unique to *P. falciparum*, or *P. vivax* specific LDH. The choice of RDT will depend on the species prevalent in that area. In most circumstances, the detection of *P. falciparum* is most important. Tests using HRP-2 are more sensitive for detecting *P. falciparum* than RDTs using pan-malarial antigens. HRP-2 antigen persists in the blood circulation 2–3 weeks after treatment and so is not useful for determining response to treatment; RDTs using pLDH are more suitable for this purpose. The best RDTs are highly sensitive and

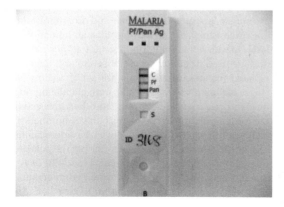

Figure 9.7 A mixed rapid diagnostic test, positive for *P. falciparum* malaria, with 3 horizontal bands showing in middle window. C=positive control; Pf=*P. falciparum* specific HRP-2 antigen; Pan=pan *Plasmodium* species LDH.

specific and can be used after little training, but are more expensive than blood films and there are concerns about stability in hot climates and their reliability in operational use.

Interpreting the results of an RDT or blood film is, in some circumstances, fraught with difficulty. In high transmission areas, asymptomatic infection is common and the presence of parasites in the blood does not equate with disease. A child with a fever and a cough with a positive malaria test may in fact have pneumonia and not be ill because of the malaria infection. This leads to over-diagnosis and over-treatment of malaria, and results in a failure to identify and treat the true cause of the illness. In low transmission countries, asymptomatic carriage is not seen, and a positive blood test is indicative of disease. To add to the difficulty, a single negative blood film does not rule out falciparum malaria as infected red cells sequester in the tissues in the later stages of the parasite's life-cycle and may not be present in the blood at the time of the test. Even if parasites are circulating, a non-immune person may become sick when the parasite density in the peripheral blood is too low to detect by microscopy or RDT. As a consequence of this, many clinicians in malaria endemic countries will choose to treat a patient for malaria on clinical grounds despite a negative blood test.

In the light of these difficulties, many malaria endemic countries have in the past adopted a policy of 'presumptive diagnosis' of malaria. A child presenting with clinical features consistent with malaria and in whom no other cause is apparent, is treated for malaria without any blood tests being performed. The clinician attending a sick child will follow a diagnostic algorithm based upon relatively simple symptoms and signs leading to the diagnosis. A policy of treatment based on presumptive diagnosis is a pragmatic answer in the face of limited resources and the diagnostic difficulties outlined above but leads to over-treatment of malaria and under-diagnosis of other potentially life threatening conditions. Now, in an era of more expensive treatment regimens, there has been a shift in policy favouring the establishment of a parasitological diagnosis over a clinical diagnosis. By 2010, 90 of the 106 (85%) of malaria-endemic countries had adopted a policy in favour of providing parasitological diagnosis rather than a presumptive diagnosis. This should reduce unnecessary use of antimalarial drugs and improve the management of patients without malaria in whom another diagnosis should be sought. In 2010, 76% of reported cases of malaria worldwide were confirmed by a diagnostic test, though the figure in sub-Saharan Africa was lower (45%) and in many countries less than 20%. In many of these countries there are insufficient staff or resources available to perform these tests on every patient with suspected malaria. Additionally, malaria is often self-diagnosed and treated by informal health care providers.

In non-endemic countries, suspected malaria is also investigated by blood film or RDTs depending on the skills available. To confidently rule out malaria infection in a febrile returning traveller, the usual practice is to perform three malaria tests over 24-48 hours.

Treatment

The aims of treatment for uncomplicated malaria are to prevent progression to severe disease and to eliminate the parasites. In severe cases, rapid reduction of parasitaemia is needed and the patient needs support until organ or tissue dysfunctions are corrected.

The ideal treatment for uncomplicated malaria is an inexpensive, single dose oral regimen with no side-effects and against which parasites would not develop resistance. None of the treatment regimens currently available satisfies all of these conditions. Antimalarial drugs vary in their regimens, tolerability, cost and efficacy. Clinical trials of different treatments usually report the adequate clinical and parasitological response (ACPR) rate which describes a successful treatment outcome; the patient is free of parasites and fever. Lower ACPR rates may be due to drug resistance or underdosing due to the use of substandard or fake drugs, vomiting or poor adherence to multidose regimens.

In addition to antimalarial drugs, supportive treatments are required to manage the complications of malaria infection. These may include the following.

- Oral or rectal paracetamol, tepid sponging and fanning.
- Intravenous fluid rehydration for hypovolaemia and acidosis. Aggressive fluid resuscitation may be detrimental in children.
- Monitoring renal function and initiating peritoneal dialysis or haemodialysis if indicated.
- Blood transfusion. In settings without a safe and readily available supply, blood should only be transfused when there are strong clinical indications; e.g. when the haemoglobin concentration is < 50 g/L (haematocrit < 15%) or at higher levels if accompanied by coma, acidosis or hyperparasitaemia.
- Anticonvulsants including rectal diazepam or lorazepam, intramuscular paraldehyde.

- Monitoring of blood glucose and correction of hypoglycaemia where necessary.
- Treating DIC if severe enough to cause bleeding; fresh whole blood, platelet-rich plasma and fresh frozen plasma may be given according to availability.
- Empirical antibiotic therapy. Concurrent Gram negative bacteraemia is recognized in children and adults with severe malaria especially those with severe anaemia or hypotensive shock. Antibiotics should also be considered in patients not responding to therapy or if sepsis or meningitis cannot be excluded.

A number of adjuvant therapies have been trialled in severe malaria with no proven benefit. These include dexamethasone, monoclonal antibodies against tumour necrosis factor, mannitol to reduce intracranial pressure and immunoglobulins.

Drugs to treat falciparum malaria

Antimalarial drugs broadly fall into five different chemical groups (Table 9.2).

Artemisinin derivatives

Artemisinin (qinghaosu) is derived from the Chinese medicinal herb quinghao (*Artemisia annua*) or sweet wormwood. In China, quinghao has been used as a treatment for fever since the 4th century AD. The parent component is artemisinin and derivatives include artesunate, artemether, arteether and droartemisinin. The artemisinins are effective against all human malaria species and multidrug-resistant *P. falciparum* and are used in the treatment of severe and uncomplicated malaria. Artemisinins are active against all stages of their parasite life-cycle, from circulating ring forms to sequestered schizonts and therefore cause the most rapid drop in circulating parasite numbers of all the antimalarial drugs; every two days artemisinins reduce the parasite load by a factor of 10^4, the parasite reduction ratio (PRR). This compares to a PRR of 10^3 for chloroquine (CQ) and sulfadoxine-pyrimethamine (SP), 10^2 for mefloquine and 10 for tetracycline. Artemisinins also kill gametocytes and this may reduce transmission rates, although probably not to an important degree in areas of high or moderate transmission, where asymptomatic infection is common and most patients will not receive treatment. Although major human toxicities were not observed using artemisinins

Table 9.2 **Classes of antimalarial drugs**

Drug group	Examples	Comments
Anti-folate combinations	Dapsone-pyrimethamine Sulfadoxine-pyrimethamine	Synergistic interaction between component drugs. Resistance is worldwide and not now recommended to treat falciparum malaria
Artemisinin derivatives	Artesunate Artemether Dihydroartemisinin	The most potent antimalarial, causing the most rapid drop in parasite count. Effective against all malaria species. Resistance now being described in parts of SE Asia
Hydroxynaphthalenes	Atovaquone-proguanil	The only compound in this class and far too expensive for widespread use. Synergistic interaction between component drugs
Quinoline derivatives	Quinine Amodiaquine Chloroquine Lumefantrine Mefloquine Piperaquine Tafenoquine	Inhibit the detoxification of haem in the parasite food vacuole. Effective against all malaria species. Resistance to CQ is worldwide
Antibiotics	Clindamycin Doxycycline	Weak antimalarial activity and only used in addition to another drug to treat malaria

in clinical trials, there have recently been reports of delayed haemolysis in some patients treated with parenteral artemisinins for severe malaria.

Artesunate is available as tablets, suppositories and a powder for preparing an intravenous solution. Rectal artesunate is being studied as a possible first-line drug for patients with severe malaria in remote areas where injections cannot be given, pending transfer to hospital. All artemisinins have very short elimination half-lives, around one hour, and if used alone the drug should be taken for seven days to ensure parasite clearance. This is operationally impractical. Shorter courses are frequently followed by recrudescence of parasites. Artemisinins are, therefore, usually used in combination with other antimalarial drugs as an 'artemisinin combination therapy' (ACT), and the treatment is taken for three days. ACT has become the first line recommended therapy for much of the world.

Quinoline derivatives

The alkaloids quinine and quinidine are derived from the bark of the Cinchona tree. This was used by native Inca tribes as a treatment for fever for hundreds of years before its 'discovery' by Jesuit missionaries. Derivatives include: chloroquine, amodiaquine, piperaquine, mefloquine, lumefantrine, halofantrine, primaquine and tafenoquine.

Quinine

Quinine is efficacious against all species of malaria, though in parts of South East Asia there is evidence of a decline in its efficacy against *P. falciparum* when used as monotherapy. Quinine is a powerful blood schizonticide and its isomer, quinidine, is equally effective but more cardiotoxic. Oral and intravenous formulations are available. As a monotherapy it should be taken three times a day for seven days, which makes it unsuitable for routine use for uncomplicated malaria. In malaria endemic areas it is usually reserved for the treatment of severe disease or when first-line therapy for uncomplicated disease has failed. In non-endemic countries like the UK, quinine is used for both severe and uncomplicated *P. falciparum* infections. Quinine has marked symptomatic adverse-effects (tinnitus, dizziness, deafness and nausea known as cinchonism) occurring in most individuals even at normal doses and may cause hypoglycaemia.

Chloroquine (CQ)

CQ has rapid antipyretic and antiparasitic effects and is taken orally once daily for three days. Its main symptomatic adverse-effect is pruritus, most commonly in individuals with coloured skin. Resistance of *P. falciparum* to chloroquine was first documented in the late 1950s in South East Asia then in Africa by the end of the 1970s and is now established in almost all malaria-endemic areas of the world. As a result, chloroquine should not be used to treat falciparum malaria though it remains the first-line treatment for infections with the other four plasmodial species. Interestingly, there is now evidence from Malawi that parasites may regain chloroquine sensitivity after several years in a human population that is not exposed to the drug. This observation has led some to suggest the intriguing possibility of recycling some of the older antimalarials as part of combination therapies.

Amodiaquine (AQ)

This 4-aminoquinoline retains some utility against CQ resistant parasites and for this reason it is increasingly being used in Africa in combination therapy with artesunate. Amodiaquine-resistant falciparum malaria is described in parts of Africa. AQ is inexpensive and is taken orally once daily for three days. It was first marketed for both the treatment and prevention of malaria. However, in the mid-1980s, severe adverse reactions in the form of hepatitis and agranulocytosis were described in travellers taking AQ as prophylaxis. As a result, the drug was withdrawn as a prophylaxis against malaria, though as a treatment it appears safe. Continued pharmacovigilance is required as there is concern that in some countries in Africa, doses will be taken several times a year to treat infections and these serious adverse reactions may be seen.

Mefloquine

Mefloquine is active against all malaria species. As a treatment it is taken as a single oral dose, but because of its cost and side-effects it is not considered a realistic treatment option for large scale use in malaria control programmes in moderate to high transmission areas. Side-effects include dizziness, disturbances of sleep and occasionally fits and psychoses and, at treatment doses, vomiting is common. Individuals with a history of convulsions or neuropsychiatric disease are advised not to use mefloquine. In South East Asia, resistance rapidly developed when mefloquine was used as a monotherapy to treat malaria.

Lumefantrine

Lumefantrine is combined with artemether in a fixed-dose tablet to make the ACT artemether-lumefantrine (Coartem™ or Riamet™). It is effective against drug-resistant falciparum malaria and the non-falciparum species. Worldwide, it is the mostly widely used ACT to treat uncomplicated malaria.

Halofantrine

Halofantrine is cardiotoxic, prolonging the QT interval and leading to arrhythmias, and is no longer recommended for the treatment of malaria.

Piperaquine

Piperaquine is a bisquinoline and is combined with dihydroartemisinin as a fixed-dose ACT treatment (Artekin™ or Euroartesim™).

Primaquine

This 8-aminoquinoline targets the liver hypnozoites of vivax and ovale malaria and is the only licensed drug for their radical cure. Primaquine taken once daily for 14 days at a dose of 30 mg for *P. vivax* (approximately 0.5–0.6 mg/kg) and 15 mg daily for *P. ovale* is highly effective especially if taken at the same time as treatment against the blood stage parasites (usually with chloroquine). The higher dose is required for *P. vivax* due to partial parasite resistance to primaquine in much of South East Asia. In patients >70 kg, the total dose can be increased to 0.6 mg/kg/day as underdosing in heavier patients has been associated with higher failure rates. Screening for glucose-6-phosphate deficiency (G6PD) deficiency should be done before administering primaquine as it causes acute haemolysis in patients with enzyme deficiency. This inherited sex-linked deficiency provides some protection against severe forms of falciparum malaria and is present in up to 30% of some populations. Different genotypes exist and so there is variability in the extent of the deficiency. For individuals living in areas with high levels of vivax or ovale transmission, reinfection is inevitable so there is no rationale for radical curative therapy and G6PD testing is not readily available in many of these countries.

In patients with severe G6PD deficiency, primaquine should be avoided. In mild to moderate deficiency a once-weekly dose of 0.75 mg/kg (around 45–60 mg) for 8 weeks can be trialled under supervision. The drug has a short half-life and if significant haemolysis occurs, it is self-limiting.

Primaquine is gametocidal. In countries with low levels of malaria transmission the addition of a single dose of primaquine (0.75 mg/kg) to a standard malaria treatment is now a WHO recommended strategy to try to reduce transmission as part of a malaria eradication programme. It can be taken without prior G6PD testing, though the safety of this approach has not been widely tested especially in Africa where there is the highest incidence of G6PD deficiency.

Tafenoquine

This 8-aminoquinoline is under evaluation as an anti-hypnozoite therapy. It has a much longer half-life than primaquine, allowing a short treatment regimen and better compliance, but it also causes haemolysis in G6PD deficient patients. The dosing regimen and effect in G6PD deficient individuals is currently being evaluated.

Antifolate drugs

These drugs inhibit parasite folic acid synthesis by competing for the active site of the parasite enzymes dihydrofolate reductase (DHFR) and dihydropteroate synthase (DHPS). Proguanil was the first of the anti-DHFR drugs to be discovered in 1945 and is structurally related to pyrimethamine, the most widely used anti-DHFR agent. Sulfa drugs, including sulfadoxine, sulfalene and dapsone, inhibit the parasite enzyme DHPS. When used alone, they have a low potency; however, when combined with anti-DHFR drugs there is synergy. This has led to their development as combination therapies; sulfalene-pyrimethamine (Metakelfin™), dapsone-pyrimethamine (Maloprim™) and sulfadoxine-pyrimethamine (SP or Fansidar™), the most widely used.

In the 1990s, in response to the emergence of CQ resistant falciparum malaria, SP replaced CQ as first-line treatment for uncomplicated malaria in many countries in Africa. SP would seem to be an ideal treatment choice for outpatient therapy – it costs less than $0.10 per adult treatment, is taken as a single oral dose and has few side-effects. However, resistance has developed quickly to SP wherever it has been used, facilitated by the long half-lives of its component parts. Despite widespread resistance, SP is still used in some countries, usually in combination with AQ or CQ, and has an important role in presumptive therapy in pregnancy (see below).

Antibiotics

Several antibiotics, including doxycycline, clindamycin and azithromycin have antimalarial activity. They reduce parasite load by a factor of 10 every 2 days and are used to augment the activity of other antimalarials. A 7-day course of doxycycline or clindamycin may be taken with quinine when decreased susceptibility to quinine is suspected.

Atovaquone

Atovaquone has weak antimalarial activity on its own but when combined with proguanil as Malarone™ has proven to be an effective treatment and prophylaxis against multidrug resistant falciparum malaria and non-falciparum species. Its high cost precludes its use in any national treatment policy in malaria endemic countries.

Resistance to antimalarial drugs

Resistance to antimalarial drugs is of huge public health importance and *P. falciparum* has developed resistance to most of the drugs currently available. The consequences of drug resistance include more cases of severe disease and death, and economic costs as a result of time off work and the need to treat resistant parasites with more expensive agents. Resistance may develop through the amplification and increased expression of specific parasite genes or by spontaneous genetic point mutations in the genes. In the presence of drug, point mutations or amplifications, which confer survival advantage to the parasite, will be preferentially selected. Mutations may arise in the drug target itself, e.g. the genes *dhfr* and *dhps*, reducing their sensitivity to the action of antifolate drugs, or resistance may arise when mutations arise in genes encoding drug transporters, resulting in a reduced concentration of drug (CQ and AQ) at its target site.

South East Asia and in particular, the Thai–Cambodian border area, is referred to as the 'birthplace' of antimalarial drug resistance. This refers to the observation that parasite drug resistance to CQ, SP and mefloquine was first observed in this area, before spreading to other parts of Asia and onto Africa. Why resistance arises first in this part of the world is not fully understood but may be due in part to the widespread use of fake or substandard drugs, and to reduced malarial immunity in Asia compared to sub-Saharan Africa. Malaria infections are usually symptomatic in that region and as a result most of the parasite population is eventually exposed to drug. Decreased sensitivity of *P. falciparum* to artemisinins has now been documented in four countries; Cambodia, Myanmar, Thailand and Viet Nam. The establishment and spread of artemisinin-resistant parasites from this area would be a public health disaster. In response to this, containment measures are now being implemented including increased surveillance, enhanced mosquito control measures and the recommendation that oral artemisinin-based monotherapies be withdrawn and replaced with ACTs.

Quinine remains efficacious in clinical trials against multidrug resistant *P. falciparum* in most parts of the world, though in parts of South East Asia there is evidence of a decline in the efficacy.

Chloroquine-resistant vivax is reported in Papua New Guinea and Indonesia, but its spread seems relatively limited. Resistance of *P. vivax* to SP is widespread. Resistant strains of *P. ovale*, *P. malariae* and *P. knowlesi* malaria have not been reported. Primaquine is the only drug currently licensed for the radical cure of vivax and ovale malaria and reduced susceptibility has been reported in the Chesson strain of *P. vivax* in South East Asia. Resistance to Malarone™ has been documented in a few case reports from Africa.

Treatment recommendations

Uncomplicated falciparum malaria

In sub-Saharan Africa, most episodes of uncomplicated malaria are treated with oral antimalarial therapy on an outpatient basis. Patients are usually less sick owing to the partial immunity built up after repeated malaria infections during childhood. In non-immune populations and severe cases, inpatient treatment is required.

In order to prevent the development of resistance, the World Health Organization (WHO) recommends combination therapy of two or more drugs with different mechanisms of action to treat falciparum malaria, a principle common to the treatment of tuberculosis and HIV. In particular the WHO recommends the use of artemisinin-based combination therapies (ACTs). The very rapid killing of asexual parasites is a property of artemisinin drugs that makes them particularly suitable for combination therapy. Taken for three days, they significantly reduce the parasite biomass for the partner drug in the combination to kill and reduce the chance that a resistant mutant will emerge. In addition, the gametocidal effects of the artemisinin may reduce help reduce onward transmission in some settings. Atovaquone-proguanil and antifolate drugs like SP are not combination therapies like ACTs as the components act synergistically together rather than independently.

Since 2006, the WHO has recommended ACTs as first-line therapy for uncomplicated malaria due to *P. falciparum*. Non-artemisinin combinations like AQ plus SP are no longer recommended. Several ACTs are available, some formulated as fixed-dose combination tablets, which is important for patient compliance. These include artemether-lu-mefantrine, artesunate-amodiaquine, artesuante-mefloquine, dihydroartemisinin-piperaquine, and artesunate-SP. The choice of ACT is guided by local resistance patterns to the partner drug. For all these combinations, the partner drug has an elimination half-life which is much longer than the artemisinin component and as a result, will be present in the blood as a monotherapy for a period of time as its concentration falls. In high transmission areas, this is a potential risk for selection of drug resistant parasites if reinfections occur during the time that drug concentrations are subtherapeutic. It remains to be seen what the impact of this will be on the long-term efficacy of ACTs.

Although there have been problems in the implementation of ACT policies in some countries due to supply and distribution difficulties, by 2010, ACTs were the first-line treatment choice in 84 countries worldwide where *P. falciparum* is endemic. ACTs are more expensive but their use has been supported financially by international funding initiatives and by pharmaceutical companies providing drugs at cost price. Total ACT demand was projected to reach 287 million treatment courses in 2011. In the WHO African Region in 2010, the number of ACTs distributed was more than twice the number of diagnostic tests, indicating that many patients continue to receive ACTs without confirmatory diagnostic testing.

Severe falciparum malaria

Intravenous artesunate has been shown to be superior to quinine for the treatment of severe malaria in adults in South East Asia, associated with a 34% reduction in mortality. The beneficial effect was most marked in those with initial parasitaemias greater than 10%. The number needed to treat to prevent one death was 13. A trial in African children with severe malaria demonstrated a 22% reduction in mortality with intravenous artesunate compared to quinine. On the basis of these data, the WHO now recommends that intravenous artesunate should be used in preference to quinine for severe falciparum malaria. Parenteral therapy should be given for at least 24 hours with step down to a full course of an ACT or oral quinine plus clindamycin or doxycycline once the patient improves.

In 2010, the WHO granted the Chinese manufacturers of intravenous artesunate 'prequalification' approval of their product. Prequalification means that the manufacturers have complied with internationally recommended standards. Previously, more stringent country or area specific regulatory approval had been required before international procurement agencies would have been able to purchase and distribute the drug; these requirements had been an impediment to the use of these drugs in many countries.

Plasmodium vivax, ovale, malariae and knowlesi

Chloroquine is the treatment of choice for the non-falciparum species, combined with primaquine if radical cure is required in vivax and ovale infections. Alternative treatments include ACTs (except artesunate-SP for vivax), quinine, atovaquone-proguanil and mefloquine. Severe cases of *P. vivax* or *P. knowlesi* infection should be treated the same as severe falciparum malaria.

Imported malaria in travellers

Treatment guidelines for imported malaria are available for several countries. These generally recommend that all patients with falciparum malaria should be admitted to hospital for treatment. Approximately 1% of all individuals with imported falciparum malaria die and predicting which patients are most likely to get severe disease or die is difficult. Patients may initially present with low parasitaemias or none of the features usually associated with severe disease and then rapidly deteriorate. Young children, the elderly and pregnant women are at particularly high risk. It is dangerous to make the assumption that patients brought up in malaria endemic areas will be immune and not suffer severe disease. Malaria immunity wanes if people are not re-exposed to malaria parasites on a regular basis so those individuals who have moved away from malaria endemic areas are also at risk of severe disease.

Artemether-lumefantrine and atovaquoneproguanil are both licensed in Europe and the USA and dihydroartemisinin-piperaquine has been registered in Europe. Mefloquine is effective for uncomplicated malaria but poorly tolerated at treatment doses and is not recommended in the UK (but is in the USA and Australia). Because chloroquine-resistant falciparum malaria is so widespread, the UK guidelines do not recommend its use for falciparum malaria; a decision made on the basis that there are several alternatives and that the risk of treating a potentially chloroquine resistant infection is too high.

Severe imported malaria is treated with intravenous quinine or intravenous artesunate if available. Intravenous artesunate is unlicensed in Europe, but in patients with high parasite counts or very severe disease, intravenous artesunate will often be used. There is no evidence to support the use of adjunctive exchange transfusion in cases of high parasitaemia. With the increasing availability of artemisinins and the rapid falls in parasite counts observed with these drugs, the theoretical benefits of exchange transfusion are now diminished such that the potential risks probably outweigh the potential benefits.

For non-falciparum malaria, chloroquine remains the treatment of choice, though artemether-lumefantrine, atovaquone-proguanil, mefloquine and quinine are also effective. Chloroquine-resistant vivax should be considered in patients who fail to respond. Primaquine should be given (after G6PD testing) concurrently with chloroquine if possible, for radical cure of vivax and ovale.

Treatment of malaria in pregnancy

Malaria in pregnancy, especially in primigravida women, is a risk factor for severe disease, maternal anaemia, prematurity and intra-uterine growth retardation. Because of these risks, many malaria endemic countries in Africa follow the WHO recommended policy of intermittent presumptive therapy (IPT). Pregnant women, irrespective of symptoms or parasitaemia, are given full treatment courses of SP or chloroquine at two or three time points during pregnancy with the aim of reducing the incidence of malaria in pregnancy and to reduce malaria-related complications. A similar approach to malaria in infancy is also recommended.

For women who present with clinical features of malaria, the most widely used treatment is quinine. Quinine may cause hypoglycaemia in late pregnancy and has a stimulatory effect on uterine muscle. However, the benefit of curing malaria in pregnancy greatly outweighs the risk of uterine excitation from therapeutic doses of the drug. Artemisinins are all teratogenic in both rats and rabbits and the WHO advises that they should be avoided in the first trimester of pregnancy unless the mother's life is at risk. In practice many women in early pregnancy have been exposed to these drugs while unaware of their pregnancy with no ill effects noted. ACTs are now recommended in preference to quinine for women in the 2nd and 3rd trimester.

Chloroquine and amodiaquine are both thought to be safe during pregnancy and in breastfeeding. There is less experience with mefloquine though there have been many hundreds of well-observed cases in which the drug has been used in pregnancy without adverse effect on mother or foetus. Doxycycline is contraindicated in pregnancy and when breastfeeding and there are few data on atovaquone-proguanil. Primaquine should also not be used as the G6PD status of the foetus is not known, and should only be used when breastfeeding if the infant is tested first.

Pharmacokinetic interactions between antimalarials and other drugs

Limited data are available on the interactions between antimalarial drugs and other drugs that are commonly co-prescribed. The liver cytochrome P450 enzymes are important in the metabolism of several antimalarials including artemether, lumefantrine and quinine. Rifampicin is potent inducer of these enzymes. Some antiretroviral agents, notably non-nucleoside reverse transcriptase inhibitors and protease inhibitors, are potent inducers and/or inhibitors. Several studies to investigate potential interactions are ongoing. One study in healthy volunteers demonstrated that co-administration of artemether-lumefantrine with efavirenz resulted in increased exposure to lumefantrine. The clinical importance of these potential interactions is at present unknown. One important interaction that has been described is an increased risk of neutropenia if amodiaquine is taken with efavirenz or zidovudine and these combinations should be avoided.

Relapse and recrudescence

In *P. falciparum* and *P. malariae* infections, episodes of illness may recur for years after the primary infection if inadequately treated or untreated due to recrudescence of small numbers of blood stage parasites. Recurrent fever may also occur in *P. vivax* and *P. ovale* due to relapse from liver hypnozoites. Relapses occur despite drug treatment to eliminate the red cell parasite stages in primary infection and can only be prevented by specific therapy to achieve a 'radical' cure with the eradication of the hypnozoites. This may however be unrealistic if the patient lives in an area where re-infection is inevitable (in fact the risks of the drug might outweigh its benefits in these circumstances).

Malaria control and eradication

In 1955 the WHO set out an ambitious plan for the worldwide eradication of malaria. The strategy relied heavily upon indoor spraying with the insecticide dichloro-diphenyl-trichloroethane (DDT) and drug treatment programmes using the drug chloroquine. This strategy was abandoned in 1969 in favour of a strategy of malaria control, reducing the malaria burden, when it became clear that worldwide eradication could not be achieved using the tools available at that time. Although the programme is viewed as having failed, malaria was eradicated from over 30 countries.

In the past few years, there has been a scale-up of malaria control measures and ambitious targets have been set to reduce the burden of malaria. This drive has been supported by huge increases in the amount of money made available by international donors, peaking at $2 billion in 2011. The Roll Back Malaria (RBM) partnership, the global coordinating body for fighting malaria, set a target to reduce malaria cases compared to 2000 in all countries by 50% by 2010 and by 75% by 2015. The cornerstones of malaria control today are malaria prevention through vector control measures, chemoprophylaxis of high risk groups and the provision of prompt, effective treatment.

The two most powerful vector control interventions are the use of long-lasting insecticide-treated bednets (ITNs) and indoor residual spraying (IRS) – the application of insecticides to the walls of homes. These interventions reduce human-vector contact and reduce the lifespan of female mosquitoes. The use of larvicidal agents in mosquito breeding areas is only beneficial if these areas are fixed and easily identified. Vector control is only effective if high coverage is achieved and sustained and the RBM target is for 'universal coverage' by 2015 with ITNs and IRS. Substantial progress has been made in the manufacture and distributions of ITNs: the percentage of households owning at least one ITN in sub-Saharan Africa is estimated to have risen from 3% in 2000 to 50% in 2011.

The roll out of ACTs has been impressive with global ACT demand projected to reach 287 million treatment courses in 2011. These drugs are undoubtedly having a significant impact on mortality and morbidity and in some situations, may reduce transmission by their gametocidal activity. IPT programmes in pregnancy are recommended in most countries with moderate or high levels of transmission. This has been shown to increase maternal haemoglobin and birth weight. Other vulnerable groups in these settings are infants and young children and the utility of IPT using ACTs is being evaluated in these groups.

We now have evidence that the huge expansion in the use of ACTs, ITNs and IRS is resulting in a measurable public health impact. The estimated incidence of malaria globally has fallen by 17% between 2000 and 2010 and malaria-specific mortality has fallen by 26%. Although the RBM target was not reached, a 50% reduction in malaria incidence was achieved by 43 countries by 2010. Optimism, not present for years in malaria control circles, has returned and some have even dared mention the 'eradication' word again. However multiple challenges remain even to maintain the achievements so far. These include keeping up with the huge demand for drugs, the widespread use of fake drugs and the decline in *P. falciparum* sensitivity to artemisinins now being reported in South East Asia. The effectiveness of ITNs decays over time, and even those impregnated with long-lasting insecticides have an estimated lifespan of only three years. Re-supplying the hundreds of millions of ITNs delivered so far will be a logistical challenge. IRS and ITNs are both critically dependent on a single class of insecticides, the pyrethroids and mosquito resistance to these has been reported in many countries. Continued monitoring for the emergence and spread of drug and insecticide resistance in different locations will be vital in the future, so that the threats of pyrethroid and artemisinin resistance can be contained.

The ultimate goal for malaria control is the development of an effective and affordable vaccine. The RTS,S/AS01 vaccine, is constructed from antigen from sporozoites fused with hepatitis B surface antigen. In field studies in Africa it has been shown to have protective efficacy rates of around 55% against all clinical episodes of malaria and 35% against severe malaria during the 12 months after vaccination in children five to 17 months of age. These trials are encouraging and partial protection may be of great importance in endemic regions. The vaccine could be available by 2015 to complement malaria control measures already in place. What we do not yet know is the duration of vaccine protection or whether further booster doses are needed. Trial data are also needed from other geographical settings. A wholly protective vaccine for those living in endemic areas remains many years distant.

Malaria prevention for travellers

Malaria prevention for travellers centres upon personal protection with repellents and nets and chemoprophylaxis with the regular administration of drugs to prevent clinical symptoms. Because falciparum has the greatest potential to cause death and is resistant to many drugs, the regimen taken is determined by the falciparum resistance pattern in the area to be visited. All the recommended falciparum chemoprophylaxis regimens will protect against the other malaria species.

Chemoprophylaxis works either by prevention of the formation of pre-erythrocytic schizonts in the liver ('causal prophylaxis') or by killing the blood stage schizonts ('suppressive prophylaxis'). Most drugs act as suppressive agents, but atovaquone-proguanil also acts as a causal chemoprophylactic agent (Fig. 9.8). Current international guidelines recommend three options for prophylaxis in countries with chloroquine-resistant falciparum; atovaquone-proguanil, doxycycline and mefloquine. These have equal efficacy in clinical trials (95–100%) but vary in side effects, dose schedule and cost. In parts of South East Asia, resistance to mefloquine precludes its use. Chloroquine-sensitive parasites predominate in parts of the Middle East and Caribbean, and in these areas chloroquine with or without proguanil can be used. Recommendations for antimalarial prophylaxis in specific geographical locations are constantly changing. Authoritative up-to-date sources such as the WHO, UK or CDC guidelines are recommended (see Further reading).

Atovaquone-proguanil (Malarone™) is a causal prophylactic, preventing development of parasites in the liver and, therefore, only needs to be taken for a week after leaving a malarious area. Doxycycline, mefloquine and chloroquine all need to be taken for 4 weeks after leaving. Primaquine is effective as a casual prophylaxis against vivax and falciparum though not licensed for this role in many countries. In addition, it kills hypnozoites in the liver, preventing late emergence of vivax or ovale infections and it is gametocidal, preventing onward transmission of all plasmodial species. It can be considered in patients with normal G6PD levels if other options are not available. In pregnancy, mefloquine is the only available option for travel to countries with CQ-resistant malaria. The UK and WHO prophylaxis guidelines advise caution using mefloquine in the first trimester, while US guidelines allow its use throughout pregnancy. Pregnant women should not take doxycycline. Atovoquone-proguanil is not recommended due to a lack of data. It is also important that all travellers to endemic areas recognize the risk of malaria and know that they should inform health personnel about their travel history, should they become unwell.

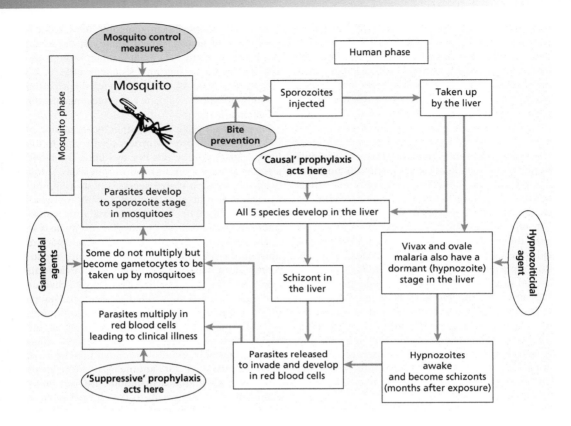

Figure 9.8 Action of preventative interventions on the malaria life cycle.

 SUMMARY

- Malaria is the most important tropical parasitic infection and one of the world's leading causes of death and morbidity. Around three billion people live in one of the 106 countries endemic for malaria.

- Five species of the genus *Plasmodium* are recognized to cause malaria in people: *P falciparum*, *P. vivax*, *P. ovale*, *P. malariae* and *P. knowlesi*.

- The consequences of malaria infection are classified into two clinical syndromes, uncomplicated malaria and severe malaria; the latter is usually associated with *P. falciparum* infection, although severe and fatal disease is also described with *P. vivax* and *P. knowlesi* infections.

- The clinical features of uncomplicated malaria are non-specific and common to each of the malaria species and to many other infections.

- Resistance to antimalarial drugs is of huge public health importance and *P. falciparum* has developed resistance to most of the drugs currently available. In order to prevent the development of resistance, the World Health Organization (WHO) recommends combination therapy of two or more drugs with different mechanisms of action to treat falciparum malaria.

Visit www.lecturenoteseries.com/tropicalmed to test yourself on this chapter using interactive MCQs.

📖 FURTHER READING

Centers for Disease Control and Prevention (USA) Many useful documents on www.cdc.gov/MALARIA/

Feacham RGA, Phillips AS, Hwang J, *et al.* (2010) Shrinking the malaria map: progress and prospects. *Lancet* **376**: 1566–78 free download from http://www.ncbi.nlm.nih.gov/pmc/articles/PMC3044848/ [First in a series of 4 useful articles about malaria epidemiology and elimination.]

UK Chemoprophylaxis Recommendations: www.hpa.org.uk/infections/topics_az/malaria/guidelines.htm
www.nathnac.org
www.travax.nhs.uk

UK treatment guidelines: www.britishinfection.org/drupal/content/clinical-guidelines

World Health Organization (2010) *Guidelines for the Treatment of Malaria*, 2nd edn. Geneva: WHO.

World Health Organization (2012) *Malaria Report.* Geneva: WHO. www.who.int/topics/malaria/en/

World Health Organization (2013) Management of severe malaria – A practical handbook. Third edition. http://apps.who.int/iris/bitstream/10665/79317/1/9789241548526_eng.pdf

10

Visceral leishmaniasis

Tim O'Dempsey
Liverpool School of Tropical Medicine

About 30 species of obligate intracellular protozoal parasites of the genus *Leishmania* are responsible for a variety of diseases in humans, collectively known as leishmaniasis. These diseases are further classified as visceral, cutaneous or mucosal according to their principal clinical presentations. A 'leishmaniac' is a person who is obsessed with these parasites.

Epidemiology

Visceral leishmaniasis (VL), also known as kala-azar (Hindi for 'black sickness'), is mainly caused by three species belonging to the *Leishmania donovani* complex, each with a characteristic regional distribution:

- *L. infantum* – Mediterranean, Middle East, Central Asia, China;
- *L. donovani* – India, East Africa;
- *L. chagasi* – South and Central America.

VL may also be caused by *L. tropica* in the Old World and *L. amazonensis* in the New World.

Over 200 million people reside in endemic areas of more than 70 affected countries. There are approximately 500 000 cases reported annually, 90% of which occur in Bangladesh, India, Nepal, Sudan and North-Eastern Brazil.

Humans are the only known reservoir of *L. donovani* in Bangladesh, India and Nepal. Humans, and possibly rodents, are thought to be the reservoir in East Africa. Wild and domestic canines are important reservoirs of *L. infantum* and *L. chagasi*. Infection occurs following the bite of an infected female sandfly (*Phlebotomus* spp. in the Old World, *Lutzomyia* spp. in the New World). Transmission may also occur via blood transfusions, infected needles or syringes, and congenitally. The incidence of VL among transplant recipients has also been increasing steadily in recent years.

In some regions, such as North-Eastern Brazil, expanding urbanization is associated with steadily increasing transmission of leishmaniasis. Globally, HIV is also contributing to the clinical reemergence of leishmaniasis. Reports of HIV co-infection currently range from 2–30% among VL patients. Pathogen proliferation and disease progression are mutually enhanced in *Leishmania* and HIV co-infection. In regions of co-endemicity, there is likely to be a shift from subclinical to clinical VL, coupled with an increased rate of transmission of VL in the general population.

Parasite and life-cycle

Leishmania amastigotes are spherical or oval bodies measuring 2–4 μm containing two distinct pieces of nuclear chromatin. The larger piece is called the nucleus, the smaller piece the kinetoplast. The sandfly becomes infected by taking up the amastigotes with its blood meal, the amastigotes being in the blood or skin of the infecting host. The amastigotes are liberated in the stomach of the sandfly and begin to multiply by simple fission, eventually forming flagellated metacyclic promastigotes, which are infectious to the new host. This process takes 1–2 weeks, depending on the species. The motile promastigotes migrate from the gut to the proboscis of the sandfly and are injected during feeding. Sandfly saliva inhibits the l-arginine-dependent nitric oxide killing mechanism of macrophages. The promastigotes are ingested unharmed by macrophages and metamorphose into

Tropical Medicine Lecture Notes, Seventh edition. Edited by Nick Beeching and Geoff Gill. © 2014 John Wiley & Sons, Ltd. Published 2014 by John Wiley & Sons, Ltd.

amastigotes. These are distributed in the reticuloendothelial system, where they lodge and multiply by binary fission.

Clinical features of visceral leishmaniasis

Clinical presentation ranges from asymptomatic or subclinical infection to acute, subacute and chronic presentations. The ratio of clinical:subclinical infections is in the range of 1:30–100. The incubation period is usually between 2 and 6 months, but ranges from 10 days to more than 10 years. Males are about three times more commonly affected than females.

Onset is usually insidious, with low-grade fever, progressive splenomegaly, hepatomegaly, lymphadenopathy (particularly in Africa), anaemia, anorexia, wasting and increased pigmentation in persons with dark skin (particularly in India).

The liver and spleen are usually firm, regular and non-tender on palpation. The spleen may reach enormous proportions, commonly extending beyond the midline and sometimes into the right iliac fossa. Patients may complain of a dragging discomfort or, less commonly, acute pain as a result of splenic infarcts. Other relatively common features include epistaxis and cough.

Patients with chronic VL may have visited traditional healers and have been subjected to medicinal cuts that subsequently become infected. Infection and ulceration of other superficial wounds is also common at the time of presentation. Intercurrent infections, such as pneumonia, bacillary or amoebic dysentery, and tuberculosis, are particularly important in patients with long-standing disease and may be the main reason for the patient seeking medical care. Other complications of VL include malnutrition, malabsorption, bleeding, nephritis and uveitis.

Some patients present acutely, with an abrupt onset of high swinging fever and other symptoms resembling malaria. Specific cutaneous lesions are uncommon at the time of original presentation in VL. Rarely, a patient may be aware of a painless papule at the site of the infective bite. Post-kala-azar dermal leishmaniasis (PKDL) may occur following treatment and is discussed below.

Case fatality rates associated with VL range from 0–50% of treated cases to 85–90% of untreated cases.

Differential diagnosis of splenomegaly

Massive spleen

- Malaria or hyperreactive malaria splenomegaly
- Portal hypertension, e.g. caused by schistosomiasis, cirrhosis, etc.
- Lymphoma, leukaemia, myelodysplasia
- Haemoglobinopathies and hereditary haemolytic anaemias
- Splenic hydatid cyst
- Still's disease
- Glycogen storage and other metabolic diseases
- Amyloidosis

Moderate spleen

- Any of the above
- Bacterial endocarditis
- Brucellosis
- Cytomegalovirus
- HIV infection
- Infectious mononucleosis
- Leptospirosis
- Lyme disease
- Relapsing fever
- Syphilis
- Toxoplasmosis
- Trypanosomiasis
- Tuberculosis
- Typhoid
- Typhus

Viscerotropic leishmaniasis

Splenomegaly and fever caused by *L. tropica* infection was noted in American troops involved in the Gulf War in the 1990s. None of these patients developed massive splenomegaly or other features typical of classical VL.

Visceral leishmaniasis and HIV co-infection

Leishmania and HIV coinfection was first recognized in 1986. HIV and VL have a mutually adverse effect on disease progression and outcome and HIV-coinfected individuals are 100–2320 times more likely to develop active VL. Most cases are thought to be caused either by reactivation of latent infection or associated with intravenous drug use (IVDU). In North-West Ethiopia 15–30% of VL patients are coinfected with HIV. IVDU-associated *L. infantum* infections are the commonest *Leishmania* and HIV coinfections in southern Europe, where, prior to the availability of combination antiretroviral therapy (cART), coinfection accounted for 25–70% of all adult cases of VL and 1.5–9% of patients with AIDS developed VL. The widespread use of cART in Europe has resulted in a reduction of incidence by 50–65%, higher survival rates, and a reduction in relapse rate.

Presentation of VL in HIV-positive patients is often atypical and may be a chance finding. Ninety per cent of cases have CD4 counts <200 × 10^6/L. Atypical clinical features include dysphagia and cutaneous or mucocutaneous lesions. Nodular or ulcerative lesions may affect the tongue, oesophagus, stomach, rectum, larynx or lungs. The course varies from asymptomatic infection to rapidly progressive and fatal disease. Symptoms may be milder and more atypical as the CD4 count falls. Visceralization of *Leishmania* spp. normally associated with cutaneous or mucocutaneous disease is being increasingly reported among HIV-infected patients throughout the world.

Prior to the use of cART, European studies indicated that 30% of patients died during or within 1 month of treatment. The mean survival was 12 months and only 16% survived for more than 3 years. Relapses commonly occurred every 3–6 months. Although cART may delay relapse, 40% of VL patients on cART will experience relapses unless receiving maintenance VL treatment, with a mean interval to first relapse of seven months. Various regimens of antileishmanial drugs, such as pentamidine, liposomal amphotericin B and miltefosine, have been proposed to reduce relapses in HIV-coinfected patients. Immune reconstitution inflammatory syndrome (IRIS) has been described in a small number of coinfected patients.

Investigations

Circumstantial evidence

Full blood count typically reveals anaemia, leucopenia and thrombocytopenia. This is partly explained by hypersplenism. However, a number of other factors may also be important including possible autoimmune mechanisms and bone marrow depression.

Diagnostic work-up should include a coagulation screen or, if unavailable, at least an estimation of the bleeding and clotting times, particularly if a splenic aspirate is planned. Bilirubin and transaminases are (usually mildly) elevated in about 20% of patients, and the alkaline phosphatase is raised in about 40%. Serum albumin is low and globulins are raised, especially IgG. Albuminuria is common but urinalysis is otherwise normal in uncomplicated disease.

The formol gel test (FGT) is a simple test that is sometimes used to provide circumstantial evidence of VL. The FGT is not specific for VL and, when positive, indicates hyperglobulinaemia, whatever the cause. Add 1 drop of concentrated formalin solution (40% formaldehyde) to 1 mL of serum in a test tube. Shake to mix thoroughly. After 20 min at room temperature, the serum becomes a firm opaque jelly (like a cooked egg white) if the test is positive.

Serological tests for antibody

Indirect fluorescent antibody test (IFAT) and enzyme-linked immunoabsorbent assay (ELISA) have sensitivities and specificities above 95%. Although these tests may not be readily available in remote areas, it is possible to collect blood spots on filter paper, which can be sent elsewhere for testing.

The direct agglutination test (DAT) is > 95% sensitive and specific, and relatively easy to perform in the field. A new, more stable version of the DAT is now available that uses freeze-dried antigen (DAT-FD). The main drawbacks are time (18 hours), cost (1–2 Euro) and clinical interpretation (may be positive in up to 30% of population in endemic areas and remains positive long after 'cure').

The fast agglutination-screening test (FAST) is a rapid (< 3 hr) test that detects antibody in serum or filter paper blood-spot samples and gives qualitative results comparable to DAT.

The rK39 test is a commercially available immunochromatographic strip that uses recombinant leishmanial antigen. This has been shown to be 100% sensitive and 98% specific in India. However, when used to test clinically suspected VL in field conditions in Sudan and Nepal, rK39 showed a lack of specificity, although a more recent version of this test has been reported to perform better. Serology may remain positive for years following successful treatment.

Serology is unreliable in immunocompromised patients and is positive in only about 50% of patients with *Leishmania* and HIV coinfection.

Parasitological evidence

The gold standard for diagnosis of VL is identification of amastigotes of *L. donovani* spp. These are most readily found in splenic aspirates (>95% positive), bone marrow (53–86%) and lymph node (>53–65%).

Amastigotes may also be detected in a peripheral blood buffy coat smear, ranging from 50% in Africa to > 90% in Bangladesh where a strong positive correlation with spleen parasite load has been demonstrated. In *Leishmania* and HIV-coinfected patients amastigotes may be detectable in the buffy coat in 50%, bone marrow in 94% and in skin lesions and other affected tissues. Amastigotes are identified using a Giemsa or other Romanowsky stain. Aspirates may also be cultured on Novy, MacNeal and Nicolle's (NNN) medium.

Polymerase chain reaction (PCR) is capable of detecting infection with a single parasite. PCR sensitivity is 82–100% for bone marrow and 72–100% for peripheral blood. A promising variety of real time PCR assays, including point of care tests, are under currently under development and are likely to greatly enhance the diagnosis and monitoring of infection and relapse, particularly in HIV-coinfected patients.

Urine antigen tests may prove useful in diagnosis and monitoring response to treatment. The detection of polypeptide fractions of K39 and K26 *Leishmania* antigen in urine of patients with visceral leishmaniasis has been shown to be 96% sensitive and 100% specific; these antigens were not detectable after 3 weeks of treatment, suggesting a good prognostic value. A latex agglutination test (KAtex; Kalon Biological, UK), that detects *Leishmania* antigens in urine has proved highly sensitive (86–100%) in two studies of HIV-coinfected patients in Spain during clinical episodes when the parasite load was high. Furthermore, the test became negative following a satisfactory clinical response to treatment which may be helpful in monitoring the efficacy of treatment and the possible occurrence of relapses. Similar results have been found among HIV-negative patients.

Performing a splenic aspirate

Splenic aspirate is a straightforward procedure, relatively painless and safe, provided that one excludes patients with a bleeding tendency and those in whom portal hypertension, a splenic hydatid cyst or vascular abnormality are considered likely in the differential diagnosis. The patient should be comfortable and lying flat with the abdomen exposed. Select an area in the middle of the long axis of the spleen. Clean the skin with an alcohol swab or other antiseptic. Using a 21 gauge needle attached to a 5 mL syringe, insert the needle subcutaneously in line with the long axis of the spleen, draw back the plunger of the syringe to the 1 mL mark to create a negative pressure and swiftly insert the needle into the body of the spleen to a depth of about 2–3 cm at an angle of about 45° to the skin and withdraw immediately while maintaining negative pressure in the syringe. The entire procedure should take only a few seconds.

Having withdrawn the needle, there may be little or nothing visible in the syringe. This is not a problem. Disconnect the needle from the syringe and draw up 2 mL of air. Reconnect the needle and carefully squirt the contents of the needle onto one or more microscope slides and make a smear. The tiny amount of tissue that appears on the slide should be sufficient for diagnostic purposes.

It is probably safest to perform splenic aspirates in a setting where the patient can remain lying down and be monitored for a few hours, and where facilities for transfusion are available if required. However, with experience, outpatient aspirates can be successfully carried out.

Management

Prior to embarking on specific chemotherapy with potentially toxic drugs, it is important to identify and treat intercurrent infections. Attention should also be given to improving the patient's nutritional status.

Pentavalent antimonials (SbV)

Sodium stibogluconate (Pentostam™) and meglumine antimonate (Glucantime™) are the drugs most commonly used as first-line treatment. These drugs are relatively expensive; however, an effective and cheaper generic version of sodium stibogluconate is now produced in India. The usual dose is 20 mg SbV/kg/day by slow intravenous infusion (the manufacturers of Pentostam™ recommend a minimum of 5 min) or intramuscularly for 20–40 days, depending on the geographical region. Side-effects include arthralgia, nausea, abdominal pain and pancreatitis. Cardiotoxicity tends to occur with high-dose regimens, particularly with prolonged use, and includes ST segment inversion, prolongation of the QTc interval and fatal arrhythmias. Toxicity, particularly pancreatitis, is increased in HIV-positive patients. Furthermore, SbV have been shown to stimulate HIV-1 replication in vitro. Mortality during treatment is four times higher with SbV than with miltefosine.

Amphotericin B

Conventional amphotericin B (AmB) is sometimes used in regions with high levels of resistance to SbV, such as Bihar, India. It is usually administered by slow intravenous infusion in 5% dextrose over 4–6 h, commencing at 0.1 mg/kg/day and gradually increasing to 1 mg/kg/day until a *total* dose of 20 mg/kg has been given. Studies in India have shown that there was no difference in infusion-related side-effects if treatment was commenced at 1 mg/kg/day. Side-effects include anaphylaxis, fever, chills, bone pain and thrombophlebitis. Hypokalaemia, renal impairment and anaemia may also occur.

Liposomal amphotericin B

Amphotericin toxicity is reduced and efficacy enhanced by lyophilization, thereby enhancing distribution in macrophages and reticuloendothelial tissues. Liposomal amphotericin B is comparatively expensive and is currently regarded as first-line treatment in Europe and the USA. Fortunately, preferential pricing has now made this drug available for first-line treatment of VL in developing countries. Liposomal amphotericin B is the least harmful option for treatment of VL in pregnancy.

The standard regimen for immunocompetent patients is 3 mg/kg/day on days 1–5, 14 and 21. However, a recent study in India showed that administration of a single infusion (5 mg/kg) or five daily infusions of 1 mg/kg cured 92% of patients. A subsequent study demonstrated a 96% cure among patients treated with a single 20 mg/kg infusion of liposomal amphotericin B, which was comparable to conventional amphotericin B treatment, less toxic and more cost-effective.

Price-subsidized liposomal amphotericin B given as a single infusion is also more cost-effective than treatment with SbV.

In immunocompromised patients with HIV, the dose of liposomal amphotericin B is 4 mg/kg/day on days 1–5 followed by 4 mg/kg/day on days 10, 17, 24, 31 and 38. The relapse rate is high, suggesting that maintenance treatment may be required.

Pentamidine

Pentamidine 4 mg/kg deep i.m. on alternate days for 5–25 weeks has been used as second-line treatment for VL. However, widespread resistance and toxicity (sudden hypotension following injection, acute hypoglycaemia, renal impairment, arrhythmias and irreversible insulin-dependent diabetes in more than 10% of patients treated) have curtailed use. Pentamidine may still have a role in preventing relapses in patients coinfected with HIV. Lower dose combination with allopurinol reduces toxicity.

Miltefosine

Originally developed as an oral antineoplastic agent, miltefosine is the first highly effective oral treatment for VL.

The recommended dose is 2.5 mg/kg up to a maximum daily dose of 150 mg for a total of 28 days. Cure rates of around 95% have been achieved in India and northern Ethiopia in HIV-negative patients, falling to 78% in HIV-coinfected patients. Relapse rates are also higher in HIV-coinfected patients. Nevertheless, daily miltefosine may have a role in preventing relapses in HIV-coinfected patients. Side-effects include gastrointestinal upset but this is rarely severe. However, miltefosine is abortifacient and teratogenic and may also reduce male fertility. Miltefosine has a long half-life (2–3 weeks) and a narrow therapeutic index, thus increasing the opportunity for the development of resistance. Combination treatment should reduce this risk (see below).

Aminosidine (paromomycin)

Aminosidine (paromomycin) at doses in the range 15–20 mg/kg/day i.m. may be used alone for 21 days or synergistically with SbV or pentamidine, thereby allowing a shorter duration of treatment when used in combination therapy with these agents (see below).

Combination treatment

Combination treatment is emerging as a means of mitigating against the development of resistance, shortening treatment duration (and possibly cost) and also as a strategy for reducing the likelihood of relapse. In areas such as Sudan, where SbV is used as first-line treatment, 'short-course' (17 days) combination treatment of sodium stibogluconate plus paromomycin showed better outcomes than standard 30 day sodium stibogluconate monotherapy. Single dose liposomal amphotericin B (AmBisome™) followed by oral miltefosine for 7–14 days has shown >95% cure rates in India. Further trials of different combination treatment regimens are now underway in a variety of locations.

Post-kala-azar dermal leishmaniasis (PKDL)

PKDL occurs following treatment of VL, within 6 months in up to 60% of patients in Sudan and within 2 years in about 10–20% of patients in India and Bangladesh. Elsewhere PKDL is uncommon, except in HIV-coinfected patients. Initially, macules and papules appear around the mouth, which gradually spread over the face and sometimes more widely over the trunk and limbs. Hypopigmented macules may resemble vitiligo. In time, nodules may develop resembling lepromatous leprosy. The papules and nodules in PKDL are usually packed with amastigotes and patients with this condition, which may persist for more than 20 years, may act as an important reservoir of infection particularly in the Indian sub-continent, where active case detection and treatment is a key transmission control measure. PKDL is commoner following VL treatment with SbV and is relatively uncommon among patients treated with miltefosine or amphotericin B. Usually, diagnosis of PKDL is made by identifying *leishmania* amastigotes in skin tissue (biopsy or aspirate). If available, PCR for detection of *leishmania* DNA from the peripheral blood buffy coat may be used to confirm the diagnosis in 40–75% of clinically suspected cases.

In Sudan, 50% of PKDL cases recover spontaneously without specific treatment, whereas in the Indian subcontinent the vast majority require treatment. If no alternative treatment is available, a further prolonged course of SbV may be required to eliminate infection. However, preliminary studies have shown that a 20-day course of liposomal amphoteracin B is more effective than SbV in Sudan and that 60–90 days of miltefosine can achieve a cure rate of over 95% at 1 year follow-up in India.

Prevention

The WHO advocates the following five-pronged approach towards reducing the incidence of leishmaniasis to a level that allows each endemic country to integrate control and surveillance activities, technically and financially, into overall health development activities:

- facilitation of early diagnosis and prompt treatment;
- support for control of sandfly populations through residual insecticide spraying of houses and use of insecticide-impregnated bednets;
- provision of health education and production of training materials;
- detection and containment of epidemics in the early stages; and
- early diagnosis and effective management of leishmania/HIV coinfections.

Eliminating or treating the reservoir host

Most success has been achieved where the domestic dog is the main reservoir, efforts being directed to catching and destroying infected dogs. Dogs with the infection look sick, lose their hair and have an enlarged spleen. France has been very active in controlling by this method. However, infected foxes invariably look healthy and are more difficult to control.

Where humans are the main reservoir, active case finding and treatment may be considered (see below). However, this is only likely to succeed if asymptomatic infections can be detected and treated safely at an acceptable cost.

There is no vaccine currently available for VL, although the future is brighter for the development and use of vaccines in disease prevention and immunotherapy.

Eliminating or avoiding the vector

Sandflies breed in dark moist habitats, such as cracks in masonry, piles of rubble, caves and in any dark protected sites such as holes in termite mounds or in outside latrines. Sandflies have a short flight range, seldom being found more than 200 m from their breeding place. They do not fly very high and are unlikely to reach people sleeping on the first floor of a building. They normally bite between dusk and dawn, and are small enough to penetrate the mesh of standard mosquito nets. Insecticide-impregnated nets may be more effective but do not prevent exposure in epidemiological settings where transmission occurs mainly away from the home (e.g. East Africa). Personal use of insect repellents or insecticide-impregnated clothing is generally not an option for people residing in endemic areas.

In India, successful control was achieved during the period when widespread insecticide spraying of houses for malaria control was in use. The resurgence of infection on an epidemic scale has occurred in several areas many years after the spraying programme was abandoned.

In epidemics and localized outbreaks, residual insecticide spraying of houses and the immediate area around the house is the most effective immediate control measure. Sandflies usually succumb to dichlorodiphenyl-trichloroethane (DDT) and their hopping flight pattern renders them particularly vulnerable. DDT is cheaper than other residual insecticides, but is unpopular because of concern about the long-term environmental impact.

In regions where dogs are an important reservoir host (Latin America, Mediterranean basin, central and Southwest Asia) the use of deltamethrin-impregnated dog-collars may be effective in reducing the burden of infection in both domestic dogs and children. (Note – the dogs wear the collars, not the children.) In Iran, the use of deltamethrine-treated dog collars has been shown to reduce the risk of infection in dogs by 54% and in children by 43%. In Brazil, more than 22 000 dogs were collared and followed up over three years. The collars were renewed regularly. The prevalence of infection among dogs fell from 12.5% in 2003 to 3.9% in 2005, and the incidence of human cases fell from 34.1 to 5.4/100 000 over the same period.

Prospects for elimination of VL from the Indian subcontinent

Several factors favour the possibility of VL elimination from the region. The disease is endemic in only a limited number of districts. Humans are the only reservoir. *Phlebotomous argentipes* is the only known vector and is restricted to areas in and around the home. A sensitive and specific rapid diagnostic field test, the rk39 ICT, can be used to improve case detection. The availability of more effective, short course treatment strategies, including cost-subsidized drugs such as liposomal amphoteracin B and miltefosine, are easier to administer and should result in higher cure rates with fewer cases of PKDL. Finally, there is strong political commitment and inter-country collaboration. The elimination initiative has adopted five main strategies:

- Early diagnosis and complete treatment of cases;
- Integrated vector management;
- Effective disease surveillance through passive and active case detection;
- Social mobilization and partnership building at all levels;
- Clinical and operational research as it is needed.

🔑 **SUMMARY**

- Visceral leishmaniasis (VL), or 'kala-azar', is caused by varying species of the *Leishmania donovani* complex. The disease is widely distributed in the tropics.

- Clinically the disease is often subacute or chronic. Fever, hepatosplenomegaly, lymphadenopathy and anaemia are common. Splenomegaly can be very large.

- There is an association between HIV infection and VL. With HIV infection VL can be more severe and clinically atypical.

- Diagnostically, splenic, bone marrow and lymph node aspirates can be very useful.

- Therapeutically, antimonial drugs such as stibogluconate remain effective, though side effects are problematic. In areas where resistance is a problem, amphotericin B and miltefosine can be useful.

💻 Visit **www.lecturenoteseries.com/tropicalmed** to test yourself on this chapter using interactive MCQs.

📖 FURTHER READING

Alvar J, Aparicio P, Aseffa A, *et al.* (2008) The relationship between leishmaniasis and AIDS: the second 10 years. *Clin Microbiol Rev* **21**: 334–59. [Excellent review of emerging clinical and epidemiological issues related to HIV and leishmaniasis coinfection.]

Davies CR, Kaye P, Croft SL, Sundar S (2003) Leishmaniasis: new approaches to disease control. *BMJ* **326**: 377–82. [Updated review of key aspects of control, and annotated educational resource list.]

Lawn SD (2007) Immune reconstitution disease associated with parasitic infections following initiation of antiretroviral therapy. *Curr Opin Infect Dis* **20**: 482–8. [Interesting review describing 24 published cases of IRIS associated with parasitic infections.]

Mondal D, Khan MDM (2011) Recent advances in post-kala-azar dermal leishmaniasis. *Curr Opin Infect Dis* **24**: 418–22. [Focuses on recent advances in diagnosis, new insights into pathogenesis and case management of PKDL.]

Mondal S, Bhattacharya P, Ali N (2010) Current diagnosis and treatment of visceral leishmaniasis. *Expert Rev Anti Infect Ther* **8**(8): 919–44. [State of the art review including > 200 references.]

Murray HW, Berman JD, Davies CR, Saravia NG (2005) Advances in leishmaniasis. *Lancet* **366**: 1561–77. [Comprehensive review that includes some excellent illustrations.]

van Griensven J, Balasegaram M, Meheus F, Alvar J, Lynen L, Boelaert M (2010) Combination therapy for visceral leishmaniasis. *Lancet Infect Dis* **10**: 184–94. [Recent review of evidence and potential for combination therapy.]

World Health Organization (2010) *Control of the Leishmaniases: Report of a Meeting of the WHO Expert Committee on the Control of Leishmaniases,* Geneva: WHO. [This new edition of the WHO reference standard reflects the latest scientific and other relevant developments in the field of leishmaniasis.]

11

Cutaneous leishmaniasis

Tim O'Dempsey
Liverpool School of Tropical Medicine

Cutaneous leishmaniasis is among the most important causes of chronic ulcerating skin lesions in the world. The organisms in the host tissues are mainly found in reticuloendothelial cells in the skin, where, as amastigotes, they multiply by simple fission. Microscopically, they cannot be distinguished from *Leishmania donovani*. The parasites, life-cycles and vectors are similar to those described for species causing visceral leishmaniasis (VL).

The clinical spectrum of disease may be classified as follows:

- cutaneous leishmaniasis (CL);
- diffuse cutaneous leishmaniasis (DCL);
- leishmaniasis recidivans (LR);
- mucocutaneous leishmaniasis (MCL), also known as mucosal leishmaniasis (ML).

It is common to attach the terms Old World or New World depending on the region in which the infection is acquired. The following species of Leishmania are commonly implicated:

- Old World: *L. tropica*, *L. major* and *L. aethiopica*; also *L. infantum* and *L. donovani*;
- New World: *L. mexicana* species complex (especially *L. mexicana*, *L. amazonensis* and *L. venezuelensis*) and *Viannia* subgenus (most notably *L.* [*V.*] *braziliensis*, *L* [*V.*] *panamensis*, *L.* [*V.*] *guyanensis* and *L.* [*V.*] *peruviana*); also *L. major*-like organisms and *L. chagasi*.

Ninety per cent of all cases of CL occur in Afghanistan, Algeria, Brazil, Pakistan, Peru, Saudi Arabia, and Syria, with 1–1.5 million new cases reported annually worldwide. Ninety per cent of all cases of ML occur in Bolivia, Brazil and Peru.

Clinical features

Cutaneous leishmaniasis (CL)

There is a variable incubation period, usually several weeks. Infections may be subclinical or clinical. Usually a papule develops at the site of infection, becomes a nodule and subsequently forms an ulcer with a central depression and raised indurated border. This may enlarge to a diameter of several centimetres and persist for months or years before eventually healing, leaving an atrophic scar. Healing time varies with different species, for example from 2–6 months (*L. major*), 3–9 months (*L. mexicana*), and 6–15 months (*L. tropica, L. braziliensis, L. panamensis*).

Some lesions do not ulcerate but persist as nodules or plaques (Figs 11.1 and 11.2). For differential diagnosis see Chapter 48.

Some patients have more than one primary lesion or may develop satellite lesions. A sporotrichoid-like nodular lymphangitis may occur (common with *L.* [*V.*] *panamensis* and *L.* [*V.*] *guyanensis*) in which there is thickening of the lymphatic channels draining the primary lesion with nodules at intervals along the path. Regional adenopathy may occur and is sometimes bubonic in nature with *L.* (*V.*) *braziliensis*. Lesion pruritus or pain, and secondary bacterial infection may also occur. Koebner phenomena and 'seeding' at sites of skin trauma, including tattoos, also may occur.

Diffuse cutaneous leishmaniasis (DCL)

The following species are usually involved:

- Old World: *L. aethiopica* – Ethiopia, Kenya;
- New World: *L. mexicana, L. amazonensis, L. venezuelensis.*

Tropical Medicine Lecture Notes, Seventh edition. Edited by Nick Beeching and Geoff Gill. © 2014 John Wiley & Sons, Ltd. Published 2014 by John Wiley & Sons, Ltd.

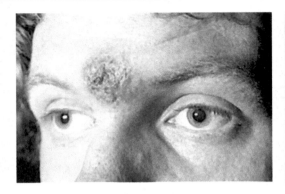

Figure 11.1 *L. tropica* lesion (Saudi Arabia).

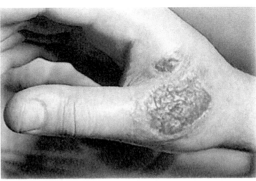

Figure 11.2 Cutaneous leishmaniasis lesion due to *L. mexicana* (Brazil).

DCL closely resembles lepromatous leprosy. A single lesion gives rise to multiple diffuse soft fleshy nodules or plaques containing enormous numbers of amastigotes. Ulceration is unusual, probably because of deficient cell-mediated immunity. There may be extensive depigmentation in the areas of affected skin, increasing the resemblance to leprosy. DCL is unlikely to resolve spontaneously and is difficult to treat.

Leishmaniasis recidivans (LR)

This relatively rare form is most frequently seen in Iran and Iraq and is also known as lupoid leishmaniasis. LR resembles lupus vulgaris and usually affects the face, sometimes invading mucous membranes. Lesions wax and wane, persisting for 20–40 years, with scarring as they heal. The combination of scarring and signs of active inflammation is characteristic of the condition.

Mucosal leishmaniasis (ML)

Also known as espundia, ML is a dreaded complication of New World CL. Most cases are caused by the *Viannia* subgenus, particularly *L. (V.) braziliensis*, *L. (V.) panamensis* and *L. (V.) guyanensis*. The onset is usually a few years after resolution of the original cutaneous lesion, but may occur while the primary lesion is still present or decades later. Haematogenous and lymphatic dispersal results in spread of amastigotes from the skin to the naso-oropharyngeal mucosa. Patients may initially complain of symptoms of chronic nasal congestion. The first perceptible lesion is often a nodule adjacent to the nostril. Granulomatous destructive lesions with chronic ulceration follow and secondary bacterial infection. After many years, the nasal septum, other nasal cartilaginous structures and palate may be destroyed, leaving a grotesque cavity in the centre of the face. Rarely, destructive lesions may occur in the urinogenital region. In endemic areas, the risk of mucosal disease following a primary cutaneous lesion is around 1–10% within 1–5 years, although there are reports of incidence rates of up to 25%.

The differential diagnosis of ML includes:

- histoplasmosis;
- leprosy;
- midline granuloma;
- neoplasms;
- paracoccidiodomycosis;
- rhinoscleroma;
- sarcoidosis ;
- syphilis;
- tertiary yaws

Cutaneous leishmaniasis and HIV coinfection

A wide range of clinical presentations, sometimes occurring simultaneously, may occur in HIV-coinfected patients, including papular, nodular, lepromatous, infiltrative, ulcerative, diffuse, psoriaform, cheloid, histioid and Kaposi's sarcoma-like lesions. Visceralization of cutaneous species may also occur. Similarly, VL species may present with cutaneous manifestations. Response to treatment may be problematic, with delayed healing and increased likelihood of recurrences. Furthermore, CL may become clinically evident or deteriorate with improved immunocompetence following commencement of cART.

Investigations

Cutaneous and diffuse cutaneous leishmaniasis

Parasitological diagnosis is usually made by biopsy of the edge of the ulcer or other lesion. The specimen obtained can be divided in portions for:

1 an impression smear (touch preparation) on a microscope slide that is then fixed with methanol and stained with Giemsa;
2 histopathology (less sensitive than impression smear);
3 culture on Novy, MacNeal and Nicolle's (NNN) medium;
4 polymerase chain reaction (PCR). PCR is particularly useful as a relatively rapid way of distinguishing *Viannia* from non-*Viannia* subgenus infections.

Other techniques that are sometimes used include needle aspirates and dermal scrapings.

Culture, isoenzyme and DNA sequencing techniques are available only in specialist centres. A new microcapillary culture technique using a monophasic medium is also used in some centres.

Leishmaniasis recidivans and mucosal leishmaniasis

Organisms are usually scanty in affected tissue, therefore PCR and culture are preferred for diagnosis. Serology is generally unhelpful but is more likely to be positive in ML than in CL. The main use of serodiagnostic methods is when CL is suspected clinically but direct diagnostic methods have failed. In endemic areas a high proportion of the population may be seropositive. False-positive results may occur with lepromatous leprosy (LL), so the distinction between DCL and LL cannot be made reliably by serology. Fortunately, bacilli are always easy to find in LL.

Leishmanin test (Montenegro test)

This is a skin test using a killed promastigote suspension as antigen (area and species specific), injected intradermally and read at 48 h, like the tuberculin test. In endemic areas a high proportion of the population will be leishmanin test-positive and may also have healed scars. The test is positive in most cases of established CL and ML. It may be negative in some cases of CL caused by *L. aethiopica* and is usually negative in DCL. A strongly positive test may be useful in diagnosing LR cases, because the routine histology from these lesions is often indistinguishable from lupus vulgaris (cutaneous tuberculosis). The test is negative in active VL but may become positive after successful treatment.

With advances in other techniques for diagnosis, the leishmanin test is seldom used in clinical practice today.

Management

Before commencing treatment, the following issues should be considered:

- the number, size, evolution and persistence of lesions;
- the location of lesion(s) (e.g. on the face);
- whether the patient is at risk of ML;
- other features (e.g. the presence of nodular lymphangitis).

Treatment of cutaneous leishmaniasis

Cosmetically unimportant lesions caused by non-destructive and non-metastasizing species usually heal spontaneously and therefore may not require active treatment.

Local, topical and physical treatments

Various local, physical and topical therapies are sometimes used, including:

- heat treatment or cryotherapy;
- topical amphotericin B (*L. major*);
- intralesional antimony therapy;
- paromomycin ointment (available in Israel).

Treatment with paromomycin may result initially in increased ulceration, so it is best avoided for ulcers on the face.

Oral treatment

The following oral agents can be used for treating relatively benign cosmetically unimportant lesions.

- *Ketoconazole* – modest activity against *L. mexicana*, *L.* (*V.*) *panamensis* and possibly *L. major.*
- *Itraconazole* – better tolerated than ketoconazole but may be less effective against the *Viannia* subgenus and *L. major.*

- *Fluconazole* – variable effectiveness against *L. major*. High dose fluconazole has been reported to be effective against *L. [V.] braziliensis* in a limited number of patients in Brazil. Treatment with 5 mg/kg/day achieved a cure rate of 75% with a mean time to healing of 7.5 weeks, whereas 8 mg/kg/day achieved 100% cure within 4–5 weeks.
- *Miltefosine* – currently being investigated for treatment of New and Old World CL and for PKDL. A number of small clinical trials have been undertaken in a variety of locations. Several trials show that miltefosine cure rate is low for certain *Leishmania* species and inferior to SbV. However, two recent trials showed higher miltefosine cure rates compared with SbV for *L. braziliensis* and *L. guyanensis*. Among Bolivian patients with ML, a small non-randomized controlled trial indicated that miltefosine was superior to amphotericin B. Miltefosine has also been used successfully in treatment of individual refractory DCL and immunosuppressed patients.

Parenteral treatment

Pentavalent antimony therapy (SbV) (i.v. or i.m.) is probably still the best option if optimal effectiveness is important.

Studies on *L panamensis* in Colombia, *L. braziliensis* in Guatemala, and *L tropica* in the USA, showed no significant difference in outcome when treatment duration with SbV 20 mg/kg/day was reduced from 20 days to 10 days.

Short-course pentamidine has been shown to be effective in Colombia where disease is predominantly caused by the *Viannia* subgenus.

Old World DCL is treated with a combination of SbV and paromomycin. Response may be poor in some parts of Ethiopia and pentamidine is used as an alternative; however, about 10% of patients are left with diabetes mellitus following treatment. New World DCL is treated with SbV.

LR may be treated with parenteral or intralesional SbV, or may respond to heat treatment.

ML treatment is of greater importance. Adequate systemic treatment of cutaneous lesions is assumed (but not proven) to decrease the risk of mucosal disease. ML is harder to treat than cutaneous lesions and becomes increasingly so as it progresses. Currently, the best treatment options are SbV 20 mg/kg i.v./i.m. for 28 days, achieving cure rates of about 75% for mild disease and 10–63% for more advanced disease. Possible alternatives to SbV are miltefosine or amphotericin B. Concomitant corticosteroids are indicated if respiratory compromise develops. A combination of oral pentoxyfylline (a TNF-α inhibitor) plus SbV for 30 days reduced the relapse rate and accelerated cure in comparison with SbV alone among patients with refractory ML in Brazil.

Choosing the most appropriate treatment for cutaneous leishmaniasis

The key questions are 'who needs parenteral treatment' and 'for how long'?

It is useful to classify clinical presentations as 'simple' or 'complex' based on the following criteria.

'Complex' : > 2–3 lesions; > 40 mm diameter; lymphatic/lymph node spread; cosmetic problems; functional problems; failure to respond to treatment as a 'simple' lesion.

Patients with complex lesions and all patients with *Viannia* subgenus species or unidentified New World species should be offered parenteral sodium stibogluconate (SSG) as first-line management (Table 11.1).

Table 11.1 **Summary of recommended first-line treatment for cutaneous leishmaniasis**

Species	Clinical presentation	
	'Simple'	'Complex'
Old World species	Intralesional, topical, physical or appropriate oral treatment.	SSG 20 mg/kg i.v. for 10–20 days
L. mexicana complex	As above	SSG 20 mg/kg i.v. for 20 days (28 days for patients with ML)
L. Viannia subgenus or unidentified New World species	SSG 20 mg/kg i.v. for 10–20 days	

Note: Clinical presentation 'Complex' if > 2–3 lesions; > 40 mm diameter; lymphatic/lymph node spread; cosmetic problems; functional problems; failure to respond to treatment as a 'simple' lesion.
SSG = sodium stibogluconate

Prevention

In general, the principles of prevention and control are the same as for VL. In the Middle East it is customary for mothers to expose cosmetically unimportant areas of their infants to sandfly bites or to deliberately inoculate them with infected material to render the child immune to that species. The development of effective vaccines is proving difficult. A vaccine using live attenuated *L. major* promastigotes has been produced which appears to be effective although its use carries a small risk of precipitating an aggressive lesion or the development of LR. There has also been some interesting work recently on the development of vaccines against sandfly saliva.

 SUMMARY

- Cutaneous leishmaniasis (CL) is a globally common cause of chronic skin ulceration.
- CL is caused by a variety of Leishmania species, and is often termed 'Old World' or 'New World', depending on geographical origin.
- Various clinical types occur, including localized, diffuse and mucocutaneous. Atypical forms can occur with HIV infection.
- Diagnosis is by smear or biopsy. Polymerase chain reaction (PCR) can be helpful.
- Treatment is complex and depends on the clinical type and infecting organism.
- Stibogluconate remains highly effective though toxic, and newer drug options are evolving.

 Visit www.lecturenoteseries.com/tropicalmed **to test yourself on this chapter using interactive MCQs.**

 FURTHER READING

Alvar J, Aparicio P, Aseffa A, *et al.* (2008) The relationship between leishmaniasis and AIDS: the second 10 years. *Clin Microbiol Rev* **21**: 334–59. [Excellent review of emerging clinical and epidemiological issues related to HIV and leishmaniasis coinfection.]

Bailey M, Lockwood D (2008) Cutaneous leishmaniasis. *Clin Dermatol* **25**: 203–11. [Excellent recent review.]

Murray HW, Berman JD, Davies CR, Saravia NG (2005) Advances in leishmaniasis. *Lancet* **366**: 1561–77. [Comprehensive review that includes some excellent illustrations.]

Reithinger R, Dujardin JC, Louzir H, Pirmez C, Alexander B, Brooker S (2007) Cutaneous leishmaniasis. *Lancet Infect Dis* **7**: 581–96. [Excellent critical review of the epidemiology, clinical pathology, diagnosis, treatment, prevention, and control of cutaneous leishmaniasis.]

World Health Organization (2010) *Control of the Leishmaniases: Report of a Meeting of the WHO Expert Committee on the Control of Leishmaniases*. Geneva: WHO. [This new edition of the WHO reference standard reflects the latest scientific and other relevant developments in the field of leishmaniasis.]

12

Tuberculosis

Bertie Squire
Liverpool School of Tropical Medicine

On 24 March 1882, Robert Koch demonstrated *Mycobacterium tuberculosis* to be the cause of the disease tuberculosis (TB). Since then, advances in human understanding of the disease have been major catalysts in the development of modern medicine. In 1993 the World Health Organization (WHO) declared tuberculosis an international emergency – an unprecedented step – international interest and funding for tuberculosis control has increased since that time, leading to the establishment, in 2000, of the Global Partnership to Stop-TB (STOP TB). As we approach the third decade of the 21st century, knowledge of the full genome of *M. tuberculosis* has led to the development of a fully automated molecular test which has unprecedented sensitivity and sensitivity for pulmonary disease. The global number of new TB cases per capita has been falling slowly since 2002, such that there were an estimated 8.8 million new cases in 2010. Although the absolute number of new TB cases has been falling since 2006, most of the world's 1.1 million TB deaths per year occur among poor populations in the developing countries of the tropics. The main clinical and public health focus of this chapter is on TB as it manifests in adulthood, but TB in childhood is an important topic which is now attracting deserved attention after many years of neglect.

Microbiology

Of the mycobacteria, *M. tuberculosis*, *M. bovis* and *M. africanum* are now known to be genetically very similar, have the highest pathogenicity, and are together referred to as the *M. tuberculosis* (MTB) complex. They are non-spore-forming, non-motile bacilli with a large cell wall content of high-molecular-weight lipids. They are aerobic but exhibit complex metabolic responses in their latent state. Growth is slow, the generation time being 15–20 h, as compared to well under 1 h for most common bacterial pathogens. Visible growth of yellow colonies in culture, on egg-based solid Löwenstein–Jensen medium, takes between 4 and 12 weeks. Growth in liquid media is faster (see below).

Bacilli of the MTB complex are referred to as tubercle bacilli, acid-fast bacilli (AFB) or acid- and alcohol-fast bacilli (AAFB) on the basis of the ability of their lipid-rich cell walls to retain the red carbol-fuchsin stain in the presence of acid and alcohol during the Ziehl–Neelsen (ZN) staining process. Under oil-immersion light microscopy the stained bacilli appear as slightly bent rods, 2–4 mm long and 0.2–0.5 mm wide. Distinguishing between the three species is impossible by microscopy and difficult by culture. Furthermore, clinical presentations of disease caused by the bacilli are similar. Therefore it is not possible to be precise about the relative contributions of the three species to the sum total of human tuberculosis disease. However, *M. tuberculosis* (MTB) is globally the most prevalent, and widely recognized to cause most of the global burden of disease, particularly in the tropics. This chapter therefore focuses on MTB and not the other less pathogenic mycobacteria, which are often referred to as mycobacteria other than tuberculosis (MOTT). Examples of MOTT include the *M. avium* complex, *M. marinum* and *M. gordonae*.

Epidemiology

Magnitude of the problem

It is estimated that one-third of the global human population is infected with MTB and the microbe is thought to cause one-quarter of avoidable adult

Tropical Medicine Lecture Notes, Seventh edition. Edited by Nick Beeching and Geoff Gill. © 2014 John Wiley & Sons, Ltd. Published 2014 by John Wiley & Sons, Ltd.

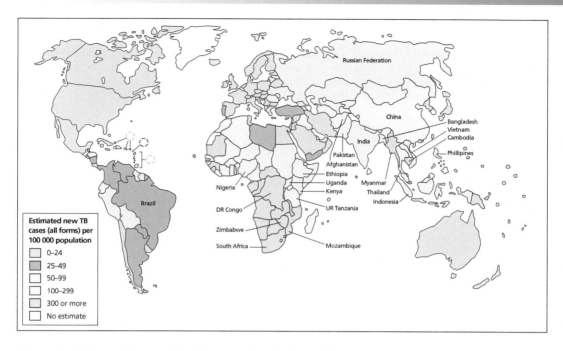

Figure 12.1 Estimated tuberculosis incidence rates (2011). *Source: Global Tuberculosis Control: WHO Report.* Geneva: WHO.

deaths in developing countries. The geographical distribution of TB is shown in Figure 12.1.

Transmission

Although transmission of *M. bovis* from cattle to humans may be important in some parts of the tropics, humans are the only reservoir of MTB infection and transmission is only possible from individuals with disease. It occurs by droplet nuclei; infectious particles of respiratory secretions aerosolized by coughing, sneezing or talking, which are sufficiently small (around 10 μm, drying to less than 5 μm diameter while airborne) to remain suspended in the air for long periods and reach the terminal air spaces if inhaled.

Infection and immunity

Once MTB droplet nuclei reach alveolar level within the lungs, the bacilli are taken up by phagocytosis into air-space macrophages. Within these cells they are processed into phagosomes which fail to acidify. In this way the bacilli avoid intracellular killing and may survive and multiply for long periods of time. Infected macrophages may therefore carry viable bacilli

in the lymphatics to regional lymph nodes or in the bloodstream to any part of the body.

Both humoral and cell-mediated immune responses are mounted against MTB and are correlated with the development of detectable delayed-type hypersensitivity (DTH) reactions. Rarely, these are manifested clinically in the form of erythema nodosum or phlyctenular conjunctivitis. More usually, DTH to MTB is detected by intradermal injection of mycobacterial tuberculin or purified protein derivatives (PPD) – the basis of the Mantoux, Tine and Heaf tests. The extent of local skin erythema, induration and blistering (in vigorous responses) are measured 48 h after injection in order to grade responses. The release of Interferon Gamma (IFNγ) by T lymphocytes in response to mycobacterial antigens has recently been exploited in the development of Interferon Gamma Release Assays (IGRA) for the detection of MTB infection (see below).

Although individuals clearly vary in their immune capacity to contain or eliminate MTB, it must be emphasized that immune responses to MTB – however generated – are generally not protective against further infection. A common misconception is that PPD skin responsiveness is correlated with the effectiveness of immunity to MTB. Although T-cell release of IFNγ is now recognized as crucial, it remains unclear what combination of cell-mediated and humoral responses to MTB is most important in conferring protective immunity, and those components responsible for the DTH responses detected by PPD skin tests are not necessarily protective.

Progression to disease

In the usual course of events, somewhere between 5% and 10% of people will develop active TB after MTB infection. About 3% develop disease within the first year with the remainder developing disease with ever-diminishing frequency thereafter. More than 90% of MTB infections, therefore, do not result in disease within a normal human lifespan.

The clinical manifestation of TB among those who develop active disease depends on two things: the state of the immune system and the location of the bulk of the MTB multiplication. In those cases where disease occurs soon after primary infection, the bacilli multiply and spread in the context of a naïve immune system. Primary forms of disease therefore occur at common thoracic sites of initial multiplication; hence pleurisy extending from an alveolar focus and cavitation in hilar lymph nodes. They also tend to disseminate to multiple sites including the central nervous system; hence tuberculous meningitis and 'miliary' tuberculosis. In disseminated disease, mini-granulomata (tubercles) develop around small numbers of bacilli which are widely distributed within tissues.

In those cases where disease occurs a long time after primary infection, either as reactivation of latent infection or as a result of reinfection with a new strain of MTB, the bacilli multiply in the context of a sensitized immune system. The associated DTH responses tend to lead to tissue destruction at the site of multiplication; hence cavitating caseous lesions, in which large numbers of multiplying bacilli are contained by an encircling rim of giant cells and granulomata – the hallmark of tuberculous pathology. These 'postprimary' lesions are most commonly in the apices of the lungs, the theory being that this location provides the most conducive combination of ventilation and perfusion for long-term latency. They may also occur at any site to which bacilli were seeded during initial multiplication around the time of primary infection.

Given sufficient time, postprimary-type disease in the lungs is likely to result in communication between the cavitating pathology and an airway. MTB bacilli can then be aerosolized in droplet nuclei

and expelled into the atmosphere when the affected individual coughs, sneezes or talks. Patients with cavitating lung disease are therefore the main sources of new MTB infections. The processes of infection and progression to disease are illustrated in Figure 12.2.

Risk factors for infection and disease

Risk factors for MTB infection fall into two broad categories:

1 those which put people in a setting in which MTB-containing droplet nuclei accumulate in the atmosphere;
2 those decreasing the ability of alveolar macrophages to incapacitate MTB once taken up.

The first category includes prolonged contact with a person or people with pulmonary TB (especially cavitating disease) and the environmental features associated with poverty. Overcrowded and poorly ventilated living and working conditions are clearly ideal for MTB transmission. As MTB is susceptible to killing on exposure to ultraviolet light, dark and humid conditions such as may be found in mines and prisons also favour transmission. The second category includes anything capable of compromising alveolar macrophage killing of MTB, such as corticosteroid therapy and HIV infection.

Risk factors for disease have in common their ability to impair cell-mediated immunity, particularly those functions dependent on T cells. Examples include HIV infection, malnutrition (particularly vitamin D deficiency) and corticosteroid therapy.

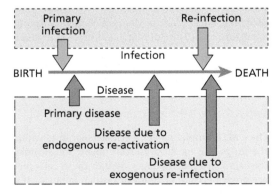

Figure 12.2 The processes of TB infection and progression to disease.

Effect of HIV on the epidemiology of TB

The superimposition of HIV infection in people with pre-existing MTB infection increases the risk of developing tuberculosis from 5–10% over a lifetime to around 15% per year. In addition to this increased risk of reactivation disease, HIV-infected people are at increased risk of acquiring new MTB infections which may also progress to disease. In those parts of the world where the prevalence of MTB infection and HIV infection overlap geographically, there has been an explosive increase in the number of TB cases, which has increased the annual risk of MTB infection for both HIV-infected and HIV-uninfected people. Both HIV infection and MTB infection tend to affect adolescents and adults in the middle decades of life; their most economically productive years. In many developing countries in the tropics, particularly in sub-Saharan Africa, these two devastating infections overlap both geographically and socially and the resultant impact on livelihoods has been appalling. TB not only arises in conditions of poverty, it is itself a poverty-generating illness.

Clinical features

Pulmonary vs. extrapulmonary disease

Pulmonary features predominate in around 85% of all TB disease presentations. Although in most instances pulmonary disease will be the only obvious pathology, it may be associated with tuberculous pathology in other organ systems. Parenchymal lung disease may extend and include pericardial disease or regional lymph node cavitation. Conversely, both pericardial tuberculosis and tuberculous lymphadenitis may occur in the absence of any concurrent pulmonary pathology and would then be classified as extrapulmonary disease. Counterintuitively, two forms of intrathoracic TB pathology are classified as extrapulmonary tuberculosis when they occur in the absence of concurrent parenchymal lung disease: mediastinal lymphadenopathy and pleurisy. This serves to emphasize that any clinical presentation in which pulmonary parenchymal disease is present is classified as pulmonary, and only patients with pulmonary disease, not extrapulmonary disease, are capable of transmitting MTB to others.

Among extrapulmonary presentations, lymphadenitis (Fig. 12.3) and pleurisy are the most common,

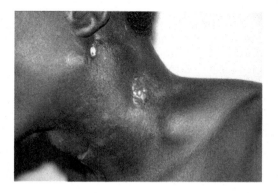

Figure 12.3 Cervical tubercuolous lymphadenitis, with ulceration of some of the nodes.

each accounting for approximately 25% of the total. Genitourinary TB is next at around 15%, followed by miliary and bone TB at around 10%. Meningeal and peritoneal TB each account for less than 5% of extrapulmonary TB disease.

Systemic symptoms

The majority of TB presentations, whether pulmonary or extrapulmonary, are insidious in onset. Varying combinations of the chronic constitutional symptoms of fevers, night sweats, weight loss and malaise (perhaps secondary to an associated anaemia of chronic disease) are common but are neither universal nor specific indicators of TB.

Symptoms of pulmonary TB

Beyond the systemic manifestations, the symptoms and signs of TB depend on the site of the major pathology. As pulmonary disease is the most common form of the disease in adults and adolescents and the priority target for public health intervention, it is the main focus for further clinical description here.

Persistent coughing of insidious onset is easily the most common symptom indicating pulmonary TB. As pulmonary pathology advances, the cough becomes more productive of mucopurulent sputum and chest pains may occur with severe coughing. However, it is important to remember that some patients with early pulmonary disease may not produce much sputum. The sputum may be streaked with blood in about 10% of cases, and this usually indicates that the cavitating pathology has led to local damage of small blood vessels. Frank or catastrophic haemoptysis can occur if the larger blood vessels become involved, but this is rare, occurring in fewer than 1% of cases.

Signs of pulmonary TB

Patients with TB may be wasted. Other than this, the signs are dependent on the site and extent of the underlying pathology. Much is often made of chest signs such as 'amphoric breathing' and consolidation. Certainly, the lung damage can be extensive and often includes signs of volume loss, including tracheal shift. The truth is that most patients with pulmonary disease have very few chest signs and, apart from detecting massive pleural effusions that need draining, the slavish pursuit of chest signs is of little use in guiding clinical management. Patients with advanced pulmonary disease in the tropics may have finger clubbing, a sign that is otherwise not often associated with TB in Europe and North America.

Clinical features of selected forms of extrapulmonary TB

Apart from tuberculous lymphadenitis (Fig. 12.3), which usually presents as a unilateral chain of matted lymph nodes that may occasionally ulcerate and discharge, extrapulmonary TB is notoriously difficult to diagnose. This is because non-specific systemic manifestations predominate in the early stages and these forms of disease have not been amenable to any investigations that come close to the immediacy and specificity of sputum smear microscopy for AFB. As pathology advances, more useful signs such as meningism, bone damage, serous effusions and fistulae may become apparent.

Effect of HIV on clinical presentations of TB

It is important to remember that there are exceptions to the simplified division of tuberculous disease into the 'primary' and 'postprimary' forms presented above. Postprimary disease may manifest itself as disseminated disease such as miliary TB if the immune system is very compromised by an additional factor such as HIV infection. Postprimary disease arising early in HIV infection, before significant immunocompromise is established, is likely to present with cavitating pathology that is indistinguishable from disease arising in HIV-uninfected individuals. However, in the later stages of HIV infection, as underlying immunocompromise becomes more severe, postprimary TB disease becomes more likely to present in a disseminated or non-cavitating form resembling primary disease. This is why extrapulmonary 'primary-like' presentations of TB, such as pleural effusions, lymphadenitis, TB meningitis, miliary TB

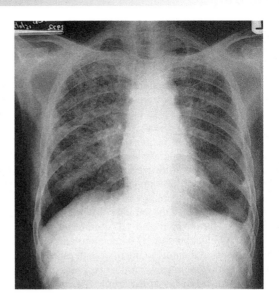

Figure 12.4 Chest X-ray of patient with miliary tuberculosis.

(Fig. 12.4) and non-cavitating pulmonary TB, are more common among HIV-infected patients.

Differential diagnosis

Pulmonary tuberculosis in the tropics has a wide differential diagnosis. Some of these, such as pulmonary paragonimiasis, nocardiosis, actinomycosis, coccidioidomycosis and melioidosis, are defined by their geographical distribution. Others, such as *Pneumocystis jirovecii* pneumonia (PCP) and pulmonary Kaposi's sarcoma (KS), occur in the context of HIV infection. The remainder, including bacterial pneumonias, lung abscess, MOTT, bronchial carcinoma, bronchiectasis, sarcoidosis, Wegener's granulomatosis and cryptogenic fibrosing alveolitis, are more universal.

The differential diagnosis of the most common extrapulmonary forms of TB, lymphadenitis and pleurisy, is mainly from neoplastic processes such as KS, lymphoma and metastatic bronchial carcinoma.

Investigations

Isolation of MTB by culture from clinical specimens is the gold standard for the definitive diagnosis of tuberculosis. However, because of the slow generation time, mycobacterial culture takes between 2 weeks (modern liquid-based culture techniques) and

12 weeks (more universal, solid-based culture techniques). This is clearly too long to be useful in guiding clinical decision-making. In addition, the laboratory infrastructure required to sustain quality-assured culture of mycobacteria is frequently unavailable in the poorer parts of the tropics.

Sputum smear microscopy for tubercle bacilli has therefore been absolutely central to the diagnosis of tuberculosis. Approximately half of all culture-proven cases of pulmonary tuberculosis produce more than the threshold 10 000 organisms per ml of sputum required for detection by microscopy. These smear-positive cases tend to have more cavitating lung disease and are more infectious than smear-negative cases. While smear microscopy is a specific test for pulmonary tuberculosis, it lacks sensitivity, particularly for early disease that has not yet cavitated. Light microscopic examination of ZN stained smears prepared direct from three sputum specimens remains the most universally available diagnostic technique in the tropics. This situation, however, is changing rapidly due to a number of advances. First, the number of specimens required and the timing of their submission has been simplified (see below). Secondly, a systematic review suggests that using auramine-phenol staining and fluorescence microscopy can increase sensitivity by an average of 10% over that achieved by ZN staining and light microscopy, without loss of specificity. Conventional fluorescence microscopes are expensive and costly to run because of the need for frequent halogen bulb changes and a consistent power supply. However, new Light Emitting Diode (LED) fluorescence microscopes can run on batteries and look set to replace light microscopes and can potentially be set up in most microscopy centres. Thirdly, automated nucleic acid amplification tests (NAAT) are now becoming available for use in primary care for the first time. Xpert MTB/RIF® was recently endorsed by the WHO. When compared against mycobacterial culture, it has a sensitivity of nearly 100% for smear-positive cases and around 70% for smear-negative cases. For both categories it has a specificity approaching 100%. In addition, Xpert MTB/RIF® can reliably detect rifampicin resistance as a proxy for multidrug resistant (MDR) TB. Xpert MTB/RIF® can be used on a desk top without laboratory isolation facilities, but is limited by the high cost of the consumables (mainly highly sophisticated cartridges) required and the requirement for an uninterrupted power supply.

The main problem in the diagnosis of tuberculosis lies with patients who have clinical features suggestive of pulmonary TB but whose sputum is negative for AFB or by Xpert MTB/RIF®. Unless there are strong clinical indicators of an alternative diagnosis, the decision on whether or not to treat for tuberculosis lies with chest radiography. Unfortunately, chest X-rays of smear-negative TB cases are notoriously difficult to interpret as the features that are most specific to TB (such as cavitation) are frequently absent. The radiological features of pulmonary TB are also particularly difficult in HIV-infected individuals, among whom an increased proportion of culture-proven cases will have a variety of atypical radiographical manifestations including lower lobe consolidation and patchy infiltrates. Films may even be normal.

PPD skin test positivity is used as a marker of MTB infection and high-grade PPD responses are correlated with the presence of active disease. However, false-positives may occur after exposure to non-pathogenic environmental mycobacteria or BCG vaccination. Similarly, false-negatives are a problem when immune responses are blunted, e.g. by HIV, measles, drugs or severe malnutrition. PPD skin testing is mainly used in the diagnosis of TB in children, in whom most disease is of primary type and only rarely smear-positive. The IGRA techniques mentioned above are more specific and sensitive in detecting latent MTB infections than PPD skin-testing. Nonetheless they still have the following disadvantages which rule them out of routine tropical practice: their place in the diagnosis of disease (rather than infection) remains controversial, they require a level of laboratory functionality that is not found in most tropical laboratories, and they are expensive.

A variety of laboratory tests indicating chronic inflammation, such as raised erythrocyte sedimentation rate and C-reactive protein, or anaemia of chronic disease may help in difficult cases but only have a limited role in the investigation of suspected TB cases in the tropics.

Management

Principles of TB chemotherapy

Tuberculosis treatment aims to:

- cure the patient of TB;
- prevent death from active TB or its late effects;
- prevent relapse of TB;
- decrease transmission of TB to others.

These aims can be achieved while preventing the selection of resistant bacilli in infectious patients through the careful use of modern chemotherapy.

Antibiotic chemotherapy for TB has been built up over the last 40 years around five first-line drugs on the basis of several randomized controlled trials and cohort studies. Four of the drugs are bactericidal (streptomycin, isoniazid, rifampicin and pyrazinamide) while the remaining one is bacteriostatic (ethambutol). Each is referred to by a single capital letter in standard descriptions of different regimens (Table 12.1, which also lists the main side-effects and doses). The bactericidal drugs act preferentially on slightly different populations of organisms (Table 12.2).

During the initial, intensive phase of chemotherapy a minimum of three drugs should be administered concurrently to reduce the more rapidly dividing bacillary load. A minimum of two drugs can be used in the continuation phase, aimed at sterilizing lesions containing fewer bacilli with slower generation times.

All modern drug regimens contain rifampicin, isoniazid and pyrazinamide and as yet there is no strong evidence that regimens shorter than 6 months' duration will reliably cure tuberculosis. Monotherapy for tuberculosis disease should never be given as it will lead to the development of antibiotic resistance.

All of the first-line drugs can be given orally except for streptomycin which requires intramuscular injection and is generally reserved for use in re-treatment regimens (see below).

Table 12.1 First-line antituberculosis drugs, standard abbreviations, dosages and adverse effects

Essential anti-TB drug (abbreviation)	Mode of action	Main adverse effect(s)	Recommended mg/kg dose (range)	
			Daily	3 times per week
Isoniazid (H)	Bactericidal	Peripheral neuropathy Hepatitis	5 (4–6)	10 (8–12)
Rifampicin (R)	Bactericidal	Hepatitis Influenza-like syndrome and thrombocytopenia[†]	10 (8–12)	10 (8–12)
Pyrazinamide (Z)	Bactericidal	Arthralgia Hyperuricaemia leading to gout	25 (20–30)	35 (30–40)
Streptomycin (S)	Bactericidal	VIII cranial nerve damage–vestibular dysfunction Nephrotoxicity	15 (12–18)	15 (12–18)
Ethambutol (E)	Bacteriostatic	Optic neuritis	15 (15–20)	30 (25–35)

[†]More common with intermittent dosage.

Table 12.2 Different populations of *Mycobacterium tuberculosis* and their susceptibility to different drugs

	In cavities	In closed caseous lesions	In macrophages
Relative number of organisms/mL	10^7–10^8	10^2–10^4	10^2–10^4
Multiplication	Active/rapid	Slow/intermittent	Slow
Medium	Neutral/alkaline	Neutral	Acid
Most useful drugs	S R H	R H	Z R H

Abbreviations: H, isoniazid; R, rifampicin; S, streptomycin; Z, pyrazinamide.

Deciding which treatment regimen to use

In principle, it is important to follow national or regional guidelines for chemotherapy. The most important first step in deciding on what treatment regimen to use is to categorize the patient according to (a) whether or not they have previously received one month or more of TB treatment and (b) the outcome of the previous TB treatment (see Table 12.3). It is therefore important to take a careful history about previous treatment before starting a patient on TB chemotherapy.

A 'trial of therapy' as a way of confirming a TB diagnosis is not recommended, unless the situation is life-threatening. In some instances, non-TB infections may respond to the broad-spectrum antibiotic effect of drugs such as streptomycin and rifampicin. There is also an increased risk of chaotic ingestion of drugs and the consequent development of drug resistance.

New patients

A single standard combination of drugs is now recommended for all new TB patients who are presumed, or known, to have drug-susceptible TB (see Table 12.4). Daily dosing is considered optimal, but three times per week dosing is also acceptable under certain conditions (see Table 12.4).

Table 12.3 Categorizing TB patients by outcome of most recent TB treatment

Category (any site of disease)		Bacteriology	Outcome of most recent prior treatment (see Table 12.5)
New		+ or −	Not applicable
Previously treated	**Relapse**	+	Cured
			Treatment completed
	Failure	+	Treatment failed
	Default	+	Defaulted
Transfer in: a patient who has been transferred from another TB register to continue treatment		+ or −	Still on treatment
Other		+ or −	All cases that do not fit the above definitions, such as patients: • for whom it is not known whether they have been previously treated • who were previously treated but with unknown outcome of that previous treatment and/or • who have returned to treatment with smear-negative PTB or bacteriologically-negative EPTB

Table 12.4 WHO-approved antituberculosis regimens for new TB patients

Intensive phase	Continuation phase	Comment
*$2HRZE$	$4HR$	Optimal
$2HRZE$	$4H_3R_3$	Acceptable alternative for any new TB patient receiving directly observed therapy
$2H_3R_3Z_3E_3$	$4H_3R_3$	Acceptable alternative provided that the patient is receiving directly observed therapy and is not living with HIV or in an HIV-prevalent setting
$2HRZE$	$4HRE$	For use in populations with known or suspected high levels of isoniazid resistance

Note: Standard code for TB treatment regimens.
There is a standard code for TB treatment regimens. Each first-line anti-TB drug has an abbreviation (shown in Table 12.1). A regimen consists of two phases. The number before a phase is the duration of that phase in months. A number in subscript (e.g. $_3$) after a letter is the number of doses of that drug per week. If there is no number in subscript after a letter, then treatment with that drug is daily.
*Preferred option.

Previously treated patients

Deciding on which regimen to use for previously treated patient depends on the availability of routine drug sensitivity testing (DST) to guide therapy of individual patients as well as the availability of reliable surveillance data on drug resistance patterns in the population as a whole. For most of the tropics the decision is between the re-treatment regimen 2HRZES/1HRZE/5HRE and an empirical regimen for multidrug resistant (MDR) TB (see below). Table 12.5 provides a guide to this important decision-making.

Multidrug-resistant (MDR) and extremely drug-resistant (XDR) TB

Wherever TB chemotherapy is delivered – especially if delivery is chaotic or disrupted – drug resistance develops and some organisms accumulate resistance to successive drugs. When resistance to both isoniazid and rifampicin are detected *in vitro*, the isolate is categorized as multidrug resistant (MDR). Patients with disease caused by such organisms are unlikely to be cured by drug regimens containing only first-line drugs. Guidelines exist for the programmatic management of such cases using the following principles:

- use at least 4 drugs highly likely to be effective;
- do not use drugs for which resistance crosses over (e.g. kanamycin and amikacin or rifabutin and rifampicin);
- eliminate drugs that are not safe for the patient;
- include drugs from groups 1–5 choosing from the hierarchy based on potency (see Table 12.6);
- be prepared to prevent, monitor and manage adverse events.

The emergence of Extremely Drug Resistant (XDR) TB in recent years is very worrying. This is defined as MDR plus resistance to both (i) any fluoroquinolone and (ii) at least one of the 3 injectable second-line drugs (see Table 12.6). This resistance pattern is virtually untreatable and has been associated with rapid progression to death in HIV-infected patients in South Africa.

The core message for all tropical practitioners is to work hard not to allow drug resistance to develop in the first place, by ensuring clinical practice within a public health framework that facilitates the DOTS strategy (see below).

Monitoring treatment

Patients with smear-positive pulmonary TB should be monitored by sputum smear examination: once at the end of the intensive phase; once during the continuation phase; and once at the end of therapy. It is unnecessary and wasteful of resources to monitor using chest radiography. For patients with smear-negative pulmonary TB and extrapulmonary TB, clinical monitoring is the usual, if somewhat unsatisfactory, way of assessing response to treatment. Routine monitoring by mycobacterial culture of sputum is rarely feasible in developing countries in the tropics.

Table 12.5 **Standard WHO regimens for previously treated patients, depending on the availability of routine drug sensitivity testing (DST) to guide the therapy of individual retreatment patients**

Drug Sensitivity Testing (DST)	Likelihood of multidrug resistance (MDR) [patient category]	
Routinely available for previously treated patients	High (failure)	Medium or low (relapse, default)
Rapid molecular-based method	DST results available in 1–2 days confirm or exclude MDR to guide the choice of regimen	
Conventional method	Empirical MDR regimen *Regimen should be modified once DST results are available*	2HRZES/1HRZE/5HRE *Regimen should be modified once DST results are available*
None	Empirical MDR regimen *Regimen should be modified once DST results or drug resistance surveillance (DRS) data are available*	2HRZES/1HRZE/5HRE for full course of treatment *Regimen should be modified once DST results or DRS data are available*

Table 12.6 Hierarchy of drugs for constructing regimens for drug resistant TB. To be guided, where possible, by the results of microbiological tests for drug sensitivity

Group 1	First-line drugs	Rifampicin, isoniazid, pyrazinamide, ethambutol
Group 2	Injectables	Streptomycin, kanamycin, amikacin, capreomycin, viomycin
Group 3	Fluoroquinolones	Ofloxacin, levofloxacin, moxifloxacin, gatifloxacin
Group 4	Oral bacteriostatic drugs	Pro/ethionamide, cycloserine, terizidone, PAS, thiacetazone
Group 5	Drugs with unclear efficacy	Clofazimine, amoxycillin/clavulanate, clarithromycin, linezolid

At the end of the intensive phase, most patients will have negative sputum smears. Such patients can then start the continuation phase of treatment. If sputum smears remain positive at this stage despite careful adherence to treatment it may indicate that the patient had a particularly heavy initial bacillary load. Rarely, this is an indication of drug-resistant TB. Whatever the reason, the initial phase should be prolonged for a third month. The patient then starts the continuation phase. If smears remain positive after a month of the continuation phase, this constitutes treatment failure and the patient should be restarted on a full course of an appropriate re-treatment regimen (see Table 12.5).

At the end of the treatment course, treatment outcomes are recorded according to one of six categories shown in Table 12.7. This allows for systematic cohort analysis and reporting of cure rates – an important part of TB control (see below).

The question of isolation

Routinely admitting smear-positive TB patients in order to 'isolate' them from the community is not an absolute requirement. In most cases, any onward community transmission of MTB from a smear-positive case will have occurred by the time the diagnosis is established and modern chemotherapy will render such patients non-infectious by the end of the second week of treatment in more than 95% of cases, provided the initial isolate is fully drug sensitive. Protecting others from infection is, on the whole, best achieved by careful chemotherapy rather than physical isolation. Admitting patients to hospital should only be necessary where the patient is severely ill and needs full hospital care and it must be remembered that a TB case is more likely to

Table 12.7 Recording standardized treatment outcomes in smear-positive pulmonary TB

Cured
Patient who is smear-negative at, or 1 month prior to, the completion of treatment and on at least one previous occasion

Treatment completed
Patient who has completed treatment but without smear microscopy proof of cure

Died
Patient who died during treatment, regardless of cause

Failure
Smear-positive patient who remained or became smear-positive again 5 months or later after commencing treatment

Defaulted
Patient whose treatment was interrupted for 2 months or more

Transferred out
Patient who has been transferred to another reporting unit and for whom the treatment outcome is not known

come into contact with individuals who are vulnerable to MTB infection (such as those infected with HIV) in hospital than in the general community. If hospital admission is necessary then this should be to a dedicated well-ventilated TB ward located away from other inpatients. Individual isolation rooms for TB patients are mostly unavailable in countries with high TB incidence. This will need to change with the increasing prevalence of drug resistant TB (see below).

Adjunctive corticosteroid therapy

Many advocate the concurrent use of high-dose corticosteroids with TB treatment for large pleural and pericardial tuberculous effusions. There are some trials indicating that this is helpful for rapid relief of symptoms and for reduction in complication rates but systematic reviews suggest that the evidence is not strong and is certainly not available for HIV-infected patients with TB. The potential disadvantages of corticosteroid therapy, including pharmacokinetic interactions with TB drugs and reactivation of other latent infections (such as strongyloidiasis), should be weighed carefully against potential benefits.

Prevention and public health aspects

The WHO-recommended DOTS strategy is the internationally recognized central approach to TB control. Bacillus Calmette–Guérin (BCG) vaccination and isoniazid preventive therapy are mentioned briefly for completeness.

BCG vaccination

The BCG vaccine has been available since the 1920s and remains a part of the vaccination schedule in most resource-poor countries. It is a live attenuated vaccine which is given intradermally. Unfortunately, there is little evidence that it provides long-lasting protection against the development of pulmonary TB. This appears to be particularly true from the trials conducted in the tropics. Nonetheless, BCG is still included in the Expanded Programme of Immunization, mainly because there is evidence that it protects against disseminated forms of TB in children. It has also been shown to be protective against leprosy and Buruli ulcer.

Isoniazid preventive therapy

The rationale behind preventive therapy is to eradicate latent infection before it develops into active disease. Several placebo-controlled trials in HIV-negative people infected with MTB have shown that daily isoniazid given for 6–12 months substantially reduces the subsequent risk of tuberculosis disease. However, preventive therapy has not been recognized as a cost-effective universal approach to TB control, but instead has been focused on individuals at increased risk of developing active disease. Such individuals are usually identified by skin testing and are either contacts of known smear-positive index cases or people who are occupationally exposed to infection (such as nurses and doctors).

A series of randomized controlled trials have indicated that isoniazid preventive therapy also reduces the risk of subsequent tuberculosis in HIV-infected individuals with latent MTB infection – at least while they continue to take the isoniazid. Significant hurdles in operationalizing this as a TB control measure remain and are discussed in Chapter 13 on HIV infection.

DOTS strategy for TB control

The objectives of TB control are to reduce mortality, morbidity and disease transmission and to prevent the development of drug resistance. The strategy recommended to meet these objectives is to provide standardized short-course chemotherapy under direct observation during the initial phase of treatment to, at least, all identified smear-positive TB cases (the sources of infection). The success of this strategy depends on the implementation of a five-point package.

1 *Direct* smear microscopy for case detection among symptomatic patients self-reporting to health services.
2 *Observation* of therapy for administration of standardized short-course chemotherapy, to ensure adherence.
3 *Treatment* monitoring through a standardized recording and reporting system, allowing continuous assessment of treatment results.
4 *Short course* chemotherapy through a system of regular drug supply of all essential antituberculosis drugs, which should be free to patients at the point of delivery.
5 Government or non-governmental organization (NGO) commitment to ensure a sustained approach to policy and funding.

Tuberculosis control activities should aim to meet two minimum targets: a cure rate of 85% and a case detection rate of 70%. The standardized outcome reporting categories described above make it possible to conduct quarterly cohort analyses of treatment outcomes and hence to report cure rates.

The controversy around direct observation of therapy and adherence

There has been considerable debate about the extent to which direct observation of therapy (DOT) is required to ensure patient adherence to therapy. In its purest form DOT (distinct from the five-point DOTS policy package) dictates that the health system should hold a given patient's TB treatment so that the patient can swallow every dose under the watchful eye of the health care worker – at least for the intensive phase. Many now accept that this system does not always make it easy for patients to adhere to every prescribed dose of treatment. If, for example, patients live far from the health care worker, they will inevitably incur considerable direct and opportunity costs in the daily travel required. Many innovative approaches to DOT have been piloted, including DOT by grocery store keepers in rural areas, workplace DOT and DOT by respected family members. The guiding principle should be to make it as easy as possible for patients to stick with therapy for the full course. The increasing use of three- and four-drug fixed-dose combinations to supplement the existing two-dose combinations of rifampicin and isoniazid should make it easier for patients to adhere (because of reduced pill burden) and harder for drug resistance to emerge.

TB, poverty and the problem of case-detection

Although TB transmission is reduced every time a smear-positive case is cured, overall reductions in prevalence and incidence depend on progress towards and beyond the 70% case detection target and this has proved more problematic than the cure rate target. Estimating the expected number of infectious cases in a given population requires full-scale community-based prevalence surveys or longitudinal cohort studies. These are expensive and time-consuming and most countries have not had the resources to undertake them. Overall, most countries do not yet have reliable data against which to measure their progress towards the case detection target or the means to measure the impact of TB control on overall TB burden of disease. The WHO does, however, produce estimates of TB incidence in its annual Global Report on TB Control. These are based on surveillance of notification trends.

The process of case detection needs close attention, especially if it is to work for those who need it most, i.e. the poor. For the time being, smear microscopy remains central in the DOTS strategy: no patients should start short-course chemotherapy unless they have had their sputum checked. The recommended approach is termed 'passive' case-finding; patients who are prompted by their symptoms to present to health facilities are then encouraged to submit a total of three sputum specimens. The process of sputum submission takes the patient a minimum of 24 h and three visits to the health facility followed by another visit to collect the results and, usually, one further visit to start treatment. These repeat visits may be impossible for particularly disadvantaged patients such as the poor and women in some traditional cultures. It is important therefore to make adequately staffed, quality-assured microscopy facilities as accessible as possible in populations with high TB incidence. In some instances this means establishing extra laboratory services (but no more than one such facility for 100 000 people, as the volume of work is then not sufficient for staff to retain skills). In other instances this means ensuring excellent logistics for transporting specimens and results between microscopy centres and collection sites. The requirement for 3 sputum specimens in order to categorize patients has been relaxed and it is now recognized that 2 specimens are sufficient, provided the quality of the smear microscopy can be assured. A recent large-scale, multicentre randomized trial has also indicated that collecting the first two specimens one hour apart provides sensitivity that is equivalent to that achieved when the specimens are collected on consecutive days. A single specimen tested by Xpert MTB/RIF® may be sufficient. All these steps towards one-stop diagnosis have great benefits for improving access by poor and disadvantaged groups.

There is increasing interest in improving case detection including moves to re-examine the potential role of 'active' case-finding for certain high-risk populations, e.g. in urban slums, prisons, and military barracks. Mass screening of populations by radiography has not been thought to be cost-effective relative to opportunist 'passive' case-finding as described above. However, it, or related approaches (sometimes called intensified case-finding), may be appropriate in some situations.

HIV and TB

One of the challenges facing developing countries in the tropics is the management of TB in populations with high HIV prevalence. HIV-infected patients who develop TB are, on the whole, more difficult to diagnose in a timely fashion. Although their TB seems curable using short-course chemotherapy, they are at increased risk of dying during and after TB therapy. This mortality appears to be multifactorial and includes late initiation of treatment. This may be partly a result of the difficulties of diagnosis but stigma and other factors also contribute. Intercurrent HIV-related complications such as bacterial and fungal infections also contribute to mortality. One randomized controlled trial in West Africa from before the era of antiretroviral therapy (ART) demonstrated that administration of co-trimoxazole prophylaxis concurrently with short-course chemotherapy can help reduce mortality in HIV-infected patients with TB.

TB programmes in the tropics are now linking up with ART programmes to ensure that all TB patients are offered HIV testing and, where possible, access to ART. Pharmacological interactions between TB drugs (notably rifampicin) and ART, cumulative drug toxicity and side-effects, and the risks of inducing immune reconstitution disease (IRD) are the key issues to take into account when combining ART and TB therapy. The most recent trial results advocate starting ART as early as possible after establishing TB therapy, in order to reduce mortality.

Although improving access to ART for all HIV-infected patients is clearly important, it must be emphasized that the most significant gains for HIV-infected patients with TB in the tropics are likely to be found through strengthening core services to improve timely diagnosis and careful clinical care.

The Stop TB Strategy

In recognition that DOTS is necessary, but not sufficient for global TB control, the Stop TB Partnership and WHO recommended a new approach in 2006, the Stop TB Strategy, to replace DOTS and to promote progress towards the TB-related Millennium Development Goals. The DOTS principles remain central to the new strategy which is summarized in Table 12.8, but makes explicit the need to engage more broadly, including approaches to drug resistant TB and TB in the context of HIV as described above.

Table 12.8 The STOP-TB Strategy (2006–2015)

- Pursue high quality DOTS expansion and enhancement
- Address TB-HIV, MDR-TB and other challenges
- Contribute to health system strengthening
- Engage all care providers
- Empower people with TB and communities
- Enable and promote research

Future developments

New diagnostics

The increasing use of automated NAAT for TB in the coming decade is likely to change many aspects of TB control. Early detection of drug resistant cases may mean that conventional monitoring of therapy by smear microscopy needs to be rethought. At the moment Xpert MTB/RIF® is only usable at clinic level where there are substantial resources, but as prices come down and true point-of-care diagnostics become available, the prospects for improved case detection are bright.

New interventions

No new drug regimen looks set to replace the current gold standard 6-month short-course chemotherapy in the short term, but there are suggestions that adding moxifloxacin to first-line regimens will enable shorter treatment regimens to be developed. There is still no obvious replacement for the BCG vaccine.

 SUMMARY

- Control of tuberculosis requires early detection and cure of infectious pulmonary cases.
- Diagnosis of pulmonary cases still relies on quality-assured sputum smear examination. Point of care tests will improve this when they become cheaper for use in resource-poor settings.
- Cure requires systematic administration of at least four drugs in the initial two-month intensive phase of treatment and at least two drugs for the remaining four or more months.
- DOTS remains central to the newer STOP-TB strategy, which advocates broader engagement across health systems.
- Co-location of TB and HIV treatment services in areas where prevalence of both infections is high helps overcome logistic and medical problems of ensuring adequate diagnosis and treatment of both infections.

 Visit www.lecturenoteseries.com/tropicalmed **to test yourself on this chapter using interactive MCQs.**

📖 FURTHER READING

Boehme CC, Nabeta P, Hillemann D, *et al.* (2010) Rapid molecular detection of tuberculosis and rifampin resistance. *New Engl J Med* **363**(11): 1005–15. [The primary reference on Xpert MTB/RIF – the first fully automated nucleic acid amplification test for TB.]

Cuevas LE, Yassin MA, Al-Sonboli N, *et al.* (2011) A multi-country evaluation of LED-fluorescence microscopy for the diagnosis of pulmonary tuberculosis. *PLOS Med* **8**(7): e1001057. doi:10.1371/journal.pmed.1001057. [An article about the use of LED microscopy which also contains useful other references to work in this field.]

Cuevas LE, Yassin MA, Al-Sonboli N, *et al.* (2011) A multi-country non-inferiority cluster randomized trial of frontloaded smear microscopy for the diagnosis of pulmonary tuberculosis *PLOS Med* **8**(7): e1000443. doi:10.1371/journal.pmed.1000443. [The primary reference for the simplified algorithm for sputum collection.]

Harries AD, Zachariah R, Corbett EL, *et al.* (2010) The HIV-associated tuberculosis epidemic – when will we act? *Lancet* **375**: 1906–19. [Excellent summary of differences and similarities of programmatic approach to both infections and their overlap.]

Lawn SD, Zumla AI (2011) Tuberculosis. *Lancet* **378**: 57–72. [Complete review.]

World Health Organization Stop TB Department (2009) *Treatment of Tuberculosis: Guidelines for National TB Programmes*, 4th edn. WHO/HTM/TB/2009.420 and *Guidelines for the Programmatic Management of Drug-resistant Tuberculosis 2011 Update*. WHO/HTM/TB/2011.6 [Available from the World Health Organization, Via Appia, Geneva, Switzerland and downloadable from www.who.int/tb/en a website that includes details of drug therapy as well as a full description of the STOP TB Strategy.]

13

HIV infection and disease in the tropics

Miriam Taegtmeyer,[1] Ralf Weigel[1] and Martin Dedicoat[2]
[1]Liverpool School of Tropical Medicine; [2]Heart of England Foundation Trust

Over 90% of new human immunodeficiency virus (HIV) infections occur in resource-poor countries. Wherever HIV is prevalent, hospitals and clinics are faced with a large and escalating burden of disease. HIV and consequent acquired immune deficiency syndrome (AIDS) is the leading cause of death in sub-Saharan Africa and the sixth biggest killer worldwide, making HIV a major tropical disease.

HIV medicine is a fast evolving field and it is hard for a textbook to be up-to-date. Specific guidelines, current seroprevalence data, epidemiological reviews, summaries, reports and updates are published regularly by the World Health Organization (WHO) and The Joint United Nations Programme on HIV/AIDS (UNAIDS). These documents and many other useful resources are available on their websites. Details of these are in the further reading.

Most countries have National AIDS Control Programmes which provide management protocols relevant to local conditions and resources. These should be followed where available. This chapter gives an overview and focuses on the clinical management of HIV infection in the tropics, where clinical progression of disease is different and available resources may be limited. Its primary target audience is the adult clinician but paediatric topics are touched on as outpatient HIV care in this setting is run in family clinics and the adult clinician may well find themselves giving care to children in this setting.

The viruses

There are two distinct types, HIV-1 and HIV-2, as well as several closely allied species. These two viruses originated in the chimpanzee and sooty mangabey, respectively. It is likely that HIV-1 and HIV-2 infected humans as a result of these primates being hunted for food. This probably happened many times before the social and environmental conditions were present to spark off the HIV epidemic. Theories linking the introduction of HIV into humans via polio vaccination campaigns in Africa in the 1950s have been disproved.

Differences between HIV-1 and HIV-2

There are clear differences between HIV-1 and HIV-2 in genomic structure and in the antibody and clinical response to infection. HIV-1 is rapidly spreading round the world and is universally distributed, whereas HIV-2 is much less common and largely restricted to West Africa. The two viruses are transmitted in the same way but HIV-2 seems less transmissible. Where HIV-1 and HIV-2 coexist, HIV-1 infection is rapidly overtaking HIV-2 in prevalence. Dual infections can occur and there is no evidence that one infection protects against the other. Both viruses cause the same immune defects and are associated with a similar disease. HIV-2 takes several years longer than

Tropical Medicine Lecture Notes, Seventh edition. Edited by Nick Beeching and Geoff Gill. © 2014 John Wiley & Sons, Ltd. Published 2014 by John Wiley & Sons, Ltd.

HIV-1 to cause significant immunosuppression or death, and diseases such as Kaposi's sarcoma do not usually occur in HIV-2 infected individuals. The main importance of HIV-2 in areas where it is prevalent is to ensure that the kits used for blood tests can detect both viruses. The rest of the chapter refers to HIV without differentiating between the two types.

HIV testing and counselling

National policy documents on HIV Testing and Counselling (HTC) are an important starting point for any programme. They define the national testing algorithms and counselling protocols and also set standards for logistics, data management and quality assurance. HIV testing should be offered as widely and to as broad a spectrum of adults as possible in hyperendemic settings, with many countries striving towards universal access. In addition, testing should be offered to all infants and children born to HIV-positive women and to children from families when another sibling or parent has HIV. Patients presenting to health care facilities for any reason in areas of high HIV prevalence should be opportunistically encouraged to test, as early diagnosis will almost certainly reduce the chance of future problems and allow antiretroviral therapy (ART) to be started before the patient becomes critically ill. In concentrated epidemics HTC programmes should focus on the key populations at higher risk of HIV infection. This refers to those most likely to be exposed to HIV or to transmit it. In most settings, men who have sex with men, transgender persons, people who inject drugs, sex workers and their clients, and sero-negative partners in sero-discordant couples are at higher risk of exposure to HIV than other people.

HTC services can be grouped by facility- or community-based services according to location and approach (see Fig. 13.1). Health facilities provide routine (opt-out) testing to pregnant women, inpatients, patients with TB or sexually transmitted infection (STI) among others through provider-initiated testing and counselling (PITC). Counsellors give a brief introduction and focus prevention messages on newly diagnosed HIV-positive individuals through tailored post-test counselling. Community settings are an opportunity for client-initiated voluntary counselling and testing (VCT) and home-based services among others. Here the counsellor offers a more client-focused, couple or family pre-test counselling session with test results accompanied by counselling, referral and linkage to facility-based treatment and care services. There is increasing interest in the scale-up of HIV self-testing in community settings.

What test to use?

Some tests are specific for HIV-1 or HIV-2, whereas others can identify both types. All are highly specific and sensitive if the manufacturer's guidelines are followed correctly; the kits are as accurate as the

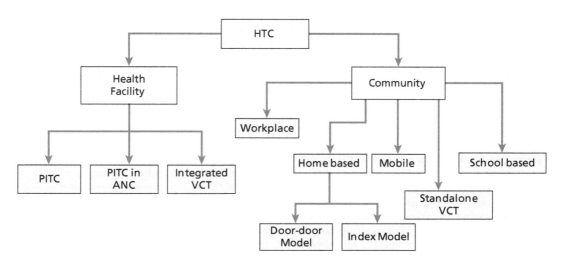

Figure 13.1 HIV Testing and Counselling (HTC) models. ANC, antenatal clinics; PITC, provider-initiated testing and counselling; VCT, voluntary counselling and testing.

laboratories or trained individuals using them. The most widely used tests identify specific anti-HIV antibodies. There is no single test that is suitable for all circumstances.

Lab-based ELISA testing is best suited for regular processing of large numbers of samples so that complete plates can be run.

Rapid ELISA tests can be performed in less sophisticated laboratories by non-laboratory staff. Many are available as single kits and so can be efficiently used when small numbers of samples need testing. Some can be stored safely at room temperature and do not require electricity. With central purchasing, unit costs can be kept quite low.

Western blots are expensive and can be difficult to interpret and standardize. The WHO no longer recommends Western blotting for confirmation, suggesting instead that, if it is necessary, the combination of ELISA with a simple or rapid assay is as reliable and much cheaper.

During acute HIV infection (AHI), also known as the seroconversion or 'window' period, antibody tests may be negative, weakly positive or discordant (where one test is positive and one is negative). If antigen tests that can accurately detect the presence of the p24 antigen are available, these can be used to diagnose AHI. Patients thought to be seroconverting should be followed up within two weeks of the first test for confirmatory testing and enrolment in care and treatment.

National HIV/AIDS programmes have specific algorithms for HIV testing which should be followed. As a minimum, a national algorithm should recommend serial testing, where every reactive result is confirmed with a second test before a positive result is given out. This may be with a second rapid test. In high prevalence countries it may be cost effective to have a parallel testing algorithm, where all positives and all negatives are automatically confirmed, as this saves cost time and effort in recalling all those with reactive results. The national reference laboratory is responsible for external quality assurance of all testing.

Special considerations arise for testing infants and young children. In infants exposed to HIV, the mother's antibodies to HIV may be apparent up to the age of 18 months. Accurate diagnostic testing for infants below this age therefore requires virological testing i.e. by polymerase chain reaction (PCR). If this is unavailable, regular clinical monitoring should take place until antibody tests can be used. Age-appropriate algorithms are essential for undertaking HIV testing in young children and should be aligned with WHO recommendations.

Epidemiology

Surveillance is carried out in order to monitor the extent of HIV infection and disease in a given region or community. In resource-poor settings, often few resources are available for epidemiological monitoring. At the start of the HIV epidemic in Africa, surveillance was only able to show gross changes in mortality and to monitor relatively crudely the arrival and subsequent spread of infection. With experience and institutional strengthening, surveillance is now much more accurate.

Specific at-risk groups include female sex-workers, clients at sexually transmitted infection (STI) clinics, workers such as migrant labourers and long-distance truck drivers, and injecting drug users. It is important to monitor these groups as they have higher prevalence rates. Other groups commonly monitored include pregnant women attending for antenatal care, blood donors, military recruits and newborn infants, although all these groups have inherent biases. Ideally, a representative population-based sample should be tested at regular intervals to accurately determine prevalence and incidence in a particular region. This provides the most valuable information, but population-based testing is difficult and expensive to organize. Disease surveillance is usually carried out in hospital and often concentrates on counting cases of AIDS as defined by the WHO in the provisional clinical case definition for Africa. HIV seroprevalence can be measured in specific groups such as hospital admissions, adults with active TB or pneumonia, or cadavers in the hospital or district mortuary.

Global seroprevalence

With rapid spread of infection (and delays in reporting and analysis) current figures quickly become out of date. By the end of 2010, UNAIDS estimated that 34 million people were living with HIV/AIDS worldwide. In that year around 2.7 million new infections occurred and about 1.8 million people died of HIV/AIDS. Sub-Saharan Africa is the region hardest hit by HIV/AIDS, accounting for 68% of all new infections and 72% of all AIDS deaths. The largest regional increases in prevalence are occurring in Eastern Europe and central Asia block countries, largely driven by injecting drug users. In Latin America the number of deaths has stabilized, partly because of the introduction of low-cost antiretrovirals (ARVs) in some countries such as Brazil. This may act as a model for other areas, although it is sobering to note that in North America and western Europe, where mortality has dropped considerably since the widespread use of antiretroviral therapy, the incidence of new infections has been stable or is increasing.

Transmission

Sexual transmission

In nearly all resource-poor countries the most significant way HIV is transmitted is sexually. While the majority of infection is via the heterosexual route there is increasing recognition of the importance of sex between men as a driver of the epidemic in Africa, Asia and other settings in the tropics. The risk of acquiring HIV after sexual intercourse is hard to quantify. There are numerous factors such as the age and sex of the individual (young women seem more susceptible, perhaps because of an immature genital tract), as well as the factors mentioned below. However, it is thought that the risk is between 0.01% and 0.1% per sexual act, depending on whether sex is vaginal or anal (which confers greater risk) and on whether there is genital trauma as a result of rape. The highest risk group for acquiring HIV are the HIV-negative partners in sero-discordant couples if there are repeated unprotected sexual exposures.

Risk factors

There are several factors that markedly increase the risk of transmission, the most important being other STIs that cause ulceration, chancroid (*Haemophilus ducreyi*) in particular, as well as primary syphilis and genital herpes simplex. STIs that cause inflammation and discharge, such as gonorrhoea, *Chlamydia* and perhaps trichomoniasis also increase the chance of sexual transmission of HIV. In women, anything that disrupts the vagina's normal flora may cause increased risk of transmission. Cervical erosion may also be a risk factor in women.

For a man, being uncircumcised is a factor that increases risk; it certainly increases the risk of acquiring other STIs. Growing evidence from randomized controlled trials in Africa suggests that male circumcision reduces the risk of HIV infection by about 60%.

Vertical transmission

In resource-poor countries, with no intervention, around 25–30% of children born to HIV-infected mothers who breastfeed may themselves become infected. Ten per cent will be infected transplacentally,

5% during delivery and around 10% as a result of breastfeeding, depending on duration.

The single most important factor for mother-to-child transmission of HIV is maternal viral load. Pregnant women with advanced disease and women who acquire HIV during pregnancy or lactation have the highest risk of HIV transmission to their child. Effective treatment of the mother with ART triple therapy can prevent both perinatal and breastfeeding transmission of HIV to infants (see "Prevention of mother-to-child transmission", p. 117).

The benefits of breast milk in reducing infant mortality from diarrhoea and pneumonia outweigh the risk of HIV transmission to the infant. The risk of transmission from breast milk can be reduced by maternal and infant ARVs and also if the introduction of complementary (mixed) feeding is delayed until after the infant has reached six months of age as the infant's gastrointestinal tract matures. Exclusive breast feeding for six months followed by continued breastfeeding and appropriate complementary feeding to meet the child's metabolic needs are recommended.

Transmission by infected blood

Two groups are at particular risk: patients receiving blood transfusions and people who inject drugs and share needles and syringes. Improperly sterilized injection equipment in hospitals and other health facilities is another (unquantifiable) risk.

Screening blood donors for HIV has greatly reduced the chance of HIV transmission through transfusion. Errors can occur in HIV testing and some donors may be in the 'window' phase with an acute infection that is not yet serologically recognizable. This can be a problem in areas of high incidence.

There is a small risk to health care workers exposed to HIV-infected blood. In a typical needlestick injury, where the skin is punctured but the inoculum is small, the risk of acquiring HIV is about 0.3%. This figure is probably much lower if the health worker takes post-exposure prophylaxis (PEP).

Pathogenesis of HIV infection

The main cell population infected by HIV is lymphocytes that carry the CD4 antigen on their surface. This is because the CD4 molecule acts as the receptor to which the virus can initially attach before entering the cell. CD4 lymphocytes are T-helper cells. The key concept in understanding the

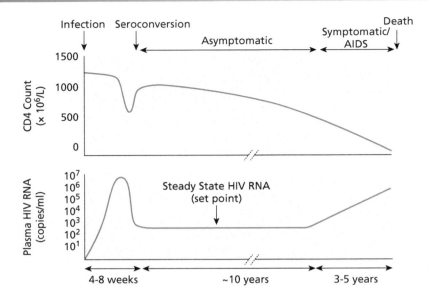

Figure 13.2 Plasma HIV viral load and CD4 cell count in HIV infection.

pathogenesis of HIV infection is the selective loss of function and progressive depletion of T-helper lymphocytes with a corresponding rise in viral load (Fig. 13.2). This is a dynamic process with millions of T cells being made daily and millions being killed daily by HIV. HIV slowly depletes the body's capacity to replace the killed T cells. The speed with which this process occurs can be predicted from the individual's viral load.

T-helper lymphocytes have an important role in the regulation of the cell-mediated immune response and also cooperate with B cells in the production of antibody. Loss of CD4 cells by HIV infection disrupts both cell-mediated and humoral immunity. This is shown by the loss of delayed hypersensitivity to such skin test (recall) antigens as purified protein derivatives (PPD) or tuberculin, and by polyclonal B-cell activation with hypergammaglobulinaemia.

Other cell populations can be infected including macrophages, which may be important reservoirs of HIV outside the blood and may carry HIV to different organs, including the central nervous system (CNS). Cytokine secretion by infected macrophages is aberrant and may have a role in chronic fever, wasting and enteropathy. Active replication of HIV is evident in lymph nodes at all stages of infection and B cells may be non-specifically activated.

Different strains of HIV may differ in virulence in the cell types that are preferentially infected. A single HIV infection can generate many different antigenic variants, which escape the control of the immune system and can be sequestered in sanctuary sites including the CNS.

Progressive immunosuppression

With the progressive destruction of one part of the immune system, a distinct form of immunosuppression develops. In the early stages of HIV, immune function is relatively preserved and the main abnormality is a much higher frequency of infections causing illness. At this stage disease presentations are clinically typical and there is normal response to standard treatment. In the later stages of HIV and in AIDS itself clinical presentations become atypical and there is a diminished response to standard therapy. As with other immune deficiency syndromes, a relatively limited number of organisms are able to exploit the specific immune defect and commonly cause disease in seropositive individuals.

It is unclear why some pathogens are so characteristic of HIV and others not. Different pathogens predominate in the early and later stages of HIV disease. A few conventional pathogens cause clinical disease in the early as well as the later stages of HIV disease. The most common pathogens occurring at any stage of infection are *Mycobacterium tuberculosis*, *Streptococcus pneumoniae* and non-typhi *Salmonella* (NTS). Common pathogens occurring in advanced infection are *Cryptococcus neoformans*, *Toxoplasma gondii*, *Pneumocystis jirovecii*, human herpes virus 8, cytomegalovirus and varicella zoster virus. Disease is caused by acute infection or by reactivation of a dormant or contained organism.

Opportunistic pathogens (relatively avirulent organisms that only usually cause disease in individuals with disrupted immune systems) are only seen in the later stages of HIV disease when much more severe immunosuppression has developed. Immune surveillance is also abnormal and specific cancers can develop such as non-Hodgkin's lymphoma, primary CNS lymphoma and Kaposi's sarcoma. Cervical neoplasia is also more common in HIV-infected women. Some of these unusual infections and malignancies are so characteristic of (late) HIV disease that they can be grouped together and used to define AIDS.

Staging HIV disease

CD4 lymphocytes are found in peripheral blood and the normal CD4 cell count in a seronegative person is about 800 to 1500×10^6/L. The absolute CD4 count is a useful way of staging HIV infection and assessing the immune status of a patient. These tests are becoming increasingly available in resource-poor settings. A count of $<200 \times 10^6$/L indicates severe immunosupression and renders a patient susceptible to a wide range of opportunistic infections, at risk of developing a life-threatening complication of HIV. The WHO currently recommends starting ART when the CD4 count is $\leq 350 \times 10^6$/L as this has increased benefits for a patients by not allowing their immune system to deteriorate to a point where they are very susceptible to infections. Some countries have even higher treatment thresholds than this. The WHO have developed a clinical staging system for HIV disease which can be used to guide clinical management of patients who are known to be HIV positive in the absence of CD4 monitoring. These stages can be used to identify patients in need of specific prophylaxis (for example with co-trimoxazole) and in need of ART. The clinical stages correspond to disease progression and may be summarized for adults and adolescents as:

- *Clinical stage 1*:
  - *Primary HIV infection:* Asymptomatic or seroconversion syndrome
  - Asymptomatic or persistent generalized lymphadenopathy (PGL)
- *Clinical stage 2*:
  - Weight loss <10% of presumed body weight
  - Recurrent respiratory tract infections (including sinusitis and ear infections)
  - Herpes zoster
  - Oral ulcers
  - Seborrhoeic dermatitis
  - Fungal nail infections
  - Angular chelitis
- *Clinical stage 3*:
  - Weight loss of >10% presumed body weight
  - Unexplained diarrhoea for >1 month

- Unexplained fever for >1 month
- Oral candida
- Oral hairy leukoplakia
- Pulmonary tuberculosis
- Severe bacterial infections (including meningitis, empyema, pneumonia, bone and joint sepsis)
- Vulvo-vaginal candidiasis for >1 month
- *Clinical stage 4*:
  - HIV wasting syndrome
  - Pneumocystis pneumonia
  - Cryptosporidiosis or cystoisosporiaisis and diarrhoea for >1 month
  - Chronic herpes simplex infection for > 1 month
  - Oesophageal candidiasis
  - Extrapulmonary tuberculosis
  - Kaposi's sarcoma
  - Cerebral toxoplasmosis
  - HIV encephalopathy
  - CMV infection
  - Cryptococcal infection
  - Atypical mycobacterial infection
  - Lymphoma

Natural history

The following account of illness caused by HIV infection highlights issues commonly encountered in the tropics. In many tropical regions problems of early disease may cause significant morbidity, whereas it is of relatively minor importance in industrialized countries. This is because of the much higher exposure in poor, overcrowded tropical communities to respiratory and diarrhoeal pathogens. There is intense exposure to TB, pneumococci and salmonellae in particular. High mortality occurs in the early stages of HIV disease from clinical problems that are easily treated and cured in centres with better facilities and resources. The time from seroconversion to death in a patient not treated with ART is very variable but the average is around 8–10 years.

Acute seroconversion illness

Initially in acute infection most adults develop a high viraemia and a marked fall in CD4 count; they are highly infectious. During seroconversion, neutralizing antibodies appear and viraemia is greatly reduced. A minority of adults experience an acute seroconversion illness which resembles glandular fever, flu or malaria. A wide range of skin rashes are seen and with transient CD4 depletion oral candidiasis and even opportunistic infections can occur. Because of the relatively non-specific features, the seroconversion illness may not be recognized unless severe. Testing for acute HIV infection may be difficult as antibody tests may remain negative for some weeks in the 'window period'. Fourth generation tests include the antigenic p24 component and may be helpful. Where antibody-only tests are available, patients should be asked to return for retesting at the end of the window period.

The immune activation phase

After seroconversion the CD4 count rapidly rises to near normal and the individual feels well. During this period, originally called the latent phase, active viral replication is taking place in the reticuloendothelial system and viral load assays can be used to quantify this. Lymph node architecture is progressively disrupted and nearly 50% of adults develop persistent generalized lymphadenopathy (PGL). This has no prognostic significance. In addition, bone and cardiovascular health are affected in this immune activation phase.

With time, the CD4 count falls and immunosuppression slowly but inevitably progresses. The rate of progression is extremely variable, but can be predicted from the viral load.

Early HIV disease

In the relatively early stage of HIV infection, when CD4 counts are only moderately reduced, individuals may start to experience specific symptoms of HIV or develop a disease typical of early HIV infection.

The HIV symptoms can be weight loss, night sweats, pruritic skin rash, unexplained fever or chronic diarrhoea. Early HIV disease can be relatively trivial, such as oral candidiasis or oral hairy leukoplakia; painful and disabling but not life-threatening, such as herpes zoster; or life-threatening bacterial or mycobacterial infections. This stage of disease was historically referred to as AIDS-related complex (ARC).

The serious early HIV diseases are pneumococcal infection (pneumonia and sinusitis), TB (pulmonary and lymphatic) and NTS infections (often bacteraemic). In general, clinical presentation is straightforward and the response to therapy good.

Late HIV disease or AIDS

The important AIDS-defining opportunistic infections in most tropical settings are cryptosporidiosis and cystoisosporiaisis in the bowel and

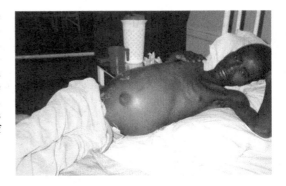

Figure 13.3 Gross ascites due to tuberculous peritonitits in a patient with advanced HIV.

cryptococcosis and toxoplasmosis in the CNS. Pneumocystis pneumonia is more important in Asia and South American settings than in Africa.

Extrapulmonary and disseminated TB (Fig. 13.3), severe bacteremic pneumococcal disease and disseminated salmonellosis are all common. Other Gram-negative septicaemias, including *Escherichia coli*, are increasingly being recognized. Mixed infections are also frequent.

Clinical problems in adults

This section describes the common and important clinical presentations of HIV disease in the tropics and discusses simple investigations, management and treatment. It is assumed that therapy is limited to a range of cheap broad-spectrum antimicrobials, and that antibiotic sensitivity testing is not routinely available. ART and associated problems are discussed separately. A much more comprehensive description of problems and their management is available on the WHO website – known as the Integrated Management of Adult Illness (IMAI).

A number of simple flowcharts and protocols for use by health care workers in primary health care clinics in the management of common HIV-related presentations may be found at the end of this chapter.

Skin conditions

The skin is the largest immunological organ. A careful examination of the skin from 'top to toe' can help in making a diagnosis of HIV infection and in clinical staging. Describing the type of the lesion, location and onset, the relation to medication and presence of itching or pain in combination with findings in other organ systems are helpful in the diagnosis. Most skin conditions are WHO stage 2 defining, but oral and persistent vulvovaginal candida infections (stage 3) qualify for ART as do oesophageal candida and Kaposi's sarcoma (both stage 4).

Papular pruritic dermatosis (PPD) is one of the most common conditions; its origin is unknown. The itchy papules are located on the back, chest, face and extremities. In dark skin, many lesions become hyperpigmented and even nodular and are often excoriated. Topical treatment with a cooling and antiseptic lotion, such as calamine can provide some relief, itching can be additionally treated with topical or systemic antihistamines. Infected lesions warrant a trial of antibiotics. An important differential diagnosis that also presents with an itchy rash is scabies. Burrows may not be visible and the distribution may be more widespread than the classical groin and finger web spaces. Treatment with benzyl benzoate or other topical antiparasitic agent needs repeating after 7 days and symptoms of itch may persist even with effective treatment. Oral ivermectin may also be used.

Fungal infections are also common. They may present as tinea (corporis, pedis, capitis) with pruritic, scaly eruptions, often with a defined edge, slowly increasing in size. If nails are infected it is called onychomycosis. Treatment with a topic antifungal may be successful, but often an oral antifungal such as griseofulvin may be required. Another commonly presenting fungal infection is seborrhoeic dermatitis. This tends to be located on the face, chest and intertriginous areas. Topical miconazole or ketoconazole combined with a topical steroid is often effective.

Viral infections present in the skin more frequently and with greater severity in immunosuppression. Herpes zoster (shingles) as a result of a reactivated varicella zoster infection is often the first sign of HIV infection (WHO stage 2) and is highly predictive of HIV positivity (Fig. 13.4). Scars from shingles (in a typical dermatomal distribution) should prompt the examiner to recommend HIV counselling and testing. Early treatment with systemic aciclovir reduces the severity and duration of the disease and severity of neuralgic pain. Other viral skin infections may also be difficult to treat in HIV infection. For example, genital warts are common and molluscum contagiosum and plane warts appear on the face. Warts are difficult to treat; local treatment with podophyllin might be successful.

Finally, drug reactions often show first on the skin. Involvement of palms, presence of a typical measles-like (morbilliform) and itchy rash or target

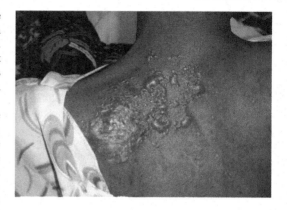

Figure 13.4 Typical dermatomal herpes zoster eruption.

lesions together with a history of drugs known to cause skin toxicity often lead to the diagnosis. Hypersensitivity reactions such as Stevens Johnson syndrome start with additional general and non-specific signs and symptoms, such as fever, nausea and vomiting and are life-threatening. Mucous membranes are involved (mouth, conjunctivae, genitals) and liver function tests are raised. ARVs causing hypersensitivity include nevirapine, abacavir and, to a lesser extent, efavirenz. Sulfur drugs (including co-trimoxazole) are a common cause of a fixed drug eruption. Thiacetazone (for TB) was associated with severe skin reactions. The key to treatment is to stop the drug and not to rechallenge with it. Intensive care may be needed in patients with hypersensitivity.

Acute cough and fever

Acute respiratory infections are amongst the most important clinical problems that occur in HIV-infected adults in the tropics, and bacterial pneumonia should always be considered in those presenting with fever and cough. Of the non-bacterial causes of pneumonia, tuberculosis should also be considered in the differential diagnosis of an acute pneumonia syndrome, with up to 10% of adult cases smear and culture positive for *Mycobacterium tuberculosis* (see Flowchart 13.1).

There is usually a short history of cough, fever and sputum production which may be purulent (or rarely rusty). Other features may be present including pleuritic pain, rigors, shortness of breath, headache (and occasionally meningism) and gastrointestinal symptoms. Many cases will have had a previous episode.

Examination findings form a spectrum, from elevated temperature and minimal chest signs to a prostrate and shocked patient gasping for air. The patient often lies on the side of the pneumonia, is sweaty, taking rapid shallow breaths and coughing frequently. Some patients may be mildly jaundiced, have meningeal irritation and confusion. Chest signs may vary from localized crackles to bronchial breathing as a consequence of dense lobar consolidation. It is important to have a high degree of suspicion as examination findings may be inconclusive.

The commonest aetiological agent is *Streptococcus pneumoniae* but other bacteria including *Haemophilus influenzae*, NTS and other Gram-negative organisms may be isolated. Mixed bacterial and mycobacterial infections are relatively common in HIV disease.

Pneumonia can be confirmed by chest X-ray but this is wasteful if physical signs are definite. Examination of sputum should usually be done, primarily to investigate for TB, but Gram staining may also be undertaken to confirm a bacterial aetiology when abundant pus cells and bacteria will be present. Treatment is the same as for HIV-negative patients: benzylpenicillin 0.6–1.2 g parenterally 6 hourly for 5–7 days for uncomplicated and routine presentations has been the traditional therapy and will be effective against pneumococci even with low levels of penicillin resistance. However, a third generation cefalosporin can be considered when available as it will provide broader antimicrobial coverage, but more importantly requires a reduced dosing frequency, making receipt of the full course of antibiotic more likely in a busy understaffed medical ward. An early switch to oral therapy should be considered as an alternative way of ensuring improved antibiotic delivery. If the patient is cyanosed, oxygen (if available) should be given by face mask; if shocked, intravenous fluids are vital.

The prognosis in HIV-related pneumonia is variable and depends on the underlying condition of the patient; overall, between 5–15% of adult patients hospitalized with pneumonia will die (see Chapter 28). Mortality is higher if patients present late with extensive disease. Poor response to therapy in the first 48 hours of treatment should lead to reconsideration of the aetiological diagnosis and a search for complications. There may be coinfection with TB or a primary tuberculous pneumonia and this should always be considered if a patient does not improve rapidly on antibacterial therapy. Pneumocystis pneumonia should be considered and treatment with high dose co-trimoxazole started particularly when there is supporting radiology. More unusual complications of common infections may need to be considered such as typhoid fever and amoebic liver abscess (although these are not specifically HIV-associated).

Of the major complications, localization of infection within an empyema is relatively common and when detected will need early drainage.

Pneumonia is a WHO stage 3 defining illness which, under current WHO guidelines, would indicate the need to commence antiretroviral therapy or, if therapy is not immediately indicated under national guidelines, the need for a CD4 count to assess eligibility. Therapy should be started as soon as possible after recovery from the pneumonia.

Chronic cough with fever

Chronic respiratory problems are common and highly associated with underlying HIV infection (see Flowchart 13.1). Most patients have pulmonary TB. The main differential diagnosis is recurrent or partly treated bacterial pneumonia, which is common in late-stage patients. Pulmonary Kaposi's sarcoma can occur with skin lesions that are usually obvious although there may only be palatal lesions, which carry a very poor prognosis. It often presents as pleural effusion, which is blood-stained when drained. Histoplasmosis can also present with a chronic cough.

Chronic cough and fever should be easy symptoms to identify; many patients have chest pain, weight loss, night sweats, weakness and haemoptysis; lower-lobe disease is frequent, with widespread crepitations; effusions and disseminated disease are much more common in HIV-infected people. TB frequently recurs so some patients will have had adequate previous therapy and represent with disease within a few months or years, due either to reinfection or reactivation.

The diagnosis of TB is more difficult to confirm by radiology or microscopy when there is underlying HIV infection. Classic upper-lobe cavitatory disease is much less common and lower-lobe consolidation is more frequent. Fewer cases are smear-positive for acid-fast bacilli. TB culture is of little help for initial patient management because the result is so delayed, but it should be performed if possible, especially in patients at high risk of multidrug resistant TB, i.e. patients who have been treated previously for TB, defaulters and certain risk groups such as prisoners. If a TB culture is taken, there must be a system in place for tracing the patient.

Patients may need to be started on TB therapy on clinical suspicion alone – a combination of cough, chest pain and constitutional symptoms has a fairly high predictive value for TB. National treatment guidelines should be followed. Patients with TB/HIV-related disease respond well to short or standard-course therapy, unless they have end-stage overwhelming disseminated or multidrug-resistant TB.

If bacterial pneumonia is suspected, a therapeutic trial of benzylpenicillin or ampicillin should be started. If no response is seen, TB therapy should then be initiated. One of the main challenges in TB therapy is to ensure good compliance and combining TB and ART services may be helpful in this respect. The challenges of managing HIV and TB coinfection are described in more detail below.

Cough and fever in children

The presentation, chronicity and differential diagnosis of cough and fever are different in children from adults. *Pneumocystis jirovecii* pneumonia (PCP) is uncommon in adults in resource-poor settings, particularly in sub-Saharan Africa, but is a major cause of mortality in HIV-exposed infants, especially those under 6 months of age. Pneumocystis pneumonia can be prevented by giving all HIV-exposed infants co-trimoxazole prophylaxis through the first 18 months of life, stopping only if they are confirmed to be HIV-negative. Treatment is with high dose co-trimoxazole. Acute, persistent and recurrent respiratory infections in children may also be caused by *S. pneumoniae, S. aureus,* cytomegalovirus and TB and these should be treated as appropriate. Up to 40% of HIV-infected children who are not taking ART develop a chronic respiratory disease called lymphocytic interstitial pneumonitis (LIP), which may be associated with finger clubbing. The treatment for LIP is ART, with steroids in severe cases. Differentiation between infection, immune reconstitution and LIP can be challenging for the adult physician and specialist advice should be sought.

High fever without focus

Fever is a frequent symptom in HIV-infected adults (see Flowchart 13.2). Careful history and examination can sometimes reveal a focus, especially in the CNS, joints or soft tissue or a cardiac murmur suggesting endocarditis. Pyomyositis is relatively common and requires drainage. Patients may have chronic middle ear disease and sinusitis, which may be the cause of the fever. Patients can have chronic symptoms such as diarrhoea, dry cough or skin lesions and then acutely develop a high swinging fever but no additional focus.

Malaria must always be excluded. Usually a high fever without focus in the tropics in a patient with underlying HIV indicates a bacterial or mycobacterial infection. Again, remember the possibility of amoebic liver abscess.

In HIV-infected patients this clinical presentation is sometimes referred to as an enteric fever-like illness and is very common. NTS as well as *Salmonella typhi* are important. Disseminated TB is increasingly recognized but *M.avium* is less common. Without blood culture, salmonella bacteraemia cannot be reliably diagnosed. In Africa about 10% of all HIV-positive adults presenting to hospital will have NTS bacteraemia and a further 5% may have other Gram-negative sepsis (including *E. coli* and classical *S. typhi*). Disseminated TB may only be diagnosed at postmortem, therefore a high index of suspicion is needed. The next problem is how to differentiate the two, and this cannot be done clinically. Blood cultures can be helpful but are hard to obtain in some settings. A positive blood culture will identify Gram-negative sepsis but a negative culture can occur if antibiotic therapy has recently been given, or it may indicate disseminated TB. Many cases of disseminated TB are anergic with minimal pulmonary lesions. *Mycobacterium tuberculosis* can take weeks to become positive in a blood culture, unlike *M. avium*. How can these sick patients be managed without any microbiology support? Experience is that, with awareness of the possibility of NTS bacteraemia, prompt broad-spectrum antibiotic therapy backed up by intravenous fluids can reduce mortality. Knowing the local antimicrobial sensitivity pattern can further reduce mortality.

The following strategy is suggested (see Flowchart 13.2): For any patient with an enteric fever-like illness, exclude a pulmonary/pleural/pericardial/lymphnode/abdominal/renal TB focus by a chest X-ray, urine microscopy, lymphnode aspirate and, if possible, ultrasound. Then concentrate on the treatment of NTS bacteraemia. First-line blind therapy can be ampicillin and gentamicin, or chloramphenicol. A quinolone would be the best choice but may not be available or affordable, but remember that oral ciprofloxacin has equivalent bioavailabilty to many intravenous antibiotics. Fluoroquinolones have some activity against mycobacteria and this can pose diagnostic problems if the patient has a partial response to therapy. Like typhoid itself, NTS bacteraemia can take several days to respond, but if there is little or no improvement after 3 or 4 days , drug resistance may be a problem. Switch to whichever first-line treatment was not used initially and consider empirical TB treatment and initiation of ART.

Chronic diarrhoea

'Slim disease' is what many people equate with African AIDS. It was the first clinical problem specifically associated with HIV infection by Ugandan investigators in 1985, and named by the local patients and their carers, who recognized a new disease in their community. Chronic diarrhoea with profound wasting is easy to identify and is associated with underlying HIV infection. Widespread metastatic disease, advanced TB, Addison's disease and untreated insulin-dependent diabetes present with wasting but not usually diarrhoea. While diarrhoea and wasting are the most obvious problems on the wards in Africa, if comprehensive studies of hospital admissions are carried out they account for only 10–20% of the HIV-related workload.

The diarrhoea is usually painless, watery and without blood or mucus. It can be variable or intermittent. Profound weight loss is clinically obvious and may be 20% or more of the premorbid weight. High fever is not typical and should suggest NTS bacteraemia or disseminated TB.

Studies from various African centres have shown a variety of stool pathogens: about 35% are parasitic infections and 10% are bacterial infections. No pathogen is identified in many cases. The hyperinfection syndrome with *Strongyloides stercoralis* does not appear to be associated with HIV infection. Noninfectious causes of diarrhoea also play a role and these include HIV enteropathy, drug reactions, alcohol excess and traditional medicines.

The current mainstay of management of patients with chronic diarrhoea is ART. This often leads to cessation of diarrhoea and rapid weight gain, although some patients continue to have diarrhoea despite ART. Blind treatments with metronidazole, albendazole or oral co-trimoxazole have also been shown to reduce diarrhoea. A therapeutic trial of each in order may be needed, depending on the setting and the available diagnostic and therapeutic options. An example flowchart may be found at the end of this chapter (see Flowchart 13.3).

Specific treatment is very limited and of variable efficacy:

- Amoebae, *Giardia* and helminths should be sought and treated with oral metronidazole when possible. Nitazoxanide has been found to be effective in treating HIV-positive patients with giardiasis that fails to respond to standard treatment.
- Some salmonellae and shigellae will respond to high-dose oral co-trimoxazole, so a trial of therapy may be indicated. However resistance to co-trimoxazole and now ciprofloxacin is increasingly common in most enteric bacterial pathogens.
- *Cystoisospora* and *cyclospora* respond to oral co-trimoxazole 160–800 mg four times daily for 7–10 days. HIV-positive patients should then receive a daily maintenance dose until a good CD4 count response to ART has been achieved.
- Cryptosporidiosis can be difficult to treat until CD4 counts are restored. Nitazoxanide may be used for treatment in HIV-related cryptosporidiosis and, because of its broad spectrum of activity, may also have a role in the 'blind' treatment of persistent diarrhoea in circumstances where diagnostic facilities are limited or absent. It is most useful in patients with higher CD4 counts. If it is not available and in the absence of ART, codeine phosphate 30 mg four times daily or loperamide in standard doses may offer some symptomatic relief.

Common parasitic gut infections in HIV and drugs active against them are listed in Table 13.1.

Oral and oesophageal candidiasis

The presentation of oropharyngeal *Candida* infection is variable. Patients initially complain of a bad

---

Table 13.1 Common parasitic gut infections in HIV and drugs active against them

	Cryptosporidiosis	Cystoisosporiaisis	Cyclosporiasis	Amoebiasis	Giardiasis
Albendazole					✓✓
Azithromycin	✓				
Ciprofloxacin		✓✓			
Co-trimoxazole		✓✓	✓✓		
Metronidazole				✓✓	✓✓
Nitazoxanide	✓✓	✓	✓	✓✓	✓✓
Paromomycin	✓			✓✓	✓✓
Rifaximin	✓	?	?	?	✓

✓✓=active, ✓=indeterminate, ?=don't know

taste. On examination you may find white plaques that leave a red area that easily bleeds after scraping. An erythematous form of candidiasis can be found on the tongue, with loss of papillae. Confluent white or red plaques that cover the entire oropharynx are a more severe form and are often very painful. Antifungal agents such as nystatin are effective when available but expensive; gentian violet mouthwashes may give some relief from milder disease. Difficulties in swallowing indicate involvement of the oesophagus. Oesphageal candidiasis can be treated with a 2-week course of fluconazole, which is often available free via a donation programme. Oral and oesophageal candidiasis are WHO stage 3 and 4 defining conditions respectively that warrant initiation of ART. For more information on painful mouth or swallowing see Flowchart 13.4.

Kaposi's sarcoma (Fig. 13.5)

Only 4% of the first 5000 reported AIDS cases in Uganda had Kaposi's sarcoma. The cancer is endemic in East Africa, and is now the most common cancer in many African countries. Kaposi's sarcoma is caused by human herpesvirus 8, but in most cases immunosupression such as HIV also needs to be present for Kaposi's sarcoma to occur.

It is usually easy to diagnose clinically. Unmistakable purple or violet raised plaques and sometimes nodular lesions can occur anywhere in the skin. The roof of the mouth is a typical site. The lesions are painless and do not itch. Other common presentations are the upper thighs, often associated with a hard oedema. Lymphadenopathy is common and may occur in the absence of skin plaques. Lesions can disseminate, particularly to the lungs. Biopsy is not necessary unless the diagnosis is uncertain.

Some patients with few lesions progress slowly and will die from other causes. Other patients progress rapidly over several months. Widespread pulmonary disease is an ominous sign. The drugs used for chemotherapy are expensive, and palliative only. Many patients with Kaposi's sarcoma respond to ART and this should be started immediately. If the patient has extensive disease that does not improve with ART, chemotherapy and radiotherapy remain an option if available.

Central nervous system disease

A wide range of conditions may present with **headache** (see Flowchart 13.5). Meningitis caused by *Cryptococcus neoformans* varies in incidence across Africa, closely related to HIV prevalence. It commonly presents as prolonged fever, headache and malaise with little neck stiffness or photophobia and there may be behavioural change, easily mistaken for psychiatric illness. Lumbar punctures in patients with cryptococcal meningitis typically reveal high opening pressures and India ink staining of CSF will pick up 80% of cases. Ideally treatment is with intravenous amphotericin B 1mg/kg daily and flucytosine for 14 days followed by fluconazole. If amphotericin is not available then high dose fluconazole (800–1200 mg) can be used as initial treatment, if necessary via a naso-gastric tube. Headache should be treated with adequate analgesia, and may also require repeated lumbar puncture to reduce intracranial pressure. ART should be initiated early which will help prevent a relapse. Patients should be given secondary prophylaxis with fluconazole for life or until their CD4 count has risen to $>200 \times 10^6/L$ for over 6 months. Unmasked cryptococcal infection is a common cause of the immune reconstitution inflammatory syndrome (IRIS) and should be considered in the differential for patients presenting with headache and/or focal signs after starting ART.

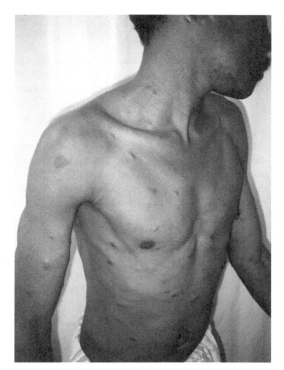

Figure 13.5 Multiple lesions of Kaposi's sarcoma in a patient with AIDS.

CNS infection with *Toxoplasma gondii* may present with focal weakness, but a relatively mild headache and an altered mental state are more common. Other signs include hemiparesis, ataxia, cranial nerve lesions, generalized in coordination, seizures and confusion. Fever is variable. Diagnosis is difficult with limited resources. One autopsy study from West Africa found evidence of cerebral toxoplasmosis in 15% of HIV-infected cadavers and was considered a primary cause of death in 10%. However, in Kenya the experience is that clinically obvious encephalitis is rare (less than 5%). Cerebral toxoplasmosis responds well to oral co-trimoxazole or sulfadoxime pyrimethamine (SP or Fansidar, 2 tablets b.d. for 6 weeks) which is more readily available than sulfadiazine and pyrimethamine. As a stage 4 defining disease, any patient with proven or suspected cerebral toxoplasmosis should be started on ART as soon as possible.

HIV causes **peripheral neuropathy** (see Flowchart 13.6) often in the lower limbs presenting as painful feet. Peripheral neuropathy due to diabetes, malnutrition and alcohol may coexist. Treatment is of the underlying cause if possible and ART can help HIV-related neuropathy. However, some ARVs such as d4T exacerbate neuropathy and should be avoided. Isoniazid can also worsen neuropathy and should always be prescribed with pyridoxine. Symptomatic treatment with analgesics and amitryptiline at night can help.

Eye disease

The ocular manifestations of HIV/AIDS include a specific microangiopathy, opportunistic infection and tumours. The specific microangiopathy of HIV manifests as multiple retinal microaneurysms and/or haemorrhages. Retinal vascular occlusion can occur. Opportunist infections can affect the lids (multiple mollusca contagiosa). Herpes simplex and herpes zoster can cause severe keratoconjunctivitis, iritis and retinal necrosis. Toxoplasmosis, syphilis, cryptococcosis and candidiasis are more severe in their clinical presentations. Ocular tumours associated with HIV/AIDS include Kaposi's sarcoma of the lid or conjunctiva, squamous cell carcinoma of the conjunctiva and lymphoma of either the conjunctiva or the retina.

Reduced vision can occur in late stage HIV infection for a number of reasons. Cytomegalovirus causes an aggressive chorioretinitis which is not uncommon, occurring at low CD4 counts (CD4 $<50 \times 10^6$/L). This causes fairly rapid but painless loss of vision. The fundoscopic appearances are white-yellow chorioretinal changes and haemorrhages (Fig. 13.6). Treatment with ganciclovir or cidofovir is very expensive and rarely available outside of major centres. ART

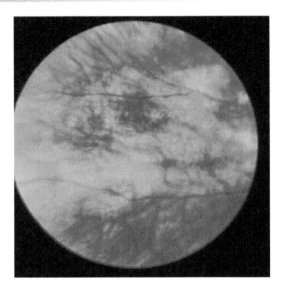

Figure 13.6 Cytomegalovirus chorioretinitis. Extensive peripheral haemorrhages and white-yellow changes.

may arrest visual loss and should be started as soon as possible

Jaundice

Jaundice can be hard to diagnose by examination, unless it has progressed to a severe stage. However, there is at least one easy way of checking for it as jaundiced patients will often have a yellow tinge under the bottom eyelid and the whites of the eyes will be yellow all over not just in small areas or streaks. Patients with jaundice may also have itchy skin, and may have dark urine. A history of recent medication, alcohol intake and current symptoms are needed as well as a thorough examination, vital signs and blood glucose. Jaundice may be due to a number of reasons, such as hepatitis, alcohol, or drugs the patient has forgotten to tell you about. A patient can be treated as non-urgent if he or she is afebrile, not drowsy and not taking any medication, and basic investigation may be performed as an outpatient. Patients should be treated as more urgent if they have developed jaundice after starting medication or if they have danger signs, such as drowsiness, fever, vomiting, high pulse rate (>100), tachypnoea (>20 per minute), or have low glucose (<3.0 mmol/L). All pregnant patients should also be treated as urgent cases. A patient with any of the danger signs should be admitted as there may be rapid progression to liver failure and death if the underlying cause is not treated.

Prophylaxis

TB chemoprophylaxis

A 6-month course of isoniazid has been shown to be effective chemoprophylaxis against TB in both HIV-positive and HIV-negative individuals. However, meta-analysis of trials indicates that this benefit is confined to individuals who have a positive reaction to tuberculin skin testing (TST) and studies on whether longer than six months is useful in high-transmission settings with ongoing risk of re-infection are conflicting. The main challenges are, firstly, proving that the patient does not have active disease and, secondly, the logistics of identifying individuals and delivering the treatment to them. The WHO recommends that in low resource settings, a TST need not be performed, and isoniazid prophylaxis should be administered to all at-risk individuals as part of the '3 Is' initiative (Intensified Case Finding, Isoniazid Preventive Therapy and Infection Control). A pragmatic approach in many settings is to focus prophylactic efforts on children who are still being breastfed by mothers who have sputum-positive disease. There is also an argument to give isoniazid prophylaxis to patients on ART who have completed TB treatment to prevent relapse but this is not widely practised.

Preventing pneumococcal disease

Protein conjugate pneumococcal vaccine has been shown to prevent pneumococcal disease in HIV-infected adults even when vaccine was given at a CD4 count below 200×10^6/L, although repeat annual vaccination may be necessary. The 23 valent pneumococcal polysaccharide vaccine does not work in this population and is not recommended by the WHO.

Co-trimoxazole prophylaxis

Following two studies in Abidjan, Côte d'Ivoire, co-trimoxazole prophylaxis is recommended for people living with HIV/AIDS in Africa. Co-trimoxazole has activity against several bacteria as well as *Cystoisospora belli*, *Pneumocystis jirovecii* and *Toxoplasma gondii*. Also it has some activity in preventing malaria. Although the Abidjan studies showed an improvement in survival and decreased morbidity in patients given co-trimoxazole, there is debate as to whether these findings are applicable to the whole of Africa, given different prevalences of drug resistance across the continent. Co-trimoxazole is generally given to all HIV-infected patients. Co-trimoxazole is also given as secondary prophylaxis to patients who have had previous cerebral toxoplasmosis or Pneumocystis pneumonia.

Preventing other infections

There are no NTS vaccines licensed for human use. Fluconazole should be used for secondary prophylaxis for patients who have had cryptococcal disease and should be considered for primary prophylaxis in patients with CD4 cell counts $<100 \times 10^6$/L who are awaiting ART.

Childhood immunization

In resource-poor countries, for infants born to HIV-infected mothers, EPI vaccines are given as usual except that two doses of measles vaccine should be given if possible at 6 and 9 months. In industrialized countries, measles vaccine is contra-indicated in severely immunosuppressed HIV-infected children. If available, Hib and conjugate pneumococcal vaccines should be given. Yellow fever is contraindicated in HIV-symptomatic infection. Complications have been described following BCG vaccination (but not from other EPI vaccines), including local disease (e.g. ipsilateral axillary lymph node disease). Approximately 1:1000 HIV-infected infants may develop disseminated BCG infection. Thus, an infant known to be HIV-infected should not receive BCG. However, this has practical implications and poses operational challenges in many low resource countries, where it requires delaying BCG until the infant's HIV status is known, using PCR at 6 weeks or later.

Antiretroviral therapy

Post-exposure prophylaxis after needle stick injury or rape (PEP)

Prophylaxis for health care staff following accidental occupational HIV exposure is available in many places and is effective at reducing transmission. When prescribing PEP after occupational exposure local protocols should be followed. Following an injury, the wound should be washed and encouraged to bleed. The source patient and the health care worker should be tested for HIV but if the test is not immediately available there should be no delay in giving prophylaxis, which should be initiated within

72 hours. A 4-week course of standard triple therapy with antiretrovirals (see below) is recommended. There are various risk assessment protocols which determine if the exposure was high or low risk, e.g. a eye splash is lower risk than a needle stick with a solid needle, which is lower risk than a needle stick with a blood-covered hollow needle. Other factors that may need to be taken into account when advising the health care worker are whether the source patient is taking ART and whether or not they have a detectable viral load or known resistant strains. Individuals taking PEP need to be told about ART side effects and to use condoms until they have a negative HIV test. Nausea, tiredness and muscle aches appear to be particularly common in PEP patients.

PEP can also be effective in reducing transmission after rape and survivors who present within 72 hours should be offered this in HIV endemic areas alongside forensic testing, counselling support, emergency contraception and STI prophylaxis. As many rapes occur out of hours, ready availability of ART in casualty departments, gynaecology wards and other delivery points ensures better access.

Public health approach to ART

Combination ART has been in widespread use in developed settings since 1996. It has unequivocally been shown to extend patients' lives and reduce opportunistic infections and malignancies. The drugs were initially very expensive but prices have dropped dramatically since 2004 and funding for large-scale ART programmes has been made available in many resource-poor countries. The model of individually tailored ART delivery used in developed countries is not feasible in resource-poor settings, where there are vast numbers of patients but limited health care infrastructure and very limited human resources. The WHO 'public health approach' to ART delivery therefore recommends using standard first-line ART regimens, often using fixed-dose combinations of drugs followed by a second-line regimen if the first fails. This approach aims to provide ART to large numbers of people in resource-poor countries, using simple protocols that allow non-specialized health care professionals to deliver ART safely. Only patients with certain problems are referred to clinicians or specialists. A limited number of ART regimens are used allowing the greatest benefit to be seen from ART in as many patients as possible. In moving forward to expand access further, the WHO recommends simplifying service provision in five areas as follows: optimize drug regimens using new formulations and better dosing; provide access to simplified diagnostics at the point-of-care for CD4

and viral load; reduce treatment-related costs; adapt delivery systems to more decentralized, integrated approaches; and, mobilize communities to be involved in managing and supporting treatment programmes.

Commonly used ART drugs and choice of regimens in resource-poor countries

There are over 20 antiretroviral drugs licensed for clinical use and many more in development. The prices of newer drugs remain high, therefore the drug regimens used in resource-poor settings tend to be older drugs that are either off patent or supplied at reduced cost. The three classes of drugs used in most standard regimens are nucleoside (or nucleotide) reverse transciptase inhibitors (NRTI), non-nucleoside reverse transcriptase inhibitors (NNRTI) and protease inhibitors (PI), which are usually boosted by the addition of a low dose of ritonavir (another PI) that maintains the dose of PIs at therapeutic levels for longer. The drugs are given in combination with 2 NRTIs forming the backbone of treatment and a third drug from another class (either an NNRTI or a boosted PI) being added. In many cases cost-effective fixed-dose combinations are given which aid adherence by reducing pill burden and lessening the chance of medication error. Below is a list of the commonly used drugs and their classes with a brief description of each. A more detailed understanding may be found in the resources listed under 'Further reading' at the end of this chapter. A summary decision-making tree may be found in Flowchart 13.7 at the end of this chapter.

Nucleoside Reverse Transcriptase Inhibitors (NRTIs)

- Zidovudine (AZT or ZDV) – one of the original ARVs. AZT has a long history of use and is relatively safe. One of the main side-effects is anaemia which can be a problem is settings where many HIV-infected patients are already anaemic.
- Stavudine (d4T) – available in fixed dose combinations and widely used in resource-poor countries. The main side effects are peripheral neuropathy and lactic acidosis. The WHO now recommends that d4T be phased out due to toxicity.
- Lamivudine (3TC) – used in most first-line regimens. Few side-effects, but resistance develops very easily. Also effective against hepatitis B.
- Emtricitabine (FTC) – similar to 3TC and also effective against hepatitis B.
- Abacavir (ABC) – more expensive than AZT and d4T. Life-threatening hypersensitivity reaction can

occur especially if a patient is rechallenged following an initial reaction. This is less common in patients of African ethnicity.

- Didanosine (ddI) – one of the original ARVs. Often poorly tolerated. Should not be given in combination with d4T. Can cause peripheral neuropathy and lactic acidosis. Is being phased out.
- Tenofovir (TDF) – the only nucleotide analogue reverse transcriptase inhibitor. Usually well tolerated. May cause renal impairment. Renal function should be measured before starting treatment and at regular intervals subsequently. Also effective against hepatitis B.

Non-Nucleoside Reverse Transcriptase Inhibitors (NNRTIs)

- Efavirenz (EFV) – well tolerated. May cause neuropsychiatric problems.
- Nevirapine (NVP) – available in fixed dose combinations. May cause severe rash and liver toxicity. If possible liver enzymes should be checked before starting NVP and shortly after. Interacts with rifampicin, making concurrent administration of antituberculosis therapy problematic.

Boosted protease inhibitors

- Lopinavir/ritonavir (PI/r) – expensive but very potent boosted protease inhibitor. Well tolerated. High barrier to resistance. Used in second-line therapy.

A note about other classes of ART

Newer drugs targeting fusion e.g. enfuvirtide (T20), CCR5 e.g. maraviroc (MRV) and integration, e.g. raltegravir (RGV) are not widely available in resource-poor settings at the time of writing, but may form part of third-line regimens in future when available more cheaply. Common ARVs are listed in Table 13.2.

To make the administration of ART as simple as possible and to preserve a patient's options for second-line therapy the limited number of drugs available are given as set regimens which vary from country to country depending on drug availability. Most national programmes designate a standard first- and second-line regimen. The first-line regimen, ideally as a fixed-dose combination, usually includes one NNRTI (e.g. EFV or NVP) plus two NRTIs, e.g. (AZT or TDF or ABC) plus (3TC or FTC). A typical second-line regimen for a patient who had failed first-line treatment would be two NRTIs not used in the first regimen and a boosted protease inhibitor.

Table 13.2 **List of common ARVs with their abbreviations**

Class	Drug	Short name	Comments
NRTI			
	Zidovudine	AZT	
	Lamivudine	3TC	Active against hepatitis B
	Stavudine	d4T	Being phased out; discontinue where possible
	Didanosine	ddI	Being phased out; discontinue where possible
	Abacavir	ABC	
	Tenofovir	TDF	Active against hepatitis B
	Emtricitabine	FTC	Active against hepatitis B Similar action to 3TC
NNRTI			
	Nevirapine	NVP	
	Efavirenz	EFV	Not used in first trimester pregnancy; used in TB-coinfected patients
	Etravirine	ETR	
PI			
	Lopinavir	LPV	
	Ritonavir	RIT	100 mg used as PI booster
	Saquinavir	SAQ	
	Atazanavir	ATZ	
	Darunavir	DRV	

Regimens for special populations

Many ARVs are safe to use during **pregnancy**, although efavirenz has in the past been avoided in the first trimester due to a hypothetical risk of teratogenicity. New WHO guidance in 2012 reviewed the available data and supported the use of efavirenz to optimize and simplify first-line treatment in pregnant women. For ART-naive pregnant women being started on treatment, the dosages of the first-line ART regimens are the same as in other adults. ART should be continued as usual during labour and the postpartum period. Particular care should be taken to screen for nevirapine-related liver toxicity and skin rash, tenofovir-induced impairment of creatinine clearance and zidovudine (AZT)-induced anaemia. AZT should not be used in women with Hb < 80 g/L. In **TB patients** efavirenz is the NNRTI of choice. Rifampicin, an important component of TB treatment, interacts with many medications, including ARVs. It decreases the blood levels of protease inhibitors by approximately 80%, of nevirapine by 30–50%, and of efavirenz by 25% depending on the genetic make-up of individual patients. In general standard dose efavirenz combined with two NRTIs is effective ART in TB patients. In **hepatitis B-coinfected** patients two NRTIs active against hepatitis B should be combined, e.g. TDF and FTC or 3TC, as these are known to slow the replication of the virus and the associated liver damage that can occur.

The 4 Ss: when to Start, Substitute, Switch and Stop treatment

HIV treatment decisions are tailored to local circumstances guided by the 'four Ss': Starting, Substituting, Switching and Stopping treatment. Table 13.3 shows suggested screening tests before initiating ART and Table 13.4 shows a suggested format for follow-up visits.

Table 13.3 Suggested screening tests before initiating ART in resource-limited settings

Test	Comment
HIV antibody test	In patients diagnosed with HIV infection outside of the treatment centre it is prudent to confirm the diagnosis of HIV
CD4 count	A CD4 count should be taken if possible to help stage the patient Also subsequent CD4 counts can be related to the baseline count
Viral load	Viral load is not essential before initiating therapy, but can be useful prognostically
Full blood count	Assess and treat anaemia. AZT should be used with caution in patients with Hb < 80 g/L, who should be monitored very closely
Renal function assessment	Renal function should be assessed by measuring electrolytes, urea and creatinine as well as urine dipstick Patients with protein or blood on dipstick should be further evaluated if possible for treatable conditions Patients with reduced glomerular filtration rate may need reduced doses of NRTIs
Liver function test	Patients with raised liver transaminases should be further evaluated for the cause, such as hepatitis or alcohol Patients given NNRTIs or PIs who have raised transaminases should be monitored closely for deterioration in liver function
Tuberculosis screening	History and examination should be performed for signs and symptoms of TB Sputum should be taken for AFB staining Further investigation such as a chest X-ray maybe required in some cases. TB can be very difficult to diagnose in patients with low (<50) CD4 counts
Hepatitis B serology	Patients with hepatitis B will benefit from ART that includes agents active against the virus such as 3TC. They are also at risk of deterioration in liver function if their ART is interrupted
Syphilis serology	Syphilis and other STIs should be sought and treated prior to starting ART
Cervical smear	The incidence of cervical abnormalities is high in HIV-infected women. Screening should only be undertaken if referral pathways are available for the management of any abnormalities detected
Pregnancy test	At each visit in women of reproductive age who are not already known to be pregnant

Table 13.4 Suggested format of routine follow visit for patients taking ART

Component	Comment
General history and examination	General enquiry about patient's health and brief examination focussing on detecting opportunistic infections such as TB (chronic cough) and STIs. This is especially important in the initial few months of therapy when side effects of therapy and immune reconstitution are more common. Measure body weight at each visit
Side-effect check	Side effects may occur early or late. It is important to be familiar with local regimens. Common examples are: AZT – anaemia; d4T – peripheral neuropathy and lactic acidosis; ddI – lactic acidosis; NVP – liver function abnormalities and rash; EFV – vivid dreams and rash
Adherence check and counselling	It is vital that patients are questioned about adherence and challenges they have faced. Pill counts can be performed. Patients should be supported and encouraged with adherence. Check other medications the patient is taking looking for possible drug interactions, e.g. NVP and rifampicin. Also ask about non-prescribed herbal remedies
Safe sex and risk behaviour check	It is important to reinforce these messages. Consistent condom use reduces onward transmission
CD4	This should be checked every 6 months. A falling CD4 count may be the first indication of failing therapy
Viral load	If available viral load estimation can show if ART is effective or not. A detectable viral load after six months of ART suggests either the patient is non-compliant or drug resistance has occurred and therapy needs to be changed
Full blood count	This should be performed monthly in patients on AZT, which may have to be stopped if anaemia occurs or worsens
Renal function assessment (electrolytes, urea and creatinine; urine dip stick)	This should be performed monthly in any patient with preexisting renal failure in case further dosage adjustment needs to be made Also renal function should be checked in patients taking TDF
Liver function assessment	This should be checked monthly in patients with preexisting liver function abnormalities and in patients taking NVP

Starting ART

When to start therapy can be based on either WHO staging alone or a combination of WHO staging and CD4 counts if available (see Flowchart 13.7). If CD4 counts are not available all patients with WHO stage 3 and 4 disease should be started on therapy. If CD4 counts are available all patients with **CD4 cell counts ≤500 × 10⁶/L** should be treated regardless of WHO stage. Patients with WHO stage 4 disease should be treated regardless of CD4 count, e.g. patients with Kaposi's sarcoma who have a high CD4 count. All patients with tuberculosis, hepatitis B or who are in serodiscordant relationships should start cART regardless of WHO stage or CD4 count.

Staging and/or CD4 count <500 × 10⁶/L are used in making decisions about **starting treatment in pregnant women.** Some countries have altered their policy to state that all pregnant women go on triple therapy ART for life if they present in pregnancy. This avoids logistical and other challenges associated with PMTCT.

There has been controversy in the past about **when to start ART in patients with TB**. Recent trials have found that starting ART reduces mortality in HIV-infected patients with TB. So all patients presenting with TB should be offered an HIV test and started on ART irrespective of CD4 count. With regard to timing a balance between the risk of immune reconstitution inflammatory syndrome (IRIS), increased pill burden and clinical benefit has to be reached. TB treatment should be initiated first, followed by ART as soon possible within the first eight weeks of treatment.

Before ART is initiated, patients undergo a series of education modules to ensure that they understand the reason for therapy, how the drugs work, the importance of compliance, how to recognize side effects and the importance of continuing to practice safe sex. The frequency of follow-up visits should follow national guidelines. Table 13.4 gives a suggested format for follow-up visits. As a rule a patient should be seen two weeks following initiation of therapy, to check for early side-effects and to reinforce treatment adherence. The patient should be seen again after a month and if there are no problems visit frequency can be increased to three monthly and in some cases six monthly intervals. Patients experiencing problems or who need careful monitoring, e.g. anaemic patients taking AZT, should be seen more frequently.

The level of monitoring depends very much on what is available. All patients should be monitored clinically and their WHO stage recorded at initiation and at subsequent visits. The patient's weight should be recorded and they should be clinically assessed at each visit for the development of opportunistic infections which may signal ART failure. Adherence to therapy should be checked.

CD4 counts, if available, are useful for helping to decide when to start therapy and also to check every six months if the patient is responding immunologically. HIV viral load estimation remains expensive and difficult to organize, although their use is increasing and dried blood spots can be used. Measuring the HIV viral load is not essential before starting therapy but is useful in assessing the success of therapy and deciding when to switch to second-line drugs if viral load is persistently detectable and > 1000 copies/ml. It may reveal treatment failure before there has been clinical disease progression and the acquisition of multiple ARV resistance mutations. Cheaper and more accessible alternatives are being developed.

Substituting drugs

Side-effects of ARVs are common. These can range from mild rashes and gastrointestinal upsets to life-threatening complications such as lactic acidosis secondary to d4T, ddI or AZT. Simple protocols should be available in all ART programmes to help health care workers decide when patients should be referred or when drugs should be substituted. If patients are warned that when starting EFZ they are likely to develop vivid dreams, they are less likely to default from treatment. Other major side-effects, such as peripheral neuropathy due to d4T or ddI, anaemia due to AZT, and lipodystrophy due to d4T should be checked for by health care workers at each visit. Lactic acidosis secondary to d4T, ddI or AZT may have an insidious onset and should be suspected in any patient on therapy for over 4 months, who develops abdominal pain, breathlessness rapidly worsening peripheral neuropathy or who becomes non-specifically unwell. Cheap point-of-care lactate meters are available.

Common reasons for substituting drugs due to side effects are rash secondary to NVP, anaemia secondary to AZT or peripheral neuropathy or lactic acidosis secondary to d4T. Patients with underlying liver disease or chronic hepatitis (B or C), should be carfully warned about the signs and symptoms of liver toxicity. If possible more hepatotoxic drugs should be avoided and liver enzymes monitored at follow-up visits. Side effects may also be a result of drug-drug interactions and all new drugs initiated in someone on ART should be checked for possible interactions. A useful website is given as a resource at the end of this chapter.

Switching regimens

Treatment is switched when the first-line regimen has failed. Failure may be defined clinically if CD4 or HIV viral load monitoring is not available, or on immunological or viral grounds. When the decision is made to switch to second-line therapy the patient should be counselled again about adherence and it should be stressed that this may well be the last effective therapy that can be offered. A search should be made for opportunistic infections as these may make the second regimen less likely to succeed and a check should be made if the patient is taking other medications including traditional remedies which may affect ART drug levels. Patients should not be rushed into therapy if they are unsure or unready to take it. Suggested second- and third-line regimens may be found in the WHO 2013 consolidated guidance.

Stopping treatment

In developed settings more ART regimens and often experimental drugs are available, so it is unusual for an individual to exhaust all therapeutic options. Sadly this is not the case in resource-poor settings, where there may be no effective therapy when second-line drugs have failed. Also, some patients may be too sick to take treatment or have severe opportunistic diseases that progress despite ART. These patients should be palliated using a home-based care or outreach team. Palliative care resources are often very limited and the availability of morphine outside of hospitals can be problematic. However, every attempt should be made to ensure that a patient can be cared for in the most humane and dignified manner possible given available resources.

Immune Reconstitution Inflammatory Syndrome (IRIS)

Immune Reconstitution Inflammatory Syndrome (IRIS), or Immune Reconstitution Disease (IRD), is common after patients start ART, especially if they have a CD4 cell count $<50 \times 10^6$/L. The pathogenesis of this disorder is thought to be due to the immune system recognizing pathogenic antigens of certain organisms such as *M. tuberculosis* and *C. neoformans* as it recovers. Patients can present with a paradoxical worsening of their clinical condition shortly after starting ART, which can be at best discouraging or at worst life threatening. The most common IRIS events are skin reactions, which often settle spontaneously or with symptomatic treatment. IRIS involving TB or cryptococcus should be treated by treating the causative organism first and steroids are often added to suppress the immune reaction. ART can usually be safely continued.

Organization of ART delivery

The organization of a country's ART progamme should be undertaken by the national department of health, which should produce country-specific protocols, often based on WHO protocols but adapted for local use. Before starting a programme it is important to ensure that: there are adequately trained staff; provision has been made to deal with staff burn out; a reliable and long-term source of medication is available; and that all parts of the health service are aware of the programme and their role in it. For example, maternity services should be aware about when and how to refer pregnant women for ART. Integration of ART services with existing programmes and other programmes related to HIV infection is sensible and can help ensure more coordinated care and tracking of referrals. Examples would include combined ART and TB clinics or Prevention of Mother to Child Transmission (PMTCT) services and ART clinics. Decentralization is recommended. Monitoring needs to be in place to ensure that the programme is working well and to pick up deficiencies that can be corrected. Programmes tend to evolve at different rates for a variety of reasons, and monitoring may identify a clinic or unit that is performing particularly well. Best practice from this area can then be implemented elsewhere.

Paediatric HIV infection

The following notes are targeted at the adult clinician working in the setting of a family clinic and are intended to provide a brief summary. For the purposes of ART prescribing, an adolescent is defined as aged 10-19 and the adult prescribing guidelines apply. The age of onset of AIDS is bimodal. Over 80% of infants

infected at or around delivery develop symptomatic HIV disease at or before 6 months of age. Others survive several years before developing AIDS and these children may have a more robust CD8 cytotoxic lymphocytic response. In resource-poor countries, many HIV-infected infants die suddenly, e.g. from pneumococcal pneumonia or septicaemia, often suddenly, before developing clinical 'AIDS'. In infants the CD4 count is not a reliable indication of disease progression.

Management of HIV in infants and children

Routine prophylaxis with co-trimoxazole from 1 month of age is given to all suspected and proven HIV-infected infants to prevent PCP as this has been shown to reduce mortality. Benefit might also relate to reduction of bacterial infections (e.g. pneumonia, sepsis, diarrhoea) and malaria as well as toxoplasmosis and cystoisosporiaisis.

In immunosuppressed/symptomatic children, ART improves growth and general well-being, reduces the risk of pneumonia and diarrhoea, and is associated with increases in CD4 cell count, haemoglobin and serum albumin. Some patients may suffer from IRIS eg, fever, worsening of the chest X-ray, effusions, lymphadenopathy and BCG reactivation. This is particularly associated with *M. tuberculosis, M. bovis and M. avium* infections and is due to an abnormal immunological response to dead or dying mycobacteria.

ART is currently recommended for **all HIV-infected children below five years of age,** irrespective of the clinical or immunological stage. ART should be initiated in all children infected with HIV five years of age and older with CD4 cell count $\leq 500 \times 10^6$/L regardless of WHO paediatric clinical stage and in all children with clinical stages 3 and 4 regardless of age and CD4 cell count. If HIV PCR is unavailable, treatment can be initiated presumptively in HIV-exposed children less than 18 months of age while a definitive diagnosis is awaited if two or more of the following conditions are present: oral thrush, severe pneumonia, severe sepsis or an AIDS indicator condition. A protease-inhibitor, e.g. ritonavir-boosted lopinavir (LPV/r), should be used as first-line ART for all children infected with HIV younger than three years (36 months) of age, regardless of NNRTI exposure. For HIV-infected children three years and older, EFV is recommended as first-line ART. Both LPV/r and EFV will be given with a backbone of two NRTI. ART coverage for children is much lower than coverage for adults. Table 13.5 gives a summary of paediatric management for the adult physician.

Table 13.5 **Summary of paediatric management for the adult physician**

Common problems	Management
Failure to thrive	Nutritional support, particularly home-based high-energy supplements and multivitamins
Fever: malaria, other infections	Paracetamol, antibiotics, antimalarials
Candidiasis	Nystatin. fluconazole for resistant thrush and oesophageal candidiasis
Dermatology: papular pruritic eruptions, infections, eczema, seborrhoea	Antibiotics (local or systemic), emolients, etc.
Diarrhoea: chronic ± blood; lactose intolerance	Oral rehydration therapy, nalidixic acid, zinc, metronidazole Low lactose milk
Otitis media: often chronic	Ampicillin or amoxicillin, dry mopping of discharge
Respiratory infections: (acute/persistent/recurrent) *S.pneumoniae, S.aureus,* PCP, CMV, TB, aspiration, IRIS	Co-trimoxazole (3 wks high dose for PCP), amoxicillin, chloramphenicol, cefotaxime or ceftriaxone, TB chemotherapy, isoniazid prophylaxis
Lymphocytic interstitial pneumonitis (LIP) (30–40% of HIV-infected children)	ART; prednisolone for 4–6 wks, then alternate days for 2-3 mths. Give only for severe LIP
Lymphadenopathy	Biopsy if in doubt-? TB, KS, non-Hodgkin's lymphoma
CNS: loss of milestones, seizures, meningitis, stroke	HIV encephalopathy, meningitis (bacterial, TB, viral or fungal*)

*For cryptococcus (India ink stain, antigen test).

Control strategies

Condom promotion and distribution is important for preventing new infections in the community as a whole, as well as in sex workers and their clients, who can be a core of HIV transmission in an area. Condoms are proven to be effective in preventing most STIs. They may not always be culturally acceptable and they rely on the male partner's cooperation. Female condoms are also effective but are cumbersome to use and may not be accepted by some partners. Provision of condoms at schools and in prisons may not be politically popular in some regions but targeting these areas is essential to prevent HIV transmission. Another difficult area is the provision of clean needles and syringes for injecting drug users both in and out of prison; this may not be legally possible in many countries.

Early treatment with ART can decrease transmission from an HIV-infected to an HIV-infected partner by 96% in sero-discordant couples and alongside consistent condom use this is one of the most effective control strategies available. However, a number of logistical, cost and implementation challenges remain before this becomes a feasible way to eliminate the HIV epidemic entirely.

Treatment of STIs has been shown to reduce HIV transmission in some studies. There is debate over the likely benefits of mass STI treatment campaigns; many areas are using syndromic management to simplify STI treatment and ensure that the important diseases are treated in a single visit.

Targeting core groups such as commercial sex workers and their clients is important but education for school children is also a high priority. Previously, sex education was not widespread in Africa and girls would not find out about contraception or STIs until they were attending antenatal programmes. Sex education and HIV awareness has to be tailored to the target audience as Western-style campaigns and materials are often inappropriate for resource-poor countries.

Circumcision, as mentioned above, provides partial protection against male acquisition of HIV and is safe if provided by well-trained health professionals in properly equipped settings. WHO and UNAIDS developed operational guidance for scaling up male circumcision services for HIV prevention and in 2010 male circumcision was being scaled up in thirteen priority countries of Eastern and Southern Africa.

Ensuring a safe blood supply is an important minimum standard in HIV prevention.

Other methods of prevention include vaginal microbicides, which have had a chequered past but are being evaluated in large prospective trials, and vaccines. Sadly, vaccines to prevent or control HIV appear to remain a long way off.

Prevention of Mother-to-Child-Transmission (PMTCT)

Historical studies have shown that NVP given as a single dose to the mother in labour and the child within 72 hours of birth can reduce HIV transmission by over 50%. The use of two ARVs such as AZT or triple therapy is even more efficacious. Antenatal services in countries with high HIV prevalence now routinely offer HIV counselling and testing and infant feeding counselling as well as ARV prophylaxis to infected women and their HIV exposed infants (see also p. 99 earlier in this chapter).

Mother-to-child-transmission of HIV can be much reduced by following the current WHO recommendations. Triple ARV prophylactic regimens covering pregnancy and the entire period of breastfeeding are key to the PMTCT strategy. For programmatic and operational reasons, particularly in a generalized epidemic setting, all pregnant and breastfeeding women with HIV should initiate ART as lifelong treatment. In some countries, HIV-infected pregnant women undergo screening for ART eligibility using clinical WHO staging criteria (Stage 3 and 4) and CD4 count measurement ($< 500 \times 10^6$/L). Eligible women start on a triple combination of 2 NRTIs and 1 NNRTI and stay on it during delivery, postpartum and beyond. Infants receive ARV prophylaxis for 4–6 weeks. Formula feeding should only be recommended if it is available, feasible, affordable, safe and sustainable (AFASS). Details of these regimens can be found in the 2013 WHO consolidated guidelines.

PMTCT remains a priority and testing is the entry point to this. At the end of 2010 UNAIDS reported that only 35% of pregnant women in low and middle income countries had had an HIV test.

 SUMMARY

- HIV testing and counselling should be readily available in many health care and community-based settings.
- Staging of HIV infection in adults and older children may be based on clinical features if CD4 cell counts and HIV viral load tests are not available.
- In resource-poor settings, national treatment programmes require simple protocols, using a limited number of defined first-line or second-line antiretroviral treatment combinations. There should be defined points at which to Start, Substitute, Switch or Stop treatment (4S).
- In such settings, simple clinical monitoring including promotion of adherence to treatment regimens can be achieved without sophisticated laboratory monitoring.
- Syndromic algorithms can guide the prevention and management of the major opportunistic infections and other HIV-related complications.
- Prevention of infection is crucial and there is growing public health evidence that treatment of all HIV-infected individuals would interrupt transmission to future generations.

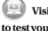 **Visit** www.lecturenoteseries.com/tropicalmed **to test yourself on this chapter using interactive MCQs.**

 FURTHER READING

Abdool Karim, SS *et al.* (2011) Integration of antiretroviral therapy with tuberculosis treatment. *NEJM* **365**: 1492–1501. [A trial looking at the timing of ART with TB treatment.]

Auvert B, Taljaard D, Lagarde E, *et al.* (2005) Randomized, controlled intervention trial of male circumcision for reduction of HIV infection risk: the ANRS 1265 Trial. *PLoS Medicine* **2**: e298. [The first trial to show the potential benefit of male circumcision in preventing HIV in Africa.]

Cohen MS, Chen YQ, McCauley M, *et al.* (2011) Prevention of HIV infection with early antiretroviral therapy. *N Eng J Med* **365**: 493–505. [Shows that ART prevents HIV transmission.]

Gilks CF, Crowley S, Ekpini R, *et al.* (2006) The WHO public health approach to antiretroviral treatment against HIV in resource limited settings. *Lancet* **368**: 505–10. [A description of the WHO's public health to large scale provision of ART in resource-poor countries with high HIV burden.]

McCarthy K, Meintjes G (2007) Guidelines for the prevention, diagnosis and management of cryptococcal meningitis and disseminated cryptococcosis in HIV-infected patients. *Southern African Journal of HIV Medicine* **3**: 25–35. [Evidence based guidelines for the management of cryptococcal disease in resource poor settings.]

Sharp P, Bailes E, Chaundhuri EE, *et al.* (2001) The origins of acquired immune deficiency syndrome virus: where and when? *Phil Trans R Soc Lond B* **356**: 867–76. [A description of the probable origins of HIV.]

World Health Organisation (2013) Consolidated guidelines on the use of antiretroviral drugs for treating and preventing HIV infection. Available at http://www.who.int/hiv/pub/guidelines/arv2013/en/index.html

Other resources

www.aidsmap.com [A constantly updated HIV/AIDS resource that features current research articles and covers HIV/AIDS conferences, there is a focus on data relevant to resource-poor settings.]

www.hiv-druginteractions.org.uk [A comprehensive and constantly updated interactive database of HIV medication interactions]

www.hivinsite.ucsf.edu/ [An extensive HIV/AIDS resource from the University of California, San Francisco.]

www.sahivsoc.org/ [Guidelines and articles on HIV treatment and prevention relevant to Southern Africa.]

www.unaids.org/en/ [A comprehensive website with general information, technical reports and annually updated statistics of the global HIV/AIDS pandemic.]

Appendix to Chapter 13

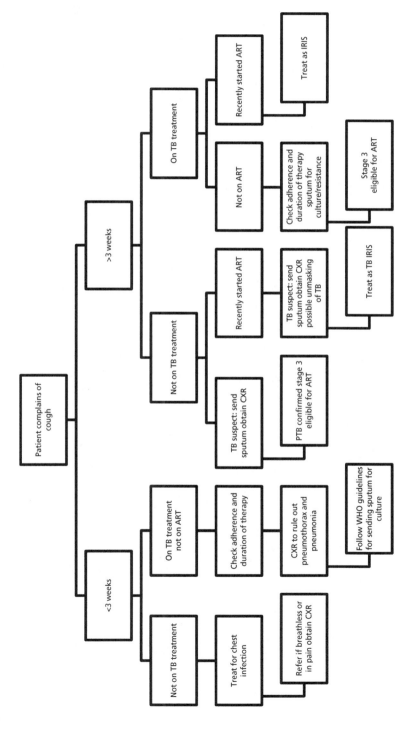

Flowchart 13.1 Cough.

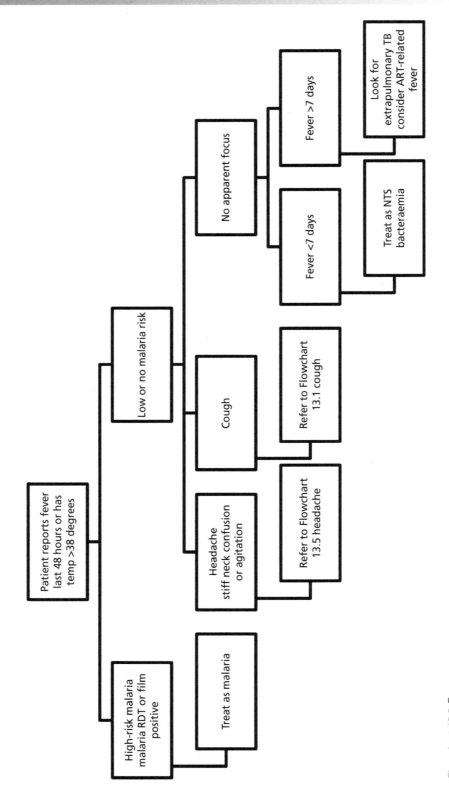

Flowchart 13.2 Fever.

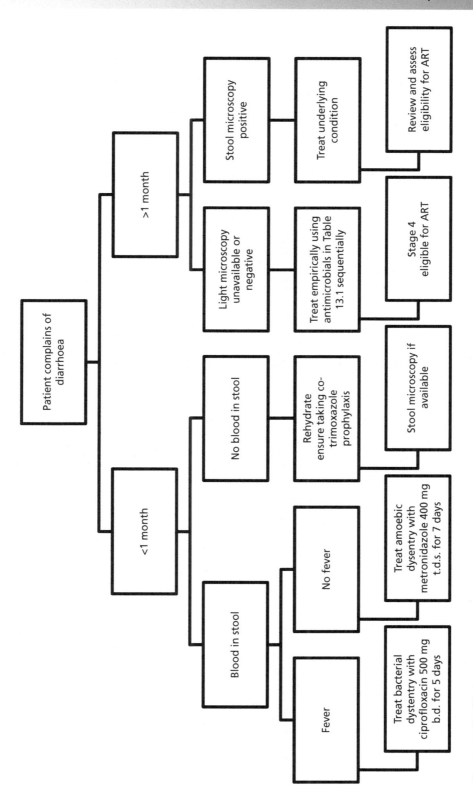

Flowchart 13.3 Diarrhoea.

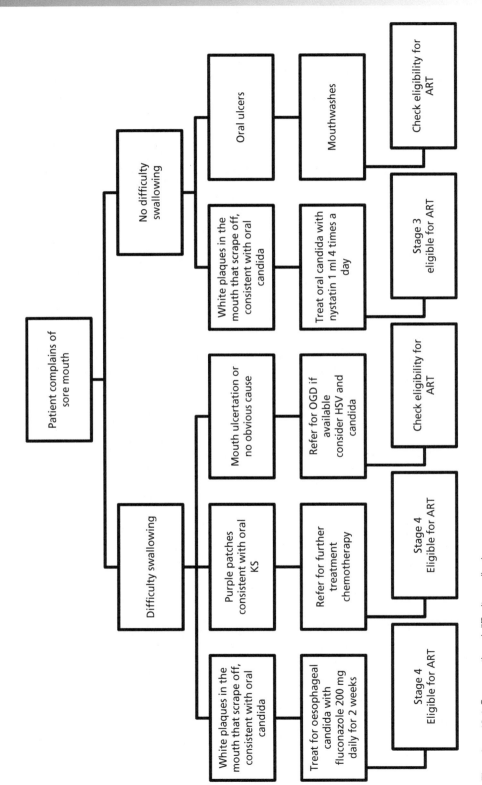

Flowchart 13.4 Sore mouth and difficulty swallowing.

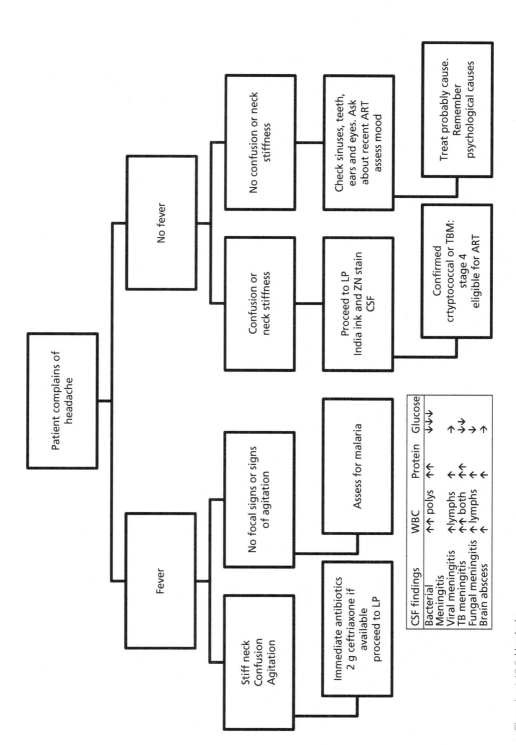

Flowchart 13.5 Headache

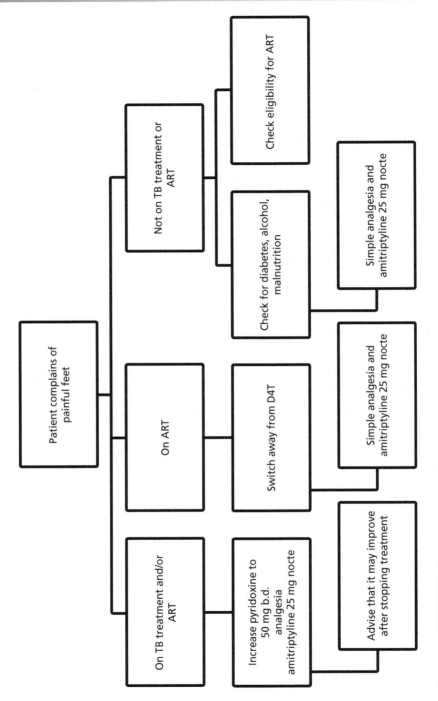

Flowchart 13.6 Painful feet.

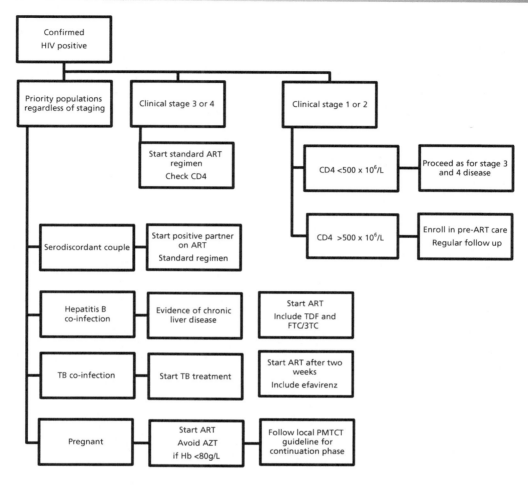

Flowchart 13.7 ART eligibility in adults (adapted from WHO Consolidated Guidelines 2013)

14

Onchocerciasis, filariasis and loiasis

Tim O'Dempsey
Liverpool School of Tropical Medicine

Introduction

Onchocerciasis and filariasis are important parasitic nematode infections affecting over 200 million of people living in the tropics and subtropics. They cause significant long-term morbidity, resulting in physical and mental suffering, disability and economic hardship. Insect vectors are important in the transmission of these parasites. Human infections occur when the insect vector feeds and introduces infective larvae which mature into adult worms and produce microfilariae, which in turn infect the insect vector.

Recently, significant progress has been made in the community control of onchocerciasis and filariasis. Mass drug administration (MDA) in mapped implementation units (mainly districts) is currently the main strategy for control. The integration of onchocerciasis, filariasis, schistosomiasis and soil transmitted helminth control programmes offers a cost-effective strategy for controlling these infections.

A major challenge facing these programmes is the elimination of adult filarial worms, which live for many years and are relatively unresponsive to standard anthelmintic agents. Recently it has become evident that adult filarial worms depend on intracellular, endosymbiotic bacteria of the genus *Wolbachia* for their development, motility and fertility. It is also evident that *Wolbachia* play a significant role in the pathogenesis of disease associated with these filarial infections. The good news is that *Wolbachia* are susceptible to tetracyclines and several other antibiotics, offering fascinating new possibilities in the management and control of filarial infections.

Loiasis affects about 25 million, transmission mainly occurring focally in tropical forested regions of West and Central Africa. Although most famous for dramatic appearances when the adult 'eye worm' journeys across the eye, loiasis is generally of less clinical importance than either onchocerciasis or lymphatic filariasis. However, coendemicity of *Loa loa* is an important consideration in planning community control of these infections because of the risk that *L. loa* encephalopathy may be precipitated by certain anthelmintic agents. *L. loa* does not have a symbiotic relationship with *Wolbachia,* and thus is not susceptible to treatment with doxycycline.

Onchocerciasis

Onchocerciasis or 'river blindness' is caused by the filarial worm *Onchocerca volvulus*. It is a major cause of blindness in tropical Africa and of skin disease throughout its distribution in Africa, Yemen and Central and South America (Fig. 14.1). Over 300 000 people, many young adults, are blind from onchocerciasis.

Life-cycle

Adult female *O. volvulus* worms are threadlike, about 40 cm long, and live in human subcutaneous tissue, sometimes coiled within fibrous nodules, where they produce living microfilariae. The microfilariae are about 350 μm long and migrate through the skin and often into the eyes. Microfilariae only develop further if they are taken up by biting blackflies of the genus

Tropical Medicine Lecture Notes, Seventh edition. Edited by Nick Beeching and Geoff Gill. © 2014 John Wiley & Sons, Ltd. Published 2014 by John Wiley & Sons, Ltd.

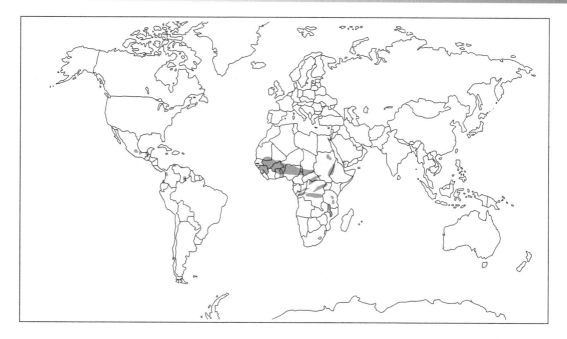

Figure 14.1 Distribution of onchocerciasis.

Simulium. These flies can transmit infection after a week or more and deposit infective larvae as they bite another person. Adult *O. volvulus* live for 12 years on average but sometimes up to 17 years and microfilariae live for about 1 year.

Epidemiology

Because *Simulium* flies breed in rapidly flowing freshwater and bite nearby, onchocerciasis mainly affects people living or working near fast-flowing rivers. The *S. damnosum* complex contains the chief vectors in Africa, and although they are found predominantly around rivers, some flies may be blown for great distances and may even reinvade other river systems that have been cleared of vectors in the past. *S. naevei* flies, which attach their eggs to crabs but do not fly far, were an important cause of onchocerciasis in Kenya in the past but this focus has been eradicated with insecticides. *Simulium ochraceum* and *S. metallicum* are vectors in the Americas and frequently breed in smaller rivers within coffee plantations.

Clinical features

Adult worms evade the host immune response and cause few symptoms. The pathology of onchocerciasis is almost entirely caused by immunological reactions to dying and dead microfilariae and their endosymbiotic *Wolbachia* which release bacterial mediators that trigger the innate immune system resulting in clinical pathology. In addition, activated eosinophils release cellular proteins that cause connective tissue damage.

The incubation period is usually about 15–18 months. Some people do not react to microfilariae and remain asymptomatic carriers for long periods. Onchocerciasis may increase risk of seroconversion in HIV-1 infections and treatment of onchocerciasis appears to be associated with reduced HIV-1 viral replication. Onchodermatitis also appears to be more severe in HIV-positive patients.

Skin (Figs 14.2–14.4)

In endemic regions, a variety of different skin manifestations are seen, usually with a significant degree of overlap.

- **Acute papular onchodermatitis (APOD)** presents with an intensely itchy, papular rash, sometimes associated with oedema.
- **Chronic papular onchodermatitis (CPOD)** is characterized by larger, pruritic, hyperpigmented papules. A localized chronic papular dermatitis, known as 'Sowda', is described in Yemen, northern Sudan and West Africa. This is

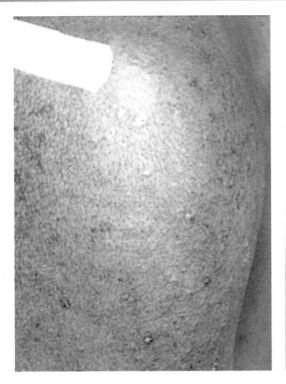

Figure 14.2 Early onchocerciasis with an itchy papular rash in a student from Cameroon.

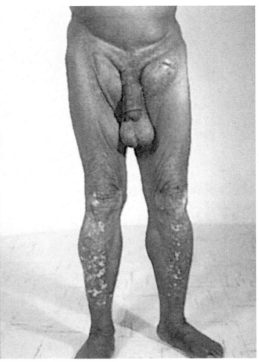

Figure 14.4 Advanced onchocerciasis (West Nigeria). There is depigmentation of the skin overlying the shins, enlargement of the inguinal lymph glands associated with laxity of the surrounding skin (hanging groins) and generalized presbydermia.

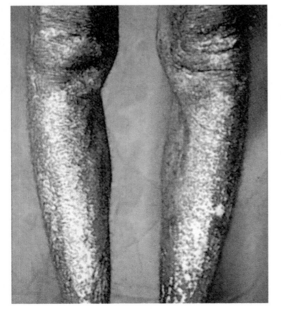

Figure 14.3 Onchocerciasis: typical depigmentation associated with grossly exaggerated skin fold pattern.

a hyperimmune response and microfilariae are scarce in skin snips.

- **Lichenified onchodermatitis (LOD)** refers to discrete or confluent, pruritic, and hyperpigmented papulonodular plaques often associated with lymphadenopathy.
- Relentless itching may give rise to excoriation and secondary bacterial infection. Healing is associated with progressive hyperpigmentation, blackening and thickening of the skin.
- **Skin atrophy and depigmentation** occur over time. Degenerative skin changes and loss of elasticity give the skin a wrinkled, prematurely aged appearance (presbydermia). Sometimes, particularly in the presence of inguinal or femoral lymphadenopathy, this may give rise to the so-called 'hanging groin' appearance. Patchy depigmentation, especially of the lower limbs, results in a characteristic 'leopard skin' appearance.

Subcutaneous nodules (Fig. 14.5)

Painless subcutaneous nodules may be palpable and are most obvious over bony prominences. These are thought to arise when adult onchocercal worms migrating subcutaneously are arrested over bony prominences and become enclosed in fibrous tissue. Nodules may measure several centimetres in diameter and contain a number of live or dead coiled female worms. Nodules are firm and at first lie free but may later become deeply attached.

- In Africa, nodules are found most readily over the pelvic brim, the sacrum, femoral greater trochanters and the medial aspects of the knees.
- In the Americas, nodules are more often found over the head.

Although nodules are likely to be clinically evident and useful diagnostically in patients with longstanding infections in highly endemic regions, this may not be the case elsewhere. In which case, ultrasound examination may be helpful in demonstrating the presence of impalpable nodules.

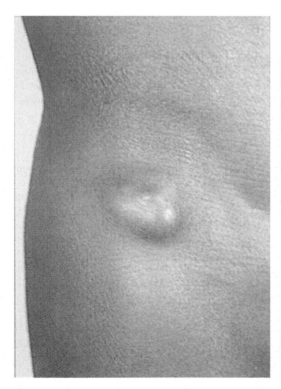

Figure 14.5 An *Onchocerca* nodule. The typical site in Africa. Many worms may be incarcerated in a multiloculated nodule.

Eye disease

Itching, redness and excess lachrymation are symptoms of early disease. Late disease leads to varying degrees of loss of vision and eventually to blindness. Microfilariae have been identified in all ocular tissues except the lens.

In Africa, two epidemiologically distinct forms of ocular onchocerciasis have been described: a mild form occurring primarily in rain forested regions in which blindness is relatively rare, and a severe form occurring in savannah regions where blindness is highly prevalent. *Onchocerca volvulus* strains in the savannah have a significantly higher *Wolbachia* DNA to nematode DNA ratio compared to forest strains, further implicating *Wolbachia* in the pathogenesis of onchocerciasis.

Anterior eye disease

- Punctate keratitis is caused by reactions to the death of microfilariae in the cornea. This may appear as a reversible, 'snow flake' opacity.
- Pannus forms as blood vessels invade the cornea from the sides and below. The pannus may cover the pupil – sclerosing keratitis – and cause blindness. This is particularly likely among heavily infected individuals in the African savannah (Fig. 14.6).

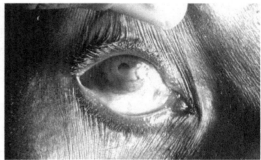

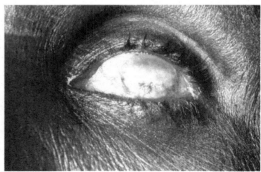

Figure 14.6 Sclerosing keratitis covering the pupil.

- Iritis leads to a loss of the pigment frill and to synechiae that cause a deformed, often pear-shaped pupil. Secondary glaucoma and cataracts occasionally result.

Posterior eye disease

- May present as widespread chorioretinitis with pigmentary changes (Fig. 14.7).
- Often accompanied by optic atrophy, which is sometimes the only finding, mainly affecting central vision.
- Various different forms of visual loss may result but a common presentation is with disabling 'tunnel vision'.

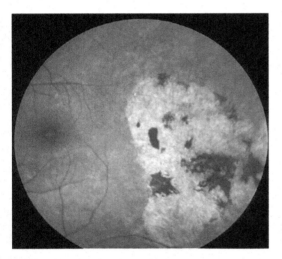

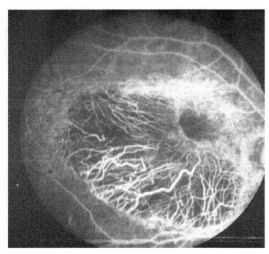

Figure 14.7 Involvement of retinal pigment epithelium in onchocerciasis

The combination of retinal and optic nerve disease, both of which are untreatable, has devastating consequences for the individual and the community. Eye disease is particularly likely when adult worms are near the eyes, therefore the risk tends to be higher with nodules on the head and upper body. Because disease progress is relatively slow, most people are blinded in middle life but with heavy infections, or more virulent strains, blindness can occur in people in their twenties.

General health

Skin disease may be socially stigmatizing and resources spent on medication may cause significant economic loss. The unrelenting itch may result in chronic sleep disturbance, depression and precipitate suicide. Although onchocerciasis does not kill directly, blind people in village communities have a shortened lifespan and onchocerciasis has led to abandonment of fertile riverside ground in some areas. Very heavy infections in childhood can impair growth. An association with convulsions has been postulated from East Africa but the evidence remains inconclusive.

Diagnosis

Skin onchocerciasis is frequently misdiagnosed as scabies; the papular eruptions of HIV infection should also be considered. History of exposure in a known focus of onchocerciasis is helpful.

Finding microfilariae

Snips of skin should be taken without blood contamination. Take snips from the vicinity of subcutaneous nodules or in Africa from the lateral aspects of the calves, thighs, the hip region or the iliac crests. In the Americas, snips from the shoulder tip or outer canthus of the eye may be more valuable because microfilariae tend to concentrate in the upper part of the body. Up to six snips may be needed to be reasonably sure that infection cannot be detected.

Techniques

1 **Skin snip.** Clean skin with alcohol and allow to dry; lift up a small piece of skin on a sharp sterile needle. Slice off a piece 1–2 mm^2 with a sterile scalpel or razor blade. The piece should be deep enough to show white dermis and capillaries should ooze blood into the site. Place the skin piece in 0.2 mL saline in the well of a microtitre plate. Fluid from the plate may be examined after

half an hour to look for active microfilariae with the low power of the microscope. If microfilariae have not appeared, the plate should be covered in clingfilm, allowed to stand for 24 h at room temperature and be re-examined for emergent microfilariae which will by then usually be immobile.

2 **Punch biopsy.** This technique is essentially the same but more elegant as it uses a Walsar corneoscleral punch to obtain the snip. However, these punches are expensive and difficult to keep sharp and sterilize.

Count the numbers of microfilariae in each skin snip. You may need to stain some to differentiate microfilariae of onchocerca from other skin or blood microfilariae. Polymerase chain reaction (PCR) techniques sometimes demonstrate microfilariae in skin snips from which no microfilariae have emerged.

3 **Slit lamp.** Use a slit lamp to look for active microfilariae in the anterior chamber of the eye after the patient has spent 5 minutes in a 'face down' position to bring the microfilariae into view.

4 **Rapid diagnostic tests.** A luciferase immunoprecipitation systems (LIPS) assay, which has been developed recently using a cocktail of four *O. volvulus* antigens, has 100% sensitivity and specificity for *O. volvulus* using a rapid 15 minute format (QLIPS). This technique also has 100% sensitivity and specificity values of 76, 84 and 93% for distinguishing *O. volvulus* from *W. bancrofti*, *L. loa* and *Srongyloides stercoralis*.

Other evidence

- **Biochemical methods.** Skin-snip microscopy is less sensitive than newer biochemical methods, including skin-snip PCR, ELISAs, EIAs, and antigen detection. Recent advances include the development of a serum antibody test card using recombinant antigen to detect *O. volvulus*–specific IgG4 in finger-prick whole-blood specimens. A triple-antigen indirect ELISA rapid-format card test also appears promising. A highly sensitive and specific urine antigen dipstick test has also recently been developed.
- **Surgery.** Subcutaneous nodules can be removed surgically to demonstrate adult worms, or aspirated with a needle to look for microfilariae.

Eosinophilia may be evident in early onchocerciasis.

One of two additional tests, now mainly of historic note, may be considered in patients with repeatedly negative skin snips, where other diagnostic techniques are unavailable:

- The Mazzotti test is sometimes useful to detect lightly infected patients but is potentially dangerous. It consists of giving diethylcarbamazine (DEC) 6 mg orally and recording the development of an itching papular skin reaction within 24 h; this may be accompanied by fever, limb oedema and even hypotension or worsening of eye damage. This test should only be used for patients with negative skin snips and normal eyes. Given that DEC is no longer recommended in the treatment of onchocerciasis and alternative diagnostic methods are now more widely available, the Mazzotti test is unlikely to be justified.

A safer variant of the Mazzotti test is the DEC patch test in which a 1 cm square of filter paper soaked in a solution of DEC is applied to the skin of the patient. If positive, this will provoke intense localized itching and inflammation at the site of application. Rarely, a full-blown Mazzotti reaction may be precipitated by a DEC patch test. Nevertheless, DEC patch testing of children aged 3–5 years has recently been advocated as an effective, low-cost method for monitoring the endemicity and transmission of onchocerciasis in Africa.

Treatment

Ivermectin, a macrocyclic lactone drug originally introduced for veterinary purposes, is now in common use for individual and mass chemotherapy of onchocerciasis. The drug kills microfilariae by immobilizing them so that they are carried away from their usual locations via the lymphatics. Therefore, in contrast to treatment with DEC, microfilaria death following ivermectin is less immediate and is less likely to provoke irreversible inflammatory responses in vulnerable organs such as the eye. Mazzotti reactions are also rare following treatment with ivermectin. However, a temporary increase in itching, papular eruptions, limb oedema, headache and fever may sometimes occur. Ivermectin has little effect on adult worms other than reducing embryogenesis. Therefore, elimination depends on repeated doses over several years. A conservative estimate is that annual treatment with ivermectin alone would need to be sustained for at least 14 years to cover the estimated life span of the adult worm.

Ivermectin is administered orally at a dose of 150 µg/kg body weight repeated every 3–6 months when treating individual patients, and at once or twice yearly intervals when used in community control programmes in Africa or the Americas respectively. Ivermectin should not be used in pregnancy or during breastfeeding although teratogenesis has not been demonstrated. Ivermectin should not be used in patients who also have heavy *L. loa* infections as fatal cases of encephalitis have occurred.

Recent reports of suboptimal responses to ivermectin in Ghana and Sudan have given rise to fears of ivermectin resistance. Although ivermectin resistant onchocerciasis has not been demonstrated definitively, this may emerge soon. Given the genetic heterogeneity of *O. volvulus* and the likelihood that resistance alleles already pre-exist, concern is growing that mass treatment with ivermectin may be transforming the population genetics in favour of ivermectin resistant *O. volvulus*.

Moxidectin, a more potent relative of ivermectin, is currently undergoing clinical trials. Moxidectin is microfilaricidal and also sterilizes or kills the adult worms and this has the potential to interrupt transmission within about 6 annual treatment rounds. However, given the similarity in mode of action, it is unlikely to be of use in the event of ivermectin resistance.

Doxycycline has been shown to kill the endosymbiotic *Wolbachia* organisms in filarial species resulting in the slow, and therefore less pathogenic, death of the parasite. A dose of 200 mg daily for 4 weeks, or 100 mg daily for 6 weeks, is effective in blocking embryogenesis and can maintain freedom from microfilariae for up to 2 years. Doxycycline also has a significant macrofilaricidal effect. A dose of 200 mg/day for six weeks kills over 60% of adult female worms and renders surviving worms sterile. Contraindications to doxycycline include age < 9 years, pregnancy and breastfeeding.

In the past nodulectomy was advised for head nodules in an attempt to reduce the likelihood of eye disease. However, this is not a guarantee of eliminating risk of eye disease because not all nodules are necessarily evident and remaining nodules would continue to produce microfilariae. Improved drug treatment has significantly improved the outlook and has reduced the justification for therapeutic nodulectomy.

Treatment of individual patients

Provided the patient does not have a high *L. loa* microfilaraemia and ivermectin (or doxycycline) is not otherwise contraindicated, the choices are as follows.

1 If the patient continues to live in endemic area, or is less than 9 years old and weighs > 15 kg: ivermectin 150 μg/kg every 3–6 months.
2 If interruption in embryogenesis and cessation of microfilariae production is desired: doxycycline 200 mg/day for 4 weeks, or 100 mg/day for 6 weeks, followed by one dose of ivermectin after 4–6 months.
3 If a strong macrofilaricidal effect is desired: doxycycline 200 mg/day for 6 weeks followed by one dose of ivermectin after 4–6 months.

So, what about patients with onchocerciasis who do have a high *L. loa* microfilaraemia? There is good news. Recently it has been shown that there is no significant additional benefit in giving a single dose of ivermectin following a course of doxycycline 200 mg daily for six weeks. Therefore, doxycycline monotherapy can be recommended for such patients.

Control

The control of onchocerciasis has progressed rapidly in the past thirty years, largely due to successful international public–private partnerships, sustained funding for regional programmes and technical advances (see also Chapter 63).

Three landmark programmes have been implemented to date as outlined below.

- The Onchocerciasis Control Programme (OCP) (1974–2002) eliminated onchocerciasis as a disease of socioeconomic and public health importance in ten countries of West Africa. Initial efforts in vector control using the organophosphate larvicide temephos proved inadequate. A major breakthrough came with Merck's donation of ivermectin, following which larviciding was abandoned in favour of regular mass chemotherapy. OCP's achievements include over 600 000 cases of blindness prevented, 40 million people protected from eye disease, infection eliminated in 1 million cases, over 400 professional staff trained, and 25 million hectares of riverine habitats and valleys have been made available for settlement, making it possible to feed 17 million people. OCP has also played a major role in strengthening health systems in West Africa.
- The African Programme for Onchocerciasis Control (APOC) (1995–present): APOC is a bigger programme than OCP and includes 19 countries, involving Ministries of Health, affected communities, international and local NGDOs, the private sector (Merck), donor countries, UN agencies, the World Bank and WHO. Community-Directed Treatment with Ivermectin (CDTI) is APOC's delivery strategy. The programme has been extended until 2015 and aims to treat over 90 million people annually in 19 countries, protecting an at risk population of 115 million, and to prevent over 40 000 cases of blindness every year.
- The Onchocerciasis Elimination Programme for the Americas (OEPA) (1991–present) has adopted an approach similar to that of APOC except that

ivermectin is administered twice a year until transmission has been interrupted. The OEPA strategy aims to reach at least 85% of the half-million persons at risk of disease. By the end of 2007, all six endemic countries (Brazil, Colombia, Ecuador, Guatemala, Mexico, and Venezuela) had established effective national programmes that met or exceeded targets in all 13 disease foci. OEPA is on target for regional elimination of ocular morbidity and interruption of transmission by 2012.

Community-directed delivery of ivermectin for 15–17 years has led to rates of transmission beneath the threshold needed for elimination in parts of Mali and Senegal and post-intervention monitoring for 18–24 months showed no further transmission. However APOC continues to face various challenges that make it difficult to achieve and maintain this level of success, including conflict, inadequate health infrastructure, and lack of resources, political commitment, necessary funding to sustain national programmes for up to 20 years. Furthermore, high risk foci of *L. loa* are currently excluded from community ivermectin programmes because of the risk of encephalopathy in individuals with high *Loa* microfilaraemias.

Significant reductions in timescales for onchocerciasis control and elimination may be possible with the development of strategies targeting *Wolbachia* using short-course antibiotics that can be safely administered to entire communities, without promoting the emergence of drug resistance among existing pathogens or damaging ecosystems.

Table 14.1 summarizes individual and community chemotherapy of onchocerciasis.

Table 14.1 **Recommended treatment strategies for mass drug distribution, individual drug administration, and morbidity control and treatment of lymphatic filariasis and onchocerciasis.**

	Mass drug administration*		Individual drug administration*	Morbidity control and treatment*
	Africa	Rest of world		
Lymphatic filariasis	IVM + ALB for at least 5 years	DEC + ALB for at least 5 years	(a) DEC (+/- ALB) 6 mg/kg single dose[1] (b) DEC 12-day course of 6 mg/kg per day in 2 or 3 divided doses; or (c) doxycycline 200 mg/day for 4 weeks followed by one dose IVM	Lymphoedema: hygiene, physiotherapy, doxycycline 200 mg/day for 6 weeks; Hydrocoele: surgical hydrocoelectomy, doxycycline 200 mg/day for 6 weeks; Tropical pulmonary eosinophilia: doxycycline 200 mg/day for 4 weeks followed by one dose IVM
Onchocerciasis	IVM every year for at least 15–17 years	IVM twice yearly until transmission has been interrupted	(a) IVM[1]; (b) doxycycline 200 mg/day for 4 weeks, or 100 mg per day for 6 weeks[2] followed by one dose IVM after 4–6 months; or (c) doxycycline 200 mg/day for 6 weeks[3] followed by one dose IVM after 4–6 months	Same as individual drug administration for onchocerciasis

[1]If patient continues to live in endemic area, or is less than 9 years of age (contraindication of doxycycline).
[2]If interruption in embryogenesis and cessation of microfilariae production is desired.
[3]If a strong macrofilaricidal effect is desired.

*Notes on drugs
ALB = Albendazole;
DEC = Diethylcarbamazine (omit if onchocerciasis co-infection or risk of serious adverse events with *Loa loa*);
IVM = Ivermectin (omit if risk of serious adverse events with *Loa loa*);

Source: Adapted from: M. Taylor *et al.* in *Lancet* 2010; 376: 1175–85.

Filariasis

Lymphatic filariasis (LF)

Filariasis, caused by *Wuchereria bancrofti* (>90% of infections worldwide), and in some areas of Asia by *Brugia malayi* or *B. timori*, affects about 120 million people and is endemic in over 80 different countries in the tropics. More than 60% of those affected live in South-East Asia and over 30% live in Africa (Fig. 14.8). While many infections are asymptomatic, a large number of people suffer acute or chronic illness including lymphoedema or elephantiasis (15 million), hydrocoele or other genital disease (25 million), acute inflammatory attacks (15 million) and chyluria (5 million). The Global Programme to Eliminate Lymphatic Filariasis (GPELF) established in 1999 aims to interrupt transmission of the parasites in all endemic countries by 2020. The strategy includes annual mass distribution of antifilarial drugs, either alone or in combination (DEC or ivermectin monotherapy, or either drug in combination with albendazole), to as many people as possible until transmission has been interrupted.

Bancroftian filariasis

Life-cycle

Adult *W. bancrofti* are threadlike worms living in the lymphatics of the groin and scrotum or sometimes those of the arm. Males measure about 4 cm long and females about 10 cm. They can live for more than 10 years and are actively reproductive for 4–6 years. Females release over 10 000 sheathed microfilariae daily. These have a lifespan of 1–2 years and appear in the peripheral blood periodically to synchronize with the biting habits of the predominant mosquito vector in the region. Nocturnal periodicity is commonest; microfilariae are usually present only during the night and disappear into the pulmonary capillaries by day. In some Polynesian islands microfilariae are found in greater numbers in daytime blood (diurnal subperiodic).

Many different mosquitoes including *Culex*, *Anopheles*, *Aedes* and *Mansonia* species may act as vectors but the chief vector in towns is *Culex quinquefasciatus* which breeds in drains and polluted water and bites at night. Filariform larvae migrate to the mouthparts of the mosquito after 10 days or more and, in contrast to malaria, are not injected directly into the bloodstream but are deposited on the skin of the new human host during feeding. They then actively invade the new host via the biting area. Thus, transmission is less efficient when compared to malaria. There is no multiplication of larvae in the mosquito.

Clinical effects

LF infections may produce a wide range of clinical effects that range from no clinical or microscopic

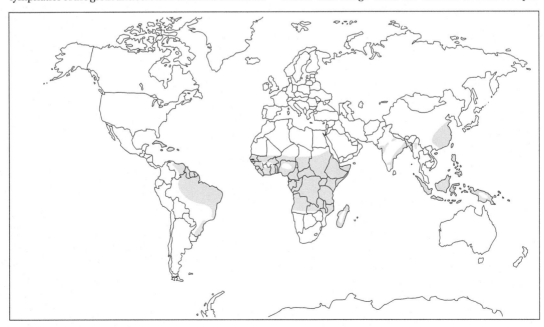

Figure 14.8 Distribution of lymphatic filariasis.

evidence of infection (asymptomatic amicrofilarae-mia), asymptomatic microfilaraemia, to filarial fever, chronic lymphatic pathology and tropical pulmonary eosinophilia (Chapter 30). Clinical symptoms may occur 8–16 months following infection, although a first episode of acute filarial fever has been described more than 15 years following exposure. Acute epi-sodes often recur several times a year. There has been considerable confusion and debate concerning the aetiology and classification of acute manifestations of LF. Recent developments, particularly with regard to the role of *Wolbachia*, have led to significant changes in our understanding of the pathogenesis of LF. In-flammatory episodes associated with LF are likely to be multifactorial involving responses to different stag-es of the parasite, secondary bacterial infection and inflammatory mediators associated with *Wolbachia*.

Clinical presentations include the following.

- Acute filarial fever without lymphadenitis which must be distinguished from other acute febrile ill-nesses in the tropics.
- Acute Filarial Lymphangitis (AFL). This occurs fol-lowing the death of adult worm (whether spontane-ous or post-treatment), resulting in a circumscribed inflammatory nodule or cord with centrifugal lym-phangitis (i.e. spreading away from the affected node). The clinical course usually mild and rarely results in residual lymphoedema. In severe cases, an abscess may develop at the site of an affected node and secondary bacterial infection may follow.
- Acute dermatolymphangioadenitis (ADLA). ADLA is characterized by intense local inflam-mation resembling cellulitis or erysipelas, often associated with secondary bacterial infection in the presence impaired lymphatic flow. This re-sults in diffuse subcutaneous inflammation which may be accompanied by ascending lymphangitis and is frequently associated with limb oedema.

  Bacteria may enter through breaks in the skin. Stasis of lymph provides excellent conditions for rapid growth of bacteria. The sufferer may com-plain of high fever, pain, swelling, nausea and vomiting. An acute episode may last about a week. Inflammation leads to damage of small lymphatic vessels, and eventually to fibrosis and progression to elephantiasis. ADLA is commoner than AFL in endemic regions and is more important as a cause of lymphoedema and elephantiasis.

The possibility that a further distinct form of acute lymphangitis and lymphoedema may occur, triggered by filarial larval stages, has also been proposed. How-ever, a case definition has not yet been agreed for this possible presentation.

Chronic LF may develop months or years after acute symptoms, or without a history of acute disease. Lymphatic obstruction leads to lymphoedema of the affected extremity and, eventually, to elephantiasis. Characteristically in the initial stages there is revers-ible pitting oedema. This gradually becomes perma-nent and the skin thickens and becomes firm. Nodular verrucose skin changes follow. Sites most commonly affected are the legs, scrotum, arms and breast. Recur-rent secondary bacterial skin infections, often strep-tococcal, may cause acute episodes of pain and fever and may be complicated by acute glomerulonephritis.

Other manifestations of LF include:

- acute epididymitis;
- chyluria, chylous diarrhoea, chylous ascites: due to rupture of dilated lymphatics; chyluria character-istically has a milky appearance, sometimes tinged pink because of the presence of red blood cells which can be seen to sediment if the urine is left to stand in a conical jar; malabsorption, particularly of fat soluble vitamins, may complicate chylous diar-rhoea;
- funiculitis (inflammation of the spermatic cord);
- hydrocoele, usually unilateral (commonest chron-ic manifestation of *W. bancrofti* filariasis);
- lymph scrotum , lymphatic fluid seeps through the scrotal skin;
- monoarthritis, glomerulonephritis.

The differential diagnosis of filariasis is wide and depends on the clinical presentation. The following should be considered.

- **Chyluria** – other causes of lymphatic obstruction, e.g. TB.
- **Elephantiasis** – chronic sidero-silicosis, Milroy's syndrome, leprosy (lepromatous), repeated strep-tococcal infection of feet.
- **Filarial fever** – malaria, other acute fevers, other recurrent fevers, acute bacterial lymphangitis.
- **Filarial lymph node enlargement** – chronic infec-tion, TB, lymphogranuloma inguinale, lymphoma, leukaemia.
- **Filarial orchitis, funiculitis, hydrocoele** – acute infection, TB, *S.haematobium*, 'surgical' causes.
- **Groin swellings** – hernias, hanging groin of oncho-cerciasis.

Brugian filariasis

Brugia malayi is a cause of filariasis in certain rural areas of Asia. There are two main forms: the noc-turnal periodic form in swampy areas from India to Korea and Japan; and the nocturnal subperiodic form in damp forests of South East Asia. The subperiodic form has an animal reservoir in monkeys, cats and pangolins. *Mansonia* species of mosquito are the major vectors although anophelines may also be involved. Clinically, brugian filariasis is less severe than bancroftian disease. Elephantiasis is usually limited to below the knees and scrotal involvement is less common.

Diagnosis and monitoring of filariasis

Eosinophilia is common during the acute stages. Parasitological diagnosis can be made on peripheral blood by means of Giemsa stained thick blood films taken at the peak of microfilarial periodicity according to the species (usually 22.00 hrs–02.00 hrs for *W. bancrofti*). However, this is relatively insensitive unless microfilaraemia is high (> 100 Mf/mL). Concentration techniques greatly improve sensitivity (e.g. Nuclepore filtration).

Staff and patients may be reluctant to undertake blood tests in the middle of the night, therefore the 'DEC provocative test' was introduced as a means of inducing parasitaemia during the day. This involved the administration of a single dose of DEC, which provokes microfilaraemia, and collection of peripheral blood after 30–60 minutes for staining and examination in the standard manner. However, DEC may cause a severe Mazzotti reaction in patients with coinfection with onchocerciasis and may precipitate an encephalopathy in patients coinfected with loiasis. With improved alternative diagnostics, the DEC provocative test is rarely necessary.

Scrotal ultrasound scanning may be useful for demonstrating live adult worms (the 'filarial dance sign') either for diagnostic purposes or for following up response to treatment.

A variety of other diagnostic techniques are now available. These include complement fixation tests for circulating *W. bancrofti* antigen such as an ELISA (TropBio-test) and a rapid finger-prick immunochromatographic card test (Amrad ICT, Binax). These tests are very sensitive and specific, diagnose adult worm infection as well as microfilariae, thus overcoming the problem of periodicity. Rapid ICT is now the preferred method for diagnosis of *W. bancrofti*. and for monitoring the success of mass drug programmes.

IgG4 (Bm 14 test for both *W. bancrofti* and *B. malayi*; Bm-RM for *B. malayi*) testing of children may be used for monitoring control programmes and for screening travellers. PCR assays have also been developed for *W. bancrofti* and *B. malayi*. Molecular xenomonitoring of parasites in pools of mosquitoes can also be used as an indicator of community transmission.

Management of filariasis

A number of anthelmintic agents are effective.

- Diethylcarbamazine (DEC) – the mainstay of treatment and prophylaxis for decades. The usual regimen is 6 mg/kg/day in two or three divided doses for 10–14 days up to a maximum total dose of 72 mg/kg. Side effects are less likely by starting with lower doses (1 mg/kg three times daily on days 1 and 2). The microfilaria count falls within a month and remains low for 6–12 months. If necessary, the course of DEC may be repeated one month after completion of the initial course. DEC has limited effect in killing the adult worms. DEC should be avoided in areas endemic for onchocerciasis or *L. loa* because of the risk of provoking a Mazzotti reaction or encephalopathy.
- Ivermectin – a dose of 150–400 µg/kg kills microfilariae but not adult worms. It is mainly used in combination treatment with DEC or albendazole.
- Albendazole – a single dose of 400 mg progressively decreases microfilaraemia over 6–12 months. Albendazole has some effect on adult worms if taken as a prolonged course.

The following general adverse reactions to anthelmintic treatment occur in decreasing order of frequency.

- Headache, fever, dizziness, anorexia, malaise, nausea, urticaria, vomiting, wheeze. General reactions and fever are positively associated with the prevalence and intensity of microfilaraemia.
- Local adverse reactions include scrotal nodules due to death of the adult worm, lymphadenitis, funiculitis, epididymitis, lymphangitis, orchitis, abscess formation, ulceration and, rarely, transient lymphoedema.

Combination treatment with anthelmintic agents is the basis for community control programmes.

- Doxycycline – Doxycycline 200 mg/day × 6 wk has been shown to be highly effective in the treatment of filariasis, producing a 99% reduction in microfilaremia at 12 months. The addition of a single dose of ivermectin after 4 weeks resulted in complete amicrofilaremia. A subsequent trial of doxycycline 200 mg/day for 8 weeks achieved similarly impressive results with almost complete elimination of microfilaria at 8-14 months, and significant reduction in the adult worm burden and presence of filaria antigenaemia. More recently, a similar macrofilaricidal effect has also been demonstrated using a six week course of doxycycline.

Doxycycline eliminates microfilariae gradually, thus avoiding adverse inflammatory events that may follow rapid destruction of parasites and release of bacterial symbionts. Adults are also gradually eliminated avoiding the development of inflammatory nodules sometimes seen with rapid death of adult worms following treatment with DEC or ivermectin. In addition, doxycycline eliminates *Wolbachia* surface protein, the inflammatory trigger for chronic disease. Use of doxycycline in the treatment of patients with LF has been shown to decrease plasma levels of lymphangiogenic factors, reduce dilation of lymphatic vessels, improve lymphoedema and reduce hydrocoele.

Treatment of individual patients

1 Provided the patient does not have a high *L. loa* microfilaraemia, the treatment options are as follows:
   (a) In the absence of coinfection with onchocerciasis, if patient continues to live in a LF endemic area, or is less than 9 years of age: DEC 6 mg/kg (+/- albendazole 400 mg) single dose treatment or a 12-day course of DEC 6 mg/kg per day.
   (b) If coinfection with onchocerciasis is present or possible: doxycycline 200 mg/day for 4–6 weeks followed by ivermectin 150–400 µg/kg.
2 If the patient has a high *L. loa* microfilaraemia: doxycycline 200 mg/day for 4 weeks.

If coinfection with *L. loa* is present, particularly if associated with a high *Loa* microfilaraemia, it is essential to reduce the microfilaraemia using albendazole prior to treatment with DEC or ivermectin. This is discussed in more detail in the section on *L. loa*.

Prevention of morbidity

Lymphoedema management involves measures to assist lymph flow including elevation, massage, exercise and bandaging of affected limbs. Elevation of the limb with massage and compression bandaging to reduce oedema is useful but is often not tolerated in the humid tropics. Doxycycline 200 mg/day for 6 weeks is also recommended for previously untreated patients.

Prevention of acute inflammatory episodes is focussed on preventing secondary bacterial infection. Careful hygiene, use of disinfectant soap and water and general skin care including early and effective treatment of any wounds or abrasions should be encouraged. Antibiotic prophylaxis with penicillin is useful if there are recurrent streptococcal infections. Surgical treatment of limb elephantiasis is not straightforward, leaves scars and is often unavailable to poor people.

Hydrocoele should be managed surgically. Doxycycline 200 mg/day for 6 weeks is also recommended for previously untreated patients.

Tropical pulmonary eosinophilia should be treated with doxycycline 200 mg/day for 4 weeks followed by ivermectin.

Control

WHO launched the Global Programme to Eliminate Lymphatic Filariasis (GPELF) in 2000. The goal is to eliminate lymphatic filariasis as a public-health problem by 2020. GPELF, APOC and OEPA implement the WHO strategy of Preventive Chemotherapy and Transmission control (PCT). PCT is a pro-poor approach built around the utilization of donated drugs. During 2000–10, over 3.4 billion treatments were delivered to a targeted population of 900 million people.

The Global Alliance for the Elimination of Lymphatic Filariasis (GAELF), was created in 2000 to support GPELF in fundraising, advocacy, communications and technical assistance. GAELF is an international public–private partnership that involving national ministries, academic institutions, NGOs, WHO, UNICEF, World Bank, donors and development agencies. Two major drug companies have been instrumental in the development of this initiative. In 1997 GlaxoSmithKline (GSK) agreed to donate albendazole for as long as it is needed to eliminate LF as a public health problem. In 1998, Merck & Co. Inc. agreed to provide ivermectin for LF in Africa in coendemic (onchocerciasis and LF) countries in association with GSK's albendazole donation for as long as necessary.

The GPELF strategy is based on two key components:

- **Mass drug administration (MDA).** Annual large-scale administration of a single dose of albendazole (400 mg) with either ivermectin (150–200 µg/kg) in areas where onchocerciasis is also coendemic, or with DEC (6 mg/kg) in areas where onchocerciasis is not endemic. MDA must be continued for 4–6 years to fully interrupt transmission. By 2010, 59 endemic countries had completed mapping, and 53 had implemented MDA, 37 of which had already completed five or more rounds of MDA in at least some of their endemic areas.

Exclusive use of DEC fortified salt for 1–2 years formed the basis for the highly successful LF elimination programme in China. However, this approach has proven challenging in other settings.

- **Morbidity management and disability prevention.** Clinical severity of lymphoedema and acute inflammatory episodes can be reduced by simple measures of hygiene, skin care, exercise, and elevation of affected limbs. The GPELF focuses on training health-care workers and communities to dispense proper care and treatment. Hydrocoele can be managed surgically.

By 2010, over 3.4 billion treatments had been delivered to a target population of almost 900 million individuals in 53 of the 81 endemic countries. Transmission of LF in at-risk populations has fallen by 43% in 10 years and the estimated economic benefit of the programme was at least US$ 24 billion for the period 2000–07.

Priorities for the second decade include the following.

1 Implementing MDA in the remaining 18 endemic countries. Many have fragile infrastructures and are in conflict or post-conflict situations. In Africa, at least 10 of these countries are coendemic for *L. loa,* which presents safety challenges when delivering MDA using currently recommended regimens.
2 Scaling up programmes to achieve full geographical coverage especially in the high-burden countries and urban environments.
3 Managing chronic morbidity more effectively. Only 33% of endemic countries had active morbidity-management programmes by 2010.

Table 14.1 summarizes individual and community chemotherapy of LF.

Vector control

LF is transmitted by five different mosquito genera: *Anopheles, Aedes, Culex, Mansonia* and *Ochlerotatus.* The different vectors have differing breeding, biting and resting characteristics.

Vector control is recommended as a possible strategy in:

1 some areas that are coendemic for *L. loa;*
2 countries where the disease burden is heaviest (e.g. Bangladesh, India, Indonesia, DRC and Nigeria) and which need to rapidly scale up MDA;
3 Pacific Island countries, where interruption of local transmission has been achieved but there is limited experience in preventing recurrence.

Where possible, malaria and LF vector control should be integrated. In appropriate circumstances, time to elimination of LF by MDA may be significantly reduced by the following vector control measures.

1 In areas of nocturnally periodic transmission, insecticide-impregnated mosquito nets can be used to protect against night-biting mosquitoes.
2 Control of mosquito breeding is helpful, particularly in towns. For example, treatment of enclosed bodies of water with a floating layer of expanded polystyrene beads can prevent mosquito breeding for at least 5 years.

Loiasis

Loa loa (the 'eye worm') is transmitted by 'red' flies of the genus *Chrysops* that inhabit tropical forests of Africa. Larvae migrate subcutaneously, maturing into 3–7 cm long adult worms over the course of about a year. Adults may survive for more than 15 years. Female worms produce microfilariae which periodically appear in the peripheral blood and can survive for up to two years. Symptoms are mainly attributable to the adult worm and include urticaria, pruritis, arthralgia and malaise. Subconjunctival migration causes intense pain and inflammation. If local anaesthetic and suitable surgical instruments are immediately available (and you and your patient are feeling brave) the worm can be removed from the eye. Trauma to the migrating adult worm, most commonly on the extremities, may provoke a localized inflammatory reaction known as Calabar swelling. Neurological complications, including a potentially fatal meningoencephalitis, are more likely to occur in patients with high microfilaraemia, particularly following the administration of anthelmintics. Proteinuria is relatively common and haematuria may also occur. Pulmonary infiltrates, pleural effusions, arthritis, lymphangitis and hydrocoele have also been described. Hypereosinophilia is common and *L. loa* has been implicated in the aetiology of endomyocardial fibrosis (EMF), although EMF is also described in association with numerous other causes of hypereosinophilia.

Diagnosis and treatment

Diagnosis may be obvious from the history, particularly if an 'eye worm' has made an appearance. Dead, calcified worms may be incidental findings on X-ray. Peripheral blood microfilaraemia peaks between 10.00 hrs and 15.00 hrs and the characteristic sheathed microfilariae measuring 250–300 μm in length can be identified in thick blood films using Giemsa or Wright stains. Concentration techniques may be helpful if films are negative. A quantative microfilarial load should be estimated as this may be useful in predicting the likelihood of an adverse reaction to treatment. Probable cases of *Loa*-related encephalopathy are defined based on threshold values for *Loa* microfilarial loads of >10 000 Mf/mL if measured before ivermectin treatment, or >1000 Mf/mL if sampled after treatment. Patients with pre-treatment microfilarial loads > 30 000 Mf/mL are at greatest risk of encephalopathy; however serious adverse effects may occur at lower levels and caution is advisable in all patients with pre-treatment microfilarial loads > 2500 Mf/mL.

Serological tests are available and may be helpful for diagnosis in travellers from endemic areas, but lack specificity and cross react with other filarial parasites and strongyloides.

Loiasis is commonly treated with DEC 2 mg/kg orally three times daily for 7–10 days. DEC has an effect on both adult worms and microfilariae. Treatment is repeated every two to three months if symptoms remain. Ivermectin 150 μg/kg as a single dose prior to treatment with DEC reduces the likelihood of a Mazzotti reaction in patients coinfected with onchocerciasis. However, treatment with DEC or ivermectin may be hazardous in patients with loiasis who have high microfilarial loads (> 2500 Mf/mL) because massive release of antigens from dying microfilariae may precipitate meningoencephalitis or renal failure. In the past, plasmapheresis has been used to reduce heavy microfilarial loads prior to treatment with DEC under steroid cover. The currently preferred strategy for managing patients with high microfilaraemia is administration of albendazole 200 mg twice daily for three weeks to gradually reduce the microfilaraemia, followed by a course of DEC or ivermectin. Prednisolone 20 mg/day, given for three days before and for three days following the start of anthelmintic treatment, may reduce the risk of encephalopathy.

Rapid Assessment Procedures for Loiasis (RAPLOA) have been developed to identify communities in Africa where individuals may be at high risk of severe adverse reactions to ivermectin. The RAPLOA development study found that the eye worm is well known in *L. loa* endemic areas and there was a clear relationship between the percentage of community members that reported a history of eye worm and the community prevalence of loiasis. A prevalence threshold of 40% was a good indicator of high-risk communities, i.e. communities where the prevalence of *L. loa* microfilaraemia was > 20%, the prevalence of high microfilarial loads (defined as > 8000 Mf/mL) was greater than 5%, or the prevalence of very high microfilarial loads (defined as > 30 000 Mf/mL) was greater than 2%.

RAPLOA has been validated as a highly sensitive and specific method for detecting high-risk communities.

Three simple questions are used in screening people aged 15 years and above:

1 Have you ever experienced or noticed worms moving along the white part of your eye?

After recording the response, the interviewer then shows a photograph of the eye worm to each respondent, guiding him/her to recognize the worm in the eye. Care should be taken to ensure that there is no confusion between eye worm and veins in the eye.

2 Have you ever had the condition in this picture?

After recording the response, the interviewer proceeds to ask the third question.

3 The last time you had this condition, how long did the worm stay before disappearing?

The respondent is classified as having a history of eye worm if the answers to the first two questions are 'yes' and the duration in question three is less than 8 days.

The Central province of Cameroon is the main focus for this problem. High-risk foci are currently excluded from ivermectin MDA programmes for the control of onchocerciasis and LF.

 SUMMARY

- Onchocerciasis, filariasis and loasis are filarial worm infections which are widely distributed in the tropics.

- Onchocerciasis or 'river blindness', is caused by *Onchocerca volvulus* transmitted by *Simulium* flies. It leads to complex skin and eye syndromes, but control programmes have greatly reduced numbers affected.

- Filariasis may be 'Wuchererian' or 'Bancroftian' and can lead to debilitating lymphoedema or elephantiasis. Mass drug administration (MDA) programmes are increasingly used to control onchocerciasis and filariasis.

- *Loa loa* (the 'Eye Worm') is characterized by visible subconjunctival adult worms. It is treated with diethylcarbamazine, ivermectin or albendazole, depending on the level of microfilaraemia.

Visit www.lecturenoteseries.com/tropicalmed to test yourself on this chapter using interactive MCQs.

FURTHER READING

Addis DG, Brady MA (2007) Morbidity management in the Global Programme to Eliminate Lymphatic Filariasis: a review of the scientific literature. *Filaria Jl* **6**: 2. [This review covers the major clinical manifestations of LF with specific reference to pathogenesis, epidemiology, economic and social impact, individual treatment and impact of mass treatment.]

Boatin BA, Richards FO (2006) Control of onchocerciasis. *Adv Parasitol* **61**: 349–94. [Detailed review describing epidemiological, biological, clinical and public health aspects of onchocerciasis.]

Hoerauf A (2006) New strategies to combat filariasis. *Expert Rev Anti Infect Ther* **4**: 211–22. [Comprehensive review including recent developments in the understanding of the pathogenesis of LF and onchocerciasis and providing clear guidelines for treatment.]

Johnston KL, Taylor MJ (2007) *Wolbachia* in filarial parasites: targets for filarial infection and disease control. *Curr Infect Dis Rep* **9**: 55–9. [Recent work on *Wolbachia* has revolutionized our understanding of the pathogenesis of filarial infections and has opened the door to novel approaches to treatment using antibiotics.]

Lancet Neglected Tropical Diseases Series (2010) http://www.thelancet.com/series/neglected-tropical-diseases [Reviews elimination and control programmes for lymphatic filariasis, onchocerciasis, schistosomiasis, and soil-transmitted helminthiasis, and describes the effect, governance arrangements, and financing mechanisms of selected international control initiatives.]

Molyneux D (2005) Onchocerciasis control and elimination: coming of age in resource-constrained health systems. *Trends Parasitol* **21**: 525–9. [Excellent description of the remarkable achievements in onchocerciasis control over the past four decades.]

Tamarozzi F, Halliday A, Gentil K, Hoerauf A, Pearlman E, Taylor MJ (2011) Onchocerciasis: the role of Wolbachia bacterial endosymbionts in parasite biology, disease pathogenesis, and treatment. *Clin Microbiol Rev* **24**: 459–68. [If you want to find out more about oncho and Wolbachia, this is the paper for you.]

Taylor M, Hoerauf A, Bockarie M (2010) Lymphatic filariasis and onchocerciasis. *Lancet* **376**: 1175–85. [Lancet Seminar provides up-to-date information on recent advances in our understanding of the pathogenesis of these diseases and the considerable progress that has been made in strategies for treatment and control.]

WHO (2011) *Progress Report 2000–2009 and Strategic Plan 2010–2020 of the Global Programme to Eliminate Lymphatic Filariasis: Halfway towards Eliminating Lymphatic Filariasis.* [Record of achievements to date and encouraging future prospects.]

15

African trypanosomiasis

David Lalloo
Liverpool School of Tropical Medicine

African trypanosomiasis is caused by species of *Trypanosoma brucei*. There are three morphologically identical parasite species:

1 *T. brucei brucei*, confined to domestic and wild animals;
2 *T. brucei gambiense*, causing gambiense sleeping sickness in West and Central Africa;
3 *T. brucei rhodesiense*, causing rhodesiense sleeping sickness in East and Southern Africa.

Transmission is by the bite of tsetse flies (members of the genus *Glossina*) and the flies are only found in Africa. In general, the infected areas are found south of the Sahara and north of the Zambezi (Fig. 15.1).

Parasites

The parasites are flattened and fusiform in shape, like slender pointed leaves, 12–35 µm long and 1.5–3.5 µm broad. They are actively motile, using a thin finlike extension from the main body, the undulating membrane, to propel themselves. The form of the parasite found in humans is the trypomastigote, in which the kinetoplast is posterior to the nucleus, and from which the flagellum arises. The flagellum runs along the free edge of the undulating membrane and usually projects in front of it, sometimes extending as far again as the creature's body.

Life-cycle

This is the same for both species. Trypomastigotes from the infected host are taken up by the tsetse fly during a blood meal. In the stomach of the fly the parasites multiply by simple fission, penetrate the gut wall and migrate to the salivary glands. There the morphology changes, the kinetoplast coming to lie just in front of the nucleus, and the parasites are now called epimastigotes (crithidia). The infective trypomastigote (the metacyclic trypanosome) is found in the saliva about 20 days after the original infecting blood meal, and the fly remains infective throughout its normal lifespan of several months.

Disease

Local effects

Metacyclic trypanosomes injected during tsetse feeding multiply in the extracellular space and lymphatics before becoming disseminated by the bloodstream. This local multiplication may cause a marked inflammatory reaction – the trypanosomal chancre.

The trypanosomal chancre appears 3 or more days after the bite and typically increases in size for 2 or 3 weeks, at the end of which time it begins to regress. The presence of a chancre is much more common in *T. b. rhodesiense* infection than in *T. b. gambiense* infection. Local lymphadenopathy may be found in the region of a bite.

Systemic effects

Multiplication of trypanosomes in the lymphatics leads to parasitaemia 5–12 days after the bite (haemolymphatic or early stage). Waves of parasitaemia are associated with fever. Parasites may then enter the central nervous system (CNS) via the choroid plexus or by transcytosis across endothelial cells to cause a lymphocytic meningoencephalitis (late stage).

Tropical Medicine Lecture Notes, Seventh edition. Edited by Nick Beeching and Geoff Gill. © 2014 John Wiley & Sons, Ltd. Published 2014 by John Wiley & Sons, Ltd.

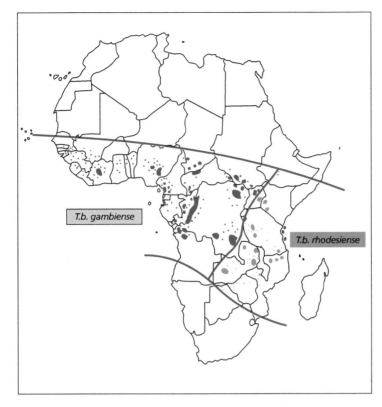

Figure 15.1 Distribution of human African trypanosomiasis.

In general, *T. b. gambiense* is better adapted to the human host than is *T. b. rhodesiense*. *Trypanosoma brucei gambiense* is therefore relatively well tolerated; the illness it causes tends to be subacute or chronic and parasitaemia may even be asymptomatic. In contrast, *T. b. rhodesiense* is normally a zoonotic infection which is transmitted to humans 'accidentally'. It causes pronounced systemic effects; parasitaemia usually causes severe incapacity and the course of the illness is relatively rapid.

Immune response and pathogenesis

The main response to trypanosomal infection is antibody production, particularly IgM. Antibody production initially controls parasitaemia, but antigenic variation in parasite surface antigens means that immune control is incomplete and this leads to successive waves of parasitaemia, which may explain the fluctuating nature of the illness. In the brain and other organs (e.g. heart or serous membranes), perivascular infiltration with lymphocytes, plasma cells and macrophages and characteristic morular cells occurs.

Microglial and astrocyte proliferation may be associated with neuronal destruction and demyelination in the brain.

Clinical picture

Trypanosoma brucei gambiense

Early stage

Fever, headache and joint pains are the main early symptoms, sometimes accompanied by fleeting areas of cutaneous oedema. A small proportion of patients with parasitaemia are asymptomatic. Lymph glands become enlarged, the most prominent glands often being in the posterior triangle of the neck (Winterbottom's sign). Odd skin rashes sometimes occur (visible only in relatively unpigmented skins), usually taking the form of areas of circinate erythema. There may be generalized pruritus, and characteristic thickening of the facial tissues giving a sad or strangely expressionless appearance. The spleen enlarges to a moderate size in many cases.

This early stage usually lasts many months, sometimes even over 2 years. Occasionally, patients with *T. b. gambiense* develop a rapidly progressive toxaemic disease that is fatal before the CNS is involved. However, most deaths occur after CNS invasion unless the patient develops an intercurrent infection.

Late stage symptoms and signs

Symptoms and signs of disturbed cerebral function predominate. Behavioural changes are common: a patient whose personal habits were previously fastidious becomes careless about appearance; his or her speech becomes coarse and temper unpredictable and he or she may behave in a socially unacceptable way. Psychiatric manifestations of agitation or delusions may become severe enough to mimic mania or schizophrenia. Sleep becomes disordered in that the patient sleeps badly at night but falls asleep during the day.

In the early evolution of this change, the patient can be readily awoken and responds by conversing fairly normally. As time goes by, sleeping periods may become longer until the patient is sleeping most of the time, and may even fall asleep while eating. At this stage, speech and motor functions in general are usually severely disturbed. Weight loss may occur because of inadequate nutrition unless the family makes strenuous efforts to help with feeding.

Focal CNS signs may develop, but there is usually more diffuse evidence of CNS disease, especially relating to extrapyramidal and cerebellar functions: widespread tremors involving the limbs, tongue and head, spasticity (mainly of the lower limbs), ataxia and sometimes choreiform movements. Convulsions are relatively uncommon. Kérandel's sign (delayed hyperaesthesia) may occur; following firm pressure on the tissues overlying a bone, there is a definite delay before the patient shows any sign of pain. In advanced cases, the tendon reflexes are often grossly exaggerated and the plantar responses may be extensor. Death usually occurs within a few months of CNS involvement becoming manifest, but may be delayed for up to a year.

Trypanosoma brucei rhodesiense

Symptoms and signs

The parasite usually produces a more acute and virulent infection than does *T. b. gambiense*, with prominent fever and systemic symptoms. Serous effusions, especially pleural and pericardial, are common and myocarditis occurs. In the early stages, *T. b. rhodesiense* may cause hepatocellular jaundice and

mild anaemia, and severe anaemia may soon develop. Both liver and spleen may be slightly enlarged, and lymph gland enlargement (seldom so prominent as in *T. b. gambiense*) is most common in the inguinal, axilliary and epitrochlear glands. *T. b. rhodesiense* may be fatal within a few weeks of the onset, often as a result of death from myocarditis before the CNS is involved.

The picture in the late stage of *T. b. rhodesiense* infection is much like that of *T. b. gambiense* but occurs early in the course of the disease and is more rapidly progressive. Clinical features of CNS involvement are similar to *T. b. gambiense*, but death is more rapid and neurological features are more pronounced than behavioural changes.

Diagnosis

Early stage disease

The diagnosis is usually made by demonstration of parasites. A number of methods may be used.

1 Examination of stained or unstained thick blood films. Films can be stained with a Romanowsky stain as for malaria or be examined wet (simply place a coverslip over a drop of blood) when the disturbance of the red cells produced by the movement of the trypanosomes can be detected using a dry $40 \times$ objective (Fig. 15.2).

2 Concentration methods are used to detect scanty parasitaemia, including microscopy of the buffy coat following centrifugation using the microhaematocrit (MHCT), the more sensitive quantitative buffy coat (QBC) technique and the minianion exchange column technique (MAEC). Microscopy

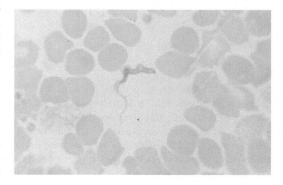

Figure 15.2 Parasite of *T.b. rhodesiense* in the blood film of a severely ill Zambian adult.

is most useful for *T. b. rhodesiense* infection. The organisms may also be isolated by inoculation into special culture media or into animals.

3 Gland puncture. This is of most use in *T. b. gambiense*; posterior cervical lymphadenopathy is common and gland aspirates may be positive when there is no peripheral parasitaemia. A needle is inserted into an enlarged node held between thumb and finger. The flow of gland juice can be improved by massaging the gland while the needle is *in situ*. The juice is then expressed on to a slide, using a syringe containing air, and examined immediately.

4 Bone marrow aspiration. This is useful in the early stages when other methods are negative.

5 The chancre. Trypanosomes can be recovered by aspiration from the chancre or from the regional glands draining the chancre if they are enlarged, before the blood is positive.

In *T. b. gambiense*, trypanosomes may be difficult to find in the blood, especially in late infections. The longer the duration of infection, the more difficult it is to find trypanosomes.

Late stage disease (CNS involvement)

This may be diagnosed clinically on the basis of neurological signs but cerebrospinal fluid (CSF) examination should be performed in all patients following one or two doses of suramin or pentamidine to clear parasitaemia (and hence reduce the risk of parasites being introduced into the CSF from the blood). The deposit from 5–10 mL of centrifuged fluid should be examined as soon as possible for motile trypanosomes or made into a smear, dried, fixed and stained with a Romanowsky stain. Late stage disease is diagnosed by the presence of trypanosomes in the CSF or by a raised CSF cell count (>5/mm^3) or increased protein level.

Immunological diagnostic methods

A number of serological methods are available. The card agglutination test for trypanosomes (CATT) is simple to carry out, and gives good results in most areas of *T. b. gambiense* but is of no value in *T. b. rhodesiense*. It is a valuable test for screening populations as the results are obtained within 30 min. Disadvantages include limited sensitivity and specificity of the antigen, as trypanosomes share antigens with several other protozoa and bacteria. The card indirect agglutination test for trypanosomes (CIATT) detects circulating antigens and has been used for the diagnosis of both *T. b. gambiense* and *T. b. rhodesiense*. This technique may also be useful to follow responses after treatment. Positive serological tests should be confirmed parasitologically before treatment.

Routine laboratory findings

A mild normochromic anaemia is common. The white blood count (WBC) is usually normal, but the erythrocyte sedimentation rate (ESR) is usually above 50 mm/h and sometimes over 100 mm/h. Serum and CSF IgM levels are usually very high.

Treatment

A number of different drugs have activity against trypanosomes. Most are relatively toxic and there is an urgent need for the development of new drugs for the treatment of sleeping sickness. Not all drugs penetrate the CSF and different drugs are therefore used for the treatment of early and late stage disease. It is important to treat coexisting infections and anaemia prior to using specific treatment: many advocate routine antihelminth and antimalarial therapy.

Early Trypanosoma brucei gambiense and Trypanosoma brucei rhodesiense infections

Suramin is the drug of choice for treating first stage *T. b. rhodesiense* infection. It is also effective in *T. b. gambiense* but pentamidine is now most commonly used to treat early *T. b. gambiense* infection. Neither of these drugs penetrate the CSF.

Suramin is administered intravenously. Following a test dose of 5 mg/kg on day 1, 20 mg/kg (max 1 g) should be given on days 3, 10, 17, 24 and 31. Suramin is usually well tolerated, but fever, nausea and proteinuria may occur. Infrequent idiosyncratic anaphylactic reactions also occur. Pentamidine can be given intramuscularly or intravenously; intravenous administration avoids painful local tissue reactions. Normal doses are 4 mg/kg/day for 7–10 days. The major reaction is syncope and hypotension; hypoglycaemia may also occur.

Late stage disease

Melarsoprol can be used for the treatment of late stage *T. b. gambiense* and *T. b. rhodesiense* infections. Eflornithine is only effective in *T. b. gambiense*.

Melarsoprol is a trivalent arsenic compound that is given intravenously and is active against blood, tissue and CNS trypanosomes. There are many different treatment schedules but it is normally administered as three or four series of three injections separated by 7 days at doses that range from 1.2 to 3.6 mg/kg (see Table 15.1 for commonly used schedule). Recent studies suggest that shorter 10-day courses (2.2 mg/kg daily) may be as effective for *T. b. gambiense*. Melarsoprol therapy is normally preceded by 1–2 doses of suramin to clear blood, lymph and tissue trypanosomes.

Melarsoprol is a toxic drug. The major side-effect is a serious encephalopathy (reactive arsenical encephalopathy), which occurs with a frequency of 2–10% and a case fatality rate of up to 50%. The danger of severe toxic effects is minimized by improving the patient's general condition, as already described. Prophylactic corticosteroids reduces the risk of an encephalopathy in *T. b. gambiense*. Other side-effects include peripheral neuropathy.

Eflornithine is used intravenously for the treatment of late stage *T. b. gambiense* infection at a dosage of 400 mg/kg/day in divided doses for 14 days. It is relatively expensive and difficult to administer but less toxic than melarsoprol. The common side-effects (gastrointestinal symptoms and anaemia) do not usually require treatment to be stopped.

Nifurtimox is a drug that has traditionally been used in Chagas, disease. Combining nifurtimox with eflornithing for treating *T. b. gambiense* allows simplification of the eflornithine regimen whilst maintaining efficacy and improving tolerability.

Monitoring cure

Patient symptoms should resolve after treatment. Despite the severity of the symptoms in advanced late cases, the degree of functional recovery after successful chemotherapy is remarkable. It may take 6 months or more for the CSF cell counts to fall below 5/mL and for normal protein concentrations to occur. Failure of these parameters to become normal may be the first indication that treatment has been unsuccessful. Full cure cannot be assumed unless a 2-year follow-up has been completed. If treatment of patients with CNS involvement has been delayed, a variable degree of neurological defect will persist. This most commonly takes the form of intellectual impairment.

Relapse

Treatment of relapse can sometimes be difficult. Relapse in *T. b. gambiense* following treatment with suramin or pentamidine is often treated with melarsoprol; eflornithine can also be used. Relapse in *T. b. rhodesiense* is usually treated with a second course of melarsoprol.

Epidemiology

Control efforts have led to a considerable reduction in the number of cases over the last fifteen years. Approximately 10 000 cases of sleeping sickness are now notified to the World Health Organization (WHO) each year; it is estimated that approximately 30 000 individuals are infected. Over 90% of cases are due to *T. b. gambiense* infection. A lack of resources and civil conflict in many of the heavily affected areas has led to an increase in cases as previously successful control programmes have broken down; more than 70% of all reported cases occur in the DRC.

Trypanosoma brucei gambiense infection

Humans are the most important reservoir of infection, although the pig and other animals are naturally infected in some parts of West Africa. Infection is spread from human to human by the bite of

Table 15.1 **Typical classical treatment schedule for an adult with late-stage *T. b. rhodesiense*.**

Day	Drug	Volume (ml)	Dose (mg/kg)
1	Suramin	2.5	5
3		5.0	10
4	Melarsoprol	0.5	0.36
5		1.0	0.72
6		1.5	1.1
14	Melarsoprol	2.0	1.4
15		2.5	1.8
16		3.0	2.2
23	Melarsoprol	3.5	2.2
24		4.0	2.9
25		5.0	3.6
31	Melarsoprol	5.0	3.6
32		5.0	3.6
33		5.0	3.6

riverine tsetse flies (*palpalis* group), which breed along the banks of rivers and lakes. Infection tends to occur where human activities bring humans into contact with the fly, such as at river crossings and sites used for the collection of water, and when fishermen come into contact with flies on the river or lake shores. Village-sized and larger outbreaks occur, sometimes amounting to epidemics. The spread of epidemics tends to be linear, following the distribution of flies along the course of rivers, or affecting islands in lakes.

Trypanosoma brucei rhodesiense infection

Trypanosoma brucei rhodesiense is usually a zoonotic infection in members of the antelope family, especially the bushbuck. It can be maintained as a zoonosis in the animal population in the absence of human cases, and is transmitted by tsetse species dwelling in savannah and woodland habitats (*morsitans* group). It is a particular hazard to those who spend long periods in enzootic areas in pursuit of their livelihood, such as hunters and honey-gatherers. Rarely, infection can occur in tourists visiting game parks.

Although *T. b. rhodesiense* cases tend to be sporadic, epidemics do occur, especially in East Africa around Lake Victoria. In these epidemics tsetse populations build up adjacent to human populations containing active cases. Domestic cattle are infected, develop a chronic parasitaemia and act as a reservoir host. The current epidemic in South-East Uganda is caused by peridomestic breeding *Glossina fuscipes* in thickets of the exotic plant *Lantana camora*.

Sleeping sickness control and surveillance

There are two major components of sleeping sickness control:

1 detection and treatment of cases;
2 vector control.

In *T. b. rhodesiense* areas, patients who present with symptoms of early parasitaemia (passive surveillance) can be treated at local rural centres: in epidemics, rapid deployment of active surveillance using blood film screening and the establishment of effective local treatment centres is important. In

T. b. gambiense areas, limited clinical symptoms in the early stages require active surveillance. Individuals can be screened using gland aspiration or rapid antigen tests (e.g. CATT).

Vector control is best achieved using insecticide-impregnated traps and targets. Sterile insect release methods may also be useful in reducing vector populations. Residual insecticide application to *Glossina* resting sites, insecticide spraying and the clearing of riverine habitat have been used in the past but resource and environmental considerations means that these can no longer be considered. In epidemic situations, treatment of the cattle reservoir by cattle trypanocides may also be a strategy for prevention of human sleeping sickness.

In all endemic areas the disease should be made notifiable to a central trypanosomiasis control unit. Specialized staff can then be sent promptly to the area and steps taken (such as active case finding and treatment) to prevent the development of an epidemic. This strategy has proved very effective in the past in Ghana, Nigeria and Uganda.

 SUMMARY

- Human African trypanosomiasis is caused by the protozoan parasites *Trypanosoma brucei gambiense* (the 'Gambian' form) and *T. brucei rhodesiense* (the 'Rhodesian' form).

- The disease is caught by tsetse fly bites. Local chancre, lymphadenopathy and fever are typical, with later central nervous system (CNS) involvement.

- The infection is slow and indolent in the *gambiense* form, but more severe and progressive in *rhodesiense* infection.

- Treatment is with suramin, and melarsoprol for CNS disease. Eflornithine is effective and less toxic, but can only be used in *gambiense* infections.

 Visit www.lecturenoteseries.com/tropicalmed **to test yourself on this chapter using interactive MCQs.**

📖 FURTHER READING

Blum J, Schmid C, Burri C (2006) Clinical aspects of 2541 patients with second stage human African trypanosomiasis. *Acta Trop* **97**: 55–64. [A comprehensive clinical description.]

Brun R, Blum J, Chappuis F, Burri C (2010) Human African trypanosomiasis. *Lancet* **375**: 148–59. [Excellent overview and source reference.]

Fèvre EM, Picozzi K, Jannin J, Welburn SC, Maudlin I (2006) Human African trypanosomiasis: epidemiology and control. *Adv Parasitol* **61**: 167–221. [A comprehensive review.]

World Health Organization (1998) *Control and Surveillance of African Trypanosomiasis*. Technical Report Series no. 881. Geneva: World Health Organization. [Advice on treatment and surveillance.]

16

South American trypanosomiasis (Chagas' disease)

David Lalloo
Liverpool School of Tropical Medicine

Parasite, life-cycle and pathogenesis

South American trypanosomiasis occurs in humans and a large number of wild and domestic animals and is widespread in Central and South America. It is caused by *Trypanosoma cruzi*, which differs from trypomastigotes of the *T. brucei* group in having a large kinetoplast. Trypanosomes in the blood of the mammalian host are taken up by triatomine bugs (reduviid, assassin bug, kissing bugs), which bite at night. All stages feed on blood but only adult bugs can fly. Organisms multiply in the hindgut of the bug as epimastigotes and develop into metacyclic trypanosomes which are excreted in the faeces of the bug during feeding. Infection is acquired by rubbing faeces of the bug into a wound or conjunctiva; infection can also be acquired by transfusion or congenital infection, or by ingesting fruit juices contaminated by triatomine bugs.

In the host, trypomastigotes multiply at the site of the bite, enter the bloodstream and enter a variety of tissue cells, particularly neuroglia and muscle cells. Parasites develop as intracellular amastigotes and form pseudocysts: rupture of these pseudocysts causes inflammation, tissue damage and further dissemination. Most pathological effects are chronic, probably related to a combination of tissue damage, neuronal loss and an autoimmune response.

Clinical features

Acute Chagas' disease

This is most common in children but may occur at any age: only one-third of individuals are symptomatic. Penetration and local multiplication of the parasite at the site of entry may cause an area of cutaneous oedema (chagoma) or orbital oedema (Romaña's sign) if entry is via the conjunctiva. A febrile reaction may occur 1–2 weeks later with the development of lymphadenopathy, hepatomegaly and splenomegaly. Rarely, death may occur at this stage as a result of cardiac damage or meningoencephalitis, especially in children. If symptomatic, the acute phase lasts for 1–3 months and resolves spontaneously.

In untreated patients, asymptomatic low-level parasitaemia may continue for many years: (indeterminate phase); 15–40% of patients will develop chronic Chagas' disease.

Chronic Chagas' disease

Chronic disease normally occurs 10–20 years after initial infection. Classical manifestations are as follows.

1 Cardiac disease. Biventricular cardiomyopathy or cardiac rhythm disturbance (often heart block).

Tropical Medicine Lecture Notes, Seventh edition. Edited by Nick Beeching and Geoff Gill. © 2014 John Wiley & Sons, Ltd. Published 2014 by John Wiley & Sons, Ltd.

2 Mega-oesophagus or megacolon as a result of destruction of the intramural parasympathetic nerve plexus. This presents as aspiration pneumonia or intractable constipation and abdominal distension.

3 Similar mega disorders of other hollow muscular viscera such as small bowel and ureter may occur resulting from nerve damage.

Immunocompromise

HIV infection or the use of immunosuppressive drugs may lead to the reactivation of latent infection causing severe myocarditis or neurological problems.

Diagnosis

Parasitological techniques

1 *Microscopy*. In the acute phase, parasites can usually be easily found on thick or thin films; centrifugation techniques increase the sensitivity.

2 *Culture*. Parasites can be cultured, but specific media and expertise are required.

3 *Xenodiagnosis*. Low-level parasitaemias can be detected by allowing uninfected bugs to feed on patients. Three to four weeks later, the bugs are dissected to look for gut infection.

4 *Biopsy*. Amastigotes may be demonstrated in pathological specimens.

Other techniques

IgM and life-long IgG responses may be detected by a number of techniques, including complement fixation test and ELISA. Cross-reactivity with other parasitic diseases and autoimmune disorders leads to poor specificity and diagnosis should be based upon at least two positive techniques. Serological tests often remain positive after parasitological cure. PCR is effective in acute infection but has limited utility in chronic disease.

Treatment

Acute stage

Nifurtimox and benznidazole suppress parasitaemia, shorten the course of the acute illness and prevent acute neurological and myocardial complications. Benznidazole is better tolerated. However, elimination of parasites and prevention of chronic disease only occurs in 50–80% of patients.

Indeterminate and chronic phase

Evaluation of the efficacy of treatment is difficult because of the limited reliability of tests for cure. Although treatment has traditionally been thought to have little effect in the intermediate phase, there is some evidence that benznidazole may be of benefit in clearing parasitaemia in some patients and may prevent progression to chronic disease. The value of parasitological treatment in chronic disease remains uncertain but may prevent progression-clinical trials are underway. Cardiac complications require symptomatic treatment and insertion of pacemakers is often necessary.

Epidemiology and control

Trypanosoma cruzi occur in a large number of mammalian species, but the most common wild hosts are rodents or small marsupials. Many species of triatomine bugs simply maintain infection amongst wild animals, but some species have become adapted to living in human dwellings, leading to human infection when infection is transmitted from domestic animals. A single adobe dwelling can harbour thousands of bugs and up to 50% of bugs may be infected. Chagas' disease can also be transmitted by transfusion and congenital infection occurs in up to 10% of seropositive women. Blood donations should be screened for evidence of infection.

Control of the disease can be achieved by the use of seroprevalence surveys to determine areas at risk and spraying of pyrethroid insecticides. Improvement in the standard of housing is also important. Elimination of cracks in mud walls or replacement of natural material roofing with iron sheets reduces available habitats for the bugs. In a number of South American countries, such activities have reduced the incidence of Chagas' disease by between 60 and 99% over the past 20 years.

SUMMARY

- *Trypanosoma cruzi* infections are transmitted by reduviid bugs. Acute infection may lead to fever, swelling at the entry site, lymphadenopathy and sometimes hepatosplenomegaly.
- Chronic disease is more common and can lead to cardiomyopathy, or bowel motility disorders such as megacolon and mega-oesophagus.
- Diagnostic methods include blood films and culture in the acute phase, serology, tissue biopsy, and even xenodiagnosis.
- Treatment is difficult. Nifurtimox and benznidazole are partially effective, but are of uncertain value in chronic disease.

Visit www.lecturenoteseries.com/tropicalmed to test yourself on this chapter using interactive MCQs.

FURTHER READING

Bern C (2011) Antitrypanosomal therapy for chronic Chagas' disease *N Engl J Med* **364**: 2527–34. [A useful summary of current issues.]

Bern C, Montgomery SP, Herwaldt BL, Rassi A Jr, Marin-Neto JA, Dantas RO, Maguire JH, Acquatella H, Morillo C, Kirchhoff LV, Gilman RH, Reyes PA, Salvatella R, Moore AC (2007) Evaluation and treatment of Chagas disease in the United States: a systematic review. *JAMA*. **298**: 2171–81. [A systematic review of the evidence in Chagas.]

Prata A (2001) Clinical and epidemiological aspects of Chagas' disease. *Lancet Infect Dis* **1**: 92–100. [Good general review of South American trypanosomiasis.]

Rassi A, Rassi A, Little WC (2006). Development and validation of a risk score for predicting death in Chagas' Heart Disease. *New Engl J Med* **355**: 799–808. [Describes clinical risk score for the severity of Chagas' heart disease.]

17

Schistosomiasis

Bertie Squire and Russell Stothard
Liverpool School of Tropical Medicine

Schistosomiasis is often known as 'bilharzia' or 'bilharziasis' after Theodor Bilharz who first described the parasite in humans and found the adult flukes in a human postmortem in Egypt in 1851. Schistosome eggs have been recovered from both Chinese and Egyptian mummies, showing that the infection was present in both of these early civilizations. Today schistosomes remain distributed throughout the tropics and flourish wherever freshwater bodies, both natural and man-made, create habitats for the appropriate snail intermediate hosts.

Three main species of schistosome affect humans with different geographical distributions (Fig. 17.1).

1 *Schistosoma haematobium* causes urogenital schistosomiasis. It is scattered throughout Africa, parts of Arabia, the Near East, Madagascar and Mauritius.
2 *Schistosoma mansoni* is mainly found in Africa and Madagascar. It was exported by the slave trade to parts of South America, the Caribbean and Arabia, where permissive snail intermediate hosts were present.
3 *Schistosoma japonicum* is found in China, the Philippines and Sulawesi. There is also a small focus in the Mekong river on the east border of Thailand caused by *Schistosoma mekongi*.

Schistosoma mansoni and *S. japonicum* cause disease of the bowel and liver. *Schistosoma intercalatum* and sister species *Schistosoma guineensis* are minor species confined to West Africa. They inhabit the veins of the lower bowel and produces terminal-spined eggs.

Parasitology

The adult flukes causing human schistosomiasis are worm-like creatures 1–2 cm long which inhabit parts of the venous system of humans. The male worm resembles a rolled leaf in having a groove on his ventral surface in which the longer, more slender female is held *in copulo*. Both sexes are actively motile. The worms sometimes live for 30 years, but their normal lifespan is probably 3–7 years.

Life-cycle

Adult females lay (non)fertilized eggs in the terminal venules of the preferred host tissues (Fig. 17.2). Their bodies obstruct the vessel and so impede the escape of eggs into the circulation. Most of the eggs penetrate the vessel wall and enter the tissues. Movements of the walls of the hollow viscus involved (as well as other factors) propel the eggs towards the lumen, from which they escape to the outside world – in the urine in the case of *S. haematobium*, and in the stools in the case of *S. mansoni* and *S. japonicum*.

The shapes of the eggs of each species are distinctive, and each contains a ciliated miracidium. This hatches out in freshwater, and swims in search of a suitable snail intermediate host. Many species of snail host are known, but in general:

1 *Schistosoma haematobium* requires an aquatic sinistral turretted snail of the genus *Bulinus*;
2 *Schistosoma mansoni* requires a flat aquatic 'rams-horn' snail, most commonly of the genus *Biomphalaria*;
3 *Schistosoma japonicum* requires a small amphibious operculate turretted snail, usually of the genus *Oncomelania*.

The miracidium penetrates the body of the snail and begins a complicated asexual replicative cycle that results, a few weeks later, in the release of minute fork-tailed cercariae into the water. As cercariae are about 200–500 μm long, they are just visible to the naked eye. They emerge from the sporocyst inside

Tropical Medicine Lecture Notes, Seventh edition. Edited by Nick Beeching and Geoff Gill. © 2014 John Wiley & Sons, Ltd. Published 2014 by John Wiley & Sons, Ltd.

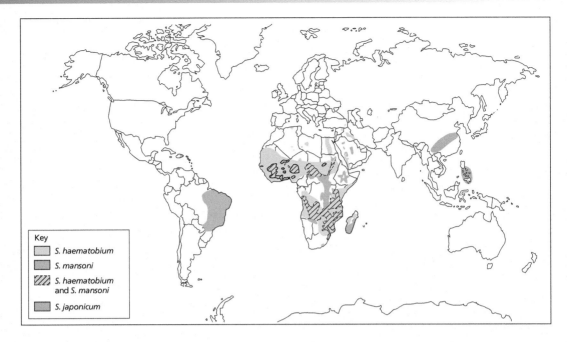

Figure 17.1 Global distribution of endemic schistosomiasis.

the snail in response to light. A snail may shed several hundred cercariae for many weeks. The cercaria is infective to the definitive host. If it finds no suitable host within 24–48 h, it dies. If it contacts human skin, however, the cercaria penetrates, sheds its tail and body, and enters the circulation with a new name – a schistosomulum. The schistosomulum reaches the liver through the lungs, by passive intravascular migration. Once in the liver, it begins to feed and grow, and in 1–3 months develops into a mature fluke in an intrahepatic portal vein. The mature males and females couple, and then migrate to their final habitats. It is easy to understand how *S. mansoni* and *S. japonicum* find the way to their homes in the lower mesenteric veins, as they have only to travel straight down the portal vein. However, it is still a mystery how *S. haematobium* eventually reaches the vesical plexus, probably via portosystemic anastomoses.

The time elapsing between cercarial penetration and the passage of eggs is the prepatent period. It can be as short as 4 weeks with *S. mansoni*, usually 12 or more weeks with *S. haematobium* and somewhere in between with *S. japonicum*. The prepatent period is sometimes very prolonged in light infections; perhaps if there are few worms in the liver, the sexes have difficulty finding each other.

Epidemiology

Magnitude of the problem

Some 300 million people are infected with schistosomes throughout the tropics, wherever freshwater bodies (particularly lakes, dams and irrigation systems) support large snail populations near concentrations of human habitation.

Requirements for transmission

1 Contamination of water with viable eggs from a reservoir host.
2 Presence in the water of susceptible snail intermediate hosts.
3 Suitable environmental conditions for development in the snail.
4 Human exposure to water containing cercariae.

Reservoir hosts

In all three schistosomes, humans are the main reservoir. Rodents, baboons, and primates may be able to maintain *S. mansoni* infection sometimes. By contrast, *S. japonicum* is more zoonotic, and many animals are

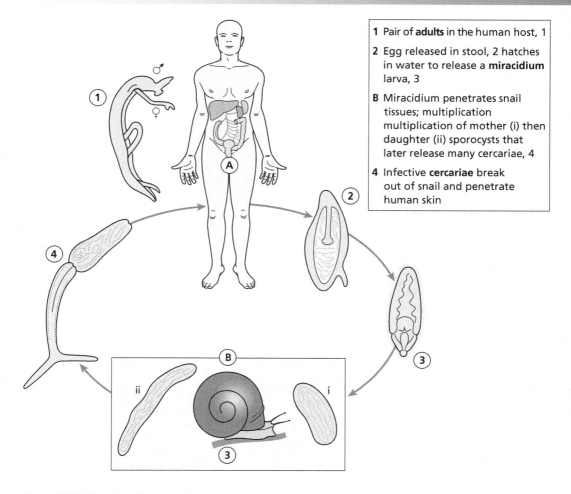

1 Pair of **adults** in the human host, 1

2 Egg released in stool, 2 hatches
in water to release a **miracidium**
larva, 3

B Miracidium penetrates snail
tissues; multiplication
multiplication of mother (i) then
daughter (ii) sporocysts that
later release many cercariae, 4

4 Infective **cercariae** break
out of snail and penetrate
human skin

Figure 17.2 Life-cycle of *S. mansoni*.

susceptible to infection, including farmed water buffalo and domestic animals such as the horse and dog.

Epidemiological patterns

In most infected communities, infection is most common and heaviest in children between 10 and 15 years old. Because children have the highest egg output and are more likely to contaminate water, they are usually the most important reservoir of infection. Exposure may be occupational, such as occurs among workers on irrigated farms and fishermen. Transmission is typically focal, and neighbouring villages may have greatly differing endemicities because of this.

Exposure and immunity

There is evidence that some degree of protective immunity to superinfection develops in schistosomiasis. It is certainly incomplete, and may depend for its maintenance on the continued presence of some living schistosomes in the body. It does not seem to be antibody-mediated, and is probably directed against the schistosomulum stage. The survival of adult worms in the circulation may be partly related to their ability to incorporate host antigens in their tegument (surface).

The log–normal distribution

In a population apparently exposed to a uniform risk of infection, some people will be found to be very heavily infected and others very lightly infected. If egg output is accepted as being related to the number of adult worms present, the distribution of worms in the population is not 'normal'. It will always be found that some of those infected have an infection with perhaps 100 times as many worms as those with the most common level of infection. If a frequency–distribution plot of egg output is carried out, the usual Gaussian curve will be seen to be distorted by having a greatly extended 'tail' to the right of the graph. The curve can be made to resemble a 'normal' curve if, instead of the egg count, the logarithm of the egg count is plotted on the x axis. This sort of distribution is called a log–normal distribution, and applies to the abundance of almost all non-replicative parasites in humans and animals.

There is no generally accepted explanation, but it could be related to the host's first exposure to infection. If the initial challenge was with a large number of parasites, at a time when no immunity existed, a large population could become established in the absence of immune opposition. On the other hand, if the first exposure was to a small number of parasites, the subsequent development of immunity could resist further infective challenges, and the total number of parasites would then remain low.

Infection in children

In hot countries, children naturally play in water. This recreational exposure is sometimes the most important source of infection but it should be remembered that infection can also take place soon after birth if domestic water supplies are contaminated with cercariae and used for infant bathing. At puberty, exposure often diminishes as modesty develops at the same time as sexual awareness. However, infection may still be acquired during activities such as personal bathing, washing clothes and utensils, and in the pursuit of irrigated farming. This change in behaviour is one factor in the tendency of the infection to diminish after puberty, but it is not the only one. Acquired immunity also appears to reduce the likelihood of a given exposure to cercariae leading to an established infection.

Progression to disease

Most people infected with schistosomiasis die of an unrelated disease. In many parts of the world, although the prevalence is high, the adverse effects of the infection are difficult or impossible to demonstrate. The notion that the infection always causes general debility and malaise, in the absence of more specific effects, is wrong. In the absence of reinfection, the tendency is for most of the worms to die within a few years and for pathology related to the eggs (see below) to resolve. However, progressive pathology does develop in those with either heavy infections or those who are re-exposed to infection over a period of many years. Meta-analyses of disability-related outcomes in endemic schistosomiasis clearly show that those infected have more anaemia, for example, than those not infected. Treatment can certainly modify the natural history of the infection and even advanced cases may show a surprising degree of improvement after chemotherapy.

Clinicopathological features

Effects of cercarial penetration

Cercariae may cause an itchy papular rash ('swimmer's itch' or 'fisherman's itch') as they penetrate the dermis. This is seldom seen in endemic areas. A conspicuous cercarial rash is more often caused by avian or other schistosomes not otherwise pathogenic in humans. It is quite common in northern Europe, North America and South East Asia.

Initial illness: acute schistosomiasis

An initial febrile illness is sometimes recognized following the first exposure. It does not develop in very light infections, and is seldom recognized in residents of endemic areas. It is mainly a problem in migrants or visitors encountering a large cercarial challenge for the first time.

The illness comes on 4 or more weeks after infection, and is usually self-limiting. The theory is that as the worms begin to lay eggs, soluble antigen (Ag) leaks out of the eggs and into the circulation. While antibody (Ab) production lags behind antigen release, moderate antigen excess prevails. This favours Ag–Ab complex formation, with the development of generalized immune complex disease. Because the antigen is soluble and distributed by the bloodstream, the effects are more general than local. The immune complex disease hypothesis probably also explains why acute schistosomiasis has been reported more frequently in *S. japonicum* where egg production per worm pair is heavier than in *S. haematobium* and *S. mansoni*.

Features of acute schistosomiasis

The condition is sometimes called Katayama fever, after the prefecture in Japan where it used to be common. Some or all of the following may occur.

- Fever
- Eosinophilia

- Diarrhoea
- Hepatomegaly
- Splenomegaly
- Cough and wheeze
- Cachexia
- Urticaria

Perhaps it is seldom recognized in children in endemic areas because immune tolerance develops *in utero*, because of transplacental passage of antigen. Spontaneous recovery may be related to restoration of Ag–Ab balance as the infection matures and antibody production increases.

Importance of the eggs: those that get away

Eggs that escape from the body enable the life-cycle to be completed. Their passage through the bladder in *S. haematobium* typically causes terminal haematuria, the cardinal symptom of the infection. At the same time, these egg-induced perforations of the bladder wall also leach serum into the urine giving rise to micro-albuminuria as typically detected by reagent strips. In heavy infections, irritation of the bladder may cause dysuria. Following a diurnal cycle, peak egg excretion of *S. haematobium* is between late morning and early afternoon and urine collected outside of these times is less likely to contain eggs. In *S. mansoni* and *S. japonicum* infections, corresponding effects may occur in the bowel: diarrhoea and blood. More commonly, the presence of a little blood is noticed in an otherwise normal stool. In most infections, no bowel symptoms are noticed. Through these mechanisms of blood loss, schistosomes contribute to the development of iron-deficiency anaemia.

Importance of retained eggs: the main pathology

The serious mischief in humans arises from tissue reaction to retained eggs. This reaction, which follows sensitization to egg antigens, is a circumoval granuloma. It results from combined humoral and cell-mediated attack on the egg, and the granuloma occupies several hundred times the volume of the egg itself. Its characteristics are epithelioid and giant cells, as well as lymphocytes and eosinophils arranged in concentric fashion around the egg. The cellular content diminishes with time, to be replaced by fibroblasts and a collagenous scar. Precipitation of Ag–Ab complex on the egg surface helps activate inflammation.

The duration of the vigorous cellular response to a single egg lasts a few weeks. If egg laying is stopped by chemotherapy, the cellular component of the granuloma usually resolves in 2 or 3 months. Not all granulomata lead to scars (Fig. 17.3). These pathological processes occur, with variations, in all the schistosome infections. They help to explain the specific features of each of the species described next.

Clinical features of *Schistosoma haematobium*

Bladder pathology and squamous cell carcinoma

Eggs become deposited in the bladder and nearby organs, not singly, but usually in clutches. This is because a female schistosome may occupy the same site for long periods, during which time she lays several hundred eggs a day. The eggs give rise to a granulomatous lesion up to several centimetres in diameter. Most commonly these fleshy lesions form in the bladder mucosa, where they simulate tumours and are called pseudopapillomas. They may be sessile (flat) or pedunculated (on stalks). Smaller deposits of eggs cause lesions a few millimetres in diameter, resembling tubercles. If bladder inflammation due to *S. haematobium* is very persistent and prolonged over many years it is associated with the development of squamous cell bladder carcinonmas.

Bladder calcification

This is common in *S. haematobium* because of calcification of the eggs, not of the bladder itself. A calcified bladder outline on X-ray may be fully compatible with normal bladder function.

Obstructive uropathy

When granulomata form near the ureteric orifices or in the ureters themselves, the ureters may become

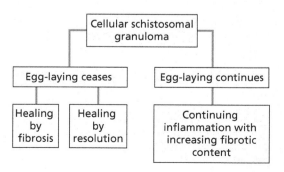

Figure 17.3 The fate of the granuloma.

obstructed. This is the cause of early obstructive uropathy. The secondary effects are hydroureter, in which the ureter becomes dilated and elongated, with varying degrees of hydronephrosis. In the most severe cases, kidney drainage may be so impaired as to cause uraemia. It used to be thought that all the changes of obstructive uropathy were irreversible, however, effective chemotherapy during the early cellular phase of the granuloma may lead to complete resolution. Longitudinal follow-up has shown that, provided reinfection does not occur, spontaneous resolution without significant scarring may also occur.

Genital schistosomiasis

Eggs from S. haematobium may be deposited at various sites throughout the urogenital system. Urethral papillomatous lesions have been reported in men and boys, and some men report changes in ejaculate consistency with or without blood in the semen. Semen microscopy in these cases often reveals eggs, but the effect on sperm counts, function and fertility have not been systematically investigated. Female genital schistosomiasis is increasingly recognized to include inflammatory lesions arising around deposited eggs in the vulva, vagina, cervix and fallopian tubes. The lower lesions can sometimes be mistaken for malignancies while the higher lesions are associated with sterility. A newly created visual atlas and classification system has been developed to grade mucosal sequelae, the lesions of which are often slow to resolve after anthelmintic treatment and are also thought to promote the transmission of HIV.

Schistosoma haematobium and the lung: schistosomal cor pulmonale

Eggs escaping from the pelvic veins into the caval circulation reach the lungs. In heavy, prolonged infections, granuloma formation may cause obstruction in pulmonary arterioles. Pulmonary hypertension, right ventricular hypertrophy and congestive heart failure may follow. Cyanosis develops from vascular shunting in the lungs.

Clinical features of Schistosoma mansoni

Most patients with S. mansoni infections have few or no symptoms. The liver is often enlarged, the spleen only in the presence of portal hypertension or during the initial illness. Severe clinical effects, except those caused by ectopic worms (see below), are only seen in heavy infections.

Pseudopolyposis of the colon

In severe S. mansoni infection, granulomata in the large gut may develop into papilloma-like outgrowths of the mucosa. They may ulcerate and bleed, and cause symptoms of dysentery. There is no proven causal relationship to colonic carcinoma, and strictures do not form.

Schistosoma mansoni and the liver: schistosomal liver fibrosis

Severe long-standing S. mansoni infections cause a characteristic liver disease, 'Symmer's pipe-stem fibrosis'. Large numbers of eggs escape from the lower mesenteric veins and reach the periportal regions, where they cause a granulomatous response that leads to gradual occlusion of the intrahepatic portal veins. Portal hypertension follows, but liver cell function is not disturbed until very late in the pathological evolution. The clinical features are:

- enlargement of liver and spleen;
- bleeding from oesophageal varices.

Patients tend to survive their bleeds much better than patients with true cirrhosis (e.g. caused by hepatitis B or alcohol), because of the well-preserved hepatocellular function. Also, because the serum albumin level is well maintained, ascites is not typical until the terminal stages of the disease. In late cases, hepatic perfusion may be so impeded that peripheral liver ischaemia occurs. Then, features of true cirrhosis may develop. When portocaval shunts are well established, the eggs of S. mansoni may bypass the liver in large numbers, and so reach the lungs. In some cases, they may be numerous enough to cause schistosomal cor pulmonale.

Clinical features of Schistosoma japonicum

This resembles S. mansoni but, for an equal number of worms, the infection is more severe. The parasite is less well adapted to humans, the circumoval granuloma is very large, and the egg output of each female worm is greater than that in S. mansoni. The initial illness (Katayama fever) may be prolonged and sometimes fatal. Many Chinese workers believe that S. japonicum can cause carcinoma of the colon, but most other experts consider the case is unproven.

Neuroschistosomiasis

Some worm pairs wander from their usual habitats and take up residence elsewhere. The chances of this happening are increased in heavy infections. The most important site for ectopic worms is the central nervous system (CNS), such as in the paravertebral venous plexus or the cerebral cortical veins. All three species may occasionally be found at these sites but this is, by comparison with pathology associated with worms in their usual sites, a rare occurrence.

In the paravertebral plexus, egg laying leads to the development of a granuloma in the constricted space of the spinal canal. The clinical syndrome is spinal cord compression or a cauda equina lesion. If treated promptly, full functional recovery may occur. When it does not, ischaemic injury may be the cause. In the brain, large localized granulomata produce symptoms and signs indistinguishable from a cerebral tumour. Diagnosis usually requires sophisticated brain imaging (see Figure 17.5).

Schistosomiasis pathology at unusual sites

Schistosomiasis cases that do not have overt antemortem pathology have been shown at postmortem to have schistosome eggs in virtually all organs, but without associated inflammation. The relation of eggs found in the brain in this way to symptoms such as epilepsy and neurosis remains speculative. The factors that lead to damaging granuloma formation in some instances but not others are not well understood. Despite this conundrum, pathology associated with schistosomal eggs has been reported on rare occasions in diverse sites including skin, peritoneum and even bone.

Investigation

Direct diagnosis

This is the only approach that can lead to a definitive diagnosis. The adult worms are inaccessible, so the aim is to find living eggs. The miracidium inside the egg dies within 4 weeks.

Schistosoma haematobium

Something about bladder wall activity means that most eggs are voided around midday. Specimens collected between 10 am and 2 pm are most likely to contain eggs. For quantitative surveys, it is very important to standardize urine collection times. Exercise has no demonstrable effect on egg output but can help dislodge emergent eggs, or friable mucosal masses, from the bladder mucosa. There is no significant or reliable concentration of eggs in any part of the urinary stream. The methods for finding eggs depend on their high specific gravity (sedimentation) or their size (filtration).

Urine sedimentation

Eggs are sedimented by natural gravity 30 min in a conical glass; the sediment is then aspirated by Pasteur pipette and examined under coverslip using lens power ×10, or by artificial gravity. Put 10 mL urine in 15 mL centrifuge tube, spin for 3 min at 1500 rpm (arm radius not critical); the deposit is then examined as before.

Living eggs are translucent, and the miracidium is recognizable. Flame cells can be seen flickering. The viability of the eggs can be checked by adding them to boiled (cool) water in a flask. Emerging miracidia are visible in light shone across the neck. Normal-looking eggs usually hatch. Opaque (calcified) eggs do not, and do not themselves signify active infection (live worms).

Urine filtration

Urine is passed through a filter by vacuum or pressure. An entire 24-h urine collection can be filtered. There are several variants of this method including a miniature membrane version that allows the eggs to be detected unstained, or stained with a drop of Lugol's iodine. Advantages of the method are that it is sensitive, accurate for counts and can provide a measure of the intensity of infection (eggs/ml of urine). Disadvantages are cost and time. In standard epidemiological surveys undertaken in endemic areas, it is possible to enumerate the number of excreted eggs into 'light' (1–49 eggs) or 'heavy' (50+ eggs) by syringe filtration of 10 ml of urine.

Schistosoma mansoni and Schistosoma japonicum

Direct smear examination is not sufficiently sensitive, e.g. for an output of 100 000 eggs per day; a stool of 200 g; a smear of 2 mg; the average count is 1 egg per smear. There is a 1 in 3 chance of finding no eggs in a patient who could be harbouring about 1000 S. mansoni worm pairs. Instead, more sensitivity is achieved through concentration techniques such as formol-ether, thiomersal, iodine and formol (TIF) glycerol sedimentation (the simplest) or a modified Kato-Katz thick smear. The Kato-Katz technique also permits a measure of intensity of infection (eggs per gramme of stool). Examination of several consecutive, concentrated stool samples may further increase sensitivity.

Biopsy techniques for all schistosomal infections

A small piece of rectal mucosa can be removed by biopsy forceps or curette under direct proctoscopic vision. It is placed on a slide under a coverslip and examined under lens power (×10). *Schistosoma haematobium* eggs are often trapped in the rectal mucosa, but may be calcified. It can be difficult to identify living eggs. Histology is not used for diagnosis as a routine. Serial sections are often needed as only the central slices of a granuloma will contain parts of the egg.

Indirect diagnosis

The main drug in use for all schistosome infections, praziquantel, is both safe and effective, so the imperative to make a definitive diagnosis before therapy (with more toxic agents) has been reduced. Although all the indirect means of diagnosis suffer more or less from a lack of specificity, treatment is increasing based on this approach.

Immunodiagnostic tests for all species

There are numerous tests for detecting circulating antischistosomal antibody including CFT, IFAT, ELISA and several others. Although the better ones correlate well with the results of direct diagnostic methods, they all suffer from the following disadvantages to a greater or lesser extent.

- They give no indication of the intensity of infection.
- They do not distinguish between past and present infection.
- They are not species specific.
- Most require high technology and are often 'in-house' methods in academic institutions, rather than commercially available for widespread use.
- They do not reliably become positive until 3 months after infection.

Immunodiagnostic tests capable of detecting the presence of circulating antigen would be of much greater use to the clinician and epidemiologist. Unfortunately, this field has not progressed to the point where tests are available for widespread use in the tropics.

Approaches to diagnosis of different clinical syndromes of schistosomiasis

Acute schistosomiasis

In the initial illness, the association of fever and eosinophilia with the other symptoms should raise the question of worms, as should the patient with diarrhoea and eosinophilia, although other worms such as *Strongyloides stercoralis*, *Capillaria philippinensis* and *Trichuris trichiura* can cause the same symptoms. In the differential diagnosis of these, direct diagnosis by examination of the stools is paramount.

Eosinophilia is not always prominent in acute schistosomiasis. In addition, acute schistosomiasis occurs at the onset of initial egg production, so eggs are rarely found in urine or stool and the antibody detection tests are not reliably positive at this stage of infection. For these reasons the diagnostic process includes elimination of other causes of fever such as malaria.

Schistosoma haematobium

In areas endemic for *S. haematobium*, the presence of haematuria (provided menstruating females are excluded) correlates well with the passage of schistosome eggs in the urine. With a dipstick-type test, provided it can detect both free haemoglobin and discrete red cells, the number of false-positives and false-negatives is very low. The false-positives are partly explained by glomerulonephritis and partly by the passage of dead eggs by patients whose worms are dead.

Radiological changes in the urinary tract may be very suggestive. Almost pathognomonic is the ring-like calcification of the bladder (Fig. 17.4),

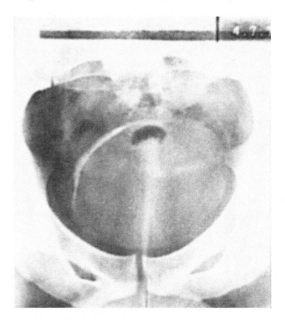

Figure 17.4 Calcified bladder in *Schistosoma haematobium* infection. Many such bladders are capable of entirely normal function, the calcification involving the eggs rather than the bladder tissues.

which may also involve the ureters, prostate and seminal vesicles. Multiple, rounded filling defects produced by pseudopapillomas in the bladder are also very typical. Ultrasonography is clearly important in detecting obstructive uropathy. Otherwise, unaccountable pulmonary hypertension in an endemic area should also arouse suspicion of schistosomiasis.

Schistosoma mansoni and Schistosoma japonicum

The presence of colonic polyps in an endemic area incriminates schistosome infection as the most likely cause, as does the syndrome of portal hypertension with normal liver function tests. Ultrasonography of the liver can been used to detect the typical pipe-stem fibrosis and alteration to liver shape and size in order to grade liver pathology.

Neuroschistosomiasis

The most useful clue, in cases with disease caused by ectopic worms or metastatic eggs, is the presence of eosinophilia. Unfortunately, eosinophilia is not invariably present, so immunodiagnostic tests may be particularly helpful. Diagnosis ususally requires sophisticated brain imaging (Fig. 17.5).

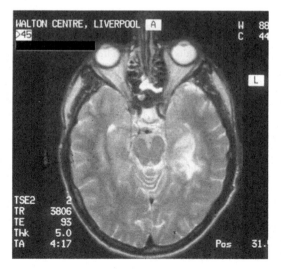

Figure 17.5 MRI scan demonstrating oedema around *S. haematobium* eggs in the left cerebral hemisphere. The clinical presentation was with motor seizures and haematuria (ova found in bladder).

Management

It is helpful to reach a definitive diagnosis with a direct test that confirms the presence of living worms before starting treatment. In practice, therapy is increasingly accepted on the basis of indirect evidence such as the results of urine dipstick detection of haematuria in an endemic country, or ELISA detection of antibody (when technology allows).

Drug treatment

All the effective anti-schistosomal drugs (with the exception of artemisinin derivatives, see below) act on adult worm pairs only, not on schistosomula. After effectively eliminating the worms, the speed of resolution of the immunopathology induced by the eggs depends on how established the tissue damage has been.

Praziquantel (Biltricide)

This isoquinoline compound currently eclipses all other chemotherapy for schistosomiasis because of its ease of administration, lack of toxicity and price. It is effective against all human schistosomes. There has been some debate about the development of resistance in areas of intense transmission in West Africa, but the case for resistance remains unproven as yet. It is given in a dosage of 40 mg/kg as a single oral dose, which is sufficient for all species. Dosing at 60 mg/kg is also licensed and used in preference for treatment of *S. mansoni* in Brazil. Side-effects include giddiness and minor gastrointestinal disturbances. No serious toxicity has been reported, but unexplained abdominal pain and short-lived bloody diarrhoea are troublesome in heavy *S. mansoni* infections. For infected children under the age of four, treatment is advised at standard 40 mg/kg dosing but tablets should be crushed or broken for ease of administration.

Other drug options

Metrifonate (active against *S. haematobium* only) and oxamniquine (active against *S. mansoni* only) are no longer in production. There is continued interest in the use of the artemisinin derivatives in both treatment for and prophylaxis against schistosomiasis – particularly in China. In laboratory models, this group of drugs appears to have some effect against schistosomula as well as adult worms, but the finding needs confirmation in the endemic setting.

Management approaches for specific presentations

In the tropics, praziquantel is most frequently used to clear adult worms in patients presenting with symptoms caused by retained eggs in tissues, or as part of mass chemotherapy (see below). The specific presentations peculiar to individuals from non-endemic areas who pick up infections during travel need mention.

Acute schistosomiasis

Praziquantel is often used in the management of this condition but the speed of its effect on symptoms is variable. On the whole, this is a self-limiting illness caused by an excess of egg antigen triggering aggressive immune responses. These will persist for a variable length of time even after the adult worms have been killed, and in severe cases adjunctive corticosteroid therapy is occasionally advocated. It is wise to give a second dose of praziquantel 3 months after the first in order to clear worms that were only maturing during the initial illness.

Asymptomatic infection

Travellers who have a one-off significant freshwater exposure (e.g. during water recreational activity such as snorkelling, windsurfing or scuba-diving) are often screened for schistosomal antibody even when they have no symptoms. It is common therefore for praziquantel treatment to be offered on the basis of a positive antibody test alone. On the whole this is a reasonable approach, but its overall effectiveness and cost-effectiveness in preventing later pathology has not been assessed and common pitfalls include:

- screening before adequate time (3 months) has elapsed since exposure;
- assuming that antibody tests can be used to monitor cure and that titres will fall to negative after treatment.

Neuroschistosomiasis

Praziquantel is used to kill the adult worms, but the offending circumoval granulomata in the nervous tissue will take a while to resolve and there is usually concern that the immunopathology will worsen on treatment. Adjunctive corticosteroid therapy is therefore the norm. In the case of cerebral involvement with epilepsy, it may take many months before anticonvulsant therapy can be withdrawn.

Monitoring treatment

It can be assumed that most light infections will be cured with a single praziquantel dose. However, when a direct diagnosis detecting viable eggs has been made, it is wise to check that egg production has ceased (in the absence of reinfection) at a 3-month follow-up.

Prevention and public health aspects

The schistosomiasis life-cycle can be interrupted at various sites. Although some sites have proved more vulnerable than others, combined approaches, where possible, have most impact but are rarely implemented in a sustained fashion.

- Contamination of water
- Intermediate host
- Human contact with infection

Reducing contamination of water

The main methods used are:

- health education;
- provision of sanitation;
- prevention of access to transmission sites;
- reduction of egg excretion by the definitive hosts (humans) by drug treatment.

Of all these measures, the one most immediately successful in most circumstances is mass chemotherapy (see below).

Attack on snails

Permanent results are possible if the habitats can be eliminated. It has been achieved in Japan and many parts of China by drainage and landfill. Temporary results are obtained with the application of poisonous chemicals (molluscicides such as niclosamide) to snail habitats. If used alone, this method is usually disappointing. The number of infected snails may not be reduced in proportion to the total snail reduction. Disadvantages include cost, the need to reapply chemicals for an indefinite period, and undesirable effects such as killing fish. It is most effective in highly controlled environments, such as irrigated agricultural estates, and when used in combination with chemotherapy.

Reducing contact with infection

The necessity for contact can be reduced by the provision of a safe water supply for washing and drinking through chlorination or filtration which will clear water of cercariae. This will not prevent recreational or occupational contact. Attempts to fence off transmission sites are usually unsuccessful. Health education is important, especially in creating the need to seek treatment post-exposure.

Mass chemotherapy

With the large-scale production of generic, off-patent praziquantel the cost per tablet has declined dramatically in recent years to not more than 4–5 US cents per 600 mg tablet. Mass chemotherapy of schistosomiasis is now receiving most support as the effective, modern approach to schistosomiasis control. It is recommended as part of a combined effort to implement the coordinated use of anthelmintic drugs in control interventions, along with mass chemotherapy for lymphatic filariasis, onchocerciasis and soil-transmitted helminths. Dosages are dispensed according to gradations on ingenious height-poles denoting half tablet divisions, which bypasses the need for functional weighing scales in small, peripheral treatment centres. The recommended treatment strategy is outlined in Table 17.1. As practical field experience is accumulating with this approach, and is being revised by WHO when to be used in elimination settings. Consensus is developing around the following potential indicators for monitoring impact:

- presence of infection (by parasitological methods);
- intensity of infection (proportion with heavy-intensity infection);
- prevalence of macrohaematuria;
- prevalence of microhaematuria;
- prevalence of anaemia;
- prevalence of ultrasound-detectable lesions (urinary tract and liver).

Future developments

New diagnostics

As with all important tropical infections, there is clearly a need for a new diagnostic tool that is as robust and specific as direct microscopy for eggs, less dependent on laboratory skill and infrastructure, and more sensitive. However, as mass chemotherapy can be conducted without definitive diagnosis, the pressure to develop this tool has diminished and there are no candidates for widespread use in developing countries. A single candidate for specific use is a point-of-care urine-dipstick (http://www.rapid-diagnostics.com) which is able to detect and quantify schistosome circulating cathodic antigen (CCA). The attraction of this is its ability to detect *S. mansoni* without recourse to stool examination but its diagnostic sensitivity for *S. haematobium* and *S. japonicum* is poor. Nonetheless, this may be a useful adjunct to the diagnostic repertoire of field-friendly diagnostic methods.

New interventions

No new drugs look set to replace the current gold standard of single dose praziquantel. Following the increasing recognition that infants and pre-school children are also at significant risk of infection, these age groups are now being targeted within control programmes and a paediatric-friendly formulation is being developed by Merck-Serona (see http://www.tipharma.com).

Table 17.1 Recommended treatment strategy for mass chemotherapy of schistosomiasis

Category	Prevalence among school-aged children	Action to be taken	
High-risk community	≥50% by parasitological methods Or ≥30% by questionnaire for visible haematuria	Treat all school-age children once a year	Also treat adults considered to be at risk (from special groups to entire communities living in endemic areas, e.g. fishermen, irrigation workers)
Moderate-risk community	≥10% but <50% by parasitological methods Or <30% by questionnaire for visible haematuria	Treat all school-age children once every 2 years	Also treat adults considered to be at risk (special risk groups only, e.g. fishermen, irrigation workers)
Low-risk community	<10% by parasitological methods	Treat all school-age children twice during their primary schooling	Praziquantel should be available in dispensaries and clinics for treatment of suspected cases

New guidelines aimed at monitoring the parasitological efficacy of praziquantel are due to be released in 2012 by the WHO. These will focus upon measuring egg reduction rate across a sample of infected patients 24 days after first treatment.

Interactions with HIV

There is increasing support for the hypothesis that schistosome infections cause increased susceptibility to infection with HIV, more rapid progression of HIV to disease, and higher risk of onward HIV transmission. Different species of schistosome vary in the size of their effects on these mechanisms but it seems *S. haematobium* is the most important promoter of transmission because it causes genital inflammation. An increased emphasis on treatment of schistosome infections as a cofactor in HIV transmission and disease progression is warranted.

With growing numbers of children receiving antiretroviral treatment in sub-Saharan Africa, it is not known if the natural histories of disease progression of either *S. haematobium* or *S. mansoni* are being altered. Similarly, the significance of drug-drug interactions of antiretroviral therapy with praziquantel are not known and will need more attention as mass drug administration campaigns are increasingly rolled out in holoendemic settings.

📖 FURTHER READING

Kjetland E, Leutscher PDC, Ndhlovu PD (2012) A review of female genital schistosomiasis. *Trends Parasitol* **28**; 58–65. [Comprehensive review describing the pathophysiology of genital schistosomiasis.]

Secor WE (2012) The effects of schistosomiasis on HIV/AIDS infection, progression and transmission. *Curr Opin HIV AIDS* **7**(3): 254–9 [Highlights the interactions of schistosomiasis and HIV-AIDS.]

Stothard JR, Sousa-Figueiredo JC, Betson M, *et al.* (2011) Closing the praziquantel treatment gap: new steps in epidemiological monitoring and control of schistosomiasis in African infants and preschool-aged children. *Parasitology* **138**; 1593–1606. [Update on the importance of paediatric schistosomiasis.]

World Health Organization website: http://www.who.int/schistosomiasis/en/index.html [Includes useful background and country-specific information, including the downloadable manual for health professionals and programme managers, WHO (2006) *'Preventive Chemotherapy in Human Helminthiasis, Coordinated Use of Anthelminthic Drugs in Control Interventions.'* ISBN 92 4 154710 3 (NLM classification: WC 800) ISBN 978 92 4 154710 9. Geneva: World Health Organization.]

 SUMMARY

- About 300 million people are affected by schistosomiasis worldwide, in association with exposure to freshwater containing the intermediate snail hosts.

- The three main species of the blood flukes causing schistosomiasis are *Schistosoma haematobium*, *S. mansoni* and *S. japonicum*.

- Clinical features result from granuloma formation and subsequent fibrosis in response to deposition of eggs in tissues such as liver, lung, the gastrointestinal tract and the urinary tract.

- There is concern about possible emergence of resistance to praziquantel, which is the main therapeutic agent.

- Complex interactions are increasingly being recognized to occur between schistosomiasis and HIV coinfections.

Visit www.lecturenoteseries.com/tropicalmed **to test yourself on this chapter using interactive MCQs.**

Leprosy

Diana Lockwood[1] and Nick Beeching[2]
[1]London School of Hygiene & Tropical Medicine; [2]Liverpool School of Tropical Medicine

Leprosy is a chronic granulomatous disease caused by *Mycobacterium leprae*. The principal manifestations of disease are anaesthetic skin lesions and peripheral neuropathy with peripheral nerve thickening. The clinical form of the disease in any individual depends on the degree of cell-mediated immunity (CMI) expressed by that individual towards *M. leprae*. Patients with high levels of CMI and elimination of leprosy bacilli develop tuberculoid leprosy, whereas those with no CMI develop lepromatous leprosy (LL). The medical complications of leprosy result from nerve damage and immunological reactions. Nerve damage should be detected early whilst it is still potentially reversible with steroid treatment. Permanent nerve damage is lifelong and causes considerable morbidity. Anti-leprosy multi drug therapy is highly effective, with a cure rate of 95%, and there is little evidence of drug resistance. Leprosy has a long history as a deforming disease and leprosy patients all over the world are frequently stigmatized and ostracized. Words such as 'leper' should be avoided and using the term Hansen's disease may reduce stigmatization.

Leprosy must be considered in the differential diagnosis for any patient who has lived in the tropics and presents with chronic skin lesions, peripheral neuropathy or apparent vasculitis.

Epidemiology

The infection is spread from human to human by droplets. There is a long clinical incubation period of 2–5 years for tuberculoid disease and 8–11 years for lepromatous disease. About 250 000 new cases per year are detected worldwide. The geographical distribution is patchy, with 62% of cases being detected in India, and Brazil, Congo, Mozambique and Nepal having the highest case rates. Age, sex and household contact are important determinants of disease. In the major leprosy endemic areas, the childhood case rate remains high, indicating ongoing transmission. HIV infection is not a risk factor for disease acquisition, and HIV-positive patients can develop all types of leprosy. Paradoxically HIV-positive patients with leprosy are a higher risk of developing Type 1 reactions and patients on ART may present with de novo leprosy as an immune reconstitution inflammatory syndrome (IRIS).

Microbiology

M. leprae is an obligatory intracellular parasite which cannot be cultivated in vitro; although it can be grown in the armadillo and in footpads of nude mice. *M. leprae* has a doubling time of 12 days and is a remarkably hardy organism, remaining viable in the environment for up to 2 months. It has a highly resistant cell wall composed of lipids, carbohydrates and proteins. Phenolic glycolipid *M. leprae* is species specific. Numerous protein antigens have been identified as important immune targets using antibody and T cell screening. The *M. leprae* genome has been completely sequenced. The organism has lost many genes and survives on only a few biochemical pathways. Only 40 genes are unique to *M. leprae*, and analysis of these genes will inform us about the unique biology of this organism.

Immune response in leprosy

The host immune response to *M. leprae* is crucial in determining either disease or immunity and the type of disease. The T cells and macrophages of the cell-mediated immune system have an important role in processing, recognition and response to *M. leprae* antigens. Antibodies to *M. leprae* antigens are produced but these do not appear to have any useful role in protection. Several stages in the immune response are recognized:

- phagocytosis of *M. leprae* by macrophages;
- presentation of *M. leprae* antigens in association with human leucocyte antigen (HLA) class II molecules;
- binding of antigen-specific T cells via the a/b T cell receptor;
- activation of T cells and production of interleukin 2 (IL-2) and T cell proliferation;
- IL-2 activates CD4, CD8, natural killer (NK) cells and macrophages;
- interferon-γ (IFN-γ) is produced and activates bactericidal mechanisms within the macrophage.

Granuloma formation results from mycobacterial persistence with continued cytokine release. The leprosy granuloma has a core of macrophages, epithelioid cells and giant cells, with lymphocytes surrounding the core, and is dependent on tumour necrosis factor a (TNF-α) from activated macrophages and T cells.

The immunological and clinical effects vary across a spectrum between two 'poles' of presentations (Fig. 18.1). In tuberculoid disease (TT), CMI is active and contains infection, so that few bacilli are found in tissues and CD4 cells and their cytokines (IL-2, IFN-γ) predominate (Th1 response). At the other pole of LL, the CMI response is poor, there are many bacilli in the tissues and responses include both CD4 and CD8 cells. CD4 cells produce few cytokines IL-4, IL-5, IL-6 and IL-10; immunoglobulin G (IgG), IgM and IgA levels are also elevated. The unresponsiveness in LL disease is

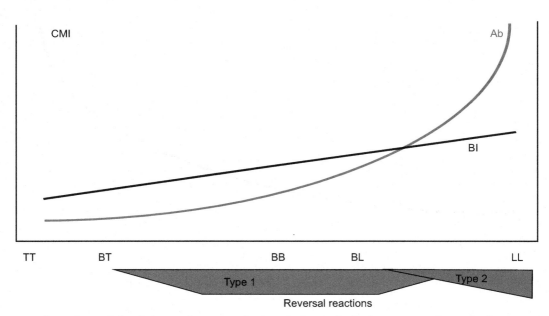

- *In the LL form of the disease,* M leprae *can be found all over the body, in nerves, skin and other tissue, because, unlike the TT localized form, it is a generalized condition.*
- *In LL macrophages ingest but do not digest the bacilli, because of a lack of CMI. They act as a convenient host in which the bacilli may even multiply, to be transported by the macrophages to all parts of the body. It has been known for up to 300* M. leprae *to be found in one macrophage.*
- *More CMI means "Upgrading" or a "Reversal" of the normal trend. On the contrary, if there is a reduction of CMI, we speak of "Downgrading" towards the lepromatous pole.*
- *Upgrading toward the tuberculoid end in reversal reactions is deleterious ie over activation of the T cells, leading to inflammation and the over expression of "protective" cytokines leading to tissue damage.*

Figure 18.1 The immunological features of the different types of leprosy. Ab, Antibody (Th2 response); BI, Bacterial Index; CMI, Cell mediated immunity (Th1 response).

because of specific T cell anergy. It may be caused by T cell non-activation, suppression or clonal deletion and also involves defective macrophage function. Borderline states (borderline tuberculoid [BT]; borderline leprosy [BB]; borderline lepromatous leprosy [BL]) are intermediate between these poles.

There is no current immunological test that can determine whether a person has protective immunity against *M. leprae*.

Clinical features

The cardinal signs of leprosy are skin lesions, which may be anaesthetic, thickened peripheral nerves and acid fast bacilli in the skin. Not all patients have all three clinical features.

Skin lesions

The most common skin lesions are macules or plaques; more rarely, papules and nodules are seen (Figs 18.2–18.5). The number of lesions indicates the ability of the CMI to limit the spread of bacilli. Tuberculoid patients have few hypopigmented lesions, while lepromatous patients have numerous sometimes confluent lesions and infiltration. Anaesthesia of lesions is most marked in TT and BT patients The few tuberculoid lesions are usually asymmetrical; more numerous lesions are often symmetrical.

Nerve damage

Damage to peripheral nerve trunks produces motor weakness in the muscles supplied and to regional sensory loss (Figs 18.6 and 18.7). The principal sites of peripheral nerve involvement are ulnar (elbow), median (wrist), radial cutaneous (wrist), common peroneal (knee), posterior tibial and sural nerves (ankle) and the facial nerve. All these nerves should be examined for enlargement and tenderness. LL patients may have a glove and stocking sensory loss. Nerve function impairment occurs before, during and after treatment. In field cohort studies, 16–56% of newly diagnosed patients have functional nerve impairment. Sensory and autonomic fibres in skin lesions are also affected producing anaeasthesia and loss of sweating. The central nervous system is not affected in leprosy.

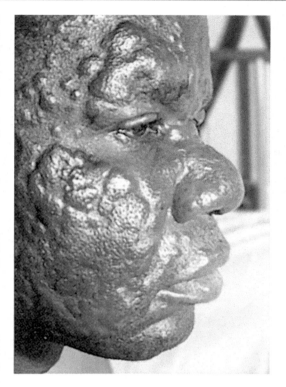

Figure 18.2 Lepromatous leprosy (LL) – nodular form.

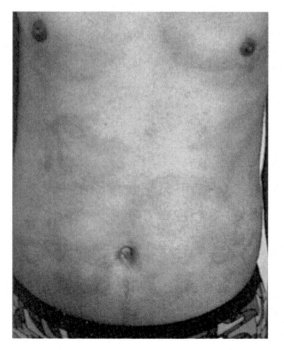

Figure 18.3 Skin lesions of borderline lepromatous (BL) leprosy.

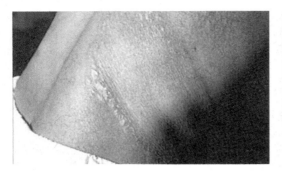

Figure 18.4 A patient from India with tuberculoid leprosy. The single lesion is anaesthetic, scaly, dry and has a raised edge.

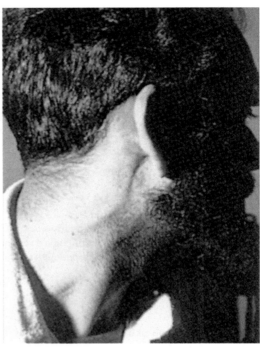

Figure 18.6 Visibly thickened posterior auricular nerve. The patient had a 'tuberculoid'-type lesion on the palm of his right hand and an associated thickening of the dorsal branch of the radial nerve.

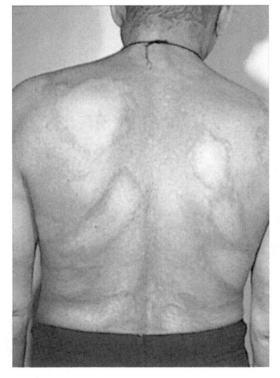

Figure 18.5 Borderline tuberculoid (BL) leprosy with numerous anaesthetic skin lesions.

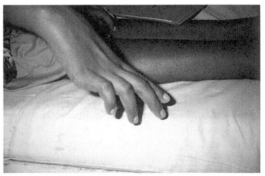

Figure 18.7 An ulnar nerve lesion in a patient from South Africa with LL.

Leprosy classification

Classification of the stage of disease helps to predict the prognosis and types of reaction that a patient may experience and also the content and duration of chemotherapy. Polar forms of disease are stable but borderline disease is unstable. BT/BL disease is associated with severe large nerve damage caused by Type 1 'reversal' reactions and neuritic reactions, and LL/BL patients suffer with erythema nodosum leprosum (ENL) (Type 2) reactions.

The Ridley–Jopling classification uses clinical and microbiological features of the patient, which mirror the immunological state (Table 18.1, Fig. 18.8).

- Skin lesions
  - Number
  - Distribution and symmetry
  - Definition and clarity
  - Anaesthesia
  - Loss of sweating and hair growth
- Peripheral nerve involvement
- Mucosal and systemic involvement
- Bacillary load

A simpler WHO field classification uses the number of skin lesions to assign patients to either paucibacillary (PB) with up to 5 skin lesions or multibacillary (MB), when more than 5 lesions are present. The number of affected nerves and the bacterial index are not used in this classification, which is used to determine type of multidrug treatment. National leprosy programmes may have their own variant of the WHO classification.

Tuberculoid leprosy

Infection is localized and asymmetrical. The skin lesions are few, hypopigmented and have sharp borders. Anaesthesia is usually present in the lesion and is often accompanied by loss of sweating. If peripheral nerve trunk involvement is present, usually only one

Table 18.1 **Classifications and features of leprosy**					
WHO Classification	Paucibacillary (PB) ←——————→	Multibacillary (MB) ←——————————————————————————→			
Bacteriological Index	0	0-1+	1-3+	3-5+	5-6+
Type of leprosy	Polar Tuberculoid	Borderline			Polar lepromatous
Ridley-Jopling Classification	TT	BT	BB	BL	LL
Skin lesions	Increasing number of skin lesions ——————————————————————————→				
Nerve lesions	Increasing number of enlarged nerves and nerve involvement ——————————————————————————→				
Stability	Stable	Unstable – may develop reactions and new nerve damage			Stable

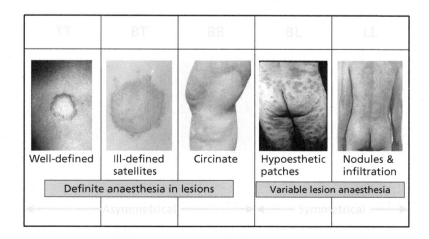

TT — Well-defined — Definite anaesthesia in lesions — Asymmetrical
BT — Ill-defined satellites
BB — Circinate
BL — Hypoesthetic patches — Variable lesion anaesthesia — Symmetrical
LL — Nodules & infiltration

Figure 18.8 Leprosy clinical spectrum

nerve trunk is enlarged and peripheral nerve trunk damage is limited. No *M. leprae* are found in the skin. True tuberculoid leprosy has a good prognosis.

Borderline tuberculoid

The skin lesions are similar to TT leprosy but are larger and more numerous. The margins are less well-defined and there may be satellite lesions. Annular lesions with a broad irregular edge and a sharply defined punched-out centre are also seen in BT leprosy. Damage to peripheral nerves is widespread and severe, usually with several thickened nerve trunks. BT patients are at risk of severe Type 1 reactions with rapid deterioration in nerve function with consequent deformities.

Borderline leprosy

BB disease is the most unstable part of the spectrum and patients usually downgrade towards LL if they are not treated or upgrade towards tuberculoid leprosy as part of a reversal reaction. There are numerous skin lesions, which may be macules, papules or plaques and vary in size, shape and distribution. The edges of the lesions may have streaming irregular borders. Nerve damage is common with involvement of several peripheral nerve trunks.

Borderline lepromatous leprosy

Borderline lepromatous leprosy is characterized by widespread, small but variable macules all over the body. With disease progression, the macules become infiltrated. Peripheral nerve involvement is widespread and often severe. Patients with BL leprosy are at risk of both reversal and ENL (Type 2) reactions.

Lepromatous leprosy

The patient with untreated polar LL may be carrying 10^{11} leprosy bacilli and the characteristic signs of LL are caused by the widespread dissemination of organisms throughout the body. The onset of disease is frequently insidious, the earliest lesions being ill-defined, widely distributed macules. Gradually, the skin becomes infiltrated and thickened and nodules develop. Thickening of facial skin gives rise to the characteristic leonine facies. Hair is lost, especially the lateral third of the eyebrows (madarosis) (Fig. 18.9). Dermal nerves are destroyed and there is sensory loss (light touch, pain and temperature) which begins at the hands and feet. Sweating is lost and this can cause profound discomfort in a tropical climate as compensatory sweating occurs in the

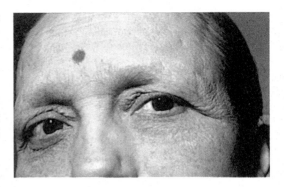

Figure 18.9 Lateral eyebrow loss or 'madarosis' in a patient with LL.

remaining intact areas. Damage to peripheral nerves is symmetrical and occurs late in disease.

Nasal collapse is now rarely seen. Testicular atrophy results from diffuse infiltration and the acute orchitis that occurs with ENL reactions. The consequent loss of testosterone leads to azoospermia and gynaecomastia. These patients are at risk of developing osteoporosis.

Other forms of leprosy

These include pure neuritic, histoid and Lucio's leprosy, and will not be considered further here.

The eye in leprosy

Blinding complications include lagophthalmos, decreased corneal sensation, acute iritis, chronic iritis and cataract. Patients at risk include those with BL and/or LL disease, those with facial patches, patients with TT disease experiencing reactions and those with disease of long duration (Table 18.2). For further details, see Chapter 62.

Diagnosis

The diagnosis of leprosy is essentially a clinical one made on finding one or more of the cardinal signs of leprosy and supported by finding acid-fast bacilli in slit skin smears.

Skin

The whole body should be inspected in a good light, otherwise lesions may be missed, particularly on the buttocks. Skin lesions should be tested for anaesthesia to light touch, pinprick and temperature.

Table 18.2 **Pathways to blindness in leprosy**

Iris	Cornea	Lid	Lens
Acute iritis (Type 2 leprosy reaction – cataract and secondary glaucoma	Anaesthetic cornea	Lagophthalmos-corneal exposure	Age-related cataract
Chronic neuroparalytic iritis – tiny pupil – night blindness	Suppurative keratitis	Chronic lacrimal sac infection	Secondary cataract
Chronic iritis – iris atrophy			

Peripheral nerve examination

The peripheral nerves should be examined for thickening and tenderness. Motor and sensory function is assessed by testing the small muscles of the hands and feet and testing sensation on the palms and soles of the feet using Semmes Weinstein monofilaments or a ball point pen. These need to be recorded in a chart and repeated monthly during treatment and continued if there is evidence of new nerve damage. (Charts for testing and recording nerve function can be obtained from the HPA Memorandum on leprosy; see Further reading.)

Wherever possible the diagnosis should be supported by a skin biopsy, which helps accurate classification. Finding dermal neural inflammation distinguishes leprosy from other granulomatous conditions. Serology is not usually helpful diagnostically because antibodies to the species-specific glycolipid PGL-1 are present in 90% of untreated lepromatous patients but only 40–50% of paucibacillary patients and 5–10% of healthy controls. PCR for detecting *M. leprae* DNA is not used as a routine diagnostic test.

Slit skin smears

The bacterial load is assessed by making a small incision through the epidermis, scraping dermal material and smearing it onto a glass slide. Several sites should be sampled (earlobes, eyebrows, edges of active lesions). The smears are then stained and acid-fast bacilli are counted. Scoring is performed on a logarithmic scale per high-power field (the bacterial index [BI]). A score of 1+ indicates 1–10 bacilli in 100 fields and 6+ indicates >1000 per field. Smears are useful for confirming the diagnosis, but are not positive in all patients and should be carried out annually to monitor response to treatment.

Differential diagnosis

A wide variety of dermatological conditions might be considered in the differential diagnosis of manifestations of leprosy, which include erythematous macules, hypopigmented macules, papules and nodules. Borderline tuberculoid leprosy is often misdiagnosed as sarcoidosis, or lupus vulgaris. Neurological problems include both mononeuropathies and polyneuropathies. Vasculitis may cause a skin rash and neuropathy. Diabetes is a common cause of peripheral neuropathy and may coexist with leprosy but does not cause nerve thickening.

Management

The management of a new leprosy patients comprises:

- treating the infection with multidrug therapy;
- detecting new nerve damage and treating with steroids if present;
- treating reactions;
- instituting care of anaesthetic hands and feet;
- support with social issues.

Educating a leprosy patient about their disease is the key to successful management and should include the following; the excellent response to multi drug treatment if a full course is completed, the risk of reactions and developing new nerve damage, the importance of treatment or compliance, and the low infectivity of most patients.

Chemotherapy

The first-line antileprosy drugs are rifampicin, dapsone and clofazimine.

Rifampicin

Rifampicin is a potent bactericidal for *M. leprae*. Four days after a single 600 mg dose, bacilli from a previously untreated lepromatous patient are no longer viable. It acts by inhibiting DNA-dependent RNA polymerase, thereby interfering with bacterial

RNA synthesis. Rifampicin is well absorbed orally. Hepatotoxicity is rarely a problem because rifampicin is only taken monthly. Because *M. leprae* resistance to rifampicin can develop as a one-step process, rifampicin should always be given in combination with other antileprotic drugs.

Dapsone

Dapsone (DDS; 4,4-diaminodiphenylsulphone) acts by blocking folic acid synthesis. It is only weakly bactericidal. Oral absorption is good. In many patients the haemoglobin drops by 10–20 g/L while taking on dapsone because it causes haemolysis and patients with G6PD deficiency are particularly at risk. The 'DDS syndrome', which is occasionally seen in leprosy, starts 6 weeks after commencing DDS and manifests as exfoliative dermatitis associated with lymphadenopathy, hepatosplenomegaly, fever and hepatitis.

Clofazimine

Clofazimine is a dye that has a weakly bactericidal action. It also has an anti-inflammatory effect and helps prevent ENL. The major side effect is skin discolouration, ranging from red to purple-black, the degree of discolouration depending on the dose and the amount of underlying leprosy infiltration. The pigmentation usually fades within 6–12 months of stopping clofazimine, although traces of discoloration may remain for years. Clofazimine also causes icthyosis on the shins and other parts of the body (Fig. 18.10). Gastrointestinal side-effects, ranging from mild cramps to diarrhoea and weight loss, may occur as a result of clofazimine crystal deposition in the wall of the small bowel.

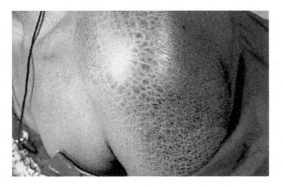

Figure 18.10 Icthyotic skin changes in a patient on clofazimine treatment.

Multidrug therapy

This has been used to treat over 16 million people since 1982. Relapse rates are low, ranging from 0% in China and Ethiopia to 2.04 per 100 person-years in India. Patients with high initial bacterial loads are at greater risk of relapse (8 per 100 person-years). So far there has been no reported drug resistance to rifampicin or clofazimine. Toxicity is limited, response is rapid and the duration of therapy is defined. Multidrug therapy (MDT) is provided free of cost to all patients through the WHO and funded by Novartis. The recommended regimens are summarized in Table 18.3 and include a component of monthly directly observed therapy and daily self-administered therapy. Ofloxacin 400 mg and minocycline 100 mg are second-line drugs that can be used to replace components of WHO-MDT if patients experience adverse effects or drug interactions. They are given as a single monthly dose.

Reactions and nerve damage

Reactions and nerve damage are immune-mediated complications of leprosy and can occur before, during and after multidrug therapy. These include Type 1 reactions, Type 2 (ENL) reactions and acute neuritis.

Type 1 reactions

These are caused by delayed hypersensitivity towards *M. leprae* antigens in skin and nerve (Fig. 18.11). Those at risk include all borderline (BT, BB and BL) patients and women in the postpartum. The peak time for reactions is during the first 2 months of treatment. Type 1 reactions occur in 30% of BL patients. Clinical manifestations include erythema, swelling and tenderness of skin lesions, and pain and tenderness of peripheral nerves with loss of sensory and motor function. Rapid severe nerve damage may occur with Type 1 reactions, so patients must be warned about symptoms and advised to return for treatment if they develop new weakness or numbness. Nearly all reactions, and especially those with nerve inflammation, must be treated with 40 mg/day prednisolone, reducing by 5 mg/day every month. Physiotherapy will be needed for affected hand, foot and eye muscles.

Erythema nodosum leprosum reaction

This is also known as a Type 2 reaction (Fig. 18.12) and is caused by immune complex deposition, T-cell dysregulation and overproduction of TNF. It affects up to 50% of LL and 10% of BL patients. There is systemic illness with malaise, fever and raised white cell count

Table 18.3 **Modified multidrug therapy regimens recommended by WHO**

Type of leprosy	Drug treatment			Duration of treatment
	Monthly supervised	and	Daily self-administered	
Paucibacillary (PB)	Rifampicin 600 mg		Dapsone 100 mg	6 months
Multibacillary (MB)	Rifampicin 600 mg		Clofazimine 50 mg	12 months
	Clofazimine 300 mg		Dapsone 100 mg	

Children

PB: Rifampicin 450 mg monthly and dapsone 50 mg daily.
MB: Rifampicin 450 mg and clofazimine 150 mg monthly, clofazimine 50 mg alternate days and dapsone 50 mg daily.

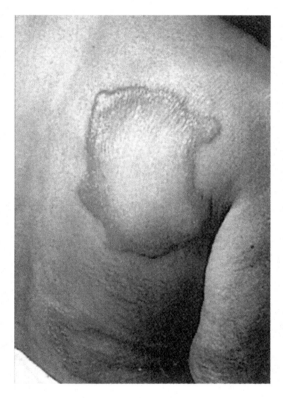

Figure 18.11 A reversal (Type 1) reaction in leprosy. The previously flat lesions suddenly become hot, painful and raised.

and erythrocyte sedimentation rate. Manifestations include widespread erythema nodosum, neuritis, iritis, arthritis, orchitis, lymphadenopathy and renal disease. ENL usually starts in the first year of chemotherapy and may relapse intermittently over several years. It is often difficult to treat. Most episodes of ENL require treatment with high-dose prednisolone (60–80mg/day) or thalidomide. Thalidomide is very effective in relieving the symptoms and signs of ENL, gives better long-term control of the reaction and avoids the adverse effects of long-term steroid treatment. However patients have to be warned about the teratogenic effects of thalidomide and women must use double contraception. Increasing the dosage of clofazimine up to 300 mg daily for 3 months may also reduce inflammatory responses. Iritis should be treated with 1% atropine and 1% steroid eye drops. Antileprosy drugs should be continued, and the patient should be reassured that the reaction will settle.

New nerve damage and neuritis

New nerve damage is that which has occurred within the last six months. Neuritis refers to acute and chronic nerve inflammation that may occur without a Type 1 or Type 2 reaction. Nerve damage may also occur as silent neuropathy which is defined as 'the development of functional deficit of a major nerve without a manifest neuritis'. Nerve function should be checked carefully during treatment so that silent neuropathy can be detected. Treatment is with 40 mg/day prednisolone as for reversal reactions, reducing slowly over a period of months. Steroid treatment is not indicated for patients who have had nerve damage for more than 6 months. Over 60% of patients who present with nerve damage at diagnosis are at risk of developing further nerve damage during and after treatment, especially during the first 12 months of treatment.

Infectivity of new patients and screening household contacts

Most leprosy patients are not infectious to others and their mycobacteria are intracellular. Untreated lepromatous patients are infectious through their nasal

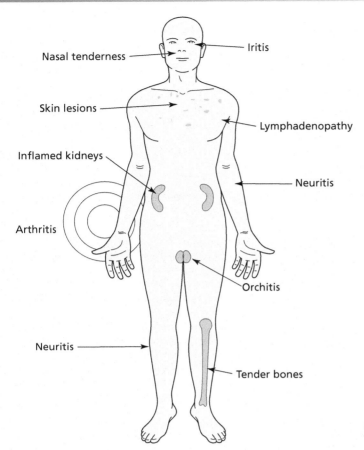

Nasal tenderness

Figure 18.12 Summary of features of Type 2 leprosy reactions

secretions. There is an increased risk of acquiring leprosy from household contact with both lepromatous and tuberculoid patients. However, the risk is low, even in endemic countries. It is impossible to distinguish between exposure to a common source and directly transmitted infection. Household contacts of new patients should be examined to check that they do not have leprosy. Children should be given BCG vaccination.

Prevention of disability

Nerve damage produces anaesthesia, dryness and muscle weakness. These three factors lead to misuse of the affected limb with resultant ulceration, infection and, ultimately, severe deformity (Fig. 18.13). Keys to prevention include regular monitoring of nerve function and recording of problems secondary to nerve dysfunction. Patients who need self-care should be identified and their understanding and implementation of this should be monitored

(Table 18.4). All patients need general training and social support; some may need surgical referral. Patients who have had reactions are also at higher risk of developing neuropathic pain.

Reconstructive surgery

Reconstructive surgery has a role in both improving function and appearance. Lagophthalmos can be ameliorated by tarsorrhaphy or temporalis muscle transfer. Appropriate tendon transfers can reduce the effects of ulnar and median nerve paralysis and improve drop foot and claw toes. Cosmetic surgery – in particular eyebrow replacement, nasal reconstruction and reduction of gynaecomastia – is important in the rehabilitation of severely deformed patients.

Women and leprosy

Women with leprosy are in double jeopardy. Not only may they develop postpartum nerve damage, but they are at particular risk of social ostracism with

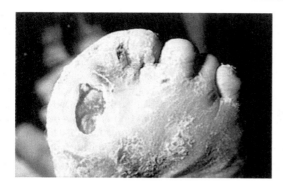

Figure 18.13 Perforating neuropathic plantar foot ulcer in a patient with LL and extensive lower limb denervation.

Table 18.4 General care of hands and feet

Self-care training
Inspect for injury
Understand why injuries happen
Soak feet and oil
Remove callus
Exercise hands and feet
Treat injuries promptly

Hands
Problems with heat/pressure/sharp objects

Feet
Plantar ulcers occur at pressure sites
Either walk less or use protective shoe insoles

Footwear
Check shoe fittings
Provide insoles
Arch supports, metatarsal pads
Orthopaedic footwear

Management of plantar ulcers
Clean wound
Bed rest, walking plaster
Check footwear
Find out why it happened

rejection by spouses and family. There is little good evidence that pregnancy causes new disease or relapse. However, there is a clear temporal association between parturition and the development of Type 1 reactions and neuritis when CMI returns to prepregnancy levels. Rifampicin, dapsone and clofazimine are safe during pregnancy, but ideally pregnancies should be planned for when leprosy is well controlled. Women may breastfeed while on multidrug therapy but should be warned that low levels of clofazimine are excreted in the breast milk and may cause some skin discoloration in the infant.

Leprosy in childhood

All types of leprosy are seen in childhood, usually after the age of 5 years. Children are at the same risk as adults of developing nerve damage and reactions, and often present with established nerve damage. Reactions should be treated with prednisolone 0.5mg/kg/day. The WHO has produced separate multidrug therapy paucibacillary (PB) and multibacillary (MB) blister packs for treating children.

Control and prevention

Vaccines

The substantial cross-reactivity between BCG and *M. leprae* has been exploited in attempts to develop a vaccine against leprosy. Metaanalyses of the effect of BCG show that it gives about 50% protection against leprosy in leprosy endemic areas. A case-control study in Venezuela showed BCG vaccination to give 56% protection to the household contacts of leprosy patients. Combining BCG and killed *M. leprae* has been tried, but two trials showed no advantage for BCG plus *M. leprae* over BCG alone. Ensuring that populations living in leprosy endemic areas have received BCG vaccination is, therefore, an important public health activity contributing to leprosy control.

Leprosy provision in general health services

For much of the 20th century, leprosy patients were detected and treated within vertical programmes dedicated to leprosy. Although these were effective, they also became inefficient as the numbers of leprosy patients declined. The management of leprosy patients is now being integrated into a range of health services including combined leprosy and tuberculosis programmes, dermatology programmes and full integration with general health services. The current WHO strategy emphasizes the importance of quality services that are accessible, patient-centred, provide free treatment with MDT, do appropriate prevention of disability and refer patients on for the management of complications. There are now huge training needs to train people to recognize leprosy. The development of referral services is also a critical need if an integrated approach is to work well.

SUMMARY

- Although the incidence of leprosy has decreased, about 250 000 new cases are diagnosed each year.
- Leprosy is a chronic granulomatous disease caused by *Mycobacterium leprae*. The principal manifestations of disease are anaesthetic skin lesions and peripheral neuropathy with peripheral nerve thickening.
- Leprosy must be considered in the differential diagnosis for any patient who has lived in the tropics and presents with chronic skin lesions, peripheral neuropathy or apparent vasculitis.
- Treatment with multidrug regimens of antibiotics for at least 6–12 months is highly effective in clearing infection.
- The key to prevention of disability is early recognition and prompt treatment of leprosy reactions, which may recur for several years after successful chemotherapy.

 Visit www.lecturenoteseries.com/tropicalmed to test yourself on this chapter using interactive MCQs.

FURTHER READING

Britton WJ, Lockwood DNJ (2004) Leprosy. *Lancet* **363**: 1209–19. [Up-to-date overview of leprosy.]

Health Protection Agency (2012) *Memorandum on Leprosy 2012*. Available from http://www.hpa.org.uk/webw/HPAweb&HPAwebStandard/HPAweb_C/1317137370741 [Updated approach to leprosy in the UK. Includes useful appendices with summary neurological assessment charts and case record forms from The Hospital for Tropical Diseases.]

International Leprosy Association (2002) Report of the International Leprosy Association Technical Forum. Evidence-based assessment of leprosy management issues. *Lepr Rev* **73** (Suppl). [Covers everything from epidemiology through diagnosis and treatment to prevention of disability.]

Kahawita IP, Walker SL, Lockwood DNJ (2008) Leprosy type 1 reactions and erythema nodosum leprosum. *An Bras Dermatol* **83**: 75–82. [Good overview of leprosy reactions and their management. Free download.]

LEPRA, Fairfax House, Causton Road, Colchester CO1 1PU, UK. [International leprosy charity, can provide posters, pamphlets, etc.]

Lockwood DN, Lambert SM (2010) Leprosy and HIV, where are we at? *Lepr Rev* **81**(3): 169–75.

Lockwood DN, Suneetha S (2005) Leprosy: too complex a disease for a simple elimination paradigm. *Bull World Health Organ* **83**: 230–5.

Rodrigues L, Lockwood DN (2011) Leprosy now: epidemiology, progress, challenges, and research gaps. *Lancet Infect Dis.* **11**(6): 464–70.

Scollard DM, Adams LB, Gillis TP, *et al.* (2006) The continuing challenges of leprosy. *Clin Microbiol Rev* **19**(2): 338–81.

Srinivasan H (1993) *Prevention of Disabilities in Patients with Leprosy: A Practical Guide*. Geneva: World Health Organization.

World Health Organization (2010) *Global Strategy for Further Reducing the Leprosy Burden and Sustaining Leprosy Control Activities 2006-2010*. Geneva: World Health Organization.

www.ilep.org.uk. ILEP (International Federation of Anti-leprosy Associations) [Website with teaching materials and links.]

www.lepra.org.uk. *Leprosy Review*. [The premier leprosy journal, free internet access.]

Part 3

Other tropical diseases

19

Amoebiasis

Tim O'Dempsey
Liverpool School of Tropical Medicine

Introduction and epidemiology

Entamoeba histolytica is an intestinal protozoan parasite with the ability to invade and cause lysis of cells. *Entamoeba histolytica* occurs worldwide, particularly in situations of poor hygiene and sanitation. Thus, infections are commonly found among people living in developing countries and immigrants or travellers from such countries. In addition, people with learning difficulties in residential institutions, men who have sex with men, and people who are immunosuppressed are also at increased risk.

The most common clinical presentation is amoebic dysentery. Extra-intestinal infections also occur, notably amoebic liver abscess (ALA). It has been shown experimentally that the majority of infections are asymptomatic and only about 20% of people who swallow cysts develop symptoms of dysentery. There are estimated to be between 40 and 50 million cases of symptomatic amoebiasis per year, resulting in 40 000–110 000 deaths.

In the past, the prevalence of infection in developing countries has been estimated to exceed 90% in some communities. This is probably an overestimate as cysts of *E. histolytica* are microscopically identical to cysts of *Entamoeba dispar* which is generally regarded as non-pathogenic, although this has recently been challenged based on DNA sequencing of material obtained from liver abscesses in Mexico. *Entamoeba dispar* is about three times as common as *E. histolytica* in developing countries and about 10 times as common in industrialized countries. Other non-pathogenic protozoa found in the human intestine include *Entamoeba moshkovskii* (which also produces cysts identical to those of *E. histolytica/E. dispar*), *Entamoeba coli*, *Entamoeba hartmanni* and *Endolimax nana*.

Other amoebae sometimes associated with disease in humans include *Entamoeba gingivalis* (periodontal disease), *Entamoeba polecki* and *Dientamoeba fragilis* (diarrhoea), *Acanthamoeba* species and *Balamuthia mandrillaris* (acanthamoebic keratitis/granulomatous amoebic encephalitis) and *Naegleria fowleri* (primary amoebic meningoencephalitis).

Parasite and life-cycle

Entamoeba histolytica is principally an infection of humans, although some monkeys also harbour the parasite. The four-nucleated cyst is ingested in food or water contaminated by human faeces. The cyst is digested in the gut releasing eight amoebic trophozoites. These live in the colon, normally on the surface of the mucosa, feeding on bacteria and other food residues. The amoebic trophozoite is variable in size, highly motile by means of its pseudopodia and characteristic flowing motion and, when invasive, usually contains ingested red cells.

The amoebae multiply in the gut by simple binary fission. As they move around the colon from right to left, the colonic contents become more solid and the actively motile amoebae stop feeding, empty their food vacuoles, become rounded and secrete a cyst wall.

The cysts are spherical, measuring 10–15 µm, and when mature contain four nuclei and sometimes a glycogen mass and a refractile chromidial bar. Amoebic cysts are passed in the formed stool of people with, usually asymptomatic, amoebiasis. The cysts can survive for prolonged periods in normal environmental conditions; e.g. for more than 12 days in cool faeces and for several weeks in water. They are killed by drying at temperatures above 50 °C, freezing below –5 °C and standard treatment of water supplies.

Under normal circumstances amoebic trophozoites are said to be non-infective; however, an epidemic of amoebic dysentery was caused by the introduction of trophozoites via an incorrectly functioning enema machine used by chiropractors in the USA and resulted in several deaths. Person–person transfer and inoculation of trophozoites into skin abrasions or mucous membranes can also occur, resulting in cutaneous amoebiasis and sexual transmission of cutaneous amoebiasis can occur by direct genital contact.

Pathogenesis

Entamoeba histolytica binds to host intestinal cells by means of a galactose-binding lectin on its surface. Following attachment, the amoeba uses pore-forming molecules called amoebapores and, possibly, phospholipidases, to disrupt the target cell, triggering a process of apoptosis, or 'cell suicide'. The amoeba then phagocytoses the dead cell and in due course the process leads to the development of mucosal ulcers with undermined edges, commonly described as 'flask-shaped' ulcers. However, this 'bind–lyse–eat' model for invasive amoebiasis may be oversimplistic. Invasion also appears to depend on cytoskeleton motility, the secretion of proteases that degrade the extracellular matrix and antibody. The host inflammatory response, including the production of cytokines and inflammatory mediators, accompanied by an influx of neutrophils, are also important in the pathogenesis of invasive amoebiasis.

Clinical studies show some evidence of mucosal immunity to recurrent infections; however protective immunity does not appear to follow an amoebic liver abscess. Acquired immunity to recurrent infection with *E. histolytica* has been shown to be linked to a mucosal immune response against a major virulence factor of the parasite, a Gal/GalNAc lectin responsible for adherence and killing of the host tissue. Small peptides derived from the galactose-binding adhesin administered by the parenteral or oral route have been shown to protect gerbils against experimental amoebic liver abscess. Therefore, the prospects for a vaccine are brightening.

Clinical features

The incubation period may range from a few days to many years. Amoebiasis is one of several 'tropical' diseases that can have a prolonged latent period and may present more than a decade following exposure.

Intestinal amoebiasis

The clinical spectrum ranges from asymptomatic infections (the majority) to fulminant amoebic colitis. The onset of invasive disease may be precipitated by another gastrointestinal infection or other illness, debility or immunosuppression. Symptoms are usually insidious with abdominal discomfort and loose stools sometimes containing mucus and blood. Patients with mild disease are relatively well with a history of a few loose stools. Investigations may reveal scanty trophozoites in faeces and a few ulcers on endoscopy. Patients with more extensive disease usually remain afebrile and ambulant despite producing 5–15 bloody stools per day containing numerous trophozoites. They are likely to have obvious rectal ulceration on endoscopy. Debilitated or immunosuppressed patients are more likely to present with rapid onset of abdominal pain, vomiting, dysuria, tenesmus and frequent bloody stools. They are likely to be febrile, dehydrated, toxic and anaemic. Abdominal tenderness may be marked and there may be evidence of peritonitis. Endoscopy is contraindicated. The most extreme presentation is that of extensive fulminating necrotizing colitis, which occurs in a minority of, usually immunocompromised, patients and is often fatal.

Complications of intestinal amoebiasis include the following.

- *Amoebic abscess* – most commonly in the liver (see below).
- *Amoeboma* – chronic inflammatory mass, single or multiple, most commonly developing in the ileocaecal region, presenting as an acute/subacute obstruction or causing an intussusception.
- *Haemorrhage* – resulting in anaemia or shock.
- *Peritonitis* – abrupt/insidious onset; may occur after the patient has commenced treatment.
- *Post-dysenteric ulcerative colitis* – mimicking classical ulcerative colitis; usually resolves slowly without specific treatment; rarely progresses to massive necrosis and toxic megacolon.
- *Skin ulceration* – usually perianal and anogenital regions, but may occur elsewhere, e.g. in surgical wounds and ileostomy/colostomy sites.
- *Stricture* – especially of the colon and rectum.

The differential diagnosis of amoebic colitis includes the following.

1 Other causes of dysentery or bloody stools such as *Shigella*, typhoid, other *Salmonella*, enteroinvasive and enterohaemorrhagic *Escherichia coli*, schistosomiasis (especially *Schistosoma mansoni* and *S. japonicum*), *Balantidium coli*, *Trichuris*

trichiura, tuberculosis, carcinoma, inflammatory bowel disease, ischaemic colitis, arteriovenous malformation and diverticulitis.

2 Any other cause of acute or chronic abdominal pain.

The differential diagnosis of an amoeboma includes tuberculosis, carcinoma, actinomycosis, an 'antibioma' or appendix mass.

Amoebic liver abscess

Trophozoites of *E. histolytica* invade the liver via the portal vein and set about destroying hepatocytes, resulting initially in the formation of microabscesses that subsequently coalesce to form multiple abscesses (25–35% of patients) or, more commonly, a single abscess (65–75% of patients) by the time the diagnosis is made. The surrounding tissue becomes oedematous with a chronic inflammatory infiltrate. Secondary bacterial infection may occur, but is unusual.

Right lobe abscesses are four times more common than those on the left. Amoebic liver abscess is about 10 times more common in males than females. All age groups may be affected, from neonates to the elderly, but ALA is most common in males aged between 20 and 40 years. Fewer than 50% have a history of dysentery within 1 month prior to presentation and many have no history of dysentery at all. A patient may present with an ALA many years after exposure, the transition from latent infection to clinical disease often being precipitated by immunosuppression or debility.

Clinical features

Patients who present in the early precoalescence stage of the development of an amoebic liver abscess may complain of low-grade fever and (usually) right upper quadrant discomfort and tenderness. This stage is sometimes referred to as 'amoebic hepatitis', a term which is perhaps misleading as it is unusual for such patients to have raised aminotransferases or bilirubin.

Most patients with ALA present when the abscess or abscesses are more 'mature' and the clinical symptoms and signs more florid. The history is usually one of gradually increasing but sometimes acute pain in the right upper quadrant of the abdomen. In some cases there is referred pain to the shoulder. Symptoms such as fever, sweats and rigors are common. In some cases the pain is localized to the lower chest wall and may be pleuritic in nature. The patient may also complain of cough and breathlessness and

have evidence of a pleural effusion, leading to a mistaken diagnosis of pneumonia. Weight loss, wasting and anaemia occur more frequently in chronic presentations and such patients may be afebrile. Most patients have tender hepatomegaly, sometimes with inflammation and oedema of the overlying tissue. There may be tenderness in the intercostal spaces (Durban's sign). Signs of a pleural effusion may be evident and the apex beat displaced, especially if the left lobe is affected. Chest X-ray frequently reveals a raised hemidiaphragm or a pleural effusion (Fig. 19.1). Jaundice is uncommon and less than half of patients with an established ALA have a raised bilirubin and transaminases, although most have a raised alkaline phosphatase. A neutrophil leucocytosis is present in around 80% of cases.

In patients with a suspicious history but without obvious tender hepatomegaly, it may be possible to elicit tenderness resulting from a deep-seated abscess by means of a gentle 'thump' over the lower rib cage. This should be regarded as something of a last resort in a situation where more sophisticated diagnostic techniques are unavailable and caution is advised if you do decide to thump your patient: (a) because your patient may thump you back (liver abscesses are usually extremely tender); and (b) worse still, the abscess may rupture.

Complications of ALA include:

- rupture through the skin or into the peritoneum, lung, pleura or pericardium (a particular risk with

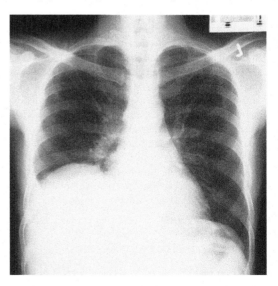

Figure 19.1 Chest X-ray of a patient with a large amoebic liver abscess, showing a grossly elevated right hemidiaphragm.

left lobe abscesses possibly resulting in cardiac tamponade);
- haematogenous seeding causing abscesses in any organ or tissue, e.g. brain, muscle, kidney or spleen.

The differential diagnosis of an ALA includes pyogenic abscess, hepatocellular carcinoma, liver secondaries, hydatid cyst, hepatitis, tuberculosis, syphilitic gumma and lung pathology.

Investigations

Microscopy

The presence of cysts only on stool microscopy is of little diagnostic value because of the problem in distinguishing between *E. histolytica* and *E. dispar*. A diagnosis of amoebic dysentery depends on finding trophozoites of *E. histolytica* containing ingested red blood cells in a fresh stool sample. Ideally, the stool sample should be examined within 15min of being produced or should be maintained at body temperature until examined. This is advised because the trophozoites lose their motility and tend to round up as the specimen cools, thus becoming more difficult to identify. Trophozoites of *E. histolytica* may also be seen in scrapings or biopsies of ulcers identified endoscopically. Non-pathogenic amoebae do not contain ingested red blood cells. In contrast to patients with bacillary dysentery, leucocytes are usually scanty in the faeces of patients with amoebic dysentery. It is rare for trophozoites of *E. histolytica* to be identified in the faeces of patients with ALA and less than half have cysts.

On aspiration, the pus from an ALA ranges in colour from pink to brown, darkening on exposure to air, and is sometimes described as resembling 'anchovy sauce' (in appearance, not odour). Characteristic trophozoites of *E. histolytica* can be identified in the pus or, more reliably, in scrapings from the wall of an ALA. Antigen detection is more sensitive. Cysts of *E. histolytica* are never found in abscesses. Leucocytes are scanty in pus obtained from an amoebic liver abscess unless there is secondary infection.

Antigen detection and polymerase chain reaction

Microscopy remains the principal method of investigation in settings with limited resources. However, stool antigen detection is more sensitive and specific and is being increasingly adopted in more affluent countries. This reliably differentiates between *E. histolytica* and *E. dispar*, but a positive test does not guarantee that *E. histolytica* is responsible for the patient's symptoms. Antigen can also be detected in pus from an ALA. Recent advances include the development of PCR assays for detection *E. histolytica* and a variety of other intestinal pathogens as discussed below.

Serology

A variety of serological tests have been developed for the diagnosis of invasive amoebiasis. Enzyme immunoassay (EIA) is now the most widely recommended and can detect E histolytica antibodies in about 95% of patients with extraintestinal amoebiasis and in 70% of those with active intestinal disease. EIA becomes negative 6–12 months following recovery. EIA may be negative in the early stages of amoebic liver abscess and should be repeated after a week if necessary.

Endoscopy

Colonoscopy is helpful in investigating patients with suspected intestinal amoebiasis in whom stool microscopy or antigen tests are negative or inconclusive. Bowel preparation with enemas or cathartics is not advised because this may interfere with the identification of the parasite. The endoscopic appearance of amoebic colitis resembles that of inflammatory bowel disease and there have been numerous examples of misdiagnosis and consequently disastrous mismanagement. Discrete patchy ulceration with a granular friable mucosa may be seen in acute cases. Larger ulcers with loosely adherent yellowish or grey 'pseudomembranes' tend to occur in more chronic disease. *Entamoeba histolytica* may invade areas of the bowel affected by other pathology, such as a carcinoma, leading to diagnostic confusion. Aspirates, scrapings or superficial biopsies from the ulcer edge should reveal motile erythrophagocytic trophozoites of *E. histolytica* if examined immediately and should also be positive when tested for antigen. The parasites are readily identified by their magenta colour in biopsy specimens using a periodic acid–Schiff stain.

Imaging

Barium enema may demonstrate areas of ulceration, stricture or a filling defect from an amoeboma; however, none of these appearances is specific for amoebiasis, and there is a risk of perforation in patients with severe disease. Ultrasound, computerized tomography (CT) and magnetic resonance imaging (MRI) are very useful in identifying a liver abscess, but cannot reliably differentiate an ALA from a pyogenic abscess. An abscess may not be evident if the patient presents in the early 'precoalescence' stage of disease, and it is worth repeating the scan after a few days if there is a high index of suspicion.

Management

Invasive amoebiasis

Treatment with one of following tissue amoebicides is usually effective.

- *Metronidazole.* Adults 800 mg three times daily orally for 5–10 days; children 35–50 mg/kg/day in three doses for 5–10 days.
- *Tinidazole.* A single oral dose of 2 g is better tolerated but more expensive. This dose should be continued for 3–6 days in more severe infections; children 50–60 mg/kg/day for 3–5 days.
- *Oral chloroquine.* 600 mg base daily for 2 days followed by 300 mg base daily for 2–3 weeks is also effective in the treatment of ALA; children 10 mg/kg/day (max. 300 mg/day base) in 2–4 divided doses for 2–3 weeks.

Eradication of cysts

One of the following luminal amoebicides is usually recommended.

- *Diloxanide furoate.* Adults 500 mg orally three times daily for 10 days; children 20 mg/kg/day in three doses for 10 days.
- *Paromomycin.* Adults and children 25–35 mg/kg/day in three doses for 7 days.
- *Iodoquinol.* Adults 650 mg three times daily for 20 days; children 30–40 mg/kg/day (max. 2 g) in three doses for 20 days.
- *Quinfamide* given in three doses of 100 mg in a single day. This regimen has been used in both adults and children; however, full prescribing information is not yet available.
- *Tetracycline* may also be used as a luminal amoebicide.

Some practical points

A 5-day course of metronidazole is usually sufficient for the treatment of amoebic dysentery and most other forms of invasive amoebiasis. In affluent settings, it is usual to follow on with a course of a luminal amoebicide. A luminal amoebicide is usually omitted in low-resource settings because of the high probability of reinfection. Reinfection, despite treatment with a luminal amoebicide, is also more likely to occur in men who have sex with men. Patients treated with tinidazole or chloroquine should also receive a luminal amoebicide.

Parenteral metronidazole is indicated for patients who are severely ill with the addition of gentamicin and a third-generation cephalosporin (if available) or ampicillin to cover secondary sepsis from bowel pathogens. Attention should also be paid to management of fluid and electrolyte disturbances, anaemia, ileus and other complications.

Surgery is recommended in cases of acute colonic perforation in the absence of diffuse colitis and in cases of ruptured amoebic appendicitis. Surgery should be avoided in patients with severe amoebic colitis because the bowel is very friable and difficult to repair or anastomose. However, patients presenting with toxic megacolon or an abdominal abscess should be managed surgically.

Amoebomas usually respond rapidly to medical treatment and failure to do so should raise suspicion of coincidental pathology, such as a carcinoma. Surgery may be indicated in cases of obstruction or intussusception.

Most patients with an uncomplicated ALA will respond to a 5-day course of metronidazole. However, it may be advisable to extend this to 10 days, particularly if a luminal amoebicide is not available. The best guide to the efficacy of treatment is the patient's clinical response. Unless indicated on clinical grounds, there is little point in repeating scans, as these are likely to remain abnormal for several months despite successful treatment.

Indications for aspiration and drainage of an ALA include failure to respond to medical treatment, impending rupture, suspected secondary bacterial infection and diagnostic uncertainty.

Management of asymptomatic individuals passing cysts depends on the clinical context and the availability of resources for diagnosis and treatment. Ideally, one should differentiate between *E. histolytica* and *E. dispar* using a stool antigen test and prescribe a luminal amoebicide for those with *E. histolytica*. This is unlikely to be possible or practical in a resource-poor setting. In these circumstances, there is little point in attempting to identify and treat such individuals, particularly as the majority have *E. dispar* and all are likely to become reinfected. It is very important to eliminate *E. histolytica* from the gut of asymptomatic patients prior to immunosuppressive treatment and such patients should receive either a 5-day course of metronidazole (or single dose of tinidazole), followed by a luminal amoebicide.

Prevention and public health aspects

Improved hygiene, sanitation and access to safe drinking water are the main issues in preventing infection with *E. histolytica*. 'Boil it, cook it, peel it or leave it' is the message for travellers.

Recent developments

Nitazoxanide, a thiazolide compound, has been shown to be well tolerated and effective in the treatment of a wide range of gastrointestinal infections in adults and children including *E. histolytica* (effective as both a tissue and luminal amoebicide), *Giardia intestinalis (G. lamblia), Blastocystis hominis, Cystoisospora belli, Cyclospora cayetanensis, Dicrocoelium dendriticum, Cryptosporidium spp., Enterocytozoon bieneusi, Trichomonas vaginalis, Balantidium coli, Ascaris lumbricoides, Strongyloides stercoralis, T. trichiura, Enterobius vermicularis, Taenia saginata, Hymenolepis nana, Fasciola hepatica, Clostridium difficile, Helicobacter pylori*, rotavirus and norovirus. Nitazoxanide is not active against aerobic bacterial pathogens such as *E. coli, Shigella, Vibrio*, and *Salmonella*.

In immunocompetent patients, a 3-day course of oral nitazoxanide is usually recommended in the following doses:

- adults and children over 12 years, 500 mg b.d.;
- children aged 4–11 years, 200 mg b.d.;
- children aged 1–3 years, 100 mg b.d.

A recent double-blind, placebo-controlled trial showed that empiric treatment with nitazoxanide reduced the duration of diarrhoea among children. However, further independent studies are required to better inform recommendations for use of this versatile drug.

PCR methods for detecting intestinal (and other) parasites are becoming increasingly available and offer excellent sensitivity and specificity compared to conventional diagnostic methods such as microscopy. A number of multiplex (detection of several pathogens simultaneously) and real-time (automated detection and quantification in real-time) PCR assays have recently been developed for screening for intestinal pathogens including *E. histolytica*.

 SUMMARY

- The two common syndromes of *Entamoeba histolytica* infection in man are intestinal amoebiasis (amoebic dysentery) and hepatic amoebiasis (amoebic liver abscess).
- Diagnosis of amoebic dysentery is ideally by finding amoebic trophozoites containing ingested red blood cells in a fresh stool sample.
- Parasites can also be found in the aspirated pus of amoebic liver abscesses, but the diagnosis is usually made clinically, if possible aided by ultrasound.
- Metronidazole remains the drug of choice, but cyst eradication also requires a luminal amoebicide such as diloxanide fuorate.

 Visit **www.lecturenoteseries.com/tropicalmed** **to test yourself on this chapter using interactive MCQs.**

📖 FURTHER READING

Aslam S, Musher DM (2007) Nitazoxanide: clinical studies of a broad-spectrum anti-infective agent. *Future Microbiol* **2**: 583–90. [Recent summary about this increasingly versatile drug.]

Haque R, Huston CD, Hughes M, Houpt E, Petri WA. Amebiasis (2003) *N Engl J Med* **348**: 1565–73. [Beautifully illustrated state-of-the-art review.]

Petri WA (2002) *Entamoeba histolytica*: clinical update and vaccine prospects. *Curr Infect Dis Rep* **4**: 124–9. [Summarizes recent findings on *E. histolytica* infection in children, differentiation of *E. histolytica* from *E. dispar*, outcome of *E. histolytica*/HIV coinfection in pregnant women in Tanzania, acquired immunity to *E. histolytica* and prospects in vaccine development.]

Stanley S (2003) Amoebiasis. *Lancet* **361**: 1025–34. [Comprehensive overview of pathogenesis, clinical and diagnostic features, and treatment.]

van Lieshout L, Verweij JJ (2010) Newer diagnostic approaches to intestinal protozoa. *Curr Opin Infect Dis* **23**: 488–93. [Update on recent developments in the laboratory diagnosis of intestinal protozoa.]

Ximénez C, Cerritos R, Rojas L, Dolabella S, Morán P, Shibayama M, *et al.* (2010) Human amebiasis: breaking the paradigm?. *Int J Environ Res Public Health* **7**(3): 1105–20. [Can *E. dispar* cause invasive amoebiasis? Find out here.]

20

Bacillary dysentery

Tim O'Dempsey
Liverpool School of Tropical Medicine

The term 'dysentery' is generally used to describe diarrhoea with visible blood and mucus. The term 'bacillary dysentery' is used interchangeably with 'shigellosis' even though numerous other bacteria also cause bloody diarrhoea, including several that are bacilli. Shigellosis occurs worldwide and is associated with poverty, crowding and lack of hygiene and sanitation.

Microbiology and epidemiology

Shigellae are non-motile Gram-negative rod-shaped bacteria, belonging to the family Enterobacteriaceae. According to current criteria for classification on the basis of DNA, Shigellae belong in the genus *Escherichia coli*. However, for historic and clinical reasons, *Shigella* has retained its identity as a separate genus.

Four groups or species are described, all but one of which include several serotypes and subtypes.

- Group A: *Shigella dysenteriae* (serotypes 1–15) tends to cause epidemics (especially *S. dysenteriae* type 1).
- Group B: *Sh. flexneri* (serotypes 1–8, with 15 subtypes) commonly causes endemic dysentery in developing countries.
- Group C: *Sh. boydii* (serotypes 120) is common on the Indian Subcontinent.
- Group D: *Sh. sonnei* (one serotype) is an important cause of dysentery in the industrialized world.

Studies in animals and epidemiological evidence in humans indicate that *Shigella* infections elicit serotype-specific immunity. Humans are the only important reservoir of infection. People who have asymptomatic infections are important as carriers. Transmission is faecal–oral via flies, food, water and person–person contact, including various sexual practices. Shigellae are notably resistant to gastric acid and a very small ingested dose, as few as 10 bacilli, may cause clinical disease. It is estimated that over 160 million clinical infections occur each year, resulting in more than one million deaths. Children aged less than five years account for 70% of cases and 60% of deaths. Dietary supplementation with zinc and vitamin A have both been shown to reduce the incidence and severity of diarrhoeal diseases, including dysentery.

Clinical features

Shigellosis principally affects the colon and, sometimes, the terminal ileum. Clinical manifestations are brought about by a combination of enteroinvasion and toxin production. Organisms invade and multiply in the mucosa causing cell death, inflammation, ulceration, haemorrhage and formation of microabscesses. Shiga toxin, an exotoxin produced by certain strains of *Sh. dysenteriae* type 1, consists of an enterotoxin causing secretory diarrhoea, a cytotoxin causing cell necrosis, and a neurotoxin that may cause central nervous system (CNS) complications in children. Shiga toxin may also be involved in the pathogenesis of haemolytic uraemic syndrome (HUS).

The incubation period usually ranges from 1 to 8 days with a median of 5 days. The clinical spectrum of shigellosis may range from asymptomatic to fulminant with fatal attacks. Many clinical episodes are mild and self-limiting, with watery diarrhoea without blood or mucus, which resolve spontaneously after a few days.

Shigella sonnei infections are usually milder, but may be severe in infants. *Shigella dysenteriae* and

Tropical Medicine Lecture Notes, Seventh edition. Edited by Nick Beeching and Geoff Gill. © 2014 John Wiley & Sons, Ltd. Published 2014 by John Wiley & Sons, Ltd.

Sh. flexneri tend to cause more severe disease with an abrupt onset of bloody, mucoid stools, cramps and tenesmus, often accompanied by fever and, sometimes, dysuria and confusion. Fever, confusion, meningism and convulsions often precede the onset of diarrhoea in young children.

Shigella dysenteriae type 1 may cause a fulminating gangrenous infection with an abrupt onset of fever, chills, rigors, vomiting and toxaemia. The patient can pass 20–60 bloody stools per day, often containing mucus and pus, and sometimes even sloughs of mucosa. Perforation is relatively rare, but severe dehydration, blood loss and sepsis can lead to acute renal failure. HUS occurs in 13% of cases of *Sh. dysenteriae* type 1, usually 1–5 days after the onset of the dysentery. Rarely, a choleraic form may occur with an abrupt onset of profuse watery diarrhoea that later becomes bloody and is associated with a high mortality.

Other complications and sequelae of shigellosis include toxic megacolon, post-dysenteric colitis, strictures, protein-losing enteropathy, granular proctitis, piles, parotitis and rectal prolapse in children. Peripheral neuropathy can also occur, particularly in children. Post-dysenteric Reiter's syndrome and symmetrical arthritis are also well-recognized sequelae.

For the differential diagnosis of bacillary dysentery see Chapter 19 (p. 178).

Investigation

The typical stool of shigellosis is often described as like 'redcurrant jelly'. Microscopically, red blood cells and pus cells are usually numerous whereas bacilli are scanty. Stool culture, even if the sample is fresh, is often difficult, and rectal swabs are more likely to be positive, particularly if directly inoculated onto appropriate culture media at the bedside. A recent advance is the development of a dipstick for rapid diagnosis of *Sh. dysenteriae* type 1. This has been shown to be effective in testing isolates from culture and awaits further trails when used directly on faecal samples. PCR assays have also been developed. Antibiotic sensitivity testing remains crucial in managing shigellosis, particularly in epidemics.

Management

Most cases can be managed supportively with oral rehydration solution. In more severe cases, intravenous fluids, such as normal saline (with or without potassium, depending on renal function) or Ringer's lactate solution will be required. Blood transfusion may be indicated, and patients with HUS may require dialysis.

The WHO recommends that all cases of bloody diarrhoea should be treated promptly with an effective antibiotic. The choice depends on local sensitivity. Multidrug resistance is now very common and widespread, especially with *Sh. dysenteriae* type 1. Empirical treatment with ciprofloxacin, or another fluoroquinolone, is currently recommended as first-line therapy. Second-line choices include pivmecillinam, ceftriaxone, or azithromycin. Antibiotic resistance is increasingly problematic. Ciprofloxacin resistance has been reported in up to 50% of cases in parts of India, and resistance to second-line antibiotics is also increasing, particularly in Asia. The possibility of secondary septicaemia from gut anaerobes and other enteropathogens should be considered in severely ill patients.

The use of antibiotics in children with dysentery caused by *E. coli* 0157:H7, which produces a Shiga-like toxin, is associated with an increased risk of development of HUS. However, at the time of writing this association has not been demonstrated among patients with shigellosis. Daily zinc supplements are recommended for 10–14 days in children aged less than five years. Vitamin A also reduces the severity of episodes of diarrhoea, including dysentery. Recently, green bananas have been shown to reduce the duration and severity of shigellosis in children.

Prevention and public health aspects

Prevention of shigellosis is very much a matter of basic hygiene and sanitation. Handwashing, preferably using soap, is very important, especially in relation to food preparation and consumption. Food and utensils should be protected from flies. At community level, provision of an adequate quantity of water is more important than the quality of water, although quality is also important, as is sanitary disposal of faeces. Epidemic shigellosis can be devastating in refugee and displaced populations. In unstable situations associated with poor hygiene and sanitation, attack rates may be greater than 30%. Severe malnutrition and extremes of age are associated with more severe disease and fatal outcome. Laboratory confirmation and antibiotic sensitivity testing is a priority. Early access to oral rehydration fluids and antibiotic treatment should be coupled with hygiene promotion and other appropriate public health measures.

The need for an effective vaccine has become more urgent with the emergence of multidrug-resistant strains of *Shigella*. Several promising candidate vaccines are currently under development but it is likely to be some time before an effective vaccine becomes widely available.

SUMMARY

- Bacillary dysentery is generally accepted as meaning acute gastroenteritis due to *Shigella* species infection.

- Clinical features include bloody diarrhoea, abdominal cramps, tenesmus and fever. Neurotoxic effects can occur in children.

- Treatment is with oral rehydration, or intravenous fluids for severe cases. Antibiotics (usually ciprofloxacin) are generally used for all but mild cases.

- Basic hygiene and sanitation are the keys to prevention and control, particularly in epidemic situations (such as refugee camps).

 Visit **www.lecturenoteseries.com/tropicalmed** **to test yourself on this chapter using interactive MCQs.**

FURTHER READING

Christopher PR, David KV, John SM, Sankarapandian V (2010) Antibiotic therapy for Shigella dysentery. *Cochrane Database Syst Rev* **8**: CD006784. [Extensive review – the bottom line is antibiotics are recommended for moderate and severe cases of shigellosis.]

Koseka M, Yoria PP, Olorteguib MP (2010) Shigellosis update: advancing antibiotic resistance, investment empowered vaccine development, and green bananas. *Curr Opin Infect Dis* **23**: 475–80. [Update on key findings in epidemiology, control and treatment of shigellosis.]

World Health Organization (2005) *Guidelines for the control of shigellosis, including epidemics due to Shigella dysenteriae 1.*
http://www.who.int/vaccine_research/documents/Guidelines_Shigellosis.pdf

21

Cholera

Paul Shears
Wirral University Teaching Hospital NHS Foundation Trust

Cholera is a bacterial infection of humans caused by *Vibrio cholerae* 01 (of classical or El Tor biotypes) and *V. cholerae* 0139, which characteristically cause severe diarrhoea and may lead to death – in those severely affected – from water and electrolyte depletion. Spread is directly from person to person by the faecal–oral route, or indirectly by infected food or water. It can spread to any part of the world and may become endemic where standards of environmental sanitation and personal hygiene are low.

Humans are the only animal reservoir of infection. However, *V. cholerae* can survive for several months in aquatic environments and transmission may be maintained from such sources. The El Tor biotype has now largely displaced classical cholera as the major pathogen of public health importance, with 0139 responsible for infection in some areas of South Asia.

ganglioside receptors of the epithelial cells. The principal pathogenic factor is the polypeptide cholera toxin released by the vibrios. Cholera toxin comprises two subunits, A and B. The B subunit attaches to the epithelial cells, and 'allows' entry of the A subunit into the cells. The A subunit 'switches on' cyclic AMP, resulting in the efflux of water, bicarbonate and electrolytes, and the clinical dehydration and electrolyte imbalance that characterizes cholera.

In 2000 the full genome of Vibrio cholerae was characterized, and the location of the genes coding for the A (ctxA) and B (ctxB) toxin sub units determined. A further regulatory gene, ToxR, has been shown to be influenced by environmental factors and may be linked to the seasonal pattern of cholera. An understanding of the pathogenic mechanism and the toxin genes has enabled the development of improved cholera vaccines.

Microbiology and pathogenesis

V. cholerae, a Gram-negative comma-shaped bacillus of the family Vibrionaceae comprises over 100 serogroups, distinguished by the composition of the oligosaccharide antigen of the cell wall. Only serogroups 01 and 0139 cause the clinical disease cholera. The classification of *V. cholerae* is important in understanding the global epidemiology of the disease, and is shown in Figure 21.1. Most current outbreaks of cholera are caused by *V. cholerae* 01 El Tor biotype, serotype Ogawa or Inaba.

The infective dose of cholera is relatively high (10^2–10^6) and infectivity is increased in achlorhydria and chronic gastritis. In the ileum, vibrios adhere to

Epidemiology

Pandemics of cholera have been described for several centuries. The current 7th pandemic began in 1961 in Indonesia, and spread relentlessly through South and East Asia, the Middle East, and in the 1970s into Africa and finally in 1990 to Latin America. The pandemic strain is *V. cholerae* 01 El Tor. In 1993 a new serotype, *V. cholerae* 0139 was reported in southern India, and has been responsible for outbreaks in Bangladesh and Thailand, though it has mostly been replaced by 01 El Tor. However, the 0139 strain is thought likely to cause the next pandemic.

In the last decade, El Tor variants have been described that have some characteristics of the classical biotype. These strains have been associated with

Tropical Medicine Lecture Notes, Seventh edition. Edited by Nick Beeching and Geoff Gill. © 2014 John Wiley & Sons, Ltd. Published 2014 by John Wiley & Sons, Ltd.

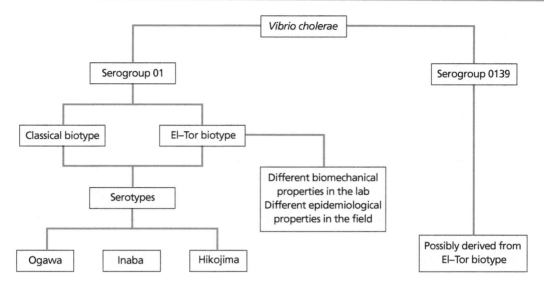

Figure 21.1 Classification of *Vibrio cholerae*.

higher severity of disease and higher case fatality rates.

Cholera is transmitted by the faecal – oral route, and occurs where sanitation and water supplies are inadequate, particularly in the poorer areas of the developing world, and in refugee and complex emergencies. Vibrios can survive for long periods in aquatic environments, and so provide a reservoir of infection when public health infrastructure is compromised. The El Tor biotype has an improved environmental survival compared to Classical, and a higher number of asymptomatic carriers:case ratio, which has contributed to its displacement of the classical biotype. Large scale epidemics have occurred in the last decade among Rwandan refugees in the Democratic Republic of Congo, in southern Sudan, Angola, Zimbabwe and Somalia. Smaller outbreaks have occurred in hospitals with limited facilities for isolation and infection control.

Following the 2010 earthquake in Haiti, there has been a major cholera outbreak among both displaced and settled populations. The responsible strain is different to that occurring in South America, and there is evidence that it may have been introduced by humanitarian assistance personnel.

Diagnosis

In outbreaks of cholera, diagnosis is usually made on clinical grounds following the WHO suspected case definition: '(a) in an area where cholera is not endemic: severe dehydration or death from watery diarrhoea in a patient aged 5 years or more; (b) in an area where there is a cholera epidemic: acute watery diarrhoea, with or without vomiting in a patient aged 5 years or more'. Laboratory investigation is required to confirm the diagnosis and to determine the serogroup and serotype for epidemiological purposes. Cholera vibrios can survive for several days in alkaline peptone water or Cary Blair medium for transport to a laboratory distant from the epidemic. Specimens are cultured at 37 °C on thiosulphate citrate bile salt sucrose (TCBS) agar. *V. cholerae* produces characteristic yellow, oxidase positive, colonies, that can be tested for agglutination with 01 or 0139 anti sera. Recently immuno-diagnostic dip sticks have been developed for the rapid diagnosis of cholera in field conditions

Treatment

Initial rehydration

Rehydration is the mainstay of cholera treatment. In severe cases with hypovolaemic shock, the restoration of blood volume is urgently needed, and this can only be achieved rapidly by intravenous infusion (see also Chapter 1). Because peripheral veins are collapsed in such patients, the initial resuscitative infusion may have to be given via the femoral or subclavian vein in adults or the internal jugular vein or intraosseus route in children.

Fluid in the initial stages is run in as quickly as possible, an initial rate of 4L/h for the first few litres is the norm in adults. The best guide to success is the return of a palpable arterial pulse. As soon as the systolic blood pressure reaches 90 mmHg, renal function usually returns. Tubular necrosis only usually develops if resuscitation is delayed.

In all patients with hypovolaemic shock, the initial fluid deficit will be at least 10% of the body weight. It is a safe rule of thumb to give one-third of the total estimated deficit in the first 20–30 min.

The type of intravenous fluid is less important than an adequate quantity. However, because patients usually have a metabolic acidosis as a result of bicarbonate loss, a deficiency of potassium and a loss of water greater than of salts, a slightly hypotonic alkaline fluid enriched with potassium is the most physiological choice.

The single fluid that meets all these needs, and is suitable both for adults and children, is Ringer's lactate solution. This contains calcium 2 mmol, chloride 111 mmol, lactate 27 mmol, potassium 5 mmol and sodium 131 mmol/L. It is suitable for both initial rehydration and maintenance therapy. Simpler solutions can be used with almost as good results, certainly in adults.

As soon as the blood volume has been restored and the pulse has returned, the drip can be moved to a more convenient site as peripheral veins reappear.

Maintenance hydration

When the patient has been resuscitated, careful monitoring of fluid intake and output must be started.

The urine output should be charted accurately, and intravenous fluid input should equal the combined volume of stool and urine, plus 500 ml added for insensible losses. Once the patient is rehydrated and able to take fluids by mouth, oral rehydration should begin, even though diarrhoea may be continuing.

Oral rehydration with glucose–electrolyte solution is used for maintenance hydration in severe cases following resuscitation, and for all milder cases from the beginning. It is cheaper than intravenous therapy, requires no special apparatus or skills and is free from the dangers of fluid overload. Its success depends on the fact that the active transport of electrolytes into the mucosal cells is glucose dependant. If glucose is not available, sucrose can be used with almost as good results, as it is rapidly split into glucose and fructose by intestinal enzymes. The WHO-recommended solution comprises, in one litre of 'clean' water; dextrose (glucose) 20 g, potassium chloride 1.5 g, sodium bicarbonate 2.5 g and sodium chloride 3.5 g. Oral rehydration should initially be given frequently and in small amounts, and can be successfully done by family members rather than health workers.

Antimicrobial agents in cholera management

Tetracycline, doxycycline and furazolidone have all been shown to reduce the volume and duration of diarrhoea, particularly in those with severe disease. The normal adult regimens are tetracycline 500 mg 6-hourly for 3 days, furazolidone 400 mg/day for 3 days, or a single dose of doxycycline 300 mg. Resistance, particularly to tetracycline, is frequently reported, and indiscriminate use of antibiotics for mild cases should be discouraged.

Control of cholera and prevention

Control involves early detection, isolation and management of cases, improvements in public health to reduce spread, and the possible use of oral cholera vaccine. Symptomatic cases are a major source of infection to household contacts, both directly, and by contaminating food and water, and in crowded refugee camps can lead to explosive epidemics. Isolation facilities for symptomatic cases will vary with the location. In hospitalized patients, single rooms and toilet facilities, and standard barrier precautions are necessary where possible, and the use of chlorine based disinfectants after discharge. Where epidemics occurr in refugee camps or crowded urban slums, locally appropriate strategies will be needed to isolate or cohort patients to reduce the risk of transmission. Facilities will be required for effective case treatment with adequate supplies of intravenous replacement fluids for severe cases and supplies of oral rehydration solution.

The challenges involved in managing large numbers of cases in the most difficult of situations have been well reported from the 1990s Rwanda refugee outbreak, where case fatality rates were reduced from over 30% to less than 5% by appropriate rehydration centres.

During outbreaks, emergency public health measures will be necessary to improve sanitation, control polluted water supplies, and improve hygiene at the household level by safe water storage, provision of soap, and appropriate education and information.

Longer-term control depends mainly on improving standards of environmental sanitation and water supply, which should be a sustained objective of international health programmes.

The role of vaccination in cholera prevention and control has become an important issue with the availability of oral cholera vaccines. The principle of these vaccines is based on an understanding of the pathogenesis and genetics of *V. cholerae*. The objective of the vaccine is to produce gut mucosal antibodies to the bacterial cell wall, and in some candidate vaccines to the B subunit of cholera toxin also.

There are currently two oral cholera vaccine types available. The whole cell B subunit vaccine (WC-rBS) contains killed 01 cells and a recombinant B sub unit, and is the vaccine available in UK. It may be considered for travellers to cholera endemic areas, particularly those who may be working with refugees or going to remote areas. An alternative vaccine has been developed in Vietnam and India, consisting of killed 01 and 0139, but not a B subunit. Trials with both vaccine types have shown good efficacy, with protection lasting up to two years.

With the availability of oral cholera vaccines, WHO has produced guidelines for their possible use in areas at risk of cholera epidemics, including mass refugee exodus or natural disasters in cholera endemic areas.

Cholera continues to be a major public health problem among poorer communities in endemic areas, and among refugees and displaced communities in complex emergencies. While new vaccines and new diagnostics may have a role to play, political and public health initiatives are essential for control.

 SUMMARY

- Humans are the only animal reservoir of cholera, which is spread directly from person to person by the faecal oral route or indirectly via infected food and water.
- Cholera is a disease of poorer areas of the world, including refugee and emergency settings, where it can cause major epidemics.
- The key aspects of clinical management are adequate assessment and oral or parenteral correction of the fluid and electrolyte losses which characterize cholera.
- Antimicrobials such as tetracyclines or furazolidone are helpful in severe cases.
- Political and public health initiatives are essential for control, in addition to the use of vaccines.

 Visit www.lecturenoteseries.com/tropicalmed to test yourself on this chapter using interactive MCQs.

FURTHER READING

Richelle C. Charles RC, Ryan ET (2011) Cholera in the 21st century. *Curr Opin Infect Dis* **24**: 472–7. [Current review.]

Sack DA, Sack RB, Nair GB, Siddique AK (2004) Cholera. *Lancet* **363**: 223–33. [Although nearly 10 years old, still an excellent overview.]

World Health Organization. *Prevention and control of cholera outbreaks: WHO policy and recommendations.* www.who.int/topics/cholera/control/en

World Health Organization. Global Response and Alert (GAR). Updated information on cholera outbreaks: www.who.int/csr/don/archive/disease/cholera/en

World Health Organization (2010) WHO position paper. Cholera vaccines. *Wkly Epidemiol Rec* 2010; 85: 117–28. www.who.int/wer/2010/wer8513.pdf

22

Giardiasis and other intestinal protozoal infections

Tim O'Dempsey
Liverpool School of Tropical Medicine

Giardiasis

Epidemiology

Giardiasis occurs worldwide, particularly in areas of poor hygiene and sanitation. Humans are the main reservoir of infection, although beavers have been implicated in outbreaks in North America. It is uncertain whether several species that occur in various domestic pets and other animals actually cause disease in humans. Most infections are acquired through drinking water contaminated with *Giardia* cysts. These are relatively resistant to chlorination and large community outbreaks have occurred from drinking chlorinated but unfiltered water. Cysts may also be ingested on food, particularly salads, and by direct faeco-oral spread, e.g. among preschool children in day-care centres or in other situations of poor hygiene and sanitation. Cysts can survive outside the body for several weeks under favourable conditions.

Parasite and life-cycle

Giardia lamblia (also known as *G. intestinalis* or *G. duodenalis*) is a flagellate protozoon that inhabits the upper small bowel. The trophozoite stage of the parasite is a flattened pear-shaped creature about 15 μm long, 9 μm wide and 3 μm thick. It is concave on its ventral surface where it attaches itself, by its sucking disc, to the intestinal mucosa, but does not invade. It has four pairs of flagella for locomotion and multiplies in the gut by binary fission. Large areas of the mucosal surface may be colonized in heavy infections.

Trophozoite adherence disrupts the intestinal brush border and interferes with enzyme activity. Attachment also stimulates an inflammatory cytokine response, resulting in secretion of fluid and electrolytes and damage to enterocytes. Trophozoites usually encyst as they pass distally along the intestine. The cyst is oval, 8–12 μm long by 6–8 μm wide, and contains four small nuclei and a central refractile axoneme. The cysts are infective as soon as passed. When swallowed by a new host, they excyst in the upper gastrointestinal tract and liberate trophozoites.

Occasionally, *Giardia* may colonize the biliary tract and – in patients with achlohydria – the stomach, usually in association with *Helicobacter pylori*.

Clinical features

The median incubation period is 7–10 days but ranges from 3 days to several months. Susceptibility to infection and disease depends on parasite and host factors. Clinical symptoms may develop after ingesting as few as 10 cysts. Most infections are asymptomatic. Clinical symptoms are more likely to develop and tend to be more severe in initial infections, and tend to be more difficult to treat in persons with impaired immunity (e.g. HIV, B cell deficiencies).

Tropical Medicine Lecture Notes, Seventh edition. Edited by Nick Beeching and Geoff Gill. © 2014 John Wiley & Sons, Ltd. Published 2014 by John Wiley & Sons, Ltd.

Symptoms are often abrupt with diarrhoea, abdominal cramps, bloating and flatulence. Often there is associated malaise, nausea and belching accompanied by a taste of rotten eggs. The diarrhoea can be variable in character, ranging from watery to greasy, but does not contain blood. Most patients have been symptomatic for several days before seeking medical help, and may have significant weight loss by the time they present. Untreated, the clinical course is variable. Many patients, often after periods of fluctuating symptoms, eventually become asymptomatic. Others continue to have persisting diarrhoea, associated with malabsorption, malnutrition and failure to thrive. In some patients, chronic diarrhoea may be partly related to lactose intolerance, which may persist despite eradication of the *Giardia*.

Differential diagnosis

The differential diagnosis includes a wide range of causes of acute and chronic non-bloody diarrhoea and other causes of malabsorption, including:

- alpha-chain disease;
- coeliac disease;
- chronic calcific pancreatitis;
- hypolactasia;
- intestinal tuberculosis;
- malnutrition;
- parasitic (capillariasis, cryptosporidiosis, cystoisosporiasis, fasciolopsiasis, strongyloidiasis);
- small bowel lymphoma;
- tropical sprue.

Investigations

The standard method of diagnosis is stool microscopy for the characteristic cysts. Passage of cysts can be intermittent and it may be necessary to examine repeated samples. Motile trophozoites are sometimes seen in saline preparations. Concentration and special staining techniques increase the sensitivity of stool microscopy and it should be possible to diagnose 50–70% of infections on examination of a single concentrated stool sample, and more than 90% of infections if three samples are examined.

A variety of new techniques are available for the rapid detection of *Giardia* antigen in stool samples, e.g. using ELISA and direct fluorescence antibody techniques. Rapid, highly sensitive and specific point of care tests are now commercially available. A panel enzyme immunoassay (EIA) has been developed for the detection of *G. lamblia*,

Entamoeba histolytica and *Cryptosporidium parvum* with sensitivities and specificities of over 95% for identification of these organisms. A number of real-time and multiplex PCR assays have also been developed.

Other methods of diagnosis include duodenal fluid aspiration and microscopy for trophozoites. Duodenal fluid can also be sampled using the 'string test' in which the patient swallows a length of string, one end of which is entwined in a gelatin capsule. The capsule dissolves and the string passes into the duodenum. Having taped the proximal end to the patient's cheek, the string is left *in situ* overnight, or with the patient fasting for 4–6 h. The string is then withdrawn, the duodenal fluid squeezed from the distal end onto a microscope slide and examined for *Giardia* trophozoites. This technique is also useful in diagnosing strongyloidiasis (Chapter 52).

Small bowel biopsy may be helpful in patients in whom an alternative or concurrent diagnosis is being considered, e.g. patients with HIV/AIDS, common variable immunodeficiency or suspected tropical sprue. The typical picture in giardiasis is of villous flattening, deepening of crypts and an increased inflammatory infiltrate in the lamina propria. *Giardia* trophozoites may also be seen in the intervillous spaces.

Management

Most patients respond to oral metronidazole 400 mg three times daily for 5 days, or 2 g/day for 3 days. Paediatric regimens are 15 mg/kg/day in three divided doses, or 40 mg/kg/day for 3 days. Tinidazole is effective as a single oral dose of 2 g for adults and 50 mg/kg (maximum 2 g) for children. Albendazole 400 mg/day for 5 days is as effective as metronidazole and better tolerated. Nitazoxanide is also effective and has proved useful in treating patients who are HIV-positive who fail to respond to standard treatment. Other drugs that are sometimes used include quinacrine, furazolidone and paromomycin. Paromomycin is not absorbed and thus is safe to use throughout pregnancy, though it is inferior to metronidazole, which may be used in the second and third trimesters.

Failure to eradicate the organism following a standard course of treatment may be because of poor compliance, reinfection or, possibly, antimicrobial resistance or underlying immunodeficiency.

Persisting symptoms despite eradication of the parasite raises the possibility of continuing lactose intolerance or that *Giardia* was a coincidental finding and the patient's symptoms are attributable to another aetiology.

Prevention and public health

Prevention is all about improving hygiene, sanitation and access to safe water. Cysts of *Giardia* are resistant to standard chlorination of water, therefore flocculation, sedimentation and filtration are of greater importance. Cysts are killed if water is boiled. Micropore filters, with or without iodine resins, are available for personal use and may be handy for travellers.

Other intestinal protozoa of importance

Cryptosporidium parvum

Parasite and life-cycle

Cryptosporidium spp. are coccidian protozoans with a worldwide distribution, found in mammals, reptiles, fish and birds. Two major, distinct species have been identified in waterborne epidemics: *C. hominis*, which is predominantly an infection of humans and *C. parvum* which infects a broader range of animals. Transmission is faeco-oral and infection most commonly occurs when the oocyst is ingested via contaminated water or food, or following person–person contact. The oocyst releases four sporozoites into the lumen of the small bowel, which invade the epithelial cells where they undergo further stages in a life-cycle that, in many ways, resembles that of malaria. *Cryptosporidium* may also invade the colon and biliary tree. *Cryptosporidium* has the ability to produce thin-walled oocysts that maintain its life-cycle within the host ('internal autoinfection'), or to produce thick-walled oocysts that are excreted in faeces. The latter are highly resistant to chlorination and small enough to pass through conventional filters. *Cryptosporidium* is notorious in causing epidemics of diarrhoea, even among communities in developed countries with access to treated water supplies. Ingestion of as few as 10 oocysts can cause symptoms in a susceptible host.

Clinical features

The incubation period for *Cryptosporidium* has not been clearly established, but usually ranges from 1 to 28 days, with an average of 7 to 10 days. *Cryptosporidium* is important in four clinical settings:

- childhood diarrhoea in developing countries;
- travellers' diarrhoea;
- protracted diarrhoea in immunocompromised patients;

- water-borne outbreaks in developed and developing countries.

Clinical features frequently include watery diarrhoea, abdominal cramps, bloating, weight loss, fever and malaise. Episodes are usually self-limiting but may become chronic or fulminant, particularly in immunocompromised patients, e.g. with HIV/AIDS, and associated biliary tract disease may also occur in this population.

Cystoisospora belli

Cystoisospora belli is a protozoan parasite with a worldwide distribution, usually acquired from faecally contaminated water or food. Disease may occur following ingestion of the mature oocyst and pathology is similar to *Cryptosporidium*. Clinical presentation is usually with watery diarrhoea, sometimes with blood and pus cells, abdominal pain and malabsorption. Unusually for a protozoan infection, eosinophilia may be present in up to 50% of patients with cystoisosporiasis. Infections are usually self-limiting but may become chronic or relapsing in immunocompromised patients.

Cyclospora cayetanensis

Cyclospora is usually acquired from faecally contaminated water, fruit or herbs. Clinically similar to *Cryptosporidium* and *Cystoisospora*, symptoms include prolonged watery diarrhoea, cramps, fever and fatigue.

Balantidium coli

The largest and probably least common protozoan pathogen of humans, *Balantidium coli*, can cause a spectrum of disease similar to that of amoebiasis, including severe, life-threatening colitis. The pig is the most important animal reservoir for human disease. Monkeys and other mammals may also be infected.

Blastocystis hominis

Although, like many of the other protozoa, *Blastocystis hominis* can infect humans without causing diarrhoea, it is now evident that it can cause acute and chronic diarrhoea, particularly in individuals who are immunocompromised.

Microsporidia

Various species of the order Microsporidia are pathogenic in humans and are increasingly recognized to be important, not only among patients with HIV and other conditions associated with immunocompromise, but also in travelers, children and the elderly. Transmission is mainly faeco-oral and a recent outbreak occurred among hotel guests after eating contaminated cucumbers. The most common pathogenic species in humans is *Enterocytozoon bieneusi*, which occurred in 7–50% of HIV-infected persons with chronic diarrhoea in the pre-ART era. Microsporidial species may invade the biliary tree and liver and may also affect other organ systems, particularly the CNS, including the eye, respiratory and genitourinary systems causing encephalitis, keratoconjunctivitis, sinusitis, pneumonia, myositis, peritonitis, nephritis, and hepatitis.

Investigations

The diagnosis of cryptosporidiosis is usually made by demonstrating acid-fast oocysts in faeces or luminal aspirates using a modified Kinyoun acid-fast stain. *Cryptosporidium* oocysts appear as round pinkish-red bodies measuring 4–6 μm. Specific antigen-detection assays are more sensitive including immunofluorescent assays, enzyme-linked immunosorbent assay (ELISA), and immunochromatographic tests.

Cystoisospora oocysts are larger and oval, measuring 10 × 30 mm. They may be visible in an unstained saline preparation and appear red with the modified acid-fast stain. Unusually for a protozoal infection, *Cystoisospora* may cause an eosinophilia.

Cyclospora oocysts are round and measure 8–10 μm. They may be seen in unstained faecal preparations and stain (variably) red with the modified acid-fast stain. They do not stain with iodine. They can be detected as blue fluorescent dots when examined in ultraviolet light.

Modified trichome stains, calcofluor or chemofluorescent stains can be used in expert hands for the diagnosis of *E. bieneusi* and other microsporidia in faeces, and electron microscopy is used in reference laboratories to confirm the identity of the organism. None of these modalities are routinely available in the tropics and underdiagnosis is the norm.

Highly sensitive and specific multiplex and real-time PCR assays are now also becoming more widely available for diagnosis of protozoal parasites.

Management

Most patients with normal immunity recover from these infections spontaneously. HIV-related cryptosporidiosis and other protozoal infections described above usually improve following the initiation of antiretroviral treatment.

Treatment of symptomatic patients with cryptosporidiosis poses problems as few of the available antimicrobials have proven and consistent efficacy. Nitazoxanide is now regarded as the drug of choice for treatment in HIV-related cryptosporidiosis and,

because of its broad spectrum of activity, may also have a role in the 'blind' treatment of persistent diarrhoea in circumstances where diagnostic facilities are limited or absent. HIV protease inhibitors (PIs) have been shown to have some effect in inhibiting proteases of certain parasites, including cryptosporidium. Therefore, the response to nitazoxanide may be enhanced with initiation of anti-retroviral combination therapy that includes a PI. A combination of azithromycin and paromomycin is recommended if nitazoxanide is not available. Nitazoxanide may also be effective against *B. hominis*, *C. belli*, *C. cayetanensis*, *E. bieneusi* and *Balantidium coli*.

Cystoisospora and *Cyclospora* respond to oral co-trimoxazole 160–800 mg four times daily for 7–10 days. HIV-positive patients should then receive a maintenance dose three times weekly. Pyrimethamine can be used if the patient is allergic to sulfonamides. Ciprofloxacin is also effective against *Cyclospora*.

B. coli usually responds to tetracycline 500 mg four times daily for 10 days. Bacitracin, ampicillin, metronidazole and paramomycin are alternatives. Surgery may be required in fulminant colitis.

B. hominis also responds to metronidazole and co-trimoxazole.

Albendazole may produce clinical improvement in patients with *E. bieneusi*, despite persistence of the parasite in stool samples and small bowel biopsies following treatment. It is more effective for treating the less common gut microsporidian *Encephalitozoon intestinalis*. Improvement also usually occurs with the introduction of antiretroviral treatment. Fumagillin has also been used for microsporidiosis but is very toxic.

 SUMMARY

- *Giardia lamblia* intestinal infection can occur worldwide. Transmission is from infected water, and diagnosis by finding typical cysts in the stool.
- Infections can be asymptomatic, or cause an acute diarrhoeal disease. However, in some cases a chronic relapsing syndrome occurs with diarrhoea, abdominal pain and sometimes malabsorption.
- Cystoisosporiasis usually responds well to oral metronidazole.
- A variety of other intestinal protozoal infections may occur; including *Cryptosporidia*, *Cystoisospora* and *Blastocystis*.
- Giardiasis and cryptosporidiosis can be particularly troublesome in HIV/AIDS.

Visit www.lecturenoteseries.com/tropicalmed to test yourself on this chapter using interactive MCQs.

FURTHER READING

Aslam S, Musher DM (2007) Nitazoxanide: clinical studies of a broad-spectrum anti-infective agent. *Future Microbiol.* **2**: 583–90. [Recent summary about this increasingly versatile drug.]

Didiera ES, Weiss LM (2011) Microsporidiosis: not just in AIDS patients. *Curr Opin Infect Dis* **24**: 490–5. [This recent review describes reports of microsporidiosis in HIV-infected individuals and, increasingly, in non-HIV-infected populations.]

Farthing MJ (2006) Treatment options for the eradication of intestinal protozoa. *Nat Clin Pract Gastroenterol Hepatol* **3**: 436-445. [Excellent review covering management of intestinal protozoal infections.]

Gardner TB, Hill DR (2001) Treatment of giardiasis. *Clin Microbiol Rev* **14**: 114–28. [Useful summary including recommendations for treatment during pregnancy.]

Tejman-Yarden N, Eckmann L (2011) New approaches to the treatment of giardiasis. *Curr Opin Infect Dis* **24**: 451–6. [Recent review focussing on recent advances in the development of new antigiardial drug candidates.]

23

Intestinal cestode infections (tapeworms) including cysticercosis

Tim O'Dempsey
Liverpool School of Tropical Medicine

Tapeworms

Tapeworms are flat segmented hermaphrodites measuring from 10 mm to 20 m. The head (scolex) attaches to the intestinal mucosa by means of suckers or hooklets. All, with the exception of *Hymenolepis nana*, require a secondary intermediate host in which the larvae develop into cysts, usually in muscle. Human infection follows consumption of cysts in undercooked meat or fish. Larval cestode infections can also occur in humans following the ingestion of the egg, the most important being cysticercosis.

Parasites and life-cycles

Taenia saginata, the beef tapeworm, is a cosmopolitan infection in which humans harbour the adult worm and cattle harbour the larval stage. Its main importance is in economic losses caused by condemnation of beef carcasses. Human infection is of social importance only. Ethiopia has the highest infection rate in the world. People acquire infection by eating undercooked meat containing cysticerci, the larval stages of the parasite encysted in the muscles of infected herbivores. The cysts evaginate in the intestine, and the head of the worm attaches itself to the mucosa of the upper third of the small intestine by its suckers. Segments called proglottids grow from the head, and new segments are added until the worm contains a chain of 1000–2000 segments.

Proglottids at the tail end of the worm develop fertilized eggs in the uterus and are called gravid segments. When mature, the gravid segments break off the chain (strobila) and leave the anus in the stool or by their own movements. Proglottids sometimes rupture in the intestine, and free eggs are also passed in the stool. The eggs that reach pasture, mainly after disintegration of the mature proglottids, are infective to cattle (and several other herbivores) when swallowed. They hatch in the bovine gut to become oncospheres, and enter the circulation where they are carried to the muscles and encyst as cysticerci. The meat is described as 'measly', and the cysticerci are easily visible to the naked eye.

Taenia saginata cysts can occur in other domestic bovines and a closely related Asian species has been shown to infect pigs, ungulates and monkeys. *Taenia solium*, the pork tapeworm, is a much less common infection than *T. saginata* but far more important because of its ability to cause severe disease in humans. Humans are the definitive host; the pig the normal intermediate host. It is found all over the world where people eat cysts in raw or undercooked pork. For this reason, intestinal infection with *T. solium* is rare in Muslims, Orthodox Jews and vegetarians. *Taenia solium* cysts also occur in dogs and cats.

Ingestion of eggs of *T. solium* can give rise to human cysticercosis, a major cause of epilepsy and other neurological disease in some parts of the world such as Central America and India. Human cysticercosis can occur regardless of religious or dietary affiliation. Human cysticercosis does not occur following the ingestion of eggs of *T. saginata*.

Beef and pork tapeworm maturation takes up to 12 weeks. A fully grown tapeworm may be 5 – 10 m long, live up to 25 years and produce about 50 000 eggs/day.

A third species of human *Taenia*, *T. asiatica*, which is also transmitted in pigs, has recently been described in Asia. Prevalence rates of up to 20% have been documented among villagers in Indonesia.

Clinical features of taeniasis

Intestinal infections are usually asymptomatic. The host may only realize that a tapeworm is on board when a proglottid segment appears in faeces or is felt as it passes through the anus. Symptoms may include loss of appetite, nausea or vague abdominal pain. Rarely, complications arise when a proglottid migrates to an unusual site, such as the appendix or pancreatic and bile ducts. Patients who are vomiting profusely for whatever reason may be further distressed by the appearance of several metres of tapeworm in the vomit.

Investigations

The eggs of *T. saginata* are indistinguishable from those of *T. solium* on routine microscopy. To make a specific diagnosis, a mature proglottid is pressed between two microscope slides and the number of lateral branches of the uterus counted. *T. saginata* has 15–20 main branches on each side, *T. solium* has 13 or fewer; but this criterion is not as reliable as once thought. The scolex, measuring about 1 mm, may be found among the smallest immature segments with the aid of a magnifying glass. The presence of hooks distinguishes the scolex of *T. solium* from that of *T. saginata*, which has no hooks. Coproantigen detection tests and PCR are also available.

Serology is sometimes used for epidemiological surveys and may be useful in the diagnosis of cysticercosis. DNA probes have also been developed to differentiate between *T. saginata* and *T. solium*.

Cysticercosis

Tissue cysts of *T. solium* are usually 1–2 cm in size and can be found in many tissues, especially subcutaneous, muscle and brain. During the initial phase of invasion and development there may be pain and swelling, accompanied by eosinophilia. Subsequently, skin nodules can sometimes be felt as movable, small, painless nodules, especially on the arms or chest. Muscle cysts eventually calcify and can be seen as calcified streaks that follow the planes of the fibres of skeletal muscle on X-ray of the forearms, psoas or thigh muscles.

The most important effect of cysticercosis is in the brain. Two forms of cysticerci are found in the CNS: intraparenchymal (cysts in the CNS tissue) and extra-parenchymal or 'racemose' (grapelike) cysts proliferating into the subarachnoid space or basal cisterns. Extraparenchymal cysticerci are uncommon in children and are associated with a poorer prognosis.

In highly endemic regions, where up to 25% of the population may be seropositive for cysticercosis, computed tomography (CT) surveys have revealed calcified cysts in 10–20% of healthy individuals. Among symptomatic cases, initially there may be a diffuse encephalitic picture. Patients with numerous parenchymal cysticerci may develop diffuse cerebral oedema, termed cysticercal encephalitis, which is more commonly seen in children. More usually, the patient presents with single or repeated seizures. Neurocysticercosis is the most important cause of epilepsy in many parts of Africa, South America and India. A small proportion of cases, more commonly with racemose cysticerci, present with features of obstructive hydrocephalus. Arachnoiditis may also occur resulting in communicating hydrocephalus and/or vasculitis. CT and magnetic resonance imaging (MRI) are needed to delineate the number, location and 'activity' of cysts in the brain. About 15–25% of patients with neurocysticercosis have a tapeworm at presentation or have a past history of tapeworm infection.

There is still controversy about the benefits and drawbacks of active antiparasitic treatment, but expert consensus is that treatment will benefit some patients with neurocysticercosis. A recent meta-analysis showed that treatment with cysticidal drugs results in better resolution of enhancing lesions and cysts, lower risk of recurrence of seizures in patients with enhancing lesions, and a reduction in the rate of generalized seizures in patients with viable cysts. Therefore, a full course anthelmintic therapy is now recommended for patients with active parenchymal neurocysticercosis.

Single-day praziquantel treatment has recently been recommended for patients who have single brain enhancing lesions and positive serology. Active parenchymal neurocysticercosis may be treated with albendazole 15 mg/kg/day in two divided doses for 8–15 days, or, as second choice, praziquantel 50–75 mg/kg/day divided in three doses for 15 days.

Viable cysts can still be found in 60–70% of patients following a course of treatment with either of these regimens, therefore repeated courses may be required. Following initial favourable reports, large scale trials of albendazole-praziquantel combination treatment are currently underway. Cimetidine 400 mg three times daily may be used to increase the levels of both albendazole and praziquantel. Dexamethasone 0.1 to 0.2 mg/kg/day in divided doses should be given before and during antiparasitic treatment to reduce the effects of inflammation around damaged cysts. Dexamethasone increases levels of albendazole and decreases levels of praziquantel. Steroids are also needed (in neurosurgical doses) for short-term management of occasional flare-ups of inflammation and cerebral oedema that occur as cysts degenerate as part of their natural history. Inactive parenchymal cysts do not require treatment with antiparasitic agents. Seizures usually respond to first-line anticonvulsant drugs. Surgical intervention, for example shunting, may be required for obstructive hydrocephalus and intracranial hypertension. If available, neuroendoscopic extraction is now recommended for intraventricular cysts. Extraparenchymal cysts, depending on number, size and location, may require repeated courses of treatment with combinations of antiparasitic drugs, steroids and, possibly, surgery (see Chapter 59).

Should we worry about undiagnosed neurocysticercosis when prescribing albendazole or praziquantel for example to individuals or in community helminth/schistosomiasis control programmes? In areas with a high prevalence of neurocysticercosis, the answer is 'yes' as neurological symptoms may be precipitated by a single dose of either of these drugs. Routine screening may not be feasible, therefore it is prudent to advise patients to seek medical advice urgently if they develop neurological symptoms (usually within a week of treatment).

Other intestinal cestode infections

Diphyllobothriasis

Diphyllobothrium latum is the most common of more than a dozen species of fish tapeworm affecting humans. Human infection follows ingestion of undercooked or raw fish or roe. Infection usually involves a single worm and most are asymptomatic or associated with vague non-specific abdominal symptoms. Megaloblastic anaemia can occur in severe cases.

Hymenolepiasis and dipylidiasis

Hymenolepis nana, the dwarf tapeworm, occurs worldwide, mainly among children. Infections are usually asymptomatic, but abdominal pain, nausea, vomiting, pruritis ani and diarrhoea – sometimes containing blood – have been described in heavy infections. Headache, dizziness, sleep and behavioural disturbances are relatively frequent and convulsions have also been reported. Autoinfection is common.

Hymenolepis diminuta, the rat tapeworm, may affect humans following ingestion of the intermediate host, commonly a weevil, flea or cockroach. Infections are usually asymptomatic and short lived.

Dipylidium caninum may infect humans, usually young infants, following accidental ingestion of a flea, the intermediate host. Infections are usually asymptomatic; however, symptoms may include abdominal pain, diarrhoea, pruritis ani and urticaria.

Management of intestinal cestode infections

A single oral dose of praziquantel (10 mg/kg) is the drug of choice for all of the above intestinal cestode infections. *Hymenolepis nana* requires 25 mg/kg as a single dose.

Niclosamide, as a single oral dose (500 mg if <11 kg; 1 g if 11–34 kg; 1.5 g if >34 kg; 2 g for adults) is also effective. Tablets should be well chewed and swallowed with plenty of water. The routine use of purgatives and antiemetics in patients with *T. solium* prior to cestocidal treatment, in order to prevent retrograde peristalsis of eggs and possible risk of cysticercosis, is not justified on the basis of clinical evidence.

Albendazole, which is used in the treatment of cysticercosis and hydatid cyst, is also effective in treating intestinal taeniasis. Nitazoxanide has also been shown to be effective in infections with *T. saginata* and *H. nana*.

Prevention and public health aspects

Control measures for taeniasis are aimed at environmental sanitation, meat inspection and adequate cooking or freezing of meat. Effective vaccines are available to prevent *T. saginata* and *T. solium* infection in livestock. A combination of community chemotherapy with niclosamide followed by population surveillance using coproantigen together with mass vaccination and chemotherapy (oxfendazole) of pigs appears to have been effective in interrupting transmission of *T. solium* in villages in Peru.

 Visit www.lecturenoteseries.com/tropicalmed to test yourself on this chapter using interactive MCQs.

> ### 🔑 SUMMARY
>
> - The main human tapeworms are *Taenia saginata* (beef tapeworm) and *Taenia solium* (pork tapeworm). Less common are *Diphyllobotrium latum* (fish tapeworm) and *Hymenolepis nana* (dwarf tapeworm).
> - Treatment of all intestinal tapeworm infections is by a single dose of praziquantel.
> - Cystercercosis is a potentially serious complication of *T. solium* infection, and in some areas is a major cause of epilepsy.
> - Neurocysticercosis can be treated with albendazole or praziquantel, but steroids (usually dexamethasone) are needed before and during anthelmintic treatment.

📖 FURTHER READING

Craig P, Akira I (2007) Intestinal cestodes. *Curr Opin Infect Dis* **20**: 524–32. [Excellent recent review summarizing the biology, clinical aspects, diagnosis, treatment and epidemiology of intestinal cestodes.]

García HH, Gonzalez AE, Evans CAE, *et al.* (2003) *Taenia solium* cysticercosis. *Lancet* **361**: 547–56. [Comprehensive review with superb illustrations and references; clear discussion of areas of controversy.]

Garcia HH, Gonzalez AE, Gilmand RH (2011) Cysticercosis of the central nervous system: how should it be managed? *Curr Opin Infect Dis* **24**: 423–7. [Recent update including developments in medical and surgical management.]

Nash, TE, Singh G, White AC, *et al.* (2006) Treatment of neurocysticercosis: current status and future research needs. *Neurology* **67**: 1120–7. [Authoritative and detailed review addressing an often controversial and difficult clinical problem.]

24

Soil-transmitted helminths

Tim O'Dempsey
Liverpool School of Tropical Medicine

The term 'soil-transmitted helminths' applies to a group of parasites whose life-cycle usually depends on a period of development outside the human host, typically in moist, warm soil. The most important of these globally are the roundworms (*Ascaris lumbricoides*), whipworms (*Trichuris trichiura*), and hookworms (*Necator americanus* and *Ancylostoma duodenale*). In some species infection occurs following ingestion of eggs that have been passed in the faeces and only become infectious having spent a period of time undergoing further development, usually in soil, for example, *A. lumbricoides*.

Penetration of the skin is the method of infection used by the hookworms. Under favourable environmental conditions, larvae hatch from eggs deposited in the soil. The larvae lie in wait in the surface layers of the soil until they come into contact with the skin of their unsuspecting host. *Strongyloides stercoralis* employs a similar *modus operandi*, but instead of eggs, larvae are passed in faeces which either can cause autoreinfection by direct penetration of the perianal skin, or go on to establish an independent life-cycle in the soil awaiting the appearance of a new host.

The prevalence and distribution of soil-transmitted helminth infections is a product of lifestyle and life-cycle. Soil-transmitted helminths do not multiply within the host. Their ability to evade the host immune response and avoid causing acute and fatal disease enables them to achieve a state of balanced parasitism that optimizes transmission. The down-regulatory immune responses induced in the host may have a fortuitous role in reducing host susceptibility to atopy and may explain why children living in regions that are highly endemic for these infections appear to be less likely to develop diseases associated with allergy, a theory known as the 'hygiene hypothesis'. Furthermore, infection with *A. lumbricoides* has been shown to dampen the immune response to a recombinant cholera toxin whereas albendazole treatment of children with ascariasis enhances the vibriocidal antibody response to the live attenuated oral cholera vaccine CVD 103-HgR.

There is also some evidence indicating that these infections may increase host susceptibility to malaria, tuberculosis and HIV. However, studies from Thailand indicate that intestinal helminth infections, particularly with *A. lumbricoides*, appear to be protective against cerebral malaria, even though such infections are also associated with an increased risk of infection with *Plasmodium falciparum*.

More than a billion people worldwide are infected with soil-transmitted helminths, often with several different species simultaneously, resulting in significant morbidity in about 300 million. The greatest burden of disease occurs among children, particularly in areas of poor hygiene and sanitation, and has a significant effect on physical and intellectual development. The World Health Organization (WHO) is currently promoting the periodic mass chemotherapy of schoolchildren and women of childbearing age in an attempt to reduce the burden of disease in vulnerable populations.

The Global Network for Neglected Tropical Diseases (NTDs), which includes international non-profit organizations, the WHO, pharmaceutical companies and ministries of health in disease-endemic countries, was established in 2006 as a major international initiative promoting an integrated NTD control strategy. The introduction of a 'rapid impact package' to treat seven of the most common NTDs (ascariasis, trichuriasis, hookworm, schistosomiasis, lymphatic filariasis, onchocerciasis and trachoma) using a combination of four drugs (albendazole/mebendazole, DEC/ivermectin, praziquantel, azithromycin) for just 50 cents per person per year (including drugs, delivery, equipment, training, health promotion,

Tropical Medicine Lecture Notes, Seventh edition. Edited by Nick Beeching and Geoff Gill. © 2014 John Wiley & Sons, Ltd. Published 2014 by John Wiley & Sons, Ltd.

monitoring and evaluation) is proving to be a highly effective public health intervention. However, there is concern that this mass-treatment approach may hasten the development of resistance to mainstay anthelmintics such as albendazole and mebendazole.

Future developments are likely to include strategies involving combination treatment with existing anthelmintics and the wider use of newer drugs with anthelmintic properties, for example nitazoxanide and tribendimidine. A promising hookworm vaccine that has been shown to be effective in animal models is currently being developed for use in humans. Prevention of infection, disease and transmission of soil-transmitted helminths in a single step by vaccination is an attractive, if ambitious, goal for the future.

Ascariasis

Epidemiology

Ascaris lumbricoides affects over 800 million worldwide with a peak prevalence and intensity of infection among children aged 3–8 years. Infection is found wherever conditions of environmental hygiene are poor.

Parasite and life-cycle

Ascaris eggs, contaminating vegetables, soil or dust, are swallowed and liberate larvae as they pass through the stomach and small intestine. The larvae penetrate the intestinal mucosa, enter the bloodstream and lymphatics and reach the lungs 4–16 days after infection. The larvae penetrate the alveoli, moult and migrate via the respiratory tract to the oesophagus and on to the small intestine, where they develop into adults, mate and start producing eggs 9–11 weeks after infection. Adults are large cream-coloured worms; males are 15–30 cm long, females 20–40 cm. They live in the small intestine and obtain nourishment from the intestinal contents. They do not suck blood or damage the mucosa significantly. Females produce up to 200 000 eggs per day. These are excreted in faeces and their ova mature into infective embryos within 1–4 weeks and may remain viable in soil for years.

The morphologically similar *Ascaris* of pigs, *A. suum*, also infects humans.

Clinical features

Ascaris pneumonitis

Fever, cough, dyspnoea, wheeze and urticaria may occur in a proportion of those infected during the migration of larvae through the lungs. Chest pain, cyanosis and haemoptysis occur in more severe cases. Ascaris pneumonitis accompanied by eosinophilia is known as Löffler's syndrome. Symptoms usually resolve spontaneously within 10 days. Pneumonitis is commoner in children and tends to be more severe on reinfection.

Clinical features resulting from adult worms

Intestinal worms are rarely noticed unless passed in the stool. Lactose intolerance and malabsorption of vitamin A and other micronutrients may sometimes occur. Worms may form a bolus in heavy infections causing intestinal obstruction, volvulus or perforation and peritonitis. Intestinal obstruction is commoner in children whereas obstruction of biliary ducts is more likely in adults. Obstruction of ducts or diverticula may cause biliary colic, cholangitis, liver abscess, pancreatitis or appendicitis, or wandering worms can make an unwelcome appearance in an endotracheal tube during anaesthesia. They have also been known to obstruct nasogastric tubes and even enter the paranasal sinuses. Even if these nomadic nematodes do not cause an obvious pyogenic peritonitis, they may continue to lay eggs, giving rise to a granulomatous peritonitis. Pneumothorax and pericarditis have also been reported.

Investigations

Ascaris pneumonitis is diagnosed on clinical grounds; the presence or absence of eggs in the stools is irrelevant. Larvae and/or eosinophils may be found in the sputum. Chest X-ray findings range from discrete densities to diffuse interstitial – or more confluent – infiltrates. Stool microscopy for eggs is usually adequate for diagnosing established infection, although stools may be negative if all the worms are male. Worms may also be found by means of barium studies, ultrasonography and endoscopy.

The Kato-Katz technique, which is a quantative method widely used for estimating the prevalence and intensity of *Schistosoma mansoni* and *S. japonicum* infections, can also be used for soil-transmitted helminths. A drawback of the Kato-Katz method is a relatively low senstitvity. FLOTAC, a newly-developed method for detecting ova of soil-transmitted helminths, which is based on the centrifugation of stool samples in a flotation solution, has been shown to be more sensitive than Kato-Katz and is also useful for diagnosing intestinal protozoal infections.

Management

- Albendazole 400 mg as single oral dose clears most infections. Heavy infections may need repeated doses for 2 or 3 days. The recommended dose in children aged 1–2 years is 200 mg.
- Mebendazole 100 mg orally twice daily for 3 days is effective. Its use in children younger than 2 years is not recommended by the manufacturer. Ectopic migration of *Ascaris* has been reported following the use of mebendazole. A single dose of 500 mg may also be effective.
- Piperazine 75 mg/kg (to a maximum of 3.5 g for adults and children >12 years and a maximum of 2.5 g for children aged 2–12 years). Side-effects are relatively common and can be serious. Therefore, piperazine should only be used if safer alternatives are unavailable.
- Pyrantel pamoate (11 mg/kg up to a maximum of 1 g) can be given as a single dose. Pyrantel and piperazine have antagonistic effects and should never be prescribed concurrently.
- Levamisole 2.5 mg/kg as a single dose may also be effective.
- Nitazoxanide is also effective.

Ascaris pneumonitis is managed symptomatically with bronchodilators and steroids if indicated. Symptoms may be exacerbated by larval death, therefore the use of antihelmintics is questionable.

Intestinal obstruction is usually managed conservatively with nasogastric aspiration, intravenous fluids and antispasmodics, followed by an anthelmintic when the obstruction has subsided. Laparotomy may be necessary if this fails or if the patient is seriously ill. It may be possible to manipulate the worms through the ileocaecal valve without having to open the bowel. Surgical or endoscopic removal of single worms blocking bile or pancreatic ducts may be necessary for patients who fail to respond to anthelmintic treatment and those with persisting pain or raised serum amylase.

Prevention and public health aspects

Improved hygiene and sanitation, access to clean water and health education are particularly important. In some communities, human excrement ('night soil') is used to fertilize vegetables and poses an obvious risk. Periodic mass chemotherapy of vulnerable schoolchildren and women of childbearing age is currently being promoted by WHO.

Hookworm

Epidemiology

Ancylostoma duodenale and *Necator americanus* are widely distributed in the tropics and subtropics, affecting approximately 600 million people worldwide. *N. americanus* predominates in the Americas, Australia, sub-Saharan Africa, South Asia and the Pacific islands, whereas *A. duodenale* is more prevalent in the Middle East, northern Africa, southern Europe, northern India and northern China. In Africa and Asia, 30–54% of moderate and severe anaemia in pregnancy is attributable to infection with hookworm. Hookworm infections commonly cause significant anaemia in all age groups, particularly if dietary iron intake is limited.

Parasites and life-cycle

Hookworms are slender tubes about 1 cm long. They have a mouth and oesophagus at the front, connected by the gut to the anus at the rear. *Ancylostoma* is larger than *Necator*. The female body is largely occupied by eggs. The teeth in *A. duodenale* and the cutting plates in *N. americanus* are used to pierce the intestinal mucosa. The mouth and pharynx are used to attach the worms to the mucosa by suction.

Hookworm eggs passed in the faeces hatch in warm moist conditions, liberating rhabditiform larvae. These develop into filariform larvae, which inhabit the surface layer of soil. Filariform larvae penetrate human skin via fissures or hair follicles and are carried in the lymphatics and venous circulation to the lungs. Here they enter the alveoli, migrate to the pharynx and then to the small intestine where they mature into adults. Adult hookworms attach themselves to the upper half of the small intestine and feed on blood. An adult *A. duodenale* may consume between 0.15 and 0.26 mL/day. *Necator americanus* consumes a relatively modest 0.03 mL/day. Blood loss also occurs at the site of attachment. Loss of plasma proteins may result in hypoproteinaemia. The journey to the intestine takes about a week. Adults are fully grown (approximately 1 cm) in 2–3 weeks and sexually mature in 3–5 weeks, after which eggs begin to appear in the faeces.

Rarely, infection with *A. duodenale* may occur following ingestion of larvae on contaminated vegetables. Infantile hookworm disease has been described in China and attributed to transmammary transmission, laying infants on contaminated soil, or using nappies made of cloth bags stuffed with infected soil.

Clinical features

Most infections are asymptomatic. Problems arise when dietary iron intake is poor or demands are high, resulting in a gradually worsening iron-deficient anaemia, sometimes associated with hypoalbuminaemia and oedema. Eventually this may lead to cardiac failure. Pregnant women, women with menorrhagia and children are at greatest risk of developing anaemia.

Other symptoms are uncommon and tend to be associated with the early stages of initial infection. 'Ground itch' may occur at the site of larval penetration and, if severe, may be associated with the development of vesicles or pustules. The serpiginous rash of cutaneous larva migrans may be seen in human hookworm infections, although this is more commonly associated with infection with dog or cat hookworm. Larval migration through the lungs may cause a pneumonitis. Occasionally, within a few weeks of a heavy infection, there may be abdominal discomfort, flatulence, anorexia, nausea, vomiting and diarrhoea, sometimes containing blood and mucus. Life-threatening gastrointestinal haemorrhage has been reported as a rare complication in young children with severe primary infections.

'Wakana syndrome' (nausea, vomiting, pharyngeal irritation, cough, dyspnoea, and hoarseness) may follow oral ingestion of *A.duodenale* larvae.

Investigations

Eosinophilia is common. Characteristic eggs can be identified by standard faecal microscopy. Concentration methods may be necessary for light infections. Culture techniques similar to those used for *Strongyloides* may also be used. Eggs may hatch in stool samples that are left for a few days before examination, liberating larvae that may be mistaken for those of *S stercoralis*, although they are morphologically distinct. Mixed infections of hookworm and *Strongyloides* may also occur.

Humans may be infected with largely non-pathogenic worms whose eggs resemble those of hookworm. The most important is *Ternidens diminutus*, a common parasite in monkeys, baboons and humans in southern Africa. The worms inhabit the large bowel, where they may cause cystic nodules. Because they suck blood, they can cause anaemia in heavy infections. Their eggs closely resemble those of the hookworm, but are larger.

Trichostrongylus worms of many species are natural parasites of herbivores in many parts of the world, and humans can become infected by ingesting the infective larvae on raw vegetables or salads. The adult worms are attached to the small intestine, but cause only slight damage and insignificant blood loss. The eggs of *Trichostrongylus* spp. have more pointed ends than the eggs of true hookworms.

Management

- Albendazole 400 mg as a single dose is usually effective.
- Mebendazole 100 mg twice daily for 3 days is commonly prescribed.
- Pyrantel pamoate 11 mg/kg (maximum 1 g) for three days is also effective.
- Levamisole 2.5 mg/kg as a single dose repeated after seven days may also be used.

Treatment for iron-deficiency anaemia may be required, preferably with oral iron. Transfusion is rarely necessary.

Prevention and public health aspects

Improved standards of hygiene and sanitation and the wearing of shoes reduce the likelihood of infection. Periodic mass chemotherapy of vulnerable schoolchildren and women of childbearing age is currently being promoted by WHO.

Interestingly, lower incidence, prevalence and intensity of infection have been noted among children who have received bacille Calmette–Guérin (BCG).

Trichuriasis

Epidemiology

Trichuris trichiura, the whipworm, has a global distribution, most prevalent in warm humid climates and infects about 600 million people worldwide.

Parasite and life-cycle

Infection occurs when eggs contaminating soil, food or fomites are swallowed. Larvae are liberated in the caecum, penetrate the crypts of Lieberkühn and migrate within the mucosa. Mature adult worms are 2–5 cm long, the thinner anterior half of the body being normally partly buried in the mucosa of the large bowel of the host (caecum, colon, rectum). They feed on tissue juices, not blood. Female worms release several thousand eggs per day. After about 2 weeks' development in warm moist soil, the eggs are embryonated and infective.

Interestingly, *T. suis*, the swine whipworm, which does not develop to maturity in humans, has been used in the management of pro-inflammatory auto-immune diseases such as Crohn's disease because of it's ability to secrete, so far undefined, molecules that create an anti-inflamatory local environment.

Clinical features

Most infections are asymptomatic. Heavy infestations may cause severe gastrointestinal symptoms resembling inflammatory bowel disease. Bleeding from the friable mucosa may result in iron-deficiency anaemia in children on poor diets. Chronic infection is associated with growth retardation. Severe *Trichuris* dysentery syndrome frequently leads to rectal prolapse.

Investigations

The diagnosis is obvious in children presenting with rectal prolapse when adult worms can be seen attached to the mucosa of prolapsed bowel. In other circumstances, the characteristic eggs may be identified in the stool. Concentration techniques can be used for light infections; however, if eggs cannot be found on direct examination, the infection is unlikely to be of clinical significance. Trichuriasis may cause a significant eosinophilia.

Management

A single oral dose of mebendazole 500 mg is more effective than albendazole 400 mg. Severe infections require either mebendazole 100 mg twice daily for 3 days, or albendazole 400 mg daily for 3 days. Single dose combination treatment using albendazole 400 mg plus ivermectin 200 micrograms/kg is also highly effective. More recently, nitazoxanide has also been shown to be effective.

Prevention

Prevention consists of simple standard methods of improved hygiene and sanitation. Periodic mass chemotherapy of vulnerable schoolchildren and women of childbearing age is currently being promoted by WHO.

Toxocariasis

Epidemiology

Young children are at greatest risk of infection with Toxocara canis and *T. cati*, parasitic roundworms of dogs and cats. Seroprevalence may exceed 80% among children in poorer communities. Sandpits in public parks fouled by dog faeces are particularly notorious as sources of infection.

Parasite and life-cycle

Infection in humans occurs following ingestion of eggs in sand or soil contaminated by dog or cat faeces. The larva from the ingested egg is released in the intestine and then goes on a prolonged safari through the tissues, lasting 1–2 years. Worms seldom develop beyond the larval stage, so do not reach maturity in the intestine. Thus, eggs are not excreted in human faeces.

Clinical features, investigations and management

Clinical disease is relatively uncommon and depends on the intensity of infection and the organs involved. There are two distinct clinical syndromes: visceral and ocular.

Visceral larva migrans

Visceral larva migrans (VLM) is caused by migrating larvae. Pneumonitis, fever, abdominal pain, myalgia, lymphadenopathy, hepatosplenomegaly, sleep and behavioural disturbances and focal or generalized convulsions can occur. Investigations commonly reveal eosinophilia, anaemia, hypergammaglobulinaemia and elevated titres of blood group isohaemagglutinins. Serological diagnosis may be established using an ELISA.

The treatment of choice for VLM is albendazole 5–10 mg/kg twice daily for 5 days in children or 400 mg twice daily for five days in adults. Alternatively, both adults and children may be treated with mebendazole 100–200 mg twice daily for 5 days. Symptomatic treatment with bronchodilators, steroids or antihistamines may also be indicated.

Ocular larva migrans

Ocular larva migrans (OLM) may occur in lighter infections. A larva invades the eye producing a granulomatous reaction, usually in the retina, resulting in visual disturbance or blindness in the affected eye. This may present as strabismus or go unnoticed. The diagnosis is sometimes made by chance on routine opthalmoscopy. The appearance is usually of chorioidoretinitis with a mass lesion, which may be mistaken for a retinoblastoma. Serology is usually negative. Antibody detection in vitreous fluid is more sensitive and specific. Patients with eye involvement seldom have eosinophilia or other evidence of generalized VLM.

Topical or systemic steroids are indicated in the management of acute OLM. There is no consistent evidence of benefit from the additional use of anti-helmintics. Steroids may also be useful in exacerbations of chronic OLM. Surgery may be required for retinal detachment, vitreous opacification or macular fibrosis.

The terms 'covert' or 'occult' toxocariasis are sometimes used in situations where serology is positive, eosinophilia is absent or low, and symptoms are absent or relatively mild and more chronic than those described in VLM. Treatment is not usually indicated for asymptomatic infections.

Prevention and public health measures

In most urban environments, children have to compete with increasing numbers of domestic pets for diminishing open spaces where they can play safely. Pet owners are advised to deworm their dogs and cats regularly and to keep them away from children's play areas. In many towns and cities protected play areas are provided for children in public parks. There are also designated areas for pet owners to exercise their animals and pet owners are legally required to clean up if their animals defaecate in a public area. Even so, when playing football in most public parks, you are as likely to be fouled by dog faeces as by a member of the opposing team.

SUMMARY

- The 'soil-transmitted helminths' are now classed as Neglected Tropical Diseases or NTDs (see Chapter 62). The most important are roundworms (ascariasis), hookworms, whipworms (trichuriasis), and toxocariasis.

- Soil-transmitted helminths are very common – over a billion people worldwide are infected, many with multiple infections.

- Most soil-transmitted helminths are easily treated with albendazole, though mebendazole is more effective for trichuriasis.

- Children are most commonly affected by soil-transmitted helminths, and mass treatment programmes have been introduced in some areas.

 Visit www.lecturenoteseries.com/tropicalmed **to test yourself on this chapter using interactive MCQs.**

FURTHER READING

Awasti S, Bundy DAP, Savioli L (2003) Helminthic infections. *BMJ* **327**: 431–3. [Concise review of rationale for global control, and role of helminths in causing cognitive impairment in children.]

Bethony J, Brooker S, Albonico M, *et al.* (2006) Soil-transmitted helminth infections: ascariasis, trichuriasis, and hookworm. *Lancet* **367**: 1521–32. [Excellent comprehensive review focusing on three of the most important helminthic infections in humans.]

Cringoli G., Rinaldi L., Maurelli MP, Utzinger J (2010) FLOTAC: new multivalent techniques for qualitative and quantitative copromicroscopic diagnosis of parasites in animals and humans. *Nat Protoc* **5**: 503–15. [Step by step guide to FLOTAC techniques.]

Lancet Neglected Tropical Diseases Series (2010) [Reviews elimination and control programmes for lymphatic filariasis, onchocerciasis, schistosomiasis, and soil-transmitted helminthiasis, and describes the effect, governance arrangements, and financing mechanisms of selected international control initiatives.] http://www.thelancet.com/series/neglected-tropical-diseases

World Health Organization. *Helminth control in school age children: a guide for managers of control programmes* – 2nd ed. (2011) [Guidance for planners and programme managers in the health and education sectors with responsibility for STH and schistosomiasis control programmes. http://whqlibdoc.who.int/publications/2011/9789241548267_eng.pdf. Information on WHO's programme for reducing the global burden of soil transmitted helminth infections can be accessed via: http://www.who.int/intestinal_worms/en/index.html]

25

Viral hepatitis

Nick Beeching
Liverpool School of Tropical Medicine

The differential diagnosis of jaundice in the tropics includes a variety of causes that are seen less often in developed countries (Table 25.1). Schistosomiasis does not usually cause jaundice, but schistosomal liver damage frequently coexists with chronic viral hepatitis. Many of the infectious causes of jaundice are common in childhood and are less likely in the differential diagnosis of a jaundiced adult in the tropics (e.g. glandular fever group, hepatitis A). The history should always include careful questioning about past and present use of alcohol, 'Western' drugs and traditional herbal remedies, many of which can be hepatotoxic. Non-alcoholic fatty liver disease is becoming increasingly important as a cause of 'cryptogenic' cirrhosis in the tropics. This chapter focuses on the effects and prevention of hepatitis A, B, C, D and E in a tropical context.

General clinicoepidemiological features

The acute syndromes produced by hepatitis A, B, D or E are indistinguishable clinically except that acute hepatitis B patients are a little more likely to experience generalized arthralgia and rashes than patients with the other viruses, and acute hepatitis C rarely causes symptoms severe enough to seek medical treatment. In all cases, a prodrome of malaise, nausea and vomiting, fever and often diarrhoea leads to a phase of jaundice with dark urine and pale faeces. This is often followed by a cholestatic phase, especially in older adults in whom the recovery period can take several months.

No drugs have been shown to alter the course of acute hepatitis caused by these viruses. This includes the ayurvedic remedy 'Liv-52', popular in the Indian Subcontinent, vitamin injections and steroids. Full supportive therapy may be required for patients with severe liver failure, which is characterized by an altered (and falling) level of consciousness, metabolic flap of outstretched hands, ascites, peripheral oedema and a rising international normalized ratio (INR) or prothrombin ratio. Such patients have a high mortality and should be transferred early to a specialist centre if possible.

The water- and food-borne viruses hepatitis A and E usually have no significant chronic sequelae or carriage state, although chronic hepatitis E is now being recognized in heavily immunosuppressed individuals. The parenterally and sexually transmitted viruses hepatitis B, C and D can cause long-term problems in those patients who go on to become chronic carriers. The effects are worse in patients with dual infection (e.g. hepatitis B plus C, or viral hepatitis and HIV) and especially with concurrent alcohol abuse, and in the tropics schistosomal hepatic fibrosis commonly coexists with chronic viral hepatitis.

Hepatitis A

Hepatitis A (HAV) is a single-stranded RNA virus, which is primarily spread by the faeco-oral route. It is so common in the tropics that almost all individuals in many developing countries will have the infection by the age of 10 years, although most will not realize this because young children rarely have significant symptoms. Adults are more likely to become jaundiced, and those over 40 years have a small risk of dying from fulminant hepatitis.

Tropical Medicine Lecture Notes, Seventh edition. Edited by Nick Beeching and Geoff Gill. © 2014 John Wiley & Sons, Ltd. Published 2014 by John Wiley & Sons, Ltd.

Table 25.1 **Some causes of jaundice in the tropics**

Prehepatic	Hepatic	Posthepatic
Haemolysis (e.g. favism with G6PD deficiency)	Viral hepatitis	Pigment gallstones
	Q fever	Hydatid in biliary tree
Haemoglobinopathies	Drugs	Ectopic ascariasis
Sepsis	Traditional medicines	*Opisthorchis/Clonorchis* infection
Malaria	Leptospirosis	Gall bladder cancer (associated with typhoid carriage)
	Yellow fever	
	Toxins, e.g. acute aflatoxin poisoning	Cholangiocarcinoma (associated with *Opisthorchis/Clonorchis*)

The incubation period is 2–6 weeks and most patients already have detectable anti-HAV immunoglobulin M (IgM) antibodies in their blood by the time they develop symptoms. Over time, the IgM antibody is lost and is replaced by a long-lasting anti-HAV IgG response, with solid immunity (i.e. second infections are very rare). Patients excrete virus from before the onset of jaundice and are infectious to others who do not wash their hands after contact.

Hepatitis A is mainly a problem for travellers to the developing world. Paradoxically, the older a 'Western' person is, the more likely they are to have had hepatitis A in childhood before sanitation was improved. However, the minority of older adults who have no immunity may have substantial morbidity or mortality if they acquire HAV during a visit to the tropics.

There are no significant clinical interactions with HIV, except that individuals with very low CD4 counts are less likely to seroconvert after hepatitis A immunization.

Prevention is very effectively provided by active immunization with hepatitis A vaccine, followed by a booster 6–12 months later to produce life-long immunity. Anti-HAV IgG levels are not measured routinely to monitor vaccine response. Passive immunity can be provided by intramuscular gammaglobulin made from sera of individuals known or presumed to be immune; however, this is rarely used in the modern era.

Some tropical countries such as Singapore and Sri Lanka have experienced such an improvement in standard of living that children are no longer exposed to HAV in childhood, but are becoming symptomatically affected at a later age. In such a setting, active immunization of the population might become appropriate but, in general, HAV vaccines have little role in the tropics except for travellers.

Hepatitis B

Hepatitis B (HBV) is a major cause of death worldwide, with 1–2 million deaths per year mainly because of the sequelae of chronic liver disease and hepatocellular carcinoma (HCC). The DNA virus replicates in the hepatocytes which then express antigens such as HBsAg (surface antigen) and HBc (core antigen) on their surface, provoking both cell-mediated (Th1) and humoral (Th2) responses. These cause liver cell destruction associated with a rise in transaminases and clinical hepatitis, followed by loss of the circulating antigens HBsAg and HBeAg, and a rise in antibodies anti-HBs, anti-HBc and anti-HBe (Fig. 25.1). Thus, the marker for current hepatitis B infection is

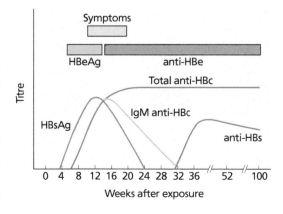

Figure 25.1 Acute hepatitis B (HBV) infection, followed by recovery.

HBsAg (and HBV DNA) in blood. A positive anti-HBc antibody test represents exposure to HBV at any time, and a positive anti-HBs antibody alone is a marker for past immunization. In some cases, immunity is insufficient to clear all the infected hepatocytes and the patient becomes a carrier, defined as having detectable hepatitis B (HBsAg) for over 6 months. Carriers with high HBV DNA levels usually have positive HBeAg tests, and 'HBeAg seroconversion' with loss of HBeAg and rise in anti-HBe antibody is a surrogate for reduced HBV DNA levels (Fig. 25.2). The presence of chronic liver disease (e.g. chronic active hepatitis) can only be determined by clinical examination, by checking liver function tests and by liver biopsy, in addition to serological tests. In future, imaging modalities tests such as the hepatic elastography (Fibroscan) may be accepted as a surrogate for liver biopsy. Point of care tests are increasingly used in the tropics to detect HBsAg, but there are concerns that their sensitivity and specificity require further validation in African settings, particularly in HIV-coinfected patients. Local quality control is essential.

Chronic carriage is currently conceptualized as going through 4 phases over a lifetime, associated with rises and falls in HBV DNA levels which are related to risk of developing HCC. During the first 'immune tolerant' phase, there are high HBV DNA levels and little immune reaction damaging infected hepatocytes, and hence normal liver function tests. During the second phase, which typically occurs in early adulthood, there is increased recruitment of cell mediated immunity, with active hepatitis which may lead to partial clearance of HBV, characterized by loss of HBeAg,

appearance of anti-HBe antibody, and reduced HBV DNA levels. However, there is wide variation in the age at which this phase commences and it may persist rather than leading to HBeAg seroconversion. A third prolonged phase follows with low-grade chronic hepatitis, and this can occasionally lead to complete clearance of hepatitis B, with loss of HBsAg and circulating HBV DNA. Finally, in some patients a 4th phase develops with rising HBV DNA levels, associated with emergence of 'precore mutant' HBeAg, increased activity in the liver and a new rise in transaminases. The patient is now more infectious and at increased risk of developing HCC. This phase may not be detected unless liver function is monitored, together with HBV DNA levels (rarely available in the tropics), as the precore mutant is not detectable by the ELISA tests used to monitor HBeAg levels.

Conditions that favour infection progressing to carriage include the neonatal state, chronic illness such as renal failure, and immunosuppression because of HIV or chemotherapy. Immunosuppressed individuals may have high levels of virus but no illness because the destruction of liver cells relies on having a strong immune response. If this is improved (e.g. by successful antiretroviral therapy or by stopping chemotherapy), patients with chronic carriage may paradoxically develop severe hepatitis.

Infants infected at the time of birth have a 90% chance of becoming carriers, this risk falling to 10% after infection at 1 year of life and to less than 5% for adults. In the Far East, Polynesia and West Africa, 30–50% of carriers are infected from their mothers at birth and most of the rest are infected by uncertain means in early childhood. This tends to cluster in families with a carrier mother. In such populations, carriage rates in adults are high (≥8%) and carriers tend to have high levels of circulating virus. In other parts of the tropics, most infections are acquired in childhood or infancy and intermediate HBsAg prevalence rates between 2 and 7% are seen in adults (Fig. 25.3, Table 25.2).

In industrialized countries, sexual transmission and shared drug injecting paraphernalia are the major routes of transmission in adulthood. Sexual transmission is important in the tropics but the major threat in this setting is nosocomial and/or iatrogenic hepatitis caused by reuse of needles and infusion sets. Other factors contributing to the spread of HBV in the tropics include traditional practices such as scarification or circumcision using non-sterile instruments, tattooing, acupuncture and barbering practices. Bedbugs (but not mosquitoes) have a small role in transmission in some settings, but control of bedbugs has little effect on reducing transmission.

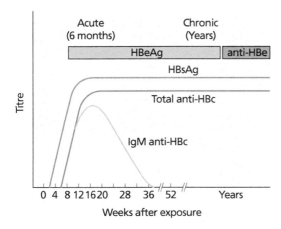

Figure 25.2 Progression of acute to chronic hepatitis B (HBV) infection (two patterns). Presence of HBeAg is used as a surrogate for high HBV DNA levels.

Table 25.2 Patterns of hepatitis B prevalence (World Health Organization definitions)

Prevalence	Adults with HBsAg (%)	Anti-HBc (%)	Incidence of infection			Location
			Infant	Child	Adult	
High	8–20	70–95	+++	++++	++	China, South East Asia, Polynesia, West Africa
Intermediate	2–7	20–60	++	+++	++	South West Asia, eastern Europe, East and Central Africa, South and Central America
Low	<2	2–6	+	−	+	North, West and Central Europe, North America, Australia

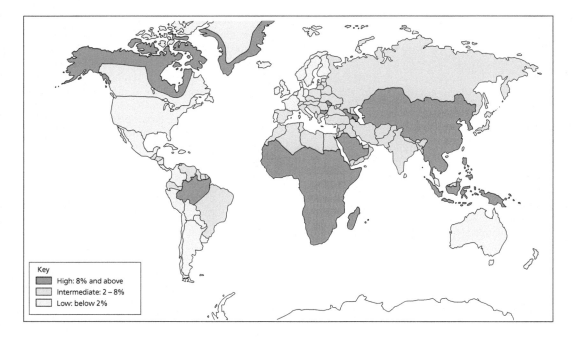

Key
High: 8% and above
Intermediate: 2 – 8%
Low: below 2%

Figure 25.3 Patterns of HBsAg endemicity as defined by WHO.

Treatment for chronic HBV is only appropriate for those with high HBV DNA levels. End points are easier to define for HBeAg-positive carriers, for whom the aim is to convert them to anti-HBe antibody positivity. A small minority subsequently lose HBsAg as well, after a delay of several years. For patients with precore mutant HBeAg, the only measurable endpoint is reduction in HBV DNA levels (or subsequent loss of HBsAg). Two approaches are currently favoured, using injectable interferons or oral nucleoside analogues. Pegylated interferon given as a weekly subcutaneous injection for 12 months will induce HBeAg seroconversion in about 30% of carefully selected patients. This option is better than high-dose interferon α (IFN-α) injections given three times a week. Both types of interferon are very expensive, carry significant side-effects and require regular injections. On the plus side, there is no emergence of resistant virus if treatment fails, and if it succeeds, the effect is usually durable and further treatment is not required. The second approach is prescription of oral nucleoside reverse transcriptase inhibitors as long-term suppressive therapy. Lamivudine was the first drug to be used, and other agents include adefovir, tenofovir and entecavir. This is a rapidly changing area, which is hampered by predictable emergence of drug resistant virus when patients take monotherapy, especially with lamivudine. Although cheaper in the medium term than interferons, with similar or slightly lower success in inducing HBeAg seroconversion, it carries significant risk of emergence of untreatable virus in those that do not respond. Further trials of double and triple therapy regimens and of new agents are in progress. All are limited by cost and side-effects, and require specialist supervision.

Treatment of HIV-coinfected patients is even more complex, as lamivudine-resistant HBV emerges very fast in HIV-positive patients who receive ART such as Triomune, a common triple regimen in sub-Saharan Africa. containing lamivudine without a second antiretroviral that also has anti-HBV activity. In resource rich settings, a typical ART regimen for such patients would include tenofovir and lamivudine or emtricitabine, but this has only recently become an option in much of sub Saharan Afica, where 10–20% of HIV-positive patients have HBV coinfection. Patients with coinfection will often experience immune reconstitution-related flares of hepatic activity after starting any form of ART and there are theoretical concerns that these could be severe if effective anti-HBV treatment is stopped at this point, leading to a rapid rise of HBV DNA concurrent with improved cell mediated immune activity. Conversely, coinfected patients who do not require ART for their HIV but require HBV treatment should not receive drugs such as lamivudine alone, as this may prejudice their future HIV treament by encouraging emergence of drug-resistant HIV. Overall, HBV is thought to upregulate HIV and vice versa, and it is likely but not established that each promotes perinatal transmission of the other virus. The significance of effects of HBV on the natural history of HIV, and response of HIV to ART, remain controversial and need further study

Hepatitis B immunization

Very effective vaccines against hepatitis B have been available for over 3 decades, containing HBsAg. This may be harvested from the plasma of chronic HBV carriers, and cheap vaccines from this source were routinely used in the tropics until recently, but are now being replaced by recombinant vaccines with support from the GAVI Alliance. The vaccine is effective in neonates and three doses of vaccine produce a long-lasting response in 80–90% of children and young adults. Vaccine schedules 'approved' for

Western licensing are usually 0, 1 and 6 months, or 0, 1, 2 and 12 months (booster fourth dose), or 0, 7 and 21 days followed by a late booster at 12 months. However, many other strategies are in use and it can be given alongside other Extended Programme on Immunization (EPI) scheduled vaccines in infancy. In Western practice it is usual to confirm seroconversion only in people at continued risk of infection, such as health care workers or partners or children of carriers. Seroconversion is defined as a rise in anti-HBs antibody > 10 units/L, 4–6 weeks after the third dose of vaccine. With or without such confirmation, a final booster vaccination 5 years later should provide life-long protection.

Factors that reduce the efficacy of active immunization include male gender, age >40 years, smoking tobacco and immunosuppression for any reason. The vaccine must be given into muscle (deltoid or thigh) and inappropriate administration into adipose tissue (e.g. buttocks) is ineffective. Active vaccination can be given at the same time as passive immunization with hyperimmune hepatitis B immunoglobulin (HBIg), a strategy that is used in some countries for extra, early protection of infants born to HBeAg-positive (high-grade) carrier mothers. Immunization of infants within 48 h of birth prevents almost all such transmissions, which is usually perinatal rather than intrauterine.

Large community-based studies in different parts of the tropics and in Italy have shown that infant or childhood vaccination programmes reduce the rate of infection by 90% or more. Most of the few who do become infected have subclinical disease, and very few become carriers. The protective effects in reducing community rates of infection, hepatitis B carriage and hepatocellular carcinoma persist for at least 15–20 years after such programmes, without further boosters being administered.

Over 150 countries have adopted policies of universal immunization against HBV. This depends on adequate supplies of affordable vaccine, which in turn requires an intact cold chain to maintain vaccine potency. In most tropical settings, the majority of infections occur in infancy or early childhood and universal infant immunization is therefore the most appropriate strategy. Subsequent boosters are not needed in tropical settings. In Western settings, in which infections predominantly occur in infants and children of carrier mothers or in adolescence and early adulthood, selective immunization of children of identified carriers may be employed. However, it is more difficult to then arrange for universal or selective adolescent or adult immunization, and most countries have opted for universal immunization in early childhood.

Hepatitis D

Hepatitis D virus (HDV, formerly delta hepatitis) resembles some plant viruses in that it is incomplete. The outer coat is derived from hepatitis B surface antigen, which means that the virus can only infect individuals who have acute hepatitis B or who are chronic HBV carriers. The virus is transmitted by the same routes as HBV and two epidemiological and clinical patterns are seen, so called 'coinfection' and 'superinfection'. Patients who are infected by hepatitis B and D viruses at the same time (coinfection) have clinical acute hepatitis that is no more severe than hepatitis B alone, and are no more or less likely to progress to chronic liver carriage and disease. More importantly, chronic HBV carriers who acquire acute hepatitis D (superinfection) are likely to develop fulminant hepatitis with a high mortality rate. In Western and tropical settings, where intravenous drug misuse is a problem, the clue to the arrival and spread of the virus is an epidemic of severe liver disease with high mortality in drug users. In tropical settings, similar epidemics are seen in previously asymptomatic HBV carriers of all ages. Such epidemics are regularly reported in South America, examples being epidemics of 'La Brea' or 'Santa Marta' fever. The epidemiological clue is the high proportion of affected patients who develop severe or fatal disease, and would be confirmed by detection of both HBV antigens and anti-HDV antibody responses. However, the latter serological tests are rarely available in a tropical setting.

As HDV only affects patients with concurrent acute or chronic HBV, it is prevented by immunization against hepatitis B and by other control measures used to prevent nosocomial or sexual transmission of hepatitis B.

Hepatitis C

Hepatitis C (HCV) is an RNA virus that is predominantly spread by blood–blood contact, and reuse of syringes and infusion equipment is responsible for high rates of hepatitis C endemicity in many parts of the tropics. Other factors encouraging blood–blood contact are also likely to be important in a tropical setting, as for HBV. Sexual and perinatal transmission of HCV is relatively inefficient but accounts for low background prevalence rates. However, the risk of sexual and perinatal transmission rises to about 10% if the 'donor' is also HIV-positive. The prevalence of anti-HCV antibodies in Egypt and parts of the Yemen is extraordinarily high, affecting over one-third of adults aged >40 years. This is because of past well-intentioned mass treatments of populations with tartar emetic for endemic schistosomiasis. The same syringes were used sequentially for many people, resulting in the largest described iatrogenic epidemic of a blood-borne virus in the world.

Hepatitis C rarely causes symptomatic acute hepatitis, but 70–80% of those infected will become chronic carriers, and there is a prolonged 'window' of antibody seronegativity of 2–3 months (ranging up to 6 months) after initial infection. Molecular methods (polymerase chain reaction, PCR) are now routinely used in Western settings to detect early infection, and to confirm the presence of viraemia in patients who are anti-HCV antibody-positive. Like HIV, HCV has different genotypic groups and a very high rate of viral turnover, leading to frequent mutations of viral quasispecies, so immunity is not solid and patients can be reinfected by HCV after successful treatment.

Chronic HCV is defined by presence of viraemia for more than 6 months, associated with abnormal hepatic histology (on liver biopsy) and/or abnormal liver function tests. Normal liver function tests do not exclude abnormal histology, so liver biopsy is often part of the full work-up of patients. The natural history is still poorly understood, and patients who have had single or few exposures to small amounts of virus seem less likely to progress. Overall, the '20' rule applies: 20% of patients initially infected will clear the virus (but still remain antibody positive). Of the remaining 80%, 20% will develop significant liver disease over 20 years. Of those with cirrhosis, up to 20% might develop HCC over a further 20 years. The most important determinant for development of serious liver disease and HCC is concurrent alcohol abuse, and the most important aspect of clinical management is to persuade chronic carriers to reduce or discontinue their alcohol intake.

Other factors that favour more rapid progression (and also resistance to treatment) include older age, male gender, infection with genotypes other than genotypes 2 or 3, and presence of stainable iron in liver biopsies. In counselling patients it is important to emphasize that many will not develop clinically apparent liver disease, and that the main risk to partners and families is sharing of needles and other sharps such as razors, nail scissors, toothbrushes, etc. In tropical settings, concurrent infection with hepatitis B and/or schistosomiasis is common and worsens the prognosis, as does HIV infection. A minority of HIV-positive individuals develop fulminant or rapidly progressive HCV for unknown reasons.

Treatment is expensive but increasingly effective. The current optimum regimens include weekly injections of pegylated (PEG) IFN-α, together with daily oral ribavirin for 6–12 months, producing viral remission in over 50% of cases. Genotypes 2 and 3 will be cured in 75% of cases by 6 months treatment, compared to about 40% of other genotypes treated for a year. Addition of protease inhibitors such as telaprevir or bocepravir to the regimen increases cure rates for genotype 1 infections to about 60–70%. Treatment can be discontinued if not effective (PCR test negativity or substantial drop in HCV RNA levels) early in the course of treatment. Similar results are obtained in HIV-coinfected patients. There are no immediate prospects for vaccination, and the only means of control is to educate health care workers and others not to reuse any kind of injection or infusion equipment. Intravenous drug misusers (most are anti-HCV antibody-positive within 3 years of starting injecting) should not share any kind of injecting equipment, including water and spoons or cookers used to dissolve drugs. Monogamous couples may choose not to start to use condoms (as the risks are small) but HCV carriers should otherwise be encouraged to use condoms with new partners. There is no evidence against breastfeeding.

Hepatitis E

Hepatitis E (HEV) is another virus spread by the faeco-oral route, usually by contamination of water supplies, with a similar incubation period and clinical outcome to HAV infection. The key difference from HAV is that immunity after natural infection is not solid, so that older children and adults can suffer repeated symptomatic infections. Large epidemics that affect people of all ages have been described in the Indian Subcontinent and central Asia for over 50 years, whereas epidemics of HAV primarily affect children. It is also well-recognized in Mexico and North Africa (Fig. 25.4) and now being diagnosed in many other areas in Africa. HEV is less common in Western countries unless there is a history of travel to the tropics or of contact with a recent traveller, but it is increasingly recognized as a cause of subclinical infection and as a cause of 'cryptogenic' acute hepatitis. Some of this is zoonotic in origin, with links to pig farming and butchering, and to consumption of undercooked pig, deer or badger meat products (e.g. smoked sausages and pâté).

HEV is endemic in the Indian Subcontinent where it accounts for the majority of symptomatic acute viral hepatitis admissions to hospital of both adults

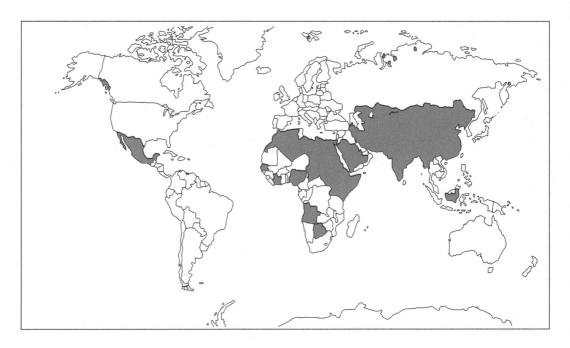

Figure 25.4 Countries with recognized hepatitis E outbreaks.

and children. Like HAV, there are usually no chronic sequelae, although progressive chronic infection has recently been described in transplant patients and HIV-positive individuals, and further clinic-epidemiological studies are essential worldwide.

The second major difference from other forms of viral hepatitis is the high incidence of fulminant hepatitis in pregnant women, with a mortality of 30–50%, particularly in the later stages of pregnancy. Perinatal transmission also occurs with a high mortality in infants who are infected.

Diagnosis is by detection of anti-HEV IgM followed by anti-HEV IgG antibodies. However, assays are not well-standardized and titres of both antibodies decline rapidly (within 1–2 years), so detection of antibodies late after infection is problematic. Passive immunization with pooled immunoglobulin from donors living in endemic areas is not effective. Very effective vaccines have been produced and tested in Nepal and China. Unfortunately, the protective immunity declines within a year or two, and the vaccine may find use in military settings but is not likely to be available for other travelers in its current formulation.

Hepatocellular carcinoma (hepatoma)

This aggressive tumour is common in the tropics, and is multifactorial in aetiology. Any patient with chronic active hepatitis is at risk, especially if cirrhosis has developed. Both chronic HBV and HCV are important causes, particularly if patients abuse alcohol. In many parts of the tropics, aflatoxins ingested in food are important epidemiologically as primary or cofactor causes, although it usually impossible to determine this in individual patients.

Patients usually present at a late stage with several months of weight loss, a painful hard irregular mass in an enlarged liver, often with ascites which may be bloodstained. Other signs of chronic liver disease may be obvious, and a 'bruit' or arteriovenous hum can be heard on auscultation over the liver. This is almost pathognomonic of hepatoma, although a 'bruit' can occasionally be heard over the liver in acute alcoholic hepatitis. Ultrasound shows diffuse infiltration of the liver by one or more tumours, often with central necrosis, which may resemble metastases from other sites. The other main differential diagnosis is acute amoebic liver abscess, which has a more acute presentation, typical ultrasound appearances, peripheral neutrophil leucocytosis and positive amoebic antibody tests. Most HCC patients have very elevated levels of alpha-fetoprotein in the serum, although this is absent in a minority. By the time that patients present with symptoms, the prognosis is very poor. Surgical removal, embolization and chemoembolization can all be attempted, and liver transplantation may be possible in some cases. In most resource-poor settings the only therapeutic option is palliation.

Prevention is by measures to control HBV and HCV infections, and countries that have initiated mass infant HBV immunization programmes have experienced marked falls in HCC incidence. Control of alcohol abuse is also important, especially in those with chronic HBV or HCV carriage.

SUMMARY

- Asymptomatic hepatitis A infection is common in many parts of the tropics, resulting in long-lasting immunity in the adult population. In countries with transitional epidemiology, less childhood exposure occurs and epidemics may occur in adults. Long-lasting protection is provided by immunization.

- Hepatitis B is preventable by immunization and countries that have introduced mass immunization programmes (usually perinatal or infant) have seen large falls in the sequelae of chronic infection including chronic liver disease, cirrhosis and hepatocellular carcinoma.

- Hepatitis C rarely causes acute disease but is a major cause of chronic liver disease in the tropics, especially in areas with uncontrolled reuse of needles and intravenous giving sets and blood transfusions. There is no vaccine.

- Chronic coinfection of hepatitis B and/or hepatitis C with HIV generally results in increased severity and earlier chronic sequelae of all infections, and adds to the complexity of therapy.

- Hepatitis E is a common cause of acute sporadic and epidemic hepatitis with high mortality in pregnant women. As immunity is not solid, infections occur in both adults and children.

- Hepatocellular carcinoma complicates chronic hepatitis and cirrhosis of any cause, especially if several causes coexist, including chronic hepatitis B or C, alcohol abuse, obesity and aflatoxin ingestion.

Visit www.lecturenoteseries.com/tropicalmed to test yourself on this chapter using interactive MCQs.

FURTHER READING AND OTHER RESOURCES

Beeching N, Dassanayake A (2011) Tropical liver disease. *Medicine* **39**(9): 556–60. doi:10.1016/j.mpmed.2011.06.002. [Short review of other tropical liver conditions with key references.]

Centers for Disease Control – National Center for Infectious Diseases. Viral hepatitis www.cdc.gov/ncidod/diseases/hepatitis/index.htm [Western-orientated patient information sheets, detailed statements of best practice, and large downloadable teaching slide sets. First source for hepatitis C.]

Fattovich G, Bortolotti F, Donato F (2008) Natural history of chronic hepatitis B: special emphasis on disease progression and prognostic factors. *J Hepatol* **48**(2): 335–52. [Review of staging and progression of hepatitis B.]

GAVI Alliance www.gavialliance.org/ [Formerly the Global Alliance for Vaccines and Immunisation, this alliance of public health institutions, industry and donors underpins development and provision of vaccines to many resource poor settings.]

Viral Hepatitis Prevention Board www.vhpb.org [Pressure group with industry funding. Large numbers of useful powerpoint presentations and region-specific reports, particularly related to epidemiology and prevention of hepatitis A and B.]

WHO website: www.who.int/csr/disease/hepatitis/resources/en/ [Excellent essays, illustrations, maps about all aspects, with extensive electronic links to online resources and full scientific referencing for those who want more information. First port of call for hepatitis A, B, D and E.]

26

Liver and intestinal flukes

Tim O'Dempsey
Liverpool School of Tropical Medicine

Food-borne trematodes include liver, lung and intestinal flukes. One-fifth of the world's population is at risk from these infections, which are endemic in at least 100 countries, half of which are among the poorest in the world. Over fifty million people are infected and there are at least 7000 deaths per year. Praziquantel is the drug of choice for most food-borne trematode infections. However, notable exceptions are *Fasciola hepatica* and *Fasciola gigantica*, for which triclabendazole is the drug of choice.

Liver flukes

Epidemiology

Fasciola hepatica and *F. gigantica* occur in sheep- and cattle-rearing areas worldwide, notably in the South American Andes, especially Bolivia where human population prevalence may exceed 90%.

Parasites and life-cycles

In common with other flukes, the life-cycles of *F. hepatica* and *F. gigantica* involve certain species of freshwater snail that are infected by miracidia liberated from eggs passed in herbivore (or human) faeces. The snails act as intermediate amplifying hosts, eventually liberating free-swimming cercariae which encyst as metacercariae on water plants.

Human infection occurs when the metacercarial cysts on raw water vegetables (e.g. watercress) are eaten, or are swallowed in contaminated water. These excyst in the duodenum, releasing larvae which penetrate the intestinal wall, and migrate via the peritoneal cavity to the liver. Having penetrated the liver capsule, they make their way to the bile ducts, where they mature into adults. Maturation in the human host takes 3–4 months. Adult flukes can survive for up to 10 years.

Clinical features

Acute symptoms caused by migrating flukes may develop 6–12 weeks after infection, including fever, malaise, abdominal pain, weight loss, urticaria and respiratory symptoms. Tender hepatomegaly may be evident. Liver enzymes are sometimes mildly elevated. Ectopic flukes can cause granuloma or abscess formation in various organs and migrating erythematous cutaneous nodules, a form of cutaneous larva migrans, may also be seen. Mature flukes in the bile ducts may initially cause fever, anorexia and abdominal pain.

Symptoms usually subside spontaneously once the adult flukes have made themselves at home. Blood loss into the bile resulting in anaemia occurs in heavy infections. Chronic symptoms include recurrent cholangitis or intermittent biliary obstruction in a minority of patients, and fatigue which can persist for more than 10 years.

Investigations

Eosinophilia is common. Ultrasound is usually normal. Computerized tomography (CT) of the liver may reveal numerous hypodense lesions, and peripheral branched hypodense hepatic lesions, best seen on CT using contrast, are relatively specific for fascioliasis. Serology may be helpful in diagnosing *F. hepatica* infections towards the end of the acute phase when eggs are still unlikely to be present in faeces.

Blood spots can be collected on filter paper for later serological testing in large-scale surveys. Serology is less reliable for *F. gigantica*. In established infections,

Tropical Medicine Lecture Notes, Seventh edition. Edited by Nick Beeching and Geoff Gill. © 2014 John Wiley & Sons, Ltd. Published 2014 by John Wiley & Sons, Ltd.

eggs may be present in faeces or in bile aspirate. Concentration techniques may be required. Fasciola excretory–secretory (FES) antigen detection in faeces is useful both in prepatent and in patent infections with *F. hepatica*.

Management

In contrast to other fluke infections, praziquantel is unreliable in the treatment of fascioliasis.

Triclabendazole, a new benzimidazole with few side-effects has become the drug of choice for treating *F. hepatica* and *F. gigantica*. A single dose of 10 mg/kg taken with food is usually effective. This may be repeated after 12 h in severe infections. Biliary colic, associated with the expulsion of dead or damaged parasites, commonly occurs 3–7 days after treatment and responds well to antispasmodic therapy. Unfortunately, cases resistant to triclabendazole have been reported in Ireland, UK and Australia.

Bithionol, 30–50 mg/kg/day in three divided doses on alternate days for 10–15 days, was the preferred treatment previously. Side-effects include mild gastrointestinal upset and pruritus.

Recently, nitazoxanide, 500 mg every 12 hours for seven days, has proven to be effective treatment for some adults with *F. hepatica*.

Prevention and public health aspects

Avoid eating potentially contaminated watercress and other water plants. Treatment of herbivores and snail control measures may sometimes be feasible. A promising vaccine is currently under development for use in sheep.

Oriental liver flukes

Epidemiology

Opisthorchis sinensis (also known as *Clonorchis sinensis*) and *O. viverrini*, affect about 20 million people in China and South East Asia. *Opisthorchis felineus*, a related species, occurs in eastern Europe and Russia. Animal hosts include domestic dogs and cats. This has important implications for control programmes.

Parasites and life-cycles

Eggs passed in human or animal faeces on contact with fresh water release miracidia that infect and multiply in certain species of freshwater snail which act as intermediate amplifying hosts. The snails eventually liberate free-swimming cercariae that, as metacercariae, encyst on susceptible species of freshwater fish.

Human infection occurs when metacercariae are consumed in raw or undercooked fish, or after ingesting metacercariae contaminating cooking surfaces and utensils. Metacercariae excyst in the small bowel, migrate along the common bile duct and colonize the biliary tree where they mature into adults within about 4 weeks. All adult oriental flukes are hermaphrodite creatures of similar appearance, lanceolate in shape, translucent and brownish in colour. In common with other flukes, they possess two suckers. *O. sinensis* is about 10–25 mm long by 3–5 mm wide. The other species are about half as big.

Clinical features

Most infections are asymptomatic. Heavy initial infections may present with an illness similar to Katayama fever. Patients with established infections may have vague right upper quadrant abdominal pain that typically occurs in the late afternoon and lasts a few hours. Patients may actually complain of feeling something moving about the liver. Other symptoms include lassitude, anorexia, flatulence, diarrhoea and fever. Hepatomegaly may be evident on examination and heavily infected patients may also be jaundiced. Some patients appear malnourished and are deficient in fat-soluble vitamins.

Recurrent bouts of ascending cholangitis, jaundice and pancreatitis can occur. Biliary cirrhosis and, rarely, cholangiocarcinoma may develop in chronic infections. Cholangiocarcinoma associated with *O. viverrini* is the most common form of liver cancer in North-Eastern Thailand, where an estimated 70% of the population are infected with the parasite. In Hong Kong, 15% of all primary liver cancers were found to be cholangiocarcinomas associated with *C. sinensis*. Genetic factors, dietary nitrosamines and aflatoxins have been implicated in the development of this malignancy.

Investigations

Diagnosis is established by identifying characteristic eggs in faeces or in biliary aspirate. Concentration techniques may be required. A number of serological tests are available with a variable range of sensitivity and specificity. A coproantigen test is now available for *O. viverrini*. Ultrasound may reveal gallstones and abnormalities of the biliary tree. Endoscopic retrograde cholangiopancreatography (ERCP) is also useful.

Management

Praziquantel is effective, either 40 mg/kg in a single dose, or 25 mg/kg three times in 24 h after meals. A 3-day course should be used for heavy infections.

Prevention and public health aspects

Health education, improving sanitation and annual treatment with praziquantel can dramatically reduce the prevalence of infection and, on the face of it, infection with oriental liver flukes should be easy to prevent by avoiding raw fish. However, food habits are very difficult to change, even with vigorous health education. It seems that once you have tasted well-prepared raw fish, the cooked item never tastes as good.

Intestinal flukes

Fasciolopsis buski, the most important intestinal fluke in humans, is widely distributed from India to South East Asia, particularly in pig-rearing communities. Metacercariae attached to edible water plants, such as the water caltrop, are ingested, excyst, attach to the mucosa of the duodenum and jejunum and develop into adults causing inflammation and ulceration.

Most infections are asymptomatic. Symptoms are more likely to occur in heavy infections, and tend to be most severe in children. These include epigastric pain, vomiting and diarrhoea, initially alternating with constipation but later becoming persistent. Wasting, oedema and ascites may also occur in severe cases. Characteristic eggs, and sometimes adult flukes, can be identified in faeces and adult flukes sometimes also appear in vomit. Echinostome species, principally found in Asia, can also infect humans causing symptoms similar to *F. buski*. Heterophyids, a group of smaller intestinal flukes affecting humans, cause milder gastrointestinal symptoms than *F. buski*. However, ectopic eggs may be deposited in other organs, e.g. the central nervous system (CNS), presenting as a space-occupying lesion, and the heart, causing myocarditis or valve damage. Praziquantel is usually effective in the treatment of intestinal flukes.

Recent Developments in Diagnosis

FLOTAC Diagnostic Techniques. A series of recently developed rapid multivalent, qualitative and quantitative copromicroscopic techniques initially developed for veterinary parasitology have recently been applied to human parasitology. Validation is currently underway for diagnosis of major nematodes, trematodes and intestinal protozoa parasitizing humans.

A range of PCR-based methods are becoming available which offer high diagnostic sensitivities and specificities, and enable the discrimination between infections caused by different trematode species.

Enhanced immunological assays are also under development in animal models, for example excretory-secretory antigen (ESA)-ELISA and monoclonal antibody (MoAb)-based sandwich ELISA tests. These are designed to improve the sensitivity and specificity of conventional immunodiagnostic assays and may soon have a role in diagnosis of human infections.

 SUMMARY

* Liver flukes include the widely distributed *Fasciola hepatica*, and the oriental fluke *Opisthorchis sinensis* (also known as *Clonorchis sinensis*). The life-cycles involve fresh water snails. Clinical features include fever, hepatomegaly and liver dysfunction.

* *Fasciolopsis buski* is the main intestinal fluke. It occurs in India and the east and may lead to chronic intestinal syndromes.

* Diagnosis is by faeces microscopy, possibly aided by PCR, or in the case of liver flukes, ultrasound. Eosinophilia is common.

* Praziquantel is the drug of choice for all fluke infections with the exception of *F. hepatica* and *F. gigantica*.

 Visit **www.lecturenoteseries.com/tropicalmed to test yourself on this chapter using interactive MCQs.**

FURTHER READING

Cringoli G, Rinaldi L, Maurelli MP, Utzinger J (2010) FLOTAC: new multivalent techniques for qualitative and quantitative copromicroscopic diagnosis of parasites in animals and humans. *Nat Protoc* **5:**

503-15. [A comprehensive review discussing the development of the FLOTAC techniques and summarizing experiences made thus far in the diagnosis of animal and human parasites.]

Fürst T, Keiser J, Utzinger J (2012) Global burden of human food-borne trematodiasis: a systematic review and meta-analysis. *Lancet Infect Dis* **12**: 210-21. [Amazingly, this is the first systematic estimate of the global burden of food-borne trematodiasis.]

Garcia HH, Moro PL, Schantz PM (2007) Zoonotic helminth infections of humans: echinococcosis, cysticercosis and fascioliasis. *Curr Opin Infect Dis* **20**: 489-94. [Recent review of these important zoonotic infections.]

Gillespie SH, Pearson RD, eds (2001) *Principles and Practice of Clinical Parasitology.* Chichester: John Wiley & Sons, Ltd, Chapters 17 and 24. [This excellent volume on clinical parasitology includes two useful chapters on food-borne trematode infections.]

Keisera J, Duthalera U, Utzinger J (2010) Update on the diagnosis and treatment of food-borne trematode infections. *Curr Opin Infect Dis* **23**: 513-20. [Discusses emerging diagnostic and therapeutic approaches.]

27

Hydatid disease

Tim O'Dempsey and Nick Beeching
Liverpool School of Tropical Medicine

Hydatid disease results from the larval stage of a small tapeworm of dogs and other canines developing in humans. The infection is a zoonosis, normally maintained in dogs and sheep or cattle in close association with humans (*Echinococcus granulosus*), or in a wild cycle such as in wild canines and rodents (*E. multilocularis*). Most human infections are with *E. granulosus* and are associated with the rearing of sheep and cattle in climatic conditions varying from tropical to subarctic. The third, and rarest species of importance in man, is *E. vogeli* which has been reported mainly in southern regions of South America.

Echinococcus granulosus (hydatid cyst disease)

Life-cycle

Infected dogs harbour the 3–6 mm adult tapeworms in their small intestine. The worms possess only three proglottids, the end one being mature. The eggs are liberated either before or after the proglottid escapes in the faeces, and contaminate pasture. When ingested by the normal herbivorous intermediate host, the oncospheres liberated in the gut enter the circulation and are trapped in the capillaries of various viscera, where they develop into cysts. A cyst is composed of a sphere of germinal epithelium containing protruding invaginations (brood capsules) and fluid. From the inner surface of the brood capsules, protoscolices develop, invaginated in much the same way as the cysticerci of *Taenia* spp. The whole structure is a hydatid cyst, and it becomes surrounded by fibrous capsule derived from the host tissue. The cyst may develop large daughter cysts in its cavity, each containing more brood capsules. The cyst continues growing for years. Brood capsules that break free from the cyst wall, and individual scolices in the cyst cavity, are called hydatid sand.

Dogs become infected by eating the contents of hydatid cysts in infected carcasses. Sheep or other herbivores become infected by swallowing the *Taenia*-like eggs passed in dog faeces. The strain of *E. granulosus* in the UK that commonly infects horses and has the foxhound as its definitive host is probably not usually pathogenic for humans. There are several other biological complexes in nature that probably do not pose the risk of human infection.

Clinical features

About 70% of cysts develop in the liver, usually the right lobe, 20% in the lungs and the rest in rarer sites. Cysts may be single or multiple. Symptoms are caused by a mass effect produced by the growing cyst, secondary bacterial infection of the cyst or because of leakage of fluid from the cyst. Hepatic cysts are initially asymptomatic until they become large. A non-tender mass may be evident on examination. If secondary bacterial infection occurs, the cyst may mimic a liver abscess. Spillage or leakage of the cyst fluid, during surgery or following rupture, can precipitate hypersensitivity reactions ranging from urticaria, pruritus and fever to fatal anaphylaxis. Secondary cysts may develop following spillage and seeding in the peritoneal cavity. Leakage from a cyst into the biliary tree may cause colic, urticaria and obstructive jaundice, sometimes complicated by secondary bacterial infection.

Most lung cysts are asymptomatic, found incidentally on a chest X-ray (Fig. 27.1). Symptomatic patients may complain of fever, dyspnoea, chest pain

Tropical Medicine Lecture Notes, Seventh edition. Edited by Nick Beeching and Geoff Gill. © 2014 John Wiley & Sons, Ltd. Published 2014 by John Wiley & Sons, Ltd.

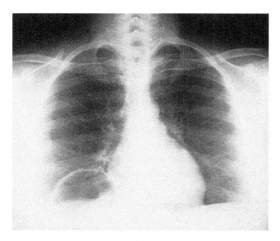

Figure 27.1 A hydatid cyst at the base of the right lung, found incidentally in an African patient.

and cough, occasionally with haemoptysis. Secondary infection may result in development of a lung abscess. Pneumothorax, empyema or a hypersensitivity reaction may occur following rupture into the lung. Seeding of pulmonary cysts is uncommon. Rupture of a cyst into a bronchus may cause the patient to cough up clear salty tasting liquid, sometimes followed by the soft white outer membrane of the cyst. A collapsed cyst may have a characteristic 'water lily' appearance on chest X-ray.

Hydatid cysts occur at a variety of other sites including spleen, bone (causing pain and pathological fracture), brain (causing convulsions or a mass effect) and eye (causing proptosis and chemosis).

Investigations

Imaging

Ultrasound is useful for abdominal cysts. X-ray, computerized tomography (CT) or magnetic resonance imaging (MRI) may be useful for detecting cysts elsewhere.

Serology

The specific immunoglobulin G (IgG) enzyme-linked immunoabsorbent assay (ELISA) antigen B-rich fraction (AgB) is the most sensitive serological test. Others include an enzyme-linked immunotransfer blot (EITB) assay and the double diffusion test for arc 5 (DD5). Current serological tests lack sensitivity for extrahepatic cysts. The DD5 may give false-positive results in patients with cysticercosis.

Others

Urine antigen detection tests are promising. Eosinophilia may follow leakage or rupture of a cyst.

Treatment

In the past, surgical removal was the preferred method of managing accessible cysts. Small cysts can be removed intact. Larger cysts should be carefully aspirated and the aspirate replaced with an equivalent volume of a scolicide, such as hypertonic saline, reaspirated after 5–10 min and the procedure repeated. Following reaspiration, the cyst cavity is opened, the membranes are removed and the cavity closed. Great care should be taken to avoid spillage of cyst fluid.

Percutaneous aspiration of cysts under ultrasound control is now used increasingly as an alternative to surgery. Following initial aspiration, hypertonic saline is injected into the cyst and reaspirated after 20 min. The procedure is summarized by the acronym PAIR (Puncture, Aspiration, Injection, Reaspiration). Indications for PAIR are as follows:

- cysts with daughter cysts, and/or with detachment of membranes;
- infected cysts;
- multiple cysts if accessible to puncture;
- non-echoic lesion > 5 cm in diameter.

PAIR is also recommended for:

- patients in whom surgery is contraindicated;
- patients who fail to respond to chemotherapy alone;
- patients who refuse surgery;
- patients who relapse after surgery;
- pregnant women.

Contraindications to PAIR are as follows:

- cysts communicating with the biliary tree;
- cysts opening into the abdominal cavity, bronchi and urinary tract;
- inaccessible or risky location of the cyst (e.g. spine, brain, heart);
- inactive or calcified lesion;
- uncooperative patients, children < 3 years.

Patients undergoing surgery or PAIR should receive albendazole, either alone or in combination with praziquantel, for 1–3 months prior to, and covering, the procedure. PAIR should be followed by an 8-week course of albendazole. Laparoscopic treatment of hydatid cysts of the liver and spleen is also effective. Antihelmintic treatment may reduce the need for surgery in patients with uncomplicated pulmonary cysts.

Albendazole is useful for patients with inoperable, widespread or numerous cysts and in patients who are unfit for surgery. The recommended regimen is now 400 mg every 12 h for adults, or 5–7.5 mg/kg every 12 h for children, for 3–24 months depending on response. Monthly treatment interruptions are no longer recommended. Albendazole absorption is enhanced if taken with fatty meals. Albendazole plus praziquantel has been shown to have greater protoscolicidal activity in animal studies and in vitro compared with either drug alone. Combined therapy has been used successfully in managing inoperable spinal, pelvic, abdominal, thoracic and hepatic hydatidosis and as an adjunct to surgery.

Prevention and Control

Large-scale programmes involving public health education and strict dog control measures have led to elimination of hydatid disease in certain regions (Iceland, Cyprus, Australia, Tasmania, New Zealand). Similar programmes have met with less success elsewhere. Recent advances include the development of a promising new recombinant vaccine (EG95) against ovine echinococcus and a vaccine against the dog tapeworm stage.

Alarmingly for Liverpool DTM&H students who enjoy weekend country rambles in Snowdonia, the prevalence of infected dogs in Wales is currently around 10–20%, having more than doubled following recent policy changes in favour of health education instead of weekly dosing of dogs with praziquantel. Remember: boil it, cook it, peel it or leave it (and don't stroke it or pet it)!

Echinococcus multilocularis (alveolar hydatid disease)

Life-cycle

Humans become infected by swallowing the eggs passed by foxes and other Canidae, possibly mainly from contaminated wild ground fruits such as bilberries and their close relatives, lingonberries and cloudberries, widely eaten in northern Europe. *E. multilocularis* transmission is confined to the northern hemisphere, with endemic foci in areas of West-central Europe, Turkey, Russia, Iran, Iraq, northern Japan (Hokkaido Island) and western and central China. A human population prevalence of 10% has been described in an intense focus in Gansu province, China. Factors with the potential of enhancing the urban infection risk for humans in the future include increasing fox populations and parasite prevalences, invasion of cities by foxes (40% of suburban and 10% of 'downtown' foxes are infected in certain European cities), the establishment of urban cycles of the parasite and the spillover of the *E. multilocularis* infection from wild carnivores to domestic dogs and cats. Various rodents are the intermediate hosts.

Clinical features

Unlike *E. granulosus*, the cyst produces daughter cysts by external and not internal budding, so it tends to invade progressively into surrounding tissues like a malignant tumour and is not contained in a well-defined fibrous capsule. It may be 30 years before a patient becomes symptomatic. The primary site of tissue invasion is usually the liver, mimicking hepatic carcinoma or cirrhosis. Metastatic lesions may occur in other tissues (lung, brain, bone) and are evident in over 10% of patients. Patients usually present with right upper quadrant pain, hepatomegaly and a palpable mass. Complications arise in around 2% of patients, either because of local invasion or as a result of metastatic lesions involving brain, lung or mediastinum. Untreated, 90% of patients die within 10 years of presentation. HIV coinfection may lead to more severe or accelerated disease progression in immunocompromised patients. Treatment with cART may enhance the response to anthelmintics.

Investigations

Ultrasound, CT, MRI and serology are useful in establishing the diagnosis. Histology provides confirmation.

Treatment

Surgical excision is preferred for the primary lesion. Pre- and post-operative treatment with albendazole is recommended. Albendazole 10–15 mg/kg is recommended post-operatively and for inoperable patients. In practice, a dose of 400 mg every 12 h is usual for adults. The optimal duration of treatment remains uncertain; patients often remain on treatment for more than 12 months. Albendazole at these doses has been used for up to 20 years; higher doses of 20 mg/kg per day have been used continuously for over 10 years. Mebendazole 40–50 mg/kg/day has also been used extensively, sometimes for up to 10 years. A 90% 10-year survival rate is possible with early diagnosis and appropriate treatment. Serology may remain positive for several years following successful treatment. If available, PET/CT may be useful in monitoring response to treatment.

 SUMMARY

- Most human hydatid disease is due to *Echinococcus granulosis*, associated with dog, sheep or cattle contact.

- Human infection can lead to the development of hydatid cysts, 70% of which are in the liver, and 20% in the lungs. Cysts are often found incidentally by X-ray.

- Treatment may involve drugs (normally albendazole), surgical removal and sometimes aspiration.

- Infections with *Echinococcus multilocularis* are less common, but lesions are less capsular and more invasive. As well as surgery, prolonged albendazole may be needed.

Visit www.lecturenoteseries.com/tropicalmed **to test yourself on this chapter using interactive MCQs.**

 FURTHER READING

Brunetti E. *et al.* (2010) Expert consensus for the diagnosis and treatment of cystic and alveolar echinococcosis in humans. *Acta Trop* **114**(1): 1–16. [Excellent review and summary of current WHO recommendations.]

Eckert J, Conraths FJ, Tackmann K (2000) Echinococcosis: an emerging or re-emerging zoonosis? *Int J Parasitol* **12–13**: 1283–94. [An excellent recent review of the epidemiology and control of human echinococcal infections.]

Kearn P (2010) Clinical features and treatment of alveolar echinococcosis. *Curr Opin Infect Dis* **23**: 505–12. [Summarizes current understanding of clinical features, knowledge on appropriate treatment, and discusses ways to improve standards of care.]

WHO (2001) *PAIR: Puncture, Aspiration, Injection, Re-Aspiration. An option for the treatment of cystic Echinococcosis.* WHO/CDS/CSR/APH/2001.6. http://www.who.int/emc-documents/zoonoses/whocdscsraph20016.html [Practical guidelines and useful images.]

28

Pneumonia

Stephen Gordon[1] and Neil French[2]

[1]Liverpool School of Tropical Medicine; [2] University of Liverpool

Pneumonia is infected consolidation of alveolar spaces. It is a leading cause of morbidity and mortality in all parts of the world particularly affecting young children and the elderly. There are an estimated 1 million deaths per year from pneumonia in African children alone. This chapter highlights the role of specific pathogens, and the difficulties of management when only limited investigational and therapeutic resources are available.

Epidemiology

Pneumonia can affect individuals of all ages but mostly affects young children and the elderly. The risk of disease exists throughout the year with seasonal variation. Rates are highest during cooler periods, with case numbers beginning to rise towards the end of the rains when malaria is also a significant problem. Pneumonia is invariably reported as a leading cause of admission to hospital in all regions of the tropics, although accurate community-based incidence data are lacking. HIV increases pneumonia risk between 5- and 10-fold; thus, between 2.2 and 3.3 million episodes of pneumonia (30–50% with HIV coinfection) can be estimated to occur in adults in Africa each year (assuming 600 million adults, 10% HIV seroprevalence). Pneumonia case fatality was 60% in the pre-antibiotic era. With effective early therapy this may be reduced to 5%. Unfortunately, case fatality rates are still reported at 15–20%, reflecting the problems of late presentation and delays in therapy, common to all resource-limited settings.

Microbiology

Streptococcus pneumoniae is the most important aetiological agent of pneumonia both in terms of frequency and severity throughout the world (Table 28.1). Preceding viral upper respiratory tract infections may be important precipitants, although the role of viruses as a primary cause of pneumonia in adults is unclear. Most importantly, patients with *Mycobacterium tuberculosis* may present with an acute pneumonic illness and can also present with a dual infection with *S. pneumoniae*. In adults, *M. tuberculosis* may be identified in as many as 8% of cases of severe acute pneumonia admitted to hospital in sub-Saharan Africa. Acute presentations of pulmonary tuberculosis in children are also well recognized.

Risk factors for pneumonia

- *Age* – small children and elderly adults are at particular risk of pneumococcal infection and in regions with high HIV prevalence this pattern is supplemented with an additional peak in incidence among adults aged 25–40 yrs.
- *Cigarette smoking* – the most important risk factor for pneumonia in immunocompetent adults is cigarette smoking with an odds ratio of 6.
- *Pregnancy* is an important risk factor for pneumonia.
- *Coexistent medical problems* – HIV infection (most important), underlying lung disease, diabetes, nephrotic syndrome, kwashiorkor, marasmus, measles and sickle cell disease/asplenia.

Tropical Medicine Lecture Notes, Seventh edition. Edited by Nick Beeching and Geoff Gill. © 2014 John Wiley & Sons, Ltd. Published 2014 by John Wiley & Sons, Ltd.

Table 28.1 Predominant aetiological agents of pneumonia listed in order of frequency according to clinical presentation

Moderate severity pneumonia (Inpatient management, not intensive care)

Common

    Streptococcus pneumoniae

    Haemophilus influenzae

Variable

    Mycoplasma pneumoniae

    Influenza type A

    Chlamydophila psittaci

    Legionella pneumophila

Rare

    Staphylococcus aureus

Most severe pneumonia (intensive care)

Common

    Streptococcus pneumoniae

    Legionella pneumophila

Variable

    Haemophilus influenzae

    Klebsiella pneumoniae (common in S Africa)

    Pseudomonas aeruginosa

    Burkholderia pseudomallei (common in SE Asia)

    Staphylococcus aureus

Rare

    Mycoplasma pneumoniae

    Chlamydophila psittaci

- *Social* – overcrowding, migrant labour, refugees, alcohol and drug abuse all increase the incidence of pneumonia.
- *Environmental* – domestic smoke from biomass fuels particularly firewood and animal dung) has been shown to increase the incidence of upper and lower respiratory tract infections in both adults and children, as have poorly ventilated dwellings and mining-associated dust exposure.

Clinical features

Symptoms of acute pneumonia

Presentation is typically acute, with a 2–3 day history of cough, fever, dyspnoea and often some pleuritic pain. In adults, purulent sputum production may not occur

for several days after antibiotic therapy is started. A more prolonged presentation may occur if the pneumonia has been partially treated or if there is underlying chronic chest disease, in particular tuberculosis. In addition to fever, cough and dyspnoea, failure to feed is an important feature in infants. Streaky haemoptysis or "rusty' sputum may occur – the latter suggestive of *S. pneumoniae* infection. Headache is common and may suggest meningitis, but this is unusual except in HIV-infected adults. Diarrhoea can occasionally be profuse and be accompanied by abdominal pain leading to confusion with acute gastroenteritis. Elderly adults may have few if any symptoms at all.

Signs of acute pneumonia

Patients usually appear unwell and may be tachycardic and febrile. Nasal flaring, use of the accessory muscles of respiration, tachypnoea and lower chest wall indrawing are particularly important to look for in children (Figure 28.1). Classically the signs of consolidation are dullness to chest percussion and bronchial breathing but in the earlier phases of pneumonia, coarse inspiratory crackles consistent with retained secretions are more common. A pleural rub may be present and does not necessarily predict complicated pleural disease. Unusual presentations include acute psychosis, confusion, hypothermia, jaundice and abdominal tenderness.

Differential diagnosis of acute pneumonia

- *Tuberculosis* – this should always be considered in poorly resolving pneumonia and is the prime concern in more prolonged presentations. Pleural effusion should always suggest this diagnosis.
- *Septicaemia* – this is very common in HIV-infected adults, either as a primary presentation or concurrently with pneumonia.
- *Metabolic acidosis including diabetic ketoacidosis* – clouded consciousness and the smell of exhaled acetone, with a more detailed history to elicit polyuria and polydipsia along with urinalysis should identify the condition.
- *Poisoning* – this should be considered when the respiratory distress is out of proportion to the pulmonary findings and there is evidence of other system involvement, particularly neurological. Important poisons are aspirin, chloroquine, petrochemicals and herbicides either intentionally or accidentally ingested or inhaled.
- *Amoebic liver abscess* – the presence of a right-sided effusion should alert the clinician to consider an amoebic problem. Rarely, consolidation may be present in the right lower lobe.

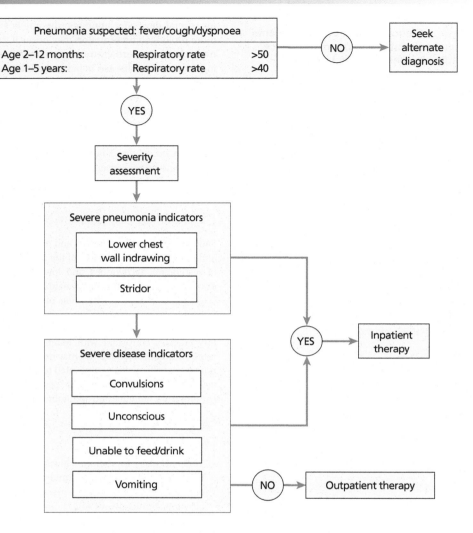

Figure 28.1 Pneumonia diagnosis and severity assessment in children. In regions with a high prevalence of bacterial pneumonia, use of respiratory rate alone will detect 80% of children who require antibiotics for pneumonia.

Investigations

In resource-poor settings, investigations should be reserved for cases in whom the diagnosis is uncertain or the management problematic.

Radiology

A chest X-ray can be used to identify pneumothoraces, lung masses, small effusions and to rule out alternate diagnoses such as pericardial effusions or pulmonary oedema which require specific therapy. Bilateral interstitial pneumonia may suggest Pneumocystis pneumonia but this radiological pattern is found with both bacterial and tuberculous infections and thus has poor diagnostic precision. When pneumonia is slow to resolve, the presence of mediastinal/hilar lymphadenopathy should stimulate a search for tuberculosis. Cavities should also point towards tuberculosis or, occasionally, anaerobic/aspiration or staphylococcal pneumonia. The presence of pleural effusions in poorly resolving pneumonia should lead to pleural aspiration and examination for empyema. A chest X-ray should not be used to confirm lobar consolidation in cases with a typical history and clear physical signs as this is often a poor use of limited resource.

Sputum Gram stain

This is a rarely used investigation as empirical antibiotic therapy is usually given. In sputum, the presence of 10–20 pus cells in a high power (×1000) field with no epithelial cells defines an adequate specimen. The presence of Gram-positive diplococci (dark purple) in association with pus cells confirms a diagnosis of pneumococcal pneumonia (see also Chapter 2). Sputum culture is not used owing to contamination with oral flora.

Sputum Ziehl–Neelsen stain

This should be carried out on all poorly resolving pneumonia and will identify 60–80% of *M. tuberculosis* infections (less in HIV endemic areas). Culture for *Mycobacterium tuberculosis*, if available, increases the diagnostic yield. If numerous pus cells are seen on Gram stain in the absence of organisms, Ziehl–Neelsen staining should be performed.

Trans-thoracic lung aspirate

This is a useful technique in children for recovering lower respiratory tract samples for staining and culture from consolidated lung. Aspirates should only be taken from consolidated lung tissue, laterally to avoid the heart. When this is done, pneumothoraces are uncommon (see also Chapter 2). In adults, this technique offers little advantage over standard blood cultures.

Pleural aspiration

Pleural effusions occur in 5–15% of cases of pneumonia. The majority will resolve with antibacterial therapy alone. Sampling of pleural fluid should always be carried out if empyema is suspected.

HIV testing

The greatly increased susceptibility of HIV-infected adults to pneumococcal infection means that pneumonia is a common first presentation of HIV infection. In regions of high HIV-prevalence the majority of pneumonia cases will be HIV-infected; rates range from 40 to 90%. Early testing is advantageous for the individual patient as cART can be planned and in some instances, HIV testing can aid diagnosis and management (e.g. suspected PCP, concurrent TB infection). HIV testing is also important to allow prevention of transmission. Adults presenting with pneumonia should be offered HIV testing.

Pulse oximetry

Pulse oximetry is now commonly available even in resource-poor settings. Cyanosis is a difficult sign to elicit and so accurate oximetry is a very useful method of appropriately allocating available oxygen. Oxygen is now also commonly available using bedside oxygen concentrators of the type used for domiciliary oxygen in developed countries.

Other microbiological tests

Blood cultures have low diagnostic sensitivity and most basic laboratories do not have appropriate facilities but recovery of an organism from blood allows confident diagnosis and determination of antibiotic sensitivity. Serology and other immune-based diagnostics (e.g. immunofluorescence for *Pneumocystis jirovecii*) are unlikely to be available.

Other investigations

Haemoglobin measurements help to identify individuals who may require blood transfusion. Biochemical assessment of renal and hepatic function are not essential but may provide prognostic information.

Management

It is an important principle in pneumonia management that **severity should guide treatment and this can be assessed at the bedside** (Figure 28.2). Indicators of poor outcome in adults are listed in Table 28.2. Vomiting or profuse diarrhoea are relative contraindications to oral therapy as antibiotic absorption may be impaired.

Outpatient therapy

Outpatient therapy is appropriate if no markers of severity are found in pneumonia (Table 28.2). Oral amoxicillin (500 mg t.d.s.) or ampicillin (500 mg q.d.s.) are effective antipneumococcal agents and are a suitable first choice. Alternative agents include co-trimoxazole, doxycycline, clarithromycin or erythromycin in patients allergic to penicillin. Individuals managed as outpatients should always be encouraged to reattend to be assessed for tuberculosis if there are persisting respiratory symptoms.

Inpatient therapy

Basic resuscitation (ensuring airway patency and adequate respiratory and circulatory activity) should

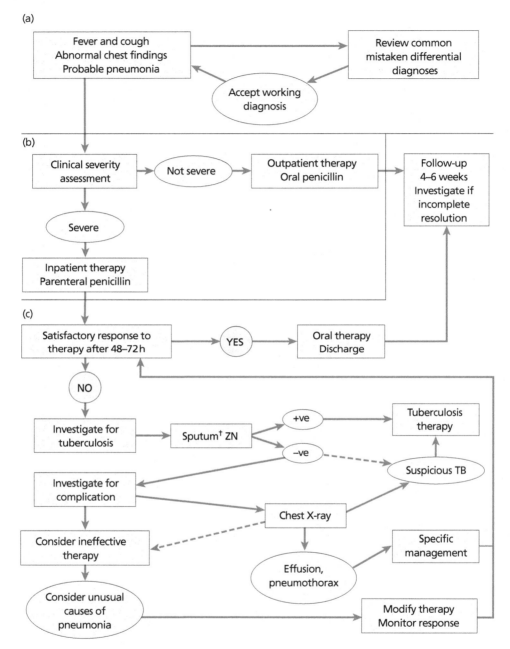

Figure 28.2 Pneumonia management: (a) establishing a presumptive diagnosis; (b) initiating empirical therapy; and (c) testing and modification of initial diagnosis by assessing response to therapy. †Sputum or pleural aspirate/lung aspirate/regional lymph node aspirate.

be rapidly followed by antimicrobial therapy. Parenteral penicillins (benzylpenicillin 1.2 g every 4–6 h or amoxicillin 0.5–1 g every 8 h) remain the agents of first choice. A macrolide, tetracycline or ciprofloxacin can be added to therapy as oral agents (parenteral preparations are unavailable or expensive) in severe disease if an atypical organism is suspected. If intravenous therapy for Gram-negative organisms (e.g. *Klebsiella* spp.) is required, then aminoglycoside therapy is appropriate (e.g. gentamicin 4–5 mg/kg).

Table 28.2 Associations of severe disease and poor outcome in adult pneumonia

Two or more factors increase chance of dying 4-fold, and 5 or more factors increase change of dying 10-fold. This scheme has the advantage of being easily applied at the bedside in resource-poor settings but has not been prospectively validated in this setting. This and other severity scores (CURB-65, CRB-65, PSI) have not yet been evaluated in resource poor settings.

Preexisting factors (history)
  Age >60 yrs
  Pre-morbid illness

Examination
  Low blood pressure and/or increased pulse
  Multilobar disease
  Increased respiratory rate (>30/min)
  Confusion

Investigation
  Low or high peripheral white cell count
  High urea
  Low PaO_2
  Bacteraemia

Ceftriaxone should be used as a second-line treatment in children with severe pneumonia with failure on the first-line treatment (WHO guidelines). Empirical antibiotic guidelines are locally defined based on antibiotic availability and known microbiological sensitivity.

Delay in presentation and treatment are important causes of death. Recent studies have demonstrated non-inferiority of health worker-managed severe pneumonia in young children by rapid administration of amoxicillin.

In addition to antimicrobial therapy, other supportive treatment should be initiated. Supplemental oxygen, clearance of respiratory secretions (by changing posture, suctioning and provision of moist air), maintenance of appropriate hydration (with intravenous fluids if necessary) and adequate pain relief (using non-opiate analgesics) may all be required. Assisted ventilation, if available, is necessary when severe respiratory muscle fatigue develops.

Complications

An appropriate response to therapy is resolution of fever within 48–72 hrs of starting antibiotics in association with an improvement in well-being and appetite. Failure of this pattern requires a reconsideration of the underlying diagnosis, therapy given and/or a search for an early complication – empyema,

suppurative pericarditis, lung abscess, pneumothorax or meningitis. The late sequelae of pneumococcal pneumonia (osteomyelitis, arthritis, endocarditis) are infrequent if appropriate antibiotics are given early. Following discharge from hospital, a follow-up visit in 4–6 weeks is advisable to ensure complete resolution of the pneumonia or further investigation for possible tuberculosis. The chest X-ray changes may take 3 months to resolve.

Prevention

Active vaccination

Polyvalent pneumococcal polysaccharide vaccines have been available for many years, but uncertainties over their effectiveness and their relative expense ($9 per dose) have limited their use. They are currently recommended for individuals with sickle cell disease but there are no other clear recommendations for use in the tropics. The vaccine is ineffective in HIV-infected adults and children under 2 years of age. The new generation protein conjugate pneumococcal polysaccharide vaccines are effective in children in Africa and are being implemented in many less economically-developed countries (LEDC) by the GAVI programme as a part of EPI. They are effective in HIV-infected African adults but not currently in routine use in this group. Protection against *Haemophilus influenzae* type b (Hib) pneumonia in children is achievable by vaccination and this is being included in the Expanded Programme on Immunization (EPI) regimen.

Chemoprophylaxis

Penicillin should be given on a daily basis to individuals with sickle cell disease or with asplenia to prevent pneumococcal infections. Daily co-trimoxazole is recommended for HIV-infected adults and children in the tropics.

Future developments

Antibiotic resistance

Penicillin resistance amongst *S. pneumoniae* is on the increase globally and represents a major threat to cheap and effective therapy of lower respiratory tract infections. At present these changes are probably of little consequence for the treatment of pneumococcal pneumonia – achievable levels of penicillin in blood and pulmonary tissue with standard dosages will be bactericidal for most of the currently 'resistant' pneumococci (unlike the situation with meningitis). Local information on bacterial sensitivity patterns is essential to plan national and district level policy.

Pneumococcal vaccines

In addition to the protein conjugate vaccines, several pneumococcal peptides (pneumolysin, pneumococcal surface proteins) are being studied as vaccine candidates or as components of the conjugate vaccines. These vaccines may be able to overcome the serotype-restricted nature of the polysaccharide vaccines and may be substantially cheaper to manufacture.

 SUMMARY

- Pneumonia is common and is strongly associated with HIV infection.
- Tuberculosis may be a coinfection in up to 10% of patients with pneumonia in sub-Saharan Africa.
- Simple severity scores can be used to predict poor outcome at the bedside, but have not been validated in tropical settings.
- Antibiotic therapy should be started as soon as possible.
- Penicillin should be adequate treatment for *Streptococcus pneumoniae*, even in the presence of moderate resistance.
- Polyvalent pneumococcal polysaccharide vaccines have little role in sub-Saharan Africa; protein conjugate polysaccharide vaccines are effective in children in this setting.

 Visit www.lecturenoteseries.com/tropicalmed to test yourself on this chapter using interactive MCQs.

FURTHER READING

Cutts FT, Zaman SM, Enwere G, *et al.* (2005) Efficacy of nine-valent pneumococcal conjugate vaccine against pneumonia and invasive pneumococcal disease in The Gambia: randomised, double-blind, placebo-controlled trial. *Lancet* **365**, 1139–46.

Klugman, KP *et al.* (2003) A trial of a 9-valent pneumococcal conjugate vaccine in children with and those without HIV infection. *N Engl J Med* **349**: 1341–8.

Scott JA, Hall AJ, Muyodi C, *et al.* (2000) Aetiology, outcome, and risk factors for mortality among adults with acute pneumonia in Kenya. *Lancet* **355**: 1225–30.

Soofi S, Ahmed S, Fox MP, *et al.* (2012) Effectiveness of community case management of severe pneumonia with oral amoxicillin in children aged 2–59 months in Matiari district, rural Pakistan: a cluster-randomised controlled trial. *Lancet* **379**: 729–37.

http://whqlibdoc.who.int/publications/2012/9789241502825_eng.pdf [free download of 2012 WHO treatment guidelines, *Recommendations for Management of Common Childhood Conditions* 2012 and evidence base.]

http://www.gavialliance.org/ [The GAVI Alliance website with country and disease specific immunization details.]

29

Lung flukes

Nick Beeching
Liverpool School of Tropical Medicine

Lung flukes of the genus *Paragonimus* are zoonoses but human infection can cause a chronic cough with haemoptysis which can easily be mistaken for tuberculosis. *Paragonimus westermani* is the most common cause of human disease.

Life-cycle

Lung flukes are hermaphrodite trematodes. The stout adults, which are about 12 mm long, live as pairs in cavities in the lungs. Large brownish eggs (85–100 × 50–60 μm) are passed in the sputum or faeces and, if they reach water, develop in about 3 weeks to release a miracidium that infects certain species of freshwater snail, in which the parasite undergoes asexual multiplication. Cercariae with knob-shaped tails emerge and encyst in freshwater crabs or crayfish.

The definitive hosts of the flukes are carnivores that eat crustacea; humans are incidental hosts infected by ingesting metacercariae in uncooked crab or crayfish meat or their juices. Human infections are most common in Asia, especially Korea where medicinal use of crayfish juice and in parts of China where eating live crabs dipped in rice wine ('drunken crabs') aid transmission (Fig. 29.1). Other species of *Paragonimus* occur in Africa and the Americas. Paragonimiasis was common during the Biafran war in Nigeria and is found in native Indians in Ecuador and Colombia.

Clinical features

Patients with acute infections may present with malaise, shivers, sweats and urticarial skin rash or abdominal pain a few days or weeks after infection.

Lung disease

- Patients present with chronic cough productive of brownish-red sputum, sometimes with haemoptysis.
- Occasionally, there is breathlessness or chest pain.
- Radiology usually shows peripheral nodules or ring shadows; sometimes there is a crescentic shadow of a fluke within the ring. CT scans are useful.
- Pleural effusions or empyema are complications.

Ectopic disease

This is caused by aberrant migration of flukes from the gut. There are many possible presentations but these include:

- abdominal pain and inflammatory masses;
- convulsions;
- cerebral tumour-like presentations;
- mental disturbance;
- migrating subcutaneous lumps (larva migrans).

Diagnosis

- Microscopy of sputum or stool. Concentrate stool using the formol-ether technique. Examine sputum for brownish flecks that may contain nests of eggs. Mucoid sputum is concentrated by adding 2–3 times the volume of 10% potassium hydroxide for 1 h and then centrifuging for 3 min at 1500 rpm. Examine the deposit using the low-power objective.
- Eggs can also be recovered by bronchoalveolar lavage.
- Serological diagnosis by enzyme immunoassay or dot enzyme immunoassay using antigens from flukes or metacercariae is available in some endemic areas.
- Radiological evidence and eosinophilia in early disease may aid diagnosis.

Tropical Medicine Lecture Notes, Seventh edition. Edited by Nick Beeching and Geoff Gill. © 2014 John Wiley & Sons, Ltd. Published 2014 by John Wiley & Sons, Ltd.

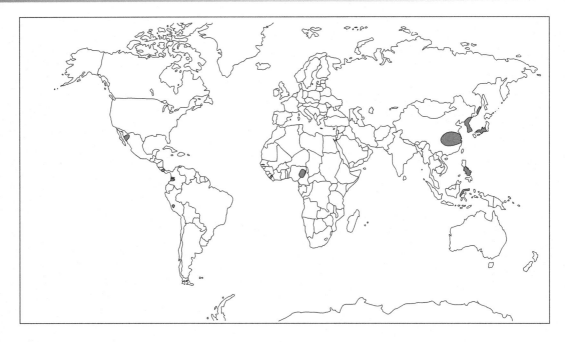

Figure 29.1 Distribution of lung fluke infections.

Treatment

Praziquantel is highly effective, given as 75 mg/kg/day in three divided doses for 2 days (150 mg/kg total dose), or as a single dose of 40 mg/kg. If available, triclabendazole is an alternative, given as 10 mg/kg once or on two successive days. Treat cautiously if cerebral disease is suspected, as a sudden increase in intracranial pressure is possible. Use dexamethasone to control cerebral oedema.

SUMMARY

* Paragonimus (fluke) infections are acquired by eating raw or undercooked crustaceans such as crabs or crayfish.
* In humans, disease localizes in the brain (especially in Asia) or lung (mainly in Africa), but ectopic disease can occur in other organs such as the colon.
* The most common chest presentation is coughing up brown-red sputum or haemoptysis and this may be mistaken for cavitatory tuberculosis.
* Chest X-ray shows nodules or ring shadows: pleural effusion or empyema occur occasionally.
* Therapy with praziquantel or triclabendazole is highly effective.

 Visit www.lecturenoteseries.com/tropicalmed to test yourself on this chapter using interactive MCQs.

FURTHER READING

Keiser J, Engels D, Büscher G, Utzinger J (2005) Triclabendazole for the treatment of fascioliasis and paragonimiasis. *Expert Opinion on Investigational Drugs* **14**: 1513–26. [Useful review of praziquantel and triclabendazole treatment of both fluke infections.]

Keiser J, Utzinger J (2009) Food-borne trematodiases. *Clin Microbiol Rev* **22**: 466–83. doi: 10.1128/CMR.00012-09 [Excellent illustrated overview of all trematodes acquired from food, including Paragonimus. Free download.]

Rosenbaum SD (2006) Paragonimiasis. Emedicine 2006 www.emedicine.com/ped/TOPIC1729.HTM [Short clinical review in Western setting with a few references, available free online.]

30

Tropical pulmonary eosinophilia

Stephen Gordon and Nick Beeching
Liverpool School of Tropical Medicine

Tropical pulmonary eosinophilia (TPE) is an asthma-like disease caused by a hyperactive immunological response to 'human' filariae, usually *Wuchereria bancrofti* or *Brugia malayi* (see also Chapter 14). Microfilariae are destroyed in the pulmonary capillaries and antigen release recruits large numbers of degranulating eosinophils that release major basic protein and other chemicals. A granulomatous reaction may eventually progress to fibrosis and permanent lung damage, possibly due to antigenic similarity between the filarial worm enzymes and proteins found on human pulmonary epithelium.

Epidemiology

TPE is found commonly in India and in parts of West Africa. The disease usually occurs in children and young adults. In other parts of the world, myeloproliferative and idiopathic eosinophilic lung disease and oesophagitis are more common.

Clinical features

Patients present with a short history of cough, wheeze and shortness of breath, worse at night and often preceded or accompanied by malaise and low-grade fever. Signs are similar to those of asthma but there is sometimes lymph node or splenic enlargement and very rarely, seventh nerve palsy or other focal neurological signs.

Investigation

Chest X-ray may be normal but often shows diffuse alveolar mottling with small 1–2 mm nodules in the middle and lower zones. Hilar adenopathy is sometimes seen and less often there is a pleural effusion or areas of hyperacute pneumonitis.

The blood shows a marked eosinophilia, usually above $3\times10^9/L$ and sometimes much higher. The erythrocyte sedimentation rate is raised. Immunoglobulin E levels are also greatly raised and tests for filarial antibodies show high titres. Microfilariae cannot usually be found in peripheral blood, even by sensitive filtration methods, but filarial antigen tests are positive.

Lung function testing shows restrictive changes and poor gas diffusion; obstructive changes are less common.

Diagnosis

Diagnosis is based on the high eosinophilia with high filarial antibody titres and the response to treatment. The differential diagnosis includes migrating helminths, especially ascariasis in children but also *Strongyloides stercoralis* or hookworms. These usually cause only temporary disability. Severe allergic asthma and allergic bronchopulmonary aspergillosis should also be considered.

Tropical Medicine Lecture Notes, Seventh edition. Edited by Nick Beeching and Geoff Gill. © 2014 John Wiley & Sons, Ltd. Published 2014 by John Wiley & Sons, Ltd.

Treatment

TPE may remit spontaneously and recurs following treatment in 20% of cases. Diethylcarbamazine (DEC) 6 mg/kg in divided doses given for 12–21 days is the standard treatment. Symptomatic response within days is usual but lung function can remain impaired for months. Albendazole 400 mg twice daily for 3 weeks may be added to a second course of DEC in those who do not respond adequately. Alternatively, doxycycline 200 mg/day for 4 weeks followed by ivermectin may be tried. In non-filarial pulmonary eosinophilia, there is a very rapid response to steroid therapy but maintenance is required to prevent relapse.

Prevention

This will only be achieved by control of *Aedes* mosquito breeding sites and reducing bites.

 FURTHER READING

Chitkara RK, Krishna G (2006) Parasitic pulmonary eosinophilia. *Semin Respir Crit Care Med* **27**: 171–84.

Vijayan VK (2007) Tropical pulmonary eosinophilia: pathogenesis, diagnosis and management. *Curr Opin Pulm Med* **13**: 428–33.

 SUMMARY

- Tropical pulmonary eosinophilia (TPE) is an asthma-like disease caused by a hyperactive immunological response to 'human' filariae, usually *Wuchereria bancrofti* or *Brugia malayi*.
- TPE is found commonly in India and in parts of West Africa. The disease usually occurs in children and young adults.
- Patients present with a short history of cough, wheeze and shortness of breath, worse at night and often preceded or accompanied by malaise and low-grade fever.
- Diagnosis is based on the high eosinophilia with high filarial antibody titres and the response to treatment.
- TPE may remit spontaneously or symptomatic response usually occurs within days of starting treatment with diethylcarbamazine. Albendazole may be added in refractory cases, or doxycycline followed by ivermectin.

Visit www.lecturenoteseries.com/tropicalmed to test yourself on this chapter using interactive MCQs.

31

Pyogenic meningitis

Nick Beeching
Liverpool School of Tropical Medicine

Bacterial meningitis is a major cause of morbidity and mortality in the tropics. It has been estimated that 1 in 250 children are affected before the age of 5 in urban West Africa (Dakar, Senegal), with up to 50% mortality. Further south in the 'meningitis belt', 1–2% of people may be affected during the cyclical epidemics of meningococcal disease that occur every 5–7 years. Viral meningitis and viral encephalitis occur in the tropics but will not be considered further here (Chapter 33).

Epidemiology

The majority of cases of pyogenic meningitis are caused by the pneumococcus *Streptococcus pneumoniae* (many serogroups), the meningococcus *Neisseria meningitidis* (serogroups A, B, C, Y, W135, X) or Haemophilus influenzae type b (Hib). The latter rarely affects patients aged over 5 years, and all three are more common in children under 2 years. These young children are an important group of patients because they are least likely to respond to polysaccharide capsule-derived vaccines that have been produced for serogroups of each of the main three bacterial species. At the extremes of age, group B streptococci and staphylococci (both *Staphylococcus aureus* and coagulase negative Staphylococci) are important in neonates, and various Gram-negative organisms are important in adults, who also become more susceptible to pneumococcal infections as age increases. The epidemiology of meningitis varies between countries and it is important to determine the usual causative organisms wherever one is practising: for example, the most common cause of bacterial meningitis in adults in Vietnam is *Streptococcus*

suis. HIV has led to a great change in the pattern of meningitis in much of Africa over the past decade, with a huge rise in invasive pneumococcal disease as well as cryptococcal meningitis and a smaller rise in tuberculous meningitis, but no specific increase in meningococcal disease. Antibiotic resistance is common in Hib throughout the world, and in pneumococci in much of the tropics. Clinically significant resistance has yet to become common in meningococci but has been reported.

Meningococcal epidemiology

Epidemics have occurred with regularity in West Africa and the Sudan for at least a century. Lapeysonnie defined the 'meningitis belt' in 1963 as an area with a high incidence and recurring epidemics between latitudes 4° and 16° north, south of the Sahara, with 300–1100 mm annual rainfall, comprising much of semiarid sub-Saharan Africa including the Sahel. This belt has high levels of seasonal endemicity with large superimposed epidemics of infection of predominantly group A meningococci at irregular intervals. This zone has been extended further south in recent years to include other countries with at least 1 month of reduced humidity (Fig. 31.1). Factors predisposing to meningococcal infection include overcrowding and poor hygiene, so that schools, urban slums, military barracks, prisons and similar large collections of people are at increased risk. Damage to the upper respiratory mucosa by tobacco or wood fire smoke, intercurrent viral infections such as influenza, or external dust (e.g. the annual dry 'Harmattan' wind in Nigeria) facilitates invasion by meningococci. While group A meningococci are usually implicated in West Africa or in previous epidemics related to the Hajj pilgrimage to Mecca, other

Tropical Medicine Lecture Notes, Seventh edition. Edited by Nick Beeching and Geoff Gill. © 2014 John Wiley & Sons, Ltd. Published 2014 by John Wiley & Sons, Ltd.

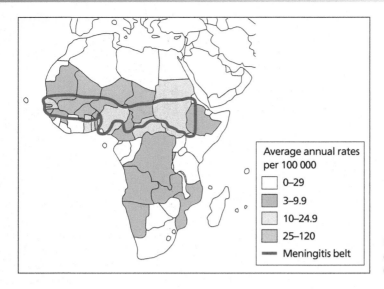

Figure 31.1 Meningococcal disease in Africa 1993–2006. (*Source*: WHO, 2008).

strains – most recently W135 (and now group X and other novel strains) – became prominent after successful vaccination against group A. In South America, epidemics of group C strains have been described but should now be preventable by vaccination. In Western countries where immunization against group C has been instituted, group B predominates and vaccines against this strain are just becoming available. There does not seem to be increased risk of meningococcal infection in HIV-positive or similarly immunocompromised patients.

Pneumococcal epidemiology

There are many serogroups of pneumococci, the predominance of which varies from country to country, so that sophisticated microbiological surveillance is required in order to confirm the relevant mixture to be included in polyvalent vaccines. Host factors common in the tropics are well-recognized to predispose to pneumococcal infection including haemoglobinopathies such as sickle and sickle-haemoglobin C (SC) disease, splenic dysfunction caused by these or because of removal after trauma, damage to the cribriform plate in the skull by trauma, and HIV infection. Recently, cyclical epidemics of specific serotypes of pneumococcal meningitis have been described, often coexisting with epidemics of meningococcal diseases. The standard of care for prevention in risk groups has been the use of polysaccharide vaccines, although the evidence base is poor and even suggests that polysaccharide pneumococcal vaccine is harmful in some HIV-positive African populations. It is likely that conjugate

vaccines will be more effective in both HIV-positive and HIV-negative groups.

Haemophilus influenzae type b epidemiology

Some countries in the tropics have virtually eliminated invasive Hib disease, including meningitis, by instituting early childhood immunization, as practised in the West. This has been shown in the Middle East and in the Gambia.

Vaccines

All three major causes of bacterial meningitis can be prevented by vaccines based on serogroup-specific antigens derived from their polysaccharide capsules. These vaccines require an intact 'cold chain' of refrigeration (<5°C) at all stages of transport from manufacturer to delivery at the point of health care. They are less immunogenic in the groups most at risk (under 2 years) and induced immunity is mainly T-cell dependent and relatively short-lived. The role of novel vaccines against serogroup B meningococci, recently licensed, needs assessment in the tropics.

New conjugate vaccines are more expensive but also more successful; proven examples are Hib vaccine and the group C meningococcal vaccine. Similar vaccines have been developed for other serogroups of meningococci (A, C, Y, W135) and for pneumococci with support from international donors. By the end of 2012, 100 million people in Africa had received MenAfriVac®, a conjugate vaccine that is greatly reducing the incidence of Group A meningococcal meningitis in that region.

Clinical features

The cardinal features of meningitis are no different in the tropics than elsewhere, and symptoms include headache, vomiting, fever, photophobia, loss of consciousness and fits, associated with the clinical signs of fever, neck stiffness and reducing level of consciousness. The index of suspicion is higher in children who may have less obvious features and who often have coexisting malaria parasitaemia. The rash of meningococcal disease develops rapidly and in darker skins may be difficult to see unless the mucosal membranes are involved – always check in the mouth and conjunctivae. In some African groups, the meningococcal rash is slightly raised and can be palpated even if it is difficult to see.

The differential diagnosis in a tropical setting is wide (Box 31.1). The most important clinical decisions are whether the patient has cerebral malaria and/or meningitis, whether there is a space-occupying lesion (often an abscess related to severe otitis media) or whether the patient has tuberculosis (TB) or cryptococcal meningitis. Examination should focus on clues to underlying predisposing factors, including broken nose, laparotomy scars (for splenectomy) and features of haemoglobinopathy suggesting pneumococcal, or HIV suggesting pneumococcal or cryptococcal meningitis. Optic fundi may show miliary TB, HIV-related retinopathy (including cytomegalovirus), haemorrhage caused by severe malaria, or tuberculomas as well as features of raised intracranial pressure in long-standing space-occupying lesions. Focal neurological signs suggest a space-occupying lesion, TB or late cryptococcal disease. Most patients with TB meningitis present with a prolonged history but some cases do present acutely, and patients with cryptococcal meningitis and HIV may have little headache and minimal or no neck stiffness.

Diagnosis

Lumbar puncture (LP) is mandatory whenever there is suspicion of meningitis. It should only be avoided if there is clear clinical evidence of a space-occupying lesion and, if omitted, the patient should be given antibiotics to cover the possibility of meningitis until it is considered safe to do an LP.

Diagnosis can be achieved with simple biochemical and microscopic tests. The patterns of white cells in cerebrospinal fluid (CSF) vary and there is considerable overlap between the groups (Box 31.2).

Box 31.1 Differential diagnosis of pyogenic meningitis

- Malaria (cerebral or otherwise)
- Typhoid
- Pneumonia
- Urinary tract infection
- Otitis media/sinusitis
- Severe paediatric gastroenteritis
- Tetanus
- Trypanosomiasis
- Brucellosis
- Rickettsial disease
- Subarachnoid haemorrhage
- Cerebral abscess or other space-occupying lesion, including tuberculoma
- Causes of lymphocytic cerebrospinal fluid (tuberculosis, cryptococcus, viral meningitis, etc.)
- Encephalitis
- Poisoning (alcohol, drugs, etc.) and other cause of coma
- Drug-induced extrapyramidal signs (phenothiazines, antiemetics)

Box 31.2 Cerebrospinal fluid patterns

Pyogenic
- Bacterial

Lymphocytic with normal glucose
- Most viruses (e.g. polio, enteroviruses, Coxsackie)
- Rickettsiae
- HIV
- Early TB
- Miscellaneous (e.g. endocarditis, neoplastic)

Lymphocytic with low glucose
- Partially treated bacterial meningitis
- Cerebral abscess
- TB
- Some viral (e.g. mumps)
- Fungal (e.g. *Cryptococcus*, *Aspergillus*)
- Brucellosis
- Syphilis
- Leptospirosis
- Trypanosomiasis

Eosinophilic
- *Angiostrongylus cantonensis*
- *Taenia solium* (cysticercosis)
- Paragonimiasis

Amoebic (rare)
- *Naegleria* spp.

Abnormalities of cells persist in the CSF for several days, even after antibiotic treatment has been started. Some viral infections, especially mumps, may have neutrophil predominance in the early stages. Biochemical tests help to distinguish these and a very high protein usually suggests bacterial infection or TB. In TB the CSF protein is sometimes high enough to form a 'spider-web' clot in the tube. The specificity of low CSF glucose for diagnosing bacterial infection is improved by comparing it to simultaneous blood glucose, especially if the patient is diabetic or has other causes of altered blood glucose levels. Urine dipsticks can be used for CSF. Stains of CSF should include Gram's stain for bacteria, which is as sensitive as latex agglutination and other antigen detection systems, Ziehl–Neelson or auramine (for TB) and India-ink stains for cryptococcal infection. Cryptococcal infection should always be considered if CSF is lymphocytic or even if there are no CSF white cells in an HIV-positive patient with suggestive symptoms. Cryptococcal antigen tests (if available) are very valuable.

Cultures for all the above organisms should be set up if facilities are available, and large volumes of CSF (10 mL) need to be taken to maximize the chances of growing *Mycobacterium tuberculosis*. Molecular tests such as polymerase chain reaction (PCR) based tests on blood or CSF are valuable in a Western setting for diagnosing meningococcal infection, particularly if the patient has already received antibiotics before arrival, but are not available in most tropical settings. Blood cultures should always be taken if facilities are available. Suggestive changes in other tests include neutrophilia in peripheral blood and a high C-reactive protein level, especially in children.

In many tropical settings, culture and more sophisticated tests are not available and Gram's staining will be negative. In such cases the features that suggest pyogenic meningitis, rather than viral meningitis or other organisms, are summarized in Table 31.1. The sensitivity and specificity, and hence usefulness at the bedside, of these features varies from area to area. In a recent study in (mainly HIV-negative) Vietnamese adults, five features were more predictive of TB meningitis compared to bacterial: age, length of history, peripheral white blood cell (WBC) count, total CSF WBC count and CSF neutrophil proportion. In a population of mainly HIV-positive adults in Malawi, patients with cryptococcal meningitis had longer histories, lower CSF WBC counts and lower proportions of neutrophils than those with bacterial meningitis.

Table 31.1 Cerebrospinal fluid changes predictive of bacterial causes if Gram's stain is negative (see also Table 3.5)

Opening pressure	High
Turbidity	Present
Total WBC	>2×10^9/L (2000/mm^3)
Neutrophils	>50% if total WBC >0.1×10^9/L (100/mm^3)
Glucose	<1mmol/L (18 mg%)
CSF: blood glucose ratio	<40%
Protein	>2 g/L (200mg%)
Gram's stain	Positive
Ziehl–Neelsen stain	Negative
India-ink stain	Negative
Culture	Positive
Antigen detection	Positive
Plus peripheral WBC	> 16 × 10^9/L

WBC, white blood cell count.

Management

The key features are to make a diagnosis, to assess severity of illness, to detect coexisting or underlying disease, and to provide both supportive and specific therapy. For pyogenic meningitis alone, empirical or pathogen-specific antimicrobials should be given as early as possible, before the LP if there is going to be any delay in the procedure. All patients should be reevaluated at least daily, especially when the CSF results become available. Patients with equivocal (lymphocytic) CSF findings are difficult; repeat LP may be required after 2–3 days. The important decision is whether to treat as TB or not, or whether the initial CSF changes were brought about by viral or partially treated bacterial meningitis or missed cryptococcal disease.

Meningococcal disease

This responds to short courses of chloramphenicol or penicillin, and will also respond to third-generation cephalosporins. Uncomplicated meningococcal meningitis has a mortality of <10% and rarely needs more than 5–7 days of parenteral treatment, and there is increasing evidence that shorter regimens are equally effective. Meningococcal septicaemia (with or without meningitis) has a mortality of >40% in most tropical settings, requiring maximal intensive care. Up to 10% of patients experience immune complex disease including uveitis, polyarthritis and pericarditis, typically in the second week of illness. This responds to inflammatory drugs, including short courses of steroids.

Uncomplicated meningitis can also be managed with single doses of Triplopen or similar mixtures of long- and short-acting penicillins, or with Tifomycin, an oily suspension of chloramphenicol administered as 2–3 g IM once only (but divided into two injections because of volume) for an adult. Tifomycin is now difficult to obtain and has largely been replaced by ceftriaxone, now that cheaper generic formulations have become available. Ceftriaxone can be given IM or IV. These regimens are useful for the management of large numbers of patients in an epidemic setting, provided that patients are reviewed daily for evidence of recovery.

Close contacts (family/household) may be given immediate chemoprophylaxis to prevent them from developing illness over the next fortnight. Suitable medications include sulfadiazine (only if the infecting strain is already known to be sensitive) but not penicillins. The usual alternative is a single dose of ciprofloxacin (15 mg/kg orally in children, 750 mg orally in adults). Other possible agents include rifampicin (20 mg/kg twice daily or 600 mg twice daily for adults, for 2 days) or ceftriaxone (50 mg/kg children or 2 g adults intramuscularly once only). 'Ring' vaccination of contacts is more appropriate in an epidemic situation (see below).

Pneumococcal disease

Antimicrobial therapy depends on local susceptibility patterns. In Papua New Guinea, much of sub-Saharan Africa and elsewhere, there may be at least moderate penicillin resistance, so that isolates need to be cultured to inform therapy, and empirical therapy should not be based on penicillin alone. In a Western setting, large doses of third-generation cephalosporins (cefotaxime or ceftriaxone) are usually adequate, and are becoming more available in tropical settings. Ceftriaxone doses such as 2 grams twice daily (IM or IV) are recommended. Otherwise, monotherapy with chloramphenicol is often the only available choice. Coexistent chloramphenicol resistance is less common, and the commonly recommended mixture of penicillin and chloramphenicol is wasteful of resources and confers no improvement in survival or reduced morbidity in survivors. Meropenem is a safe (but expensive) alternative in proven chloramphenicol and penicillin-resistant cases, or vancomycin can be used. Pneumococcal meningitis has a mortality

of over 50% in many tropical settings and in sub-Saharan Africa the majority of these patients are also HIV-positive. Up to 40% of survivors will have significant neurological deficits. Treatment should last for at least 10 days for uncomplicated disease and may need to extend beyond 14 days in difficult cases.

Haemophilus influenzae disease

Found mainly in young children, clinically significant resistance to ampicillin and/or amoxicillin and to benzyl penicillin is present in about 50% of cases. Less marked chloramphenicol resistance is present in up to 10% of tropical cases. The treatment of choice is a third generation cephalosporin or chloramphenicol alone. Empirical ampicillin cannot be used until the patient's own isolate is known to be sensitive. Chemoprophylaxis of contacts is not usual in tropical settings.

Empirical therapy

Unless there is good epidemiological (current epidemic) and clinical (typical rash) evidence to suggest meningococcal disease, the average adult or child with pyogenic meningitis has to be managed to cover the main three bacterial pathogens, including cover for *Salmonella* spp. in younger children. Monotherapy with chloramphenicol or a third-generation cephalosporin is the treatment of choice. In resource-poor settings with multiresistant pathogens, it has been shown that two doses of Tifomycin 48 h apart are as effective for inpatient treatment as parenteral ampicillin plus chloramphenicol for over a week, in terms of hospital mortality and serious sequelae in survivors. Ceftriaxone has now replaced this in most settings.

Patients at extremes of age need extra cover for other pathogens, e.g. anti-staphylococcal cover such as flucloxacillin, and/or antipseudomonal cover for neonates (e.g. gentamicin). Patients with possible intracerebral abscess should receive metronidazole to cover anaerobes as well as chloramphenicol or third generation cephalosporins.

Use of steroids

Complications of bacterial meningitis are common and severe (Box 31.3). In parts of West Africa they may account for over one-third of cases of deafness. There has been controversy over the years about using high-dose steroids to prevent this. Previous studies showed that post-meningitis deafness could be reduced by dexamethasone given to

> **Box 31.3 Complications of bacterial meningitis**
>
> - Cranial nerve palsy
> - Hemiplegia
> - Deafness
> - Subdural empyema
> - Abscess
> - Late hydrocephalus

Western children with Hib meningitis treated with cephalosporins. The benefit was balanced by some morbidity from gastrointestinal haemorrhage, and subsequent studies of steroid use in children in low HIV prevalence settings in the tropics have generally shown harm or no benefit. One large study in Egypt showed that adults and children with pneumococcal meningitis (not meningococcal or Hib) had reduced mortality and subsequent deafness if given dexamethasone. In northern Europe, only adult patients with proven or suspected pneumococcal meningitis were thought to benefit from high-dose dexamethasone (40 mg/day intravenously for 4 days), given shortly before the first dose of antibiotics. Similar benefit was observed in patients with *S. suis* meningitis in Vietnam (a low HIV prevalence setting) despite late presentation and prior administration of antibiotics to some patients.

However, two large prospective trials have shown neither benefit nor harm from the use of high dose dexamethasone in Malawi as an adjunct for treating pyogenic meningitis in children or adults with a high prevalence of HIV, many of whom presented late for hospital treatment. High-dose dexamethasone is expensive and extra resources are required to administer it in a tropical setting. There is no evidence to support its use in definite or probable meningococcal disease or in most patients who have already received antibiotics of some sort in low HIV prevalence settings. A recent meta-analysis that included tropical trials concluded that there was no role for the use of steroids in any subgroup with pyogenic meningitis, particularly in tropical settings. Unfortunately the early promise shown by glycerol as an alternative in children has not been fulfilled in a trial in adults in Malawi, which was stopped early due to worse outcomes in the glycerol group.

In Vietnam, high doses of dexamethasone reduced mortality from tuberculous meningitis, but increased the number of survivors with severe disability.

Epidemic control (meningococcus)

The World Health Organization (WHO) has developed the definition of an 'alert threshold' for an epidemic of meningococcal meningitis as an incidence of >15 cases per 100 000 population for 1 week. This equates to 2 or more cases in one week in a refugee camp of 10 000 people. Other features that should alert the clinician are a shift in the average age of patients affected, from younger than 5 years to teenagers or older, especially if in a high-risk situation (e.g. refugee camp or in the 'meningitis belt' during the dry season). If more than 3 years have elapsed since the last epidemic, the alert threshold is reduced to 10 cases per 100 000 (Table 31.2).

Early recognition is the key to management (Box 31.4). This should be followed by maximal attempts to confirm the diagnosis by culturing the organism to determine its antimicrobial sensitivities (to guide chemoprophylaxis) and serogroup (to guide vaccination). If facilities to do this are not routinely available, outside assistance is required. This is needed anyway to support enhanced surveillance and to enable provision of adequate supplies of drugs, vaccines, etc. Once an outbreak is declared, a decision must be made on how to get publicity to the affected population and how to conduct surveillance. Health care workers and educated lay persons need to be briefed, using simple case definitions for triaging the worried well as well as the sick at designated assessment centres, and clinical management protocols need to be prepared to guide treatment of patients. The numbers may be large enough to require buildings to be made over specifically for this purpose.

Epidemics of group A disease can be controlled by vaccination – there is ample evidence to support this. The effectiveness depends on both early recognition of an outbreak, and on rapid mass administration of the appropriate vaccine. Mass chemoprophylaxis can

Table 31.2 Meningococcal epidemiology

	Endemic	Epidemic
Incidence/100 000	<10	10–1000
Carrier:case ratio	High	Low
Secondary infections	Rare	Frequent
Peak age	<5	5–15
Usual serogroup	B or C	A, C or W135

Box 31.4 **Management of meningococcal epidemics**

Early recognition ('threshold' 15 cases/100 000 population/week)

Identify organism
- Confirm clinical diagnosis, get CSF from cases
- Establish strain and antibiotic sensitivity

Alert peripheral staff
- Diagnostic algorithms and case definitions
- Treatment algorithms

Alert authorities
- Surveillance schemes
- Temporary treatment centres

Prevent major outbreak
- Mass chemoprophylaxis
- Mass vaccination

also be used if the organism is sulfa-sensitive, or if a decision is made to use fluoroquinolone, but this is often not practical in a large population.

SUMMARY

- Pyogenic meningitis is common in tropical settings, especially in the 'meningitis belt' in sub-Saharan Africa.
- The associated high mortality and morbidity can be reduced by early diagnosis and treatment.
- Except in meningococcal disease, antimicrobial resistance is common and in most settings empirical broad spectrum coverage needs to include parenteral third generation cephalosporins such as ceftriaxone.
- There is no evidence of benefit of dexamethasone or other steroid in pyogenic meningitis in the tropics, although they do reduce mortality in tuberculous meningitis.
- The WHO has produced a useful resource pack to assist in recognition and management of outbreaks of meningococcal meningitis.
- Recent roll-out of new conjugate vaccines is reducing the incidence of meningococcus group A disease in West Africa and this is a model for future immunization programmes.

Visit www.lecturenoteseries.com/tropicalmed to test yourself on this chapter using interactive MCQs.

 FURTHER READING

British Infection Association. http://www.britishinfection.org/drupal/content/clinical-guidelines [UK oriented algorithm for management of adult meningitis, that can be adapted for local use]

Greenwood B (2006) Pneumococcal meningitis epidemics in Africa. *Clin Infect Dis* **43**: 701–2. [Overview of changing epidemiology of pneumococcal meningitis in Africa.]

Meningitis Vaccine Project. http://www.meningvax.org/index.php [Full list of resources.]

Molesworth AM, Cuevas LE, Connor SJ, Morse AP, Thomson MC (2003) Environmental risk and meningitis epidemics in Africa. *Emerg Infect Dis* **9**(10): 1287–93. [Article free online. History & geography of meningococcal epidemics in Africa, nice maps.]

Novak RT *et al.* (2012) Serogroup A meningococcal conjugate vaccination in Burkina Faso: analysis of national surveillance data. *Lancet Infect Dis* **12**: 757–64. [Probable dramatic reduction in Group A meningococcal disease in Burkina Faso after complete population coverage with new conjugate vaccine in late 2010. Now being rolled out across the meningitis belt.]

Santaniello-Newton A, Hunter PR (2000) Management of an outbreak of meningococcal meningitis in a Sudanese refugee camp in Northern Uganda. *Epidemiol Infect* **124**: 75–81. [Case fatality rate of 13% and attack rate of 0.3% (group A meningococcus). They had better experience than other authors and estimated vaccine protective effect to be approximately 83%. The biovalent (A+C) vaccine they used had to be given subcutaneously. They emphasize the need for early epidemic recognition and immunization campaign.]

Scarborough M, Thwaites GE (2008) The diagnosis and management of acute bacterial meningitis in resource-poor settings. *Lancet Neurol* **7**: 637–48. [Comprehensive review from experienced authors with both African and Asian viewpoints.]

Stephens DS, Greenwood G, Brandtzaeg P (2007) Epidemic meningitis, meningococcaemia, and *Neisseria meningitidis*. *Lancet* **369**: 2196–2210. [Superb summary of all aspects of meningococcal disease.]

van de Beeke D *et al.* (2010) Adjunctive dexamethasone in bacterial meningitis: a meta-analysis of individual patient data. *Lancet Neurol* **9**: 254–6. [Steroids don't work for acute bacterial meningitis, especially in sub-Saharan Africa with high HIV prevalence and late presentations.]

van de Beek D, Brouwer MC, Thwaites GE, Tunkel AR (2012) Advances in treatment of bacterial meningitis. *Lancet* **380**: 1693–1702. doi: 10.1016/S0140-6736(12)61186-6. [Recent review of current situation – see also the associated articles on diagnosis and vaccines.]

World Health Organization. www.who.int/topics/meningitis/en/ [World Health Organization website. Source of latest country-specific information and guidelines for diagnosis and treatment, links to Meningitis Vaccine Project and other materials, e.g. those below.]

World Health Organization (2007) Standardized treatment of bacterial meningitis in Africa in epidemic and non epidemic situations. http://www.who.int/csr/resources/publications/meningitis/WHO_CDS_EPR_2007_3.pdf

World Health Organization (2010) Managing meningitis epidemics in Africa. A quick reference guide for health authorities and health-care workers. http://whqlibdoc.who.int/hq/2010/WHO_HSE_GAR_ERI_2010.4_eng.pdf

32

Cryptococcal meningitis

David Lalloo
Liverpool School of Tropical Medicine

Organism and epidemiology

Cryptococcal disease is caused by the yeast-like fungus Cryptococcus neoformans. There are three varieties: var. *gattii*, var. *grubii* and *var. neoformans*. Vars *grubii* and *neoformans* occur worldwide and are found in the environment related to avian droppings. Var. *gattii* occurs predominantly in the tropics and is much harder to find in the environment, but occurs in association with eucalypt trees.

Cryptococcal disease occurs in both immunocompetent and immunocompromised hosts. Infection is acquired by inhalation and predominantly causes pulmonary disease or cryptococcal meningitis (CM). In the tropics prior to the AIDS epidemic, var. *gattii* caused CM in immunocompetent individuals. However, most cases of cryptococcal disease in the tropics now occur in patients with HIV infection and are caused by var. *grubii* or *neoformans*. CM occurs in HIV-infected individuals throughout the tropics, predominantly in those with CD4 cell counts of less than 100×10^6/L. It is estimated that there are over 700 000 cases of invasive cryptococcal disease in Africa annually and it is one of the most common identified causes of death in HIV-infected Africans.

Clinical features

Cryptococcosis presents as pneumonia, cryptococcal meningitis or disseminated disease. Pneumonia is less common, often asymptomatic or mild and may resolve spontaneously. A small number of immunocompromised patients have a rapidly progressive pulmonary illness. CM presents as a subacute or chronic meningitis with headache, fever and alteration in mental state, often of several weeks' duration. The disease mimics tuberculous meningitis and may be indistinguishable clinically. Clinical signs include fever, cranial nerve palsies and visual disturbance associated with papilloedema; neck stiffness is relatively uncommon. Disseminated infection occurs in advanced immunosuppression, often presenting as fever. Skin lesions may occur and may contain the organism.

Diagnosis

A high index of suspicion should be maintained in those with HIV infection and unexplained fever or headache. Lumbar puncture classically demonstrates a raised cerebrospinal fluid (CSF) protein and white cell count with a predominant lymphocytosis, although the cell count and protein can be normal in early CM or if the patient is very immunosuppressed. The lumbar opening pressure is commonly raised. Cryptococci can be seen after Gram staining or simply demonstrated in the CSF by the addition of a few drops of India ink (Fig. 32.1). This outlines the capsule of the organism and makes it easier to distinguish the organism from white cells. India ink staining is positive in up to 70% of patients. The organism can also be cultured from the CSF, blood or, occasionally, skin lesions. Latex agglutination tests can detect cryptococcal polysaccharide antigen (CrAg) with a high sensitivity in the CSF or the blood and may be very useful if culture facilities are not available- newer lateral flow assays are even more sensitive.

Tropical Medicine Lecture Notes, Seventh edition. Edited by Nick Beeching and Geoff Gill. © 2014 John Wiley & Sons, Ltd. Published 2014 by John Wiley & Sons, Ltd.

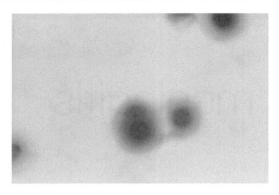

Figure 32.1 Budding yeast-like organisms of *Cryptococcus neoformans* in the cerebrospinal fluid stained with Gram's stain.

Treatment

Optimum treatment of CM is amphotericin B (1 mg/kg/day) in combination with flucytosine (100 mg/kg/day) for 2 weeks followed by fluconazole 400–800 mg daily for a further 8 weeks. However, there are often practical difficulties in the administration of amphotericin in resource-poor settings because of its renal toxicity and the need to monitor renal function. Shorter regimens are currently being evaluated. Fluconazole (1200 mg daily, with or without flucytosine) may be used as initial therapy and is much easier to administer than amphotericin, but may take longer to sterilize the CSF and has been associated with higher relapse rates. Use of intravenous pre-hydration and potassium supplementation reduces the toxicity of amphotericin.

Relapse is common in HIV patients following successful initial treatment and ART initiation is one of the most important interventions for this group: the optimum timing of ART initiation is unknown. Initiation of antiretroviral therapy after successful treatment may be associated with cryptococcal immune reconstitution syndrome which can be difficult to distinguish from relapse. Secondary prophylaxis with fluconazole (200 mg/day) is effective in preventing relapse and needs to be continued for life or until the CD4 count has risen to above 200×10^6/L for several months following antiretroviral therapy.

Many patients with CM have raised intracranial pressure, which is associated with a poor prognosis. There is strongly suggestive evidence that repeated lumbar punctures reduce the intracranial pressure and improve outcome. No other intervention has been shown to be effective in the reduction of intracranial pressure. In the absence of treatment of CM, the disease is uniformly fatal. Even with treatment, case fatality rates can be as high as 50% in some parts of the tropics.

Prevention

A positive CrAg in HIV-positive individuals prior to commencing ART is highly predictive of subsequent cryptococcal disease. In high prevalence areas, routine screening and fluconazole treatment of CrAG-positive patients prior to ART is recommended. In patients with CD4 cell counts $<100 \times 10^6$/L, fluconazole prophylaxis is appropriate if a delay before initiation of ART is anticipated.

 SUMMARY

- Cryptococcal meningitis in the tropics now mostly occurs in HIV-infected patients, predominantly in those with particularly low CD4 cell counts.
- Cryptococcosis can present as pneumonia or disseminated disease, as well as meningitis.
- Typically in cryptococcal meningitis, the cerebrospinal fluid (CSF) is under high pressure, with a raised protein level and lymphocytosis. *Cryptococci* may be seen with Gram or India ink staining.
- Optimum treatment is with combined amphotericin B and flucytosine for 2 weeks, followed by more prolonged (e.g. 8 weeks) fluconazole. Even with such treatment, mortality is high.

 Visit www.lecturenoteseries.com/tropicalmed to test yourself on this chapter using interactive MCQs.

FURTHER READING

Bicanic T, Harrison TS (2005) Cryptococcal meningitis. *Brit Med Bull* **72**: 99–118. [Good review on clinical and therapeutic aspects.]

World Health Organization (2011) Rapid advice: Diagnosis, prevention and management of cryptococcal disease in HIV-infected adults, adolescents and children. http://www.who.int/hiv/pub/cryptococcal_disease2011/en/ [Useful clinical guidelines.]

33

Encephalitis

Tom Solomon[1] and Rachel Kneen[2]
[1]University of Liverpool; [2]Alder Hey Children's Foundation NHS Trust

Encephalitis (inflammation of the brain parenchyma) is strictly speaking a pathological diagnosis that should only be made with histological evidence at autopsy or from brain biopsy. Because of the obvious practical limitations of this, clinical definitions are often used. Most patients present with the triad of fever, headache and encephalopathy (reduced level of consciousness). Many also have focal neurological signs and seizures. However, patients occasionally present simply with abnormal behaviour, which may be mistaken for psychiatric illness.

Causes of encephalitis

Encephalitis can be caused by many viruses, other organisms and autoimmune processes (Table 33.1) However, viruses transmitted by insects (arboviruses; Chapter 40) make encephalitis especially common in the tropics.

Arboviral encephalitis

The arboviruses that cause neurological disease in humans come principally from three viral families (see Fig. 40.1). The most important are the flaviviruses, especially Japanese encephalitis virus. Flaviviruses exist in enzootic cycles, being transmitted by mosquitoes (in warm climates) or ticks (in cooler northern climates); most humans are coincidentally infected 'dead end' hosts. In addition, alphaviruses and bunyaviruses cause central nervous system (CNS) disease in the Americas.

Japanese encephalitis

Japanese encephalitis is the most important cause of epidemic encephalitis worldwide. There are an estimated nearly 70 000 cases annually with more than 10 000 deaths. More than half the survivors have severe neurological sequelae.

Epidemiology

The virus is transmitted naturally between birds by *Culex* mosquitoes, especially *Culex tritaeniorhynchus*, which breeds in rice paddy fields. Peri-domestic animals (especially pigs) act as amplifying hosts, and subsequently humans become infected (Fig. 33.1). In southern tropical areas the disease is endemic, in northern temperate zones it occurs in summer epidemics (Fig. 33.2). The geographical area affected is expanding, possibly because of increasing irrigation projects, and spread by birds. In endemic areas of rural Asia the virus is ubiquitous and almost all children are infected, but only a small proportion develop disease.

Clinical features

Following a non-specific febrile illness, which may include coryza, cough, vomiting, diarrhoea and headache, patients develop a reduced level of consciousness. This may be heralded by convulsions; status epilepticus is common. Focal neurological signs include upper and lower motor neurone signs; a 'Parkinsonian syndrome' with tremor, cogwheel rigidity and mask-like facies; rigidity spasms, flexor and extensor posturing, and other signs of raised

Tropical Medicine Lecture Notes, Seventh edition. Edited by Nick Beeching and Geoff Gill. © 2014 John Wiley & Sons, Ltd. Published 2014 by John Wiley & Sons, Ltd.

Table 33.1 Infectious causes of encephalitis

Arthropod-borne viruses (often epidemic and geographically localized)
Flaviviruses (Japanese encephalitis, West Nile)
Alphaviruses (Venezuelan and Eastern equine encephalitis)
Bunyaviruses (La Crosse encephalitis)

Non-arthropod-borne viruses (mostly sporadic and non-geographically localized)
Herpes viruses (herpes simplex virus types 1 and 2, varicella zoster virus, Epstein–Barr virus)
Enteroviruses (Coxsackie, echovirus, enterovirus type 71)
Paramyxoviruses (measles, mumps, Nipah)
Rabies (Chapter 36)
Human immunodeficiency virus

Acute disseminated encephalomyelitis
Occurs several weeks after an acute infection (often viral) or vaccination

Other infectious causes of encephalitis
Usually distinguishable from viral encephalitis, either because of their slower onset, or because they are associated with other features (e.g. multiorgan failure, rash)
Trypanosomiasis, especially *Trypanosoma brucei rhodesiensis*
Toxoplasma occasionally presents with diffuse encephalitis
Amoebic meningoencephalitis, especially *Naegleria fowleri*
Typhus, especially African tick typhus (*Rickettsia africae*) and scrub typhus in Asia (*O. tsutsugamushi*)
Secondary syphilis, and other spirochaetes (e.g. relapsing fevers)

intracranial pressure. Other patients present with aseptic meningitis, febrile convulsions or a polio-like acute flaccid paralysis. The differential diagnosis includes other causes of encephalitis and non-viral causes of CNS disease (see Table 3.1).

Investigations

Typically, lymphocytes are present in the CSF (5–100/mm^3), with a normal glucose level and slightly elevated protein (0.5–1 g/L). However, the CSF may be normal if taken too early or too late in the disease. IgM antibodies appear in the serum and CSF after the first few days of illness and can be detected by ELISA or rapid diagnostic kits. Virus is sometimes isolated from CSF or brain tissue at postmortem, or detected by PCR in the CSF. Computerized tomography (CT) or magnetic resonance imaging (MRI) may show characteristic midbrain changes.

Management

This is discussed at the end of this chapter.

Prevention and public health

Vaccines against Japanese encephalitis include:

- a live attenuated vaccine which is safe and efficacious, and has been used in China for many years (SA-14-14-2);
- an inactivated vaccine based on this strain (IC51, marketed as "Ixiaro");
- a chimeric vaccine in which the structural proteins of the Chinese vaccines are inserted into the yeallow fever 17D 'backbone'(Chimerivax-JE, marketed as "IMOJEV").

Additional locally produced inactivated tissue culture derived vaccines are also available in some countries in Asia.

Vector control measures such treating rice paddy fields with neem cake (a natural insecticide) and intermittent irrigation of rice paddies to prevent *Culex* breeding probably have no major role in control. Individual protective measures include avoiding mosquito bites (easier for visitors than residents) and using DEET-containing spray, bed nets and protective clothing.

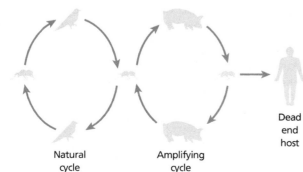

Natural cycle   Amplifying cycle

Dead end host

Figure 33.1 The transmission cycle of Japanese encephalitis virus. The virus is transmitted naturally between aquatic birds by *Culex* mosquitoes. During the rainy season, when there is an increase in the number of mosquitoes, the virus 'overflows' into pigs and other peri-domestic animals, and then into humans, from whom it is not transmitted further.

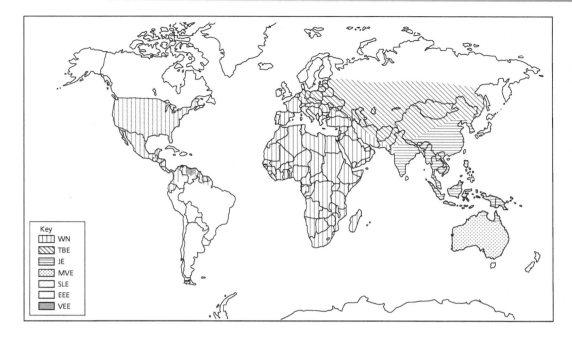

Figure 33.2 Map showing the approximate global distribution of CNS arboviruses. In North America Western equine encephalitis has a similar distribution to St Louis encephalitis (SLE), and La Crosse has a similar distribution to West Nile (WN). EEE, Eastern equine encephalitis; JE, Japanese encephalitis; MVE, Murray valley encephalitis; TBE, tick-borne encephalitis; VEE, Venezuelan equine encephalitis.

West Nile virus

This is a flavivirus widely distributed throughout Africa, Asia, the Middle East, southern Europe, and has recently spread to North America. It is transmitted between water fowl by *Culex pipiens*. West Nile virus was previously considered to be a cause of fever–arthralgia–rash syndrome, with occasional CNS disease. The virus appeared in the USA in 1999, and rapidly spread across the continent. Vaccines are in development, though whether any will prove to be commercially viable is uncertain.

St Louis encephalitis virus

This is a flavivirus found in the Americas. It previously caused large epidemics (3000 cases/year) but now only around 100 cases/year. It may be a good example of how arboviral disease can be controlled if there is enough money for sentinel surveillance and vector control (spraying).

Tick-borne encephalitis virus

The disease caused by this virus has many synonyms, e.g. Russian spring–summer encephalitis. The organism is a flavivirus transmitted between rodents and other small mammals by *Ixodes* ticks. It is also transmitted by ingesting infected goat's milk. The disease is found in a wide area from eastern Europe to the Far East and particularly affects forestry workers and hikers, who present 1–2 weeks after a tick bite. It is a biphasic illness with a high fever for 1 week followed by an afebrile period, then a meningoencephalitis or myelitis with upper limb, respiratory and bulbar flaccid paralysis. The CSF often shows neutrophils, and a peripheral leucocytosis and elevated erythrocyte sedimentation rate (ESR) may mimic bacterial meningitis. A formalin-inactivated vaccine is available.

Murray Valley encephalitis virus

This is a flavivirus causing encephalitis in Australia and Papua New Guinea.

Equine encephalitis viruses

Venezuelan, Eastern and Western equine encephalitis viruses are mosquito-borne alphaviruses transmitted between birds and/or small mammals by *Culex*, *Aedes* and *Culiseta* mosquitoes. They cause epidemics of encephalitis in horses and humans in the Americas.

La Crosse virus

A bunyavirus transmitted between chipmunks and squirrels, principally by *Aedes* mosquitoes. It causes up to 200 cases of encephalitis in the USA annually but has a low case fatality rate.

Management of patients with encephalitis

There is no specific antiviral treatment for most forms of viral encephalitis. Aciclovir is effective for herpes simplex virus type 1 and related viruses. In the West it is therefore given as soon as encephalitis is suspected. In the tropics, where other causes are more common, aciclovir is often reserved for cases that are atypical for the common local arboviral cause (e.g. wrong age, wrong season) or for cases with typical radiological changes of herpes. Ideally, encephalitis patients in a coma should be sedated and ventilated on an intensive care unit. This allows airway protection, maximum medication to control seizures and hyperventilation to reduce raised intracranial pressure but this is often not possible.

Whatever the viral cause, attention must be paid to the complications of encephalitis.

- *Pneumonia* – often caused by aspiration. Treat with broad-spectrum antibiotics.
- *Seizures* – sometimes these may be subtle motor seizures: look for twitching of a digit, the mouth or

eye. Confirm with electroencephalogram if possible. Treat seizures with diazepam. Treat status epilepticus with phenytoin (using a cardiac monitor) or phenobarbital (see Chapter 59).

- *Raised intracranial pressure* – there may be elevated CSF opening pressure at lumbar puncture. Look for clinical signs of brainstem herniation syndromes (Chapter 3). Nurse patients at 30° with the neck straight, give osmotic diuretics (e.g. mannitol), hyperventilate.
- *Malnutrition* – despite nasogastric feeding, very common in patients who are ill for more than a few days.
- *Bedsores* – minimized by good nursing care. Placing rubber gloves (inflated with water) between the knees and below the heels can help prevent some sores.
- *Contractures* – encourage the family to keep joints supple; use splints (improvised if necessary) to keep joints in position.

 SUMMARY

- Encephalitis can be caused by many viruses, other organisms and autoimmune processes. Viruses transmitted by insects (arboviruses) make encephalitis especially common in the tropics.
- Japanese encephalitis (JE) is the most important cause of epidemic encephalitis worldwide. There are an estimated 70 000 cases annually with more than 10 000 deaths. More than half the survivors have severe neurological sequelae.
- Effective vaccines are available to prevent Japanese encephalitis.
- There is no specific antiviral treatment for most forms of encephalitis. Aciclovir (for herpes encephalitis) is often reserved for use in atypical cases of encephalitis in regions where JE and other arboviruses are prevalent.
- Effective management of encephalitis includes managing common complications such as pneumonia, seizures, raised intracranial pressure, malnutrition, bed sores and contractures.

 Visit **www.lecturenoteseries.com/tropicalmed** **to test yourself on this chapter using interactive MCQs.**

FURTHER READING

Halstead SB, Thomas SJ (2011) New Japanese encephalitis vaccines: alternatives to production in mouse brain. *Expert Rev Vaccines* **10**(3): 355–64. [Review.]

Kneen R, Michael BD, Menson E, *et al.* (2012) Management of suspected viral encephalitis in children – Association of British Neurologists and British Paediatric Allergy, Immunology and Infection Group national guidelines. *J Infect* **64**(5): 449–77. Epub 2011 Nov 18.

PATH (2005). *Japanese Encephalitis Clinical Care Guidelines.* http://www.path.org/vaccineresources/files/JE_clinical_care_guidelines_PATH.pdf [Practical guidelines from PATH for use in resource-poor settings.]

Solomon T, Michael BD, Smith PE, *et al.* (2012) Management of suspected viral encephalitis in adults –Association of British Neurologists and British Infection Association National Guidelines. *J Infect* **64**(4): 347–73. Epub 2011 Nov 18. [Comprehensive British guidelines on diagnosis and management of adult and children with suspected or proven encephalitis, with many tables and algorithms. Free downloads from British Infection association website at http://www.britishinfection.org/drupal/content/clinical-guidelines.]

34

Acute flaccid paralysis

Tom Solomon[1] and Rachel Kneen[2]

[1]University of Liverpool; [2]Alder Hey Children's Foundation NHS Trust

Acute flaccid paralysis is defined as weakness in one or more limbs, or the respiratory or bulbar muscles, resulting from damaged lower motor neurones. Poliomyelitis was the most important cause, but since it has declined other causes have become more important.

Classically, in acute flaccid paralysis there is weakness with reduced tone (flaccid weakness) and reduced or absent reflexes. Differentiating from upper motor neurone weakness is usually straightforward, but it should be remembered that acute spinal shock (e.g. caused by trauma) can initially cause flaccid paralysis before spasticity develops.

Pathophysiology and clinical presentations

Broadly speaking, there are two pathophysiological processes that cause acute flaccid paralysis (Fig. 34.1). These are direct viral damage of lower motor neurone cell bodies in the anterior horn of the spinal cord (e.g. polio, other enteroviruses, flaviviruses); and a para- or post-infectious immunologically mediated process damaging the motor nerves, and often sensory nerves (e.g. Guillain–Barré syndrome), sometimes caused by antibodies directed against the gangliosides (glycolipids in the nerve cell membranes). Recognizing the clinical features of these two patterns helps in determining the likely cause (Table 34.1).

Anterior horn cell damage causing acute flaccid paralysis

Polio

Infection with this enterovirus can be asymptomatic, can cause a mild non-specific febrile illness, viral meningitis or paralytic poliomyelitis, which can be spinal or bulbar. Paralytic poliomyelitis is biphasic, with a non-specific fever followed by a brief afebrile period before the central nervous system (CNS) is invaded. This is heralded by further fever and an acute-onset asymmetrical flaccid paralysis of one or more limbs, which may be painful. Since the World Health Organization campaign to eradicate polio using the oral polio vaccine, the number of cases dropped from more than 350 000 cases in 1988 to approximately 1900 cases in 2002. Most of these came from South Asia (India, Pakistan and Afghanistan), West Africa (mainly Nigeria) and Central Africa (mainly Democratic Republic of Congo). Subsequently the number of cases rose again; for example in 2004 there were 1255 confirmed cases from 16 countries. The setbacks occurred in parts of the Asian subcontinent and Africa because of difficulty immunizing in areas of ongoing conflict, poor compliance with immunization because of mistrust in some communities, natural disasters disrupting infrastructure, and issues over financing the programme. By June 2012, just three countries had endemic disease: Nigeria, Pakistan and Afghanistan. The hope is that the declaration of polio eradication as a 'programmatic emergency' by the World Health Organization, plus additional funding, will finally see this disease eradicated.

Tropical Medicine Lecture Notes, Seventh edition. Edited by Nick Beeching and Geoff Gill. © 2014 John Wiley & Sons, Ltd. Published 2014 by John Wiley & Sons, Ltd.

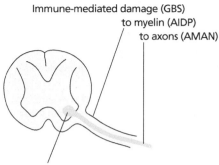

Immune-mediated damage (GBS)
to myelin (AIDP)
to axons (AMAN)

Direct viral damage of anterior horn cells
Polio, enteroviruses, echovirus,
Coxsackie virus
JEV, other flaviviruses

Figure 34.1 Pathophysiology of acute flaccid paralysis. Immune-mediated Guillain–Barré syndrome (GBS) occurs in two forms: in acute inflammatory demyelinating polyneuropathy (AIDP) the myelin is damaged; in acute motor axonal neuropathy (AMAN) the motor axons are targeted. Viruses such as polio and Japanese encephalitis virus (JEV) cause paralysis by directly attacking the lower motor neurones (the anterior horn cells).

Enterovirus 71

Enterovirus 71 has caused epidemics of acute flaccid paralysis in recent years (especially in Asia), often in association with hand, foot and mouth disease. Large outbreaks occur in some countries every 3–4 years. Many other enterovirus, Coxsackie virus and echovirus serotypes occasionally cause acute flaccid paralysis.

Japanese encephalitis virus

Japanese encephalitis virus, West Nile and other flaviviruses typically cause meningoencephalitis, but flaviviruses can also present with a pure flaccid paralysis that can be clinically similar to polio (Chapter 33).

Immune-mediated causes of acute flaccid paralysis

Guillain–Barré syndrome is now recognized as a group of disorders classified according to the predominant type of nerve injury (axonal or demyelinating) and the main nerve fibres involved (motor, sensory, cranial). Different antiganglioside antibodies are associated with different diseases.

Acute inflammatory demyelinating polyneuropathy (AIDP, or 'classical' Guillain–Barré syndrome)

This typically presents several weeks after a febrile illness with back pain, then symmetrical ascending flaccid paralysis and sensory changes. Recovery is usual. Treat rapidly progressing symptoms with intravenous immunoglobulin if available.

Acute motor axonal neuropathy (AMAN, or Chinese paralytic syndrome)

This typically follows diarrhoea caused by *Campylobacter jejuni*. Symmetrical weakness is present with no sensory changes. Residual weakness is common. Occurs in summer epidemics in China.

Other causes

- Any exposure to toxins?
- Any tick bites (tick paralysis is a slowly ascending paralysis that recovers when the tick is removed)?
- Consumption of poorly preserved food (botulinum toxin)?

Table 34.1 **Clinical features to distinguish causes of acute flaccid paralysis**

	Direct viral damage to anterior horn cells (e.g. polio)	Immune-mediated damage to peripheral nerves (e.g. Guillain–Barré syndrome)
Paralysis onset	During (or straight after) febrile illness	Several weeks after febrile illness
Pattern of paralysis	Asymmetrical	Symmetrical
Time to reach maximum weakness	Short (e.g. 2–3 days)	Long (e.g. 7–14 days)
Sensory involvement	No	Often (depending on exact disease)
CSF	Increased lymphocytes (e.g. 100/mm³)	Increased protein (e.g. 1 g/L, especially late in the disease)
Pain	Often limb muscle pain	Often back pain

- Exposure to rabid animal (paralytic rabies)?
- History of a severe sore throat with neck swelling (diphtheritic neuropathy)?

Nerve conduction studies

Where available, nerve conduction studies may help distinguish further.

- *Anterior horn cell damage* – motor amplitude is reduced because motor cell bodies have been damaged.
- *Classical Guillain–Barré syndrome* (autoimmune demyelinating polyneuropathy) – motor and sensory nerves have reduced conduction velocities and delayed distal latencies because demyelinated nerves conduct more slowly.
- *AMAN* (Chinese paralytic syndrome) – motor amplitudes are reduced because motor axons have been damaged.

 SUMMARY

- Acute flaccid paralysis is defined as weakness in one or more limbs, or the respiratory or bulbar muscles, resulting from damaged lower motor neurones.
- Classically, there is weakness with reduced tone (flaccid weakness) and reduced or absent reflexes.

- Poliomyelitis remains an important cause in a few countries where immunization programmes have been interrupted.
- Epidemics of acute flaccid paralysis due to enterovirus 71 occur in Asia.
- Immune mediated causes (Guillain–Barré syndrome) must be distinguished from these viral infections and other causes such as rabies, tick paralysis, diphtheria and botulism.

 Visit www.lecturenoteseries.com/tropicalmed to test yourself on this chapter using interactive MCQs.

📖 FURTHER READING

Bolton CF (1995) The changing concepts of Guillain–Barré syndrome. *New Engl J Med* **333**: 1415–16. [Good explanation of acute motor axonal neuropathy as a form of Guillain–Barré syndrome.]

Minor PD (2012) The polio-eradication programme and issues of the end game. *J Gen Virol* **93**: 457–74. Epub 2011 Nov 29. [Review of final stages of eradication]

Solomon T, Willison H (2003) Infectious causes of acute flaccid paralysis. *Curr Opin Infect Dis* **16**: 375–9. [Annotated review of main infectious causes.]

35

Spastic paralysis

Tom Solomon
University of Liverpool

Spastic paralysis is caused by damage to the upper motor neurones, and is characterized by weakness with increased tone, brisk reflexes and extensor plantars.

Causes and anatomy

Some of the important causes of spastic paralysis are shown in Fig. 35.1. The upper motor neurones can be affected anywhere along the corticospinal tract, but the associated features give a clue as to the site of damage as follows.

- A pure spastic paraparesis with no sensory changes is usually caused by damage in the brain where sensory and motor pathways are far apart (e.g. spastic diplegia in cerebral palsy, or frontal meningioma).
- In the spinal cord, sensory pathways lie close to the motor pathways and so are often also affected by any pathology. Look for dorsal column signs (loss of light touch, vibration and joint position sensation) and a sensory level.
- Intrinsic cord lesions are usually painless.
- Extrinsic lesions causing spinal cord compression often also press on the sensory roots as they leave the spinal cord, and thus cause pain in the distribution of those roots (radicular pain).

Assessment of the patient with spastic paralysis

Important features to determine include the following.

- Speed of onset – rapid in vascular disease, more prolonged in inflammatory, infectious and compressive disease.
- Past and current medical problems – cerebral palsy, tuberculosis, HIV, macrocytic anaemia.
- Urinary hesitancy, frequency or retention (the latter is a late feature).
- Constipation, incontinence, reduced anal tone and sensation.
- Presence of pain – extrinsic lesions compressing spinal roots cause radicular pain (e.g. tumours); abscesses give back pain and local tenderness.
- Examine for a gibbus of Pott's disease (see below), or naevus/hairy patch of spinal dysraphism (spina bifida occulta).
- Sensory level – nipples are T4, umbilicus is T10.

Important tropical causes of spastic paralysis

Tuberculosis

Tuberculosis (TB) causes spastic paralysis in one of three ways.

1 TB of the vertebral bones leads to collapse (Pott's disease) and secondary cord compression (a bony prominent sharp kyphosis caused by a collapsed vertebra is known as a gibbus).
2 Chronic TB meningitis leads to secondary arteritis and cord infarction.
3 A tuberculoma compresses the cord directly. When the nerve roots are involved there is an associated painful radiculopathy, and bladder dysfunction.

Many patients have a personal or family history of TB or evidence of the disease elsewhere. Investigate with a tuberculin test, erythrocyte sedimentation

Tropical Medicine Lecture Notes, Seventh edition. Edited by Nick Beeching and Geoff Gill. © 2014 John Wiley & Sons, Ltd. Published 2014 by John Wiley & Sons, Ltd.

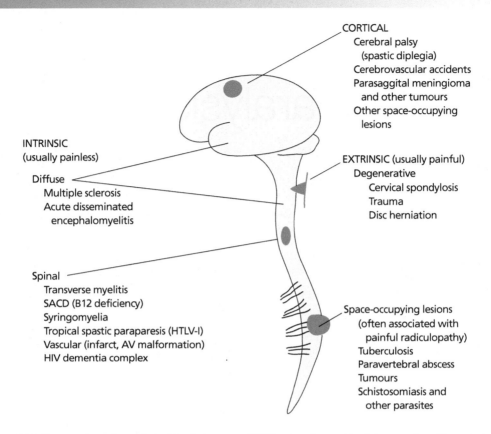

CORTICAL
Cerebral palsy
(spastic diplegia)
Cerebrovascular accidents
Parasaggital meningioma
and other tumours
Other space-occupying
lesions

INTRINSIC
(usually painless)

Diffuse
Multiple sclerosis
Acute disseminated
encephalomyelitis

EXTRINSIC (usually painful)
Degenerative
Cervical spondylosis
Trauma
Disc herniation

Spinal
Transverse myelitis
SACD (B12 deficiency)
Syringomyelia
Tropical spastic paraparesis (HTLV-I)
Vascular (infarct, AV malformation)
HIV dementia complex

Space-occupying lesions
(often associated with
painful radiculopathy)
Tuberculosis
Paravertebral abscess
Tumours
Schistosomiasis and
other parasites

Figure 35.1 Causes of spastic paralysis. AV, arteriovenous; SACD, subacute combined degeneration of the spinal cord.

rate (ESR), chest X-ray, spinal X-ray, computerized tomography (CT) or magnetic resonance imaging (MRI) scanning if possible. Treatment consists of antituberculous therapy, plus surgery if appropriate.

Spinal epidural abscess

Spinal epidural abscess is most frequently caused by *Staphylococcus aureus*. Patients present with the triad of fever, backache/tenderness and radicular pain, followed by rapidly progressive spastic paraparesis, sensory loss and bowel and bladder dysfunction. There is usually a peripheral leucocytosis, elevated ESR and mild cerebrospinal fluid (CSF) pleocytosis with an increased protein level. An X-ray may show soft tissue changes and associated vertebral osteomyelitis. On myelography, the flow of contrast medium is blocked. MRI is the investigation of choice. Patients should be treated with emergency surgical drainage and antibiotics.

Transverse myelitis

Transverse myelitis is an acute inflammation of the spinal cord. Presentation is rapid and often a sensory level is present. It can be associated with many common infectious agents including many viruses and some bacteria (particularly *Mycoplasma pneumoniae*). It can also occur after most vaccinations. For many patients, it will be a monophasic illness and no cause may be found, however some patients will go on to develop multiple sclerosis or Devic's neuromyelitis optica and others may have a connective tissue disorder. Tropical infections that are associated with transverse myelitis include HIV (see below), schistosomiasis, syphilis, dengue, scrub typhus, leptospirosis and *Borrelia burgdorferi*.

HIV myelopathy

HIV myelopathy is a progressive myelopathy and is a frequent finding in patients with the AIDS–dementia complex. There is usually spasticity with increased or decreased reflexes, ataxia, incontinence and dorsal column signs. The MRI scan is usually normal, but at autopsy there is vacuolation of the spinal cord white matter, especially in the posterior and lateral columns of the thoracic cord. HIV myelopathy is thought to be caused directly by HIV-1 invasion. Other causes of myelopathy in AIDS include lymphoma, *Cryptococcus* and herpes viruses.

Subacute combined degeneration of the spinal cord (SACD)

This is caused by vitamin B_{12} deficiency resulting from poor diet or impaired absorption secondary to tropical sprue, *Diphyllobothrium latum* infection (fish tapeworm), gastrointestinal surgery or as part of pernicious anaemia. The disease leads to a mixture of upper motor neurone deficit (corticospinal tract damage), sensory deficit caused by dorsal column involvement and peripheral neuropathy, sometimes with optic neuropathy and dementia. Classical findings are extensor plantars with absent knee jerks. Neck flexion causes shooting pains down the arms (Lhermitte's sign). There is usually a macrocytic anaemia. The disease is treated with intramuscular vitamin B_{12} injections 1000 mg/day for 6 days, then reducing to a maintenance dose (Chapter 57).

Tropical spastic paraparesis

Tropical spastic paraparesis is found in the Caribbean, Seychelles, equatorial Africa, Japan and parts of the Americas. Most cases are caused by human T lymphotrophic virus type 1 (HTLV-1), transmitted sexually, by exposure to blood products or by breast milk. Hence it is also know as HTLV-1 associated myelopathy. It is more common in females than males. The disease presents with progressive spastic paraparesis, impaired vibration and joint position sensation and bowel and bladder dysfunction. Corticosteroids may be helpful, but there have been no randomized controlled trials.

 Visit www.lecturenoteseries.com/tropicalmed **to test yourself on this chapter using interactive MCQs.**

 SUMMARY

- Spastic paralysis is caused by damage to the upper motor neurones anywhere along the corticospinal tract, and is characterized by weakness with increased tone, brisk reflexes and extensor plantars. Associated features give a clue to the site of damage.

- Tuberculosis is an important cause in the tropics via several mechanisms: secondary cord compression after vertebral collapse; chronic TB meningitis with arteritis and infarction; direct cord pressure from a tuberculoma.

- Spinal epidural abscess, usually caused by *Staphylococcus aureus*, is characterized by local back pain and rapid progression, and requires urgent surgery as well as antibiotics.

- HIV myelopathy is a progressive myelopathy and is a frequent finding in patients with the AIDS–dementia complex. Other HIV-related causes include lymphoma and opportunistic infections such as Cryptococcus.

- Tropical spastic paraparesis is found in the Caribbean, Seychelles, equatorial Africa, Japan and parts of the Americas. Most cases are caused by human T lymphotrophic virus type 1 (HTLV-1).

FURTHER READING

Croda MG, de Oliveira AC, Vergara MP, *et al.* (2008) Corticosteroid therapy in TSP/HAM patients: the results from a 10 years open cohort. *J Neurol Sci* **269**: 133–7.

Thwaites G, Fisher M, Hemingway C, *et al.* (2009) British Infection Society guidelines for the diagnosis and treatment of tuberculosis of the central nervous system in adults and children. *J Infect* **59**: 167–87. [Comprehensive British guidelines on British Infection Association website, free download from http://www.britishinfection.org/drupal/content/clinical-guidelines]

Tompkins M, Panuncialman I, Lucas P, Palumbo M (2010) Spinal epidural abscess. *J Emerg Med* **39**: 384–90. [Review.]

36

Rabies

Tom Solomon[1] and David Lalloo[2]
[1]University of Liverpool; [2]Liverpool School of Tropical Medicine

The rabies virus is a bullet-shaped RNA rhabdovirus that is widely prevalent among warm-blooded animals in many tropical countries. Worldwide, dogs are the main transmitters of rabies to humans: bats are involved in North America, certain South American countries, some areas of Europe and, more recently, Australia. Between 35 000 and 50 000 people die from rabies each year, with most deaths occurring in Asia.

On reaching the brain of an infected animal, the rabies virus spreads along peripheral nerves to reach the skin and the lachrymal and salivary glands. An animal bite with virus-laden saliva is therefore the usual mode of infection, although the disease can also be acquired by salivary contamination of cuts, abrasions and mucous membranes, and occasionally by inhalation. Rarely, rabies has been transmitted by corneal transplants taken from donors dying from unrecognized rabies. The risk of rabies in a person bitten by a rabid animal varies widely up to 50%, depending on the site and nature of the bites and the animal species.

Rabies in the dog

This is usually furious: the dog rushes around emitting a high-pitched bark, and biting not only people but also objects. The animal may paw at its mouth, as if trying to dislodge a foreign body and salivate excessively. It nearly always dies within 15 days of becoming infective. This fact is made use of when a dog that has bitten someone is impounded. If the dog is alive 15 days after the bite, it is very unlikely to have been infective when it bit.

Dogs can be given a high degree of protection against rabies by an attenuated live vaccine.

Rabies in other animals

Dogs, foxes, wolves and jackals are the major reservoirs of rabies in most parts of the world, and cats can also transmit infection, usually themselves suffering from a paralytic illness typical of 'dumb rabies'. In South America and the Caribbean, bats are very important vectors and cause enormous economic losses because of death of cattle from paralytic rabies. Bats can also cause human disease, not only from their bites but also from the inhalation of aerosolized bat secretions by speleologists exploring caves, mainly in the Americas.

Clinical features in humans

Once inoculated, the rabies virus travels centripetally along peripheral nerves to reach the spinal cord and brain. The incubation period is related to the inoculum size and the time taken to reach the brain: generally it is 2–8 weeks but may range between 9 days and a year or more. The incubation period is proportional to the distance the virus has to travel and therefore tends to be shorter in children, and after bites on the face and neck.

The disease may be heralded by pain, paraesthesiae or pruritus in the bitten area; these occur in 30–80% of cases. The illness proper usually begins abruptly with fever, insomnia, anxiety and other psychological disturbances. In the encephalitic (furious) form of the disease the patient suffers from intermittent episodes of confusion, agitation and aggression verging on mania, with intervening periods of calm and lucidity. Copious secretion of ropy saliva is characteristic and the patient may literally 'froth at the mouth'.

Tropical Medicine Lecture Notes, Seventh edition. Edited by Nick Beeching and Geoff Gill. © 2014 John Wiley & Sons, Ltd. Published 2014 by John Wiley & Sons, Ltd.

Painful spasms of the throat muscles, often precipitated by attempts to swallow, are accompanied by 'hydrophobia', an overwhelming terror of drinking. Spasms often become more widespread, to involve the diaphragm and respiratory muscles: they may be accompanied by spitting, grimacing, vomiting, opisthotonos and seizures. Spasms may also be precipitated by air blowing on to the face (aerophobia). Death usually occurs within a week, with respiratory and bulbar paralysis.

Some 20% of patients suffer from a paralytic form of rabies. There is an ascending sensorimotor neuropathy with ocular, cranial and laryngeal palsies and sphincter disturbances: fasciculation may be seen in muscles. Hydrophobia is rare.

Diagnosis

Diagnosis during life

In most cases the diagnosis will be made on the characteristic clinical picture: laboratory tests for virus detection may not be available and currently lack sensitivity. Immunofluorescence of corneal impression smears or skin biopsies can detect viral antigen, especially late in the illness. Skin biopsies are taken from the nape of the neck so as to contain hair follicles and peripheral nerves. Attempts to culture virus from saliva, cerebrospinal fluid (CSF) or biopsies may not succeed in the later stages of illness because of the presence of neutralizing antibodies. Diagnostic antibody tests do not become positive until about the eighth day and are difficult to interpret in vaccinated patients.

Rapid diagnostic methods based on nucleic acid amplification are being developed and look very promising: viral RNA can be detected in saliva and CSF as early as the second day of illness.

Postmortem diagnosis

Because of cross-infection hazards a postmortem should only be performed if absolutely necessary. Staff should be immunized and must wear protective clothing and visors.

Immunofluorescence of fresh brain is the technique most widely used to demonstrate viral antigen. Rabies virus can be detected using tissue culture and mouse inoculation. Polymerase chain reaction (PCR) methods can also be applied. Histology, which is not routinely performed, shows a diffuse meningoencephalitis with extensive neuronal destruction and the presence of Negri inclusion bodies within brain cells.

Treatment

Rabies is almost invariably fatal and the disease causes great suffering. The main aim of treatment is to relieve symptoms with heavy sedation such as a mixture of a phenothiazine, a barbiturate and diamorphine. Intensive care with a cocktail of antiviral drugs has been reported to save a small number of patients with bat-derived rabies virus; however, many subsequent attempts with similar regimens have failed.

Precautions with rabies patients

The patient's saliva is potentially infectious. Everyone in contact with the patient should be protected using barrier nursing, with the addition of visors. Staff should receive rabies immunization (four intradermal injections of 0.1 mL of human diploid cell vaccine, each given into a different limb on the same day).

Postexposure treatment

The aim is to eliminate or neutralize rabies virus during the incubation period. Management is aided by asking the patient 10 key questions (Table 36.1).

First aid treatment

Wash and flush the wound vigorously with soap and water, detergent, or water alone. Then apply ethanol (700 mL/L) tincture or aqueous solution of iodine, or

---

Table 36.1 **Ten questions to ask the patient**

1 Was the person bitten, or licked on an open wound or mucous membranes by an animal?
2 Where on the body was the bite/lick?
3 Where did the incident take place and on what date?
4 What species was the animal?
5 Is rabies known or suspected in the species? In the area?
6 Is there a known and contactable owner?
7 (a) Was the animal behaving normally at the time?
  (b) Had it been vaccinated?
  (c) Is the animal being held under observation?
8 If the animal was a dog or a cat did it become ill while under observation?
9 If the animal has died, does laboratory examination of the animal's brain confirm rabies?
10 Has the bitten person previously received rabies vaccine? How much does the person weigh (relevant to rabies immune globulin dosage)?

0.1% quaternary ammonium compounds (with the latter, remove all traces of soap first).

Immediate treatment by or under the direction of a physician

1 Treat as in first aid treatment above, then:
2 If indicated (Table 36.2), use topical rabies immune globulin around the wound (see below).
3 Postpone suturing of wound; if suturing is necessary, use immune globulin locally.
4 Where indicated, institute antitetanus procedures and administer antibiotics and drugs to control infections other than rabies.

Postexposure immunization (see Table 36.2)

Active immunization

Purified inactivated cell culture or duck embryo vaccines are recommended as they are potent and safe. Costs can be reduced by intradermal administration. Two-site and eight-site intradermal regimens have been recommended by the WHO; a newer 4-site regimen may be more convenient. Whichever vaccine is used, it must be started as early as possible after exposure and should never be withheld whatever time has elapsed.

Passive immunization

Rabies immune globulin (RIG) should be given for high-risk exposures (Table 36.2) unless the patient has been previously fully immunized. The dose is 20 IU/kg body weight using human RIG and 40 IU/kg using equine RIG. Up to half the dose is given by infiltration in and around the wound and the rest given by intramuscular injection at a site separate from the first dose of vaccine. If RIG is initially unobtainable, it may be given up to day 7. Equine RIG may cause allergic reactions and the usual precautions against anaphylaxis must be taken. Serum sickness occurs in 1–6% of patients, usually 7–10 days after injection. At the time of writing this preparation is not being manufactured.

Postexposure vaccine regimens

The following vaccines are recommended by the World Health Organization (WHO).

- Human diploid cell vaccine (HDCV).
- Purified Vero cell vaccine (PVRV).

Table 36.2 Treatment according to nature of exposure

| Nature of exposure | Status of biting animal (irrespective of previous vaccination) | | Recommended treatment |
	At time of exposure	During 15 days*	
1 Contact, but no lesions; indirect contact; no contact	Rabid		None
2 Licks of the skin; scratches or abrasions; minor bites (covered areas of arms, trunk and legs)	Suspected as rabid	Healthy	Start vaccine. Stop treatment if animal remains healthy for 15 days*
		Rabid	Start vaccine; administer rabies immune globulin if appropriate upon positive diagnosis and complete the course of vaccine
	Rabid; wild animal, or animal unavailable for observation		Vaccine + rabies immune globulin, according to previous immunization history
3 Licks of mucosa; major bites (multiple or on face, head, finger or neck)	Suspect or rabid domestic or wild animal, or animal unavailable for observation		Vaccine + rabies immune globulin, according to previous immunization history. Stop treatment if animal remains healthy for 15 days*

*Observation period applies to dogs and cats. Ten days recommended by WHO.
Source: UK Department of Health, 2000.

- Purified primary chick embryo cell vaccine (PCECV).
- Purified duck embryo vaccine (PDEV).

WHO recommended schedules

1 Intramuscular administration (into the deltoid, never the buttock). For use with all recommended vaccines. One dose of vaccine on days 0, 3, 7, 14 and 28. Alternatively, two doses on day 0 (one into each deltoid), one dose on day 7 and one on day 21.
2 Two-site intradermal method ('2-2-2-0-1-1'). For use with PVRV, PCECV and PDEV. Days 0, 3 and 7: one intradermal dose given at each of two sites over the deltoid. Days 28 and 90: one intradermal dose given at one site on the upper arm. The intradermal dose is one-fifth of the intramuscular dose.
3 Eight-site intradermal method ('8-0-4-0-1-1'). For use with HDCV and PCECV. Day 0: 0.1mL of vaccine at each of eight sites (deltoid, lateral thigh, suprascapular region and lower quadrant of abdomen). Day 7: 0.1 mL of vaccine at each of four sites (deltoid and thighs). Days 28 and 90: 0.1 mL of vaccine at one site (deltoid).
4 An updated Thai Red Cross Regimen, approved by the WHO/DCGI India, involves injection of 0.1 mL of reconstituted vaccine per ID site and on two such ID sites per visit on Days 0, 3, 7 and 28 (2-2-2-0-2).

Nerve tissue vaccines

These are less potent and are more likely to cause neuroparalytic complications. Suckling mouse brain (SMB) vaccine is often used in Latin America. Subcutaneous doses are usually given daily for 7 days, with booster doses at 10, 20 and 90 days. Vaccines prepared in fixed sheep and goat brains (e.g. Semple vaccine) carry an appreciable risk of postvaccinal encephalitis or polyneuritis.

Need for flexibility

These vaccination recommendations are intended only as a guide. Modification of standard procedures may be justifiable in areas of low rabies endemicity or where there is no indication of rabies infection in the animal species involved. Local expert advice should be obtained whenever possible. Vaccine use in the immunocompromised needs further investigation.

Pre-exposure immunization

This is recommended for travellers to endemic areas and those at special risk (e.g. veterinarians and animal handlers). Three doses of a cell culture or PDEV are given on days 0, 7 and 28. The vaccines may be given intramuscularly or intradermally; doses according to manufacturers' instructions. The antibody response may be impaired by concomitant chloroquine administration, particularly if the intradermal route is used.

Prevention of rabies

In endemic areas this depends upon the mass immunization of dogs, import controls and the elimination of strays. Unvaccinated dogs (those not wearing a collar with a vaccination tag) should be regularly caught and destroyed. The best results are obtained by professional dogcatchers using bait. Attempts to control dogs by soldiers armed with assault rifles are invariably unsuccessful and dangerous.

 SUMMARY

- Between 35 000 and 50 000 people die from rabies each year, with most deaths occurring in Asia. The main animals transmitting to humans are dogs or bats.
- The risk of rabies in a person bitten by a rabid animal varies widely up to 50%, depending on the site and nature of the bites and the animal species.
- The incubation period is proportional to the distance the virus has to travel from the bite site to the brain and therefore tends to be shorter in children and after bites on the face and neck.
- Rabies is almost invariably fatal and the disease causes great suffering. The main aim of treatment is to relieve symptoms.
- Rabies can be prevented after bites by prompt wound toilet in addition to adequate post-exposure immunization. People at risk, e.g. veterinarians or travelers in remote settings, should be immunized in advance of possible exposure.

Visit www.lecturenoteseries.com/tropicalmed to test yourself on this chapter using interactive MCQs.

📖 FURTHER READING

Anon (1999) Human rabies prevention: United States, Recommendations of the Advisory Committee on Immunization Practices (ACIP). *Morbid Mortal Week Rep* **48** (RR–1): 1–21. [Largely concerned with USA practice, this discusses rabies epidemiology in bats, terrestrial carnivores and other wild animals. Extensively referenced.]

Department of Health (2000) *Memorandum on Rabies Prevention and Control.* London: Department of Health. [Contains useful information on all aspects of rabies control: immunization, patient management, postmortem precautions and veterinary action.]

Health Protection Agency. Many useful guidelines on pre travel immunization and assessment and immunization after animal exposure can be found on the Health Protection Agency website at http://www.hpa.org.uk/Topics/InfectiousDiseases/InfectionsAZ/Rabies/Guidelines/of

Warrell MJ (2012) Intradermal rabies vaccination: the evolution and future of pre- and post-exposure prophylaxis. *Curr Top Microbiol Immunol* **351**: 139–57. [Expert source reference.]

Willoughby RE, Kelly ST, Hoffman GM, *et al.* (2005) Survival after treatment of rabies with induction of coma. *New Engl J Med* **352**: 2508–14. [Description of a rare case of successful rabies treatment, though with neurological damage.]

World Health Organization (1997) *WHO Recommendations on Rabies Postexposure Treatment and the Correct Technique of Intradermal Immunization Against Rabies.* Geneva: World Health Organization WHO/EMC/ZOO.96.6. [Essential reading, this gives straightforward advice on first aid, pre- and postexposure immunization and the use of rabies immune globulin.]

37

Tetanus

David Lalloo
Liverpool School of Tropical Medicine

Bacteriology and pathogenesis

Tetanus is caused by *Clostridium tetani*, a Gram-positive obligate anaerobe with a terminal spore, which is ubiquitous in the environment, particularly in soil. Spores are highly resistant to light and temperature; clinical disease occurs when spores are inoculated into wounds. Most cases of tetanus are related to acute injuries. Spores germinate under anaerobic conditions at the site of a wound and the growing bacteria produce two toxins: tetanolysin and tetanospasmin. Tetanospasmin undergoes proteolytic cleavage and binds and enters the presynaptic terminal. There, tetanospasmin cleaves the protein that allows fusion of synaptic vesicle with the membrane and thus prevents transmitter release. Tetanospasmin is able to travel retrogradely via axons to cell bodies and cross synapses, thus reaching the spinal cord, brain and autonomic nervous system. It primarily affects inhibitory glycine or γ-aminobutyric acid (GABA) neurones, leading to increased firing and lack of normal relaxation and causing the classical spasms of tetanus.

Clinical manifestations

The incubation period varies according to the site of injury and is shorter in severe disease, with an average incubation of 8 days for severe disease. There are several classical clinical subtypes, which reflect the main site of action of toxin.

Generalized tetanus

This is the most common clinical form. It often commences with trismus ('lock jaw') in which the patient is unable to open their mouth or risus sardonicus, a grimace caused by spasm of facial muscles. The predominant feature is of repeated spasms which may involve the neck, thorax, abdomen or extremities. Generalized spasms with opisthotonos also occur. Spasms are precipitated by external or internal stimuli, may last for minutes and are painful as full consciousness is retained. Respiratory compromise may occur because of involvement of the glottis or diaphragm. The disease may continue to progress for up to 10 days after the first symptoms.

In severe tetanus, autonomic dysfunction may occur after several days. Hypertension, tachycardia, arrhythmias and hyperpyrexia may all occur and can be extremely difficult to manage. Recovery may take up to 4 weeks: case fatality rates can reach 60%, with death usually occurring because of respiratory or autonomic involvement.

Neonatal tetanus

This is usually caused by infection of the umbilical stump. The risk of infection is related to the length of stump, the care and cleanliness with which the cord is ligated and cut and the cleanliness of the environment. Neonatal tetanus only occurs in the children of non-immune mothers. Symptoms and signs occur 1–10 days postpartum. Initially, generalized weakness and floppiness of the baby are noticed, with irritability and an inability to suck and feed. Subsequently, spasms, opisthotonos and hypersympathetic states occur. Up to 90% of affected infants die and mental retardation is common in survivors.

Tropical Medicine Lecture Notes, Seventh edition. Edited by Nick Beeching and Geoff Gill. © 2014 John Wiley & Sons, Ltd. Published 2014 by John Wiley & Sons, Ltd.

Localized tetanus

This is usually a mild form in which rigidity is limited to muscles near the site of injury. Weakness of the muscles may also occur because of the action of the toxin at the neuromuscular junction. Symptoms may be mild and persist for months. If the diagnosis is not made, progression to the generalized form may occur.

Cephalic tetanus

This is the rarest form and occurs in head injuries or with middle ear infection. The incubation period is normally 1–2 days and the major clinical manifestations are caused by involvement of cranial nerves with facial paresis, dysphagia and extraocular palsies. This form can also progress to generalized tetanus.

Diagnosis

The diagnosis is usually made clinically. Bacteriology is of little help, the organism is often not found and a positive wound culture for *C. tetani* does not prove that the organism is toxin-producing and causing disease. Blood and cerebrospinal fluid (CSF) findings are usually normal. The differential diagnosis is limited but includes dental abscesses, strychnine poisoning, dystonic reactions, hypocalcaemia and seizures in adults and metabolic or neurological causes of posturing in neonates.

Treatment

Tetanus should be treated by the administration of tetanus immunoglobulin (human tetanus Ig 150 IU/kg i.m. or equine tetanus Ig 10^4–10^6IU i.m.). There is evidence that there might be additional benefit from intrathecal administration of tetanus Ig, but this is rarely given in practice. If tetanus immunoglobulin is not available, commercially produced human normal immunoglobulin preparations contain anti-tetanus antibodies and may be used instead. The recommended dose is 250–500 ml i.v. for an adult (equivalent to about 5000–10 000 IU). Wounds should be débrided to prevent further germination of spores. Metronidazole (preferred) or benzylpenicillin should be given to prevent multiplication of bacteria. Much of the care is supportive. External stimulation should be reduced to prevent precipitation of spasms: patients should be nursed in a quiet, dim environment. The airway should be protected; endotracheal intubation or tracheostomy is often necessary. Spasms can be treated by the use of high doses of benzodiazepines; baclofen is also effective. Some patients require paralysis with non-depolarizing neuromuscular junction blockers. The treatment of autonomic instability is difficult as manifestations can alter quite rapidly. Labetolol or verapamil may be useful for the management of hypertension; atropine or pacing may be needed for bradycardias and sympathomimetics and fluids are sometimes necessary to treat hypotension. Intravenous magnesium reduces the need for muscle relaxants and drugs to control cardiovascular manifestations.

Neonatal tetanus is treated in a similar fashion to generalized tetanus.

Epidemiology and prevention

Although tetanus occurs worldwide, it is predominantly a problem of tropical and developing countries, being particularly common in the Philippines, Vietnam, the Asian Subcontinent, Indonesia and Brazil. Over 90% of the deaths occur under the age of 5. Approximately 60 000 deaths occur annually from neonatal tetanus; this reflects a greater than 90% reduction in the number of deaths since the 1980s through the use of maternal vaccination, and better obstetric practice and care of the cord.

Tetanus is a vaccine-preventable disease. Immunization with tetanus toxoid is very effective. Children should receive vaccination with tetanus toxoid as part of the routine diphtheria, tetanus and pertussis (DTP) immunization and receive boosters aged 4–7 and in adolescence. A single booster in adulthood leads to lifetime protection. For those first vaccinated in adulthood, routine booster doses should be given at 10 yearly intervals following primary immunization: five doses in total protects for life, although if tetanus-prone injuries occur, a booster should be given if not immunized within the last 5 years. A single dose of tetanus toxoid in pregnancy leads to protective titres in a proportion of mothers and neonates: non-immunized mothers should ideally receive two doses four weeks apart during pregnancy.

SUMMARY

- *Clostridium tetani* is widely distributed, and infection occurs via spores entering wounds, and producing neurotoxins.
- Classical tetanus is associated with painful muscular spasms (including trismus, opisthotonus and risus sardonicus). Autonomic dysfunction can also occur.
- Diagnosis is usually clinical. Treatment is with tetanus immunoglobulin, and antibiotics (penicillin or metronidazole) to prevent further spore germination.
- Tetanus is vaccine-preventable, and tetanus toxoid is highly effective.

 Visit **www.lecturenoteseries.com/tropicalmed** **to test yourself on this chapter using interactive MCQs.**

 ## FURTHER READING

Farrar JJ, Yen LM, Cook T, *et al.* (2000) Tetanus. *J Neurol Neurosurgery Psychiatry* **69**: 292–301. [A useful review of the subject.]

Sanya EO, Taiwo SS, Olarinoye JK, *et al.* (2007) A 12 year review of cases of adult tetanus managed at the University College Hospital, Ibadan, Nigeria. *Tropical Doctor* **37**: 170–2. [Gives a good insight into the current clinical spectrum of adult tetanus.]

38

Brucellosis

Nick Beeching
Liverpool School of Tropical Medicine

Brucellosis (Malta fever, Rock fever) is one of the classical zoonoses (infections of animals transmitted to humans). It is an important cause of fever in many parts of the world and is often underdiagnosed because of lack of laboratory facilities. This is increasingly recognized in India and neighbouring countries, and in some Pacific settings.

Epidemiology

Brucellae are Gram-negative coccobacilli. At least six species infect a wide variety of land-based mammals and new species have recently been described in marine mammals such as whales and seals. Three species are responsible for most human infections:

1 *Brucella abortus*, usually a disease of cattle, is prevalent in Africa, the Indian Subcontinent and temperate zones;
2 *Brucella melitensis*, whose normal ruminant host is sheep and goats but is also found in camels, is particularly prevalent in countries around the Mediterranean, the Middle East and Central and South America;
3 *Brucella suis*, whose natural host is pigs, is still a problem in the USA.

Brucella canis (natural host dogs) can rarely infect humans. The organisms are intracellular and can remain hidden in the reticuloendothelial system so that clinical incubation periods after infection range from several weeks to months. Despite this, brucellosis does not appear to be more common or more severe in patients with HIV. In animals, they are important causes of epididymitis, abortion and infertility, but host animals may appear symptomless.

Humans acquire infection from ingesting milk or dairy products such as laban, lassi, buttermilk and cheeses that have not been pasteurized. The products of abortion and placentae from infected animals are highly infectious and farmers and veterinarians can easily become infected by aerosol transmission from the products of conception. Rarely, human brucellosis can be acquired via breast milk, sexual transmission or transfusion of blood products. Veterinarians and farmers sometimes have localized skin disease caused by direct contact with infected animal products. Brucellosis is not transmitted by eating the meat of infected animals unless it is eaten raw and has been externally contaminated. In endemic settings, brucellosis is mainly a problem for the rural poor. Brucellosis has been eliminated from much of northern Europe, where cases are related to travel and immigration from endemic areas.

Clinical features

The symptoms of brucellosis are of recurrent prolonged bouts of fever. If specific treatment is not given, undulating patterns of fever may last for several weeks, followed by an afebrile period and then relapse. Approximately half of all cases are associated with focal musculoskeletal symptoms, which may be the only clinical clue that differentiates brucellosis from other causes of fever such as typhoid, Q fever, malaria, etc. In an endemic area, it is the first clinical diagnosis for any patient who presents with fever and difficulty in walking. Fever is worse at night and may be associated with profuse sweating. Patients are depressed, anorexic and lethargic, although the onset of these symptoms is often insidious. A small proportion

Tropical Medicine Lecture Notes, Seventh edition. Edited by Nick Beeching and Geoff Gill. © 2014 John Wiley & Sons, Ltd. Published 2014 by John Wiley & Sons, Ltd.

present with more pronounced neuropsychiatric disorder or low-grade meningoencephalitis, and 5–10% of men have orchitis which must be distinguished from mumps. Patients often have a dry cough, mimicking the presentation of typhoid. Epistaxis is an unusual but well-recognized presentation because of associated thrombocytopaenia, but other features of bleeding disorder such as haematemesis or malaena are very unusual.

The overall pattern of presentation varies with the age of the patient and the infecting species. *B. abortus* infections have a more insidious onset, are more likely to affect the axial skeleton and to become chronic. *B. melitensis* tends to have a more acute onset and is more likely to affect peripheral joints as well as the vertebrae. Children often present with fever and a single clinically affected joint, typically the hip or knee, and this may be mistaken for rheumatic fever or septic arthritis. *B. suis* infections have an acute presentation complicated by focal deep tissue abscesses.

Patients look unwell and are lethargic but do not look as toxic as those with enteric fever. The temperature is almost invariably raised but often returns to normal during a 24-h cycle. Up to 10% have cervical or other lymphadenopathy, which must be differentiated from glandular fever, HIV or tuberculous (TB) adenitis. One-quarter have mild to moderate splenomegaly. The chest is usually clear, even if the patient has a cough. Individual joints may show signs typical of septic arthritis with swelling, heat, tenderness and effusions. There may be local tenderness, especially on movement of vertebrae or sacroiliac joints, but deformity of the back or long tract neurological signs are very unusual and suggest TB rather than brucellosis. Brucellosis is rarely fatal unless complicated by endocarditis (~1% of cases), but causes prolonged debilitation and loss of productivity.

Diagnosis

The full blood count shows low white blood cells (WBCs) with lymphopenia and mild thrombocytopenia. Occasionally, there is more pronounced reduction of platelets and haemoglobin. Mild elevation of alkaline phosphatase and transaminases is common. Blood culture is the most reliable method of confirming the diagnosis, but will only be positive in about two-thirds of *B. melitensis* cases and less than one-third of cases caused by *B. abortus*. If modern 'signalling' blood culture systems are used, they usually become positive within a week but culture should be prolonged to 3 weeks to detect late positives. If basic culture facilities are all that are available, cultures should be prolonged to at least 6 weeks, with most of the positives occurring between days 7 and 21. Laboratory staff must be told that brucellosis is a possibility, both so that cultures are prolonged and so that they are aware of the significant hazard that *Brucella* poses to laboratory workers because of the risk of aerosol spread.

A single bone marrow culture has a better yield than three sets of blood cultures and is occasionally useful in patients with pyrexia of unknown origin (PUO) who have been given antibiotics. Synovial fluid should be cultured for *Brucellae* in any case of septic arthritis in an endemic area, and aspirates or biopsies from abnormal tissues such as lymph nodes or liver should also be cultured. Cerebrospinal fluid (CSF) usually shows mild elevations of lymphocytes and proteins, and organisms may be cultured.

Serological tests are still based on the old (Wright's) standard agglutination test (SAT). *Brucella* antigen supplied with the kit is added to successive dilutions of patient serum, and if visible agglutination occurs the test is positive. These tests are notoriously affected by the 'prozone phenomenon', which causes false-negative results. This occurs because patients with brucellosis have immunoglobulin A (IgA) antibodies, which interfere with agglutination at low dilutions, and the blocking effect is only overcome at increasing serum dilutions. Thus, the result might be negative at dilutions of 1/40, 1/80, 1/160 and 1/320 and positive only at 1/640. Many inexperienced laboratories will only dilute serum to 1/160 and therefore miss the true positives.

As with all serological tests, a fourfold rise in titre between acute and convalescent samples (10–14 days later) is strongly suggestive of brucellosis, but this result is too delayed to guide the immediate management of patients with fever. In endemic areas, many patients have had previous exposure to brucellosis and have low titres of antibodies already, so the diagnostic 'cut-offs' for a single sample to be positive have to be set higher, typically at 1/160 or 1/320. In a non-endemic area, or for an expatriate who has recently been exposed for the first time in an endemic area, a titre of 1/80 would be strongly predictive of brucellosis. About 10% of blood culture-positive patients have negative serological results at first presentation, so a negative result does not entirely rule out brucellosis.

The SAT is affected by the antigen used and many different commercial kits are available. Some provide antigens for both *B. abortus* and *B. melitensis* but there is much cross-reaction and one cannot reliably distinguish these infections on the basis of serology alone. Mercaptoethanol can be added to patient serum to dissociate IgM and therefore indicate if IgG predominates (more suggestive of chronic infection), but this is only moderately reliable. The SAT has been adapted in some reference laboratories to be performed in microtitre trays, the so-called MAT. All these tests cross-react with some other Gram-negative bacteria (*Yersinia, Vibrio cholerae*) and recent cholera immunization.

Enzyme-linked immunoabsorbent assay (ELISA) tests have also been developed and are used in some laboratories, but are not internationally standardized and are more expensive. Rose Bengal serological tests, designed for animal diagnosis, are used as screening tests on human sera in many tropical settings, but their specificity and sensitivity have not been fully validated for this purpose. Urinary dipsticks to detect antibodies are sensitive but not widely used, and assays for circulatory or urinary antigen remain experimental. Molecular techniques (polymerase chain reaction; PCR) to detect DNA are sensitive but are still not standardized for routine clinical diagnostic use.

Tissues such as bone, lymph node or liver contain non-caseating granulomata but the distinction from tuberculous granulomata is not always easy. Radiological bone changes are also seen later; typically, erosions at the edge of joints or the end-plates of vertebrae, with associated sclerosis. Marked bony destruction is unusual and is more suggestive of TB. Isotope bone scans show hotspots in affected bones and joints and frequently reveal further foci of infection that are asymptomatic. The clinical and radiological features that discriminate between spine involvement with TB or brucellosis are shown in Table 38.1.

Treatment

Three questions guide management, once a presumptive or definite diagnosis has been made.

1 Is the disease acute (duration <1 month) or relapsing or chronic (>6 months)?
2 Is there focal disease of bone or joints?
3 Has tuberculosis definitely been excluded?

Adults with acute non-focal disease should be treated for a minimum of 6 weeks. Patients with focal disease and/or chronic disease require 3 months of treatment. Monotherapy should not be used because, although clinical illness responds in the short term, early relapse occurs in more than 30% of cases. At least two antibiotics should be used for all cases. Patients in whom tuberculosis has not been excluded have to be treated for both infections simultaneously or should be given antimicrobials to which only brucellosis responds (i.e. streptomycin or rifampicin should not be used).

The time-honoured combination of an oral tetracycline for 6–12 weeks plus 1g/day streptomycin intramuscularly for 2–3 weeks is the gold standard. The preferred form of tetracycline is now 100 mg doxycycline twice daily as it is easier to take and less likely to cause renal toxicity. Modern aminoglycosides such as gentamicin (5 mg/kg/day for 10–14 days) can be substituted for streptomycin, but the optimal duration of therapy has not yet been confirmed. Pending further trials, the

Table 38.1 **Radiology of spine: differences from tuberculosis**

	Brucellosis	**Tuberculosis**
Site	Lumbar + others	Dorsolumbar
Vertebrae	Multiple or contiguous	Contiguous
Discitis	Late	Early
Body	Intact until late	Morphology lost early
Canal compression	Rare	Common
Epiphysitis	Anterosuperior (Pedro-Pons' sign)	General: upper + lower disc region, centre, subperiosteal
Osteophyte	Anterolateral (parrot beak)	Unusual
Deformity	Wedging uncommon	Anterior wedge (gibbus)
Recovery	Sclerosis of whole body	Variable
Paravertebral abscess	Small, well localized	Common + discrete loss transverse process
Psoas abscess	Rare	More likely

WHO recommends 14 days of gentamicin (7 days is known to be insufficient). An alternative regimen is doxycycline with rifampicin, both given for 6 weeks or 3 months. The relapse rate after 6 weeks of this regimen is >10% compared to ~5% with doxycycline/streptomycin, and some national programmes discourage use of rifampicin for this purpose, reserving it for tuberculosis and leprosy treatment. Co-trimoxazole in high doses (three tablets twice a day for large adults) can be used but can cause anaemia and drug rashes, and should be supplemented with daily folic acid. It provides a good alternative to tetracyclines in young children when given with a second antibiotic, but in adults, co-trimoxazole plus doxyxcycline is more effective than co-trimoxazole plus rifampicin. There is some evidence that children (<12 years) are adequately treated by 3 weeks rather than 6 weeks of therapy.

Pregnant women should not receive tetracyclines and are usually given rifampicin alone or with 2 tablets co-trimoxazole twice daily (avoid, or add folate supplements, in the first trimester). The triple combination of doxycycline, rifampicin and gentamicin is superior to a double regimen and should be used for all infections with complications such as severe spondylitis, endocarditis or meningitis. Further drugs such as ceftriaxone may be added, and patients with endocarditis often need valve replacement as well. Fluoroquinolones have been disappointing for routine treatment but some physicians add them as a third drug in difficult cases. Azithromycin does not appear to be useful.

Follow-up

Patients should be seen at 3 and 6 weeks to encourage adherence to antibiotic therapy. The most useful features are improvement in general mood and health, with return of appetite and weight. Serology is not very useful as it follows a variable pattern for months to years after successful treatment and does not predictably rise to warn that relapse is imminent. Relapse is conventionally defined as a further episode of brucellosis occurring less than 6 months after the first. This is usually a result of failure to take adequate antibiotics for long enough rather than being due to drug resistance, and should be treated with a further 3-month course of two antibiotics as for a first episode; some would insist on including streptomycin or gentamicin for retreatment, in order to be sure the drugs have

been taken. Chronic brucellosis is difficult to define serologically and difficult to distinguish from chronic fatigue syndrome, depression or malingering. Immunity after brucellosis is not solid in humans, who may suffer from repeated infections. No vaccine is available for human use.

Public health aspects

Brucellosis is controlled by simple measures that require political commitment. The first is education of the public to eat or drink only pasteurized milk and dairy products and to discourage the practice of eating uncooked liver or meat, but this is often difficult to achieve in the face of tradition. Animal herds can be protected by administration of live vaccines, and such control has also been shown to reduce the incidence of human infection. Control of infected herds or flocks is usually based on 'test and slaughter' (i.e. if any animal in the herd tests positive, the whole herd is slaughtered). The public will only comply with such measures if they are offered adequate financial compensation.

 SUMMARY

- Brucellosis is one of the classical zoonoses (infections of animals transmitted to humans), and human disease is eradicated by adequate veterinary control programmes.
- Humans usually acquire infection from ingesting milk or dairy products that have not been pasteurized or by inhalation of aerosols containing organisms, e.g. on farms (from dried products of conception of aborted animals) or in diagnostic laboratories.
- It is an important cause of fever in many parts of the world and is often underdiagnosed because of lack of laboratory facilities.
- Almost half those affected have focal musculoskeletal symptoms in addition to fluctuating fever over weeks.
- Therapy requires at least 6 weeks of treatment with at least two antimicrobials, primarily to reduce the risk of subsequent relapse.

Visit www.lecturenoteseries.com/tropicalmed **to test yourself on this chapter using interactive MCQs.**

📖 FURTHER READING

Centers for Disease Control. Brucellosis: frequently asked questions. http://www.cdc.gov/brucellosis/ [Useful general detail on the web, including patient handouts and updated information of all sorts.]

Dean AS, Crump L, Greter H, *et al.* (2012) Clinical manifestations of human brucellosis: a systematic review and meta-analysis. *PLoS Negl Trop Dis* **6**(12): e1929. [Two recent reviews in the public domain.]

Dean AS, Crump L, Greter H, *et al.* (2012) Global burden of human brucellosis: a systematic review of disease frequency. *PLoS Negl Trop Dis* **6**(10): e1865.

Franco MP, Mulder M, Gilman RH, et al. Human brucellosis. *Lancet Infect Dis* 2007;7:775-786. http://www.ncbi.nlm.nih.gov/pubmed/18045560 [Nice overview of all aspects]

Health Protection Agency (HPA) for general information and detail of deliberate release from British perspective www.hpa.org.uk/

Skalsky K, Yahav D, Bishara J, *et al.* (2008) Treatment of human brucellosis: systematic review and meta-analysis of randomized controlled trials. *BMJ* **336**: 701–4. [Best of several recent metanalyses on treatment with most references on supplementary website.]

World Health Organization (WHO) www.who.int/entity/zoonoses/diseases/brucellosis/en/index.html [Has some information. The most useful recent publication *Brucellosis in animals and humans* (WHO 2006), a comprehensive document on all aspects of brucellosis, is available at www.who.int/csr/resources/publications/Brucellosis.pdf]

39

Typhoid and paratyphoid fevers

Chris Parry
Liverpool School of Tropical Medicine

Typhoid and paratyphoid fevers are illnesses caused by *Salmonella enterica* serovar Typhi and serovars Paratyphi A, B and C. They cause a systemic septicaemic illness which is also called enteric fever. The many salmonellas, which usually cause gastroenteritis, occasionally also cause an enteric fever-like illness, especially severe in patients with HIV infection and pre-school children in sub-Saharan Africa.

Typhoid and paratyphoid are most common where standards of personal and environmental hygiene are low and only to this extent are these diseases tropical. There are estimated to be 27 million cases of typhoid fever worldwide each year with more than 200 000 deaths. The incidence is more than 100/100 000 population/year in the Indian Subcontinent and South East Asia, and 10–100/100 000 population/year in other resource-poor countries in Asia, Africa, the Caribbean, Central and South America. In endemic areas, the disease is most common in children and young adults (aged 2–35 years).

Organisms

The organisms are Gram-negative bacilli of the Enterobacteriacae. All possess somatic (O) and flagellar (H) antigens. *S. enterica* ser. Typhi and ser. Paratyphi C possess a surface (Vi) antigen that coats the O antigen and potentially protects it from antibody attack. *S. enterica* ser. Typhi and ser. Paratyphi A and B infect only humans. *S. enterica* ser Paratyphi C may also affect a variety of animals.

Mode of infection

Infection is usually by ingestion, with transmission in water (mainly *S. enterica* ser. Typhi) and food. Ingestion of 10^5 *S. enterica* ser. Typhi organisms may cause a relatively low attack rate with a long incubation period. Increasing the infecting dose to 10^9 organisms raises the attack rate to 95% and greatly shortens the incubation period. Conditions causing low gastric acidity allow a lower inoculum to cause infection. The most important reservoirs of infection are asymptomatic convalescent or chronic human carriers. Food-handlers, who are also carriers, are a potentially important source of transmission.

Typhoid fever

After ingestion, the organisms attach and then penetrate the small intestinal mucosa, and are transported by the lymphatics to mesenteric lymph glands. There they multiply, and enter the bloodstream via the thoracic duct and are carried to the bone marrow, spleen, liver and gallbladder. At these sites the bacilli are able to survive and multiply inside macrophages. Eventually, the bacteria are rereleased into the bloodstream and this second bacteraemia corresponds to the onset of symptoms.

There is a secondary invasion of the bowel via the infected bile. Macrophages collect in large numbers in the intestinal lymph follicles, particularly the Peyer's patches in the ileum. The strong inflammatory

Tropical Medicine Lecture Notes, Seventh edition. Edited by Nick Beeching and Geoff Gill. © 2014 John Wiley & Sons, Ltd. Published 2014 by John Wiley & Sons, Ltd.

response in the Peyer's patches may lead to hyperplasia, necrosis and ulceration in 7–10 days if the inflammation does not resolve. Involvement of blood vessels may lead to bleeding and, if the whole thickness of the bowel is involved, perforation follows.

Elsewhere in the body, foci of inflammation with macrophages and lymphocytes, so-called typhoid nodules, are scattered in various organs, especially the liver, spleen, marrow and lymph glands. More diffuse organ involvement also occurs, affecting the myocardium, kidney and lung. Late in the disease there may be abscess formation, most often affecting bone, brain, liver or spleen. Serious disease of the brain, lung and kidneys is not invariably accompanied by typhoid nodule formation, and the assumption is that some unidentified toxin must be the cause.

The natural course of the untreated disease is very variable. In a classical case, fever has returned to normal at the end of the third week and repair processes then begin. However, in some cases, fever and symptoms last for only a few days (particularly in preschool children) and in others may continue for many weeks. Death most commonly results from perforation, haemodynamic shock associated either with intestinal haemorrhage or severe toxaemia with altered consciousness, and occasionally from other complications such as meningitis.

Clinical picture

The average incubation period is about 14 days, but can vary from less than a week to more than 3 weeks. The only almost constant symptom is fever. The onset is usually gradual, and rigors are unusual. Fever increases day by day in the first week, often with an evening rise. A high and sustained fever (39–40 °C) then continues for another week or more, falling by lysis in the third or fourth week.

Patients with typhoid usually feel very unwell, with malaise, generalized aches and pains, and anorexia. Abdominal pain or discomfort, headache, diarrhoea or constipation and a non-productive cough are common symptoms.

Physical signs

These depend not only on the severity of the illness but on the length of time the patient has been ill. In patients who seek medical aid early, there has usually been no significant dehydration from diarrhoea, and the patient often looks relatively well and is mentally alert. In contrast, the patient who presents after 2 weeks of illness is often very toxic, mentally stuporose and gravely dehydrated. The high fever may be accompanied by hepatomegaly, splenomegaly (often tender), mental changes including apathy, signs of bronchitis and meningism.

Rose spots are usually only seen with ease in fair-skinned patients. They are found from day 7 onwards and take the form of pink macules, usually scanty and found mainly on the trunk. They fade on pressure from a glass slide. In occasional patients, the pulse rate is disproportionately slow compared with the fever, and may not reach 100 b.p.m. even when the temperature is 40 °C (so-called relative bradycardia).

Complications

These may develop as the illness progresses, and can follow a clinically mild attack. The clinician must remember that typhoid patients may present with the complication rather than with the symptoms of typhoid fever, and these patients are often difficult to diagnose. The most important complications are as follows, with the first three the most common.

- *Perforation.* This typically occurs in the third week. Toxic patients may show few signs of peritonitis, except for abdominal distension, increasing toxaemia and a rising pulse. Surgery is preferable to conservative management, and excision or segmental resection is safer than simple suturing, because the gut wall immediately surrounding the perforation may be too friable to hold sutures. Antibiotic therapy should be broadened to cover gastrointestinal organisms contaminating the peritoneum.
- *Haemorrhage.* Patients may have repeated small bleeds that resolve without specific treatment. Massive bleeding is typically a complication of the third week. Surgery is seldom needed provided that blood transfusion is available.
- *Severe toxaemia.* Some patients have severe disease characterized by delerium, obtundation, stupor, or coma often accompanied by haemodynamic shock (not caused by gastrointestinal haemorrhage). For unexplained reasons, this complication has been reported more frequently in Indonesia, Papua New Guinea and West Africa than in other countries.
- *Haemolytic anaemia.* This may occur in patients with glucose-6-phosphate dehydrogenase (G6PD) deficiency; typhoid depresses G6PD levels in normal as well as in deficient patients.
- *Typhoid lobar pneumonia.* This is a rare complication of the second and third week. Rusty sputum is not produced.
- *Meningitis.* This may be the only obvious manifestation of typhoid, when it resembles any other pyogenic meningitis. It usually occurs in young children.

- *Renal disease.* This may present as renal failure or an acute nephrotic syndrome, and is probably an immune-complex nephritis. Recovery after successful chemotherapy is usual.
- *Typhoid abscess.* This is a late complication that can occur almost anywhere, especially in the spleen, liver, brain, breast and skeletal system.
- *Skeletal complications.* These are mainly suppurative arthritis and osteomyelitis. Both may be greatly delayed in onset. Zenker's degeneration of muscle or polymyositis may occur.
- *Other complications or sequelae.* Many are described including suppurative parotitis, acute cholecystitis, deep venous thrombosis, psychiatric disturbance and Guillain–Barré syndrome.

Diagnosis

Culture

Culture of the organism is the best way to confirm the diagnosis, but the technology to do this is often lacking in those hospitals in developing countries that most need it. Blood culture is the most useful, particularly in the first and second week. The average number of bacteria in the blood is low, so an adequate volume of blood should be taken for culture to increase the likelihood of a positive result. Bone marrow culture gives a higher culture positive rate, probably because the concentration of organisms is 10-fold higher than in the blood, and may even yield a positive culture after chemotherapy has been started. A string capsule used to sample duodenal contents can yield positive cultures, but in practice this method is not widely used. Aspirates from rose spots, cerebrospinal fluid (CSF) or pus from abscesses may also yield positive cultures. Stool culture does not definitively confirm the diagnosis, as the patient may be a chronic carrier. Faecal and urine cultures are mainly of value for the detection of carriers.

Serodiagnosis

The Widal test, which measures agglutinating antibodies to the somatic (O) and flagellar (H) antigens, is widely used. Although the test is relatively cheap and straightforward to perform, it lacks specificity and sensitivity. In endemic areas low levels of antibodies are detectable in the healthy population, presumably because of prior exposure to the organisms and other non-typhoid salmonellae that share O and H antigens, and H antibody titres can remain high for a long time after typhoid immunization. In typhoid patients, titres often rise before the clinical onset, making it very difficult to demonstrate the diagnostic fourfold rise between initial and subsequent specimens. Furthermore a significant number of culture-positive patients develop no rise in titre at all. However, if the test is interpreted intelligently, bearing all these facts in mind, a significant number of patients will be correctly diagnosed by the Widal test, when all other methods have failed. Interpretation of the result is helped by knowledge of the background levels of antibodies in the local healthy population.

A number of rapid diagnostic tests are commercially available but most suffer from a similar lack of sensitivity and specificity as the Widal test. New antibody tests that detect different antigens to those used in the Widal test and the currently available rapid diagnostic tests are being developed and appear promising.

Other laboratory findings

The white blood cell (WBC) count is usually within the normal range, as is the differential count, but there may be leucopenia or leucocytosis and relative lymphocytosis is common. Biochemical tests usually show only minor changes, such as slight elevation of transaminases and bilirubin. A considerable elevation of indirect bilirubin is often associated with haemolytic anaemia in patients with G6PD deficiency and in children. In severe cases, albuminuria is almost invariable. There may be evidence of disseminated intravascular coagulopathy (DIC), although this rarely causes a clinical problem.

Treatment

The mainstay of treatment is effective antimicrobial chemotherapy. In endemic areas many patients are managed as outpatients with oral antibiotics. Severely ill patients who may be mentally uncooperative require admission to hospital, good nursing care and careful supportive medical care, including attention to fluid and electrolyte balance.

Chemotherapy (Table 39.1)

Chloramphenicol used to be acknowledged everywhere as the drug of choice, with amoxicillin or co-trimoxazole as effective alternatives. However, in recent years, multidrug-resistant (MDR) isolates of *S. enterica* ser. Typhi and ser. Paratyphi A resistant to all three antibiotics have been widely reported in

Table 39.1 **Choice of antibiotic to treat typhoid fever**

Antibiotic	Dosage	Frequency	Route	Duration (days) Non-severe	Duration (days) Severe or complicated	Side effects
Chloramphenicol	50–100 mg/kg/day Reduce dose 30 mg/kg/day when fever ceases	4	o (i.m./i.v.)	14–21	14–21	Bone marrow depression
Amoxicillin	75–100 mg/kg/day	3	o/i.m./i.v.	14	14	
Co-trimoxazole (trimethoprim-sulfamethoxazole)	8 mg/kg/day trimethoprim + 40 mg/kg/day sulfamethoxazole	2–3	o/i.m./i.v.	14	14	Nephrotoxic Allergy Not for children <2 years
Ciprofloxacin*	20 mg/kg/day	2	o/i.v.	5–7	10–14	
Ofloxacin*	15 mg/kg/day	2	o/i.v.	5–7	10–14	
Gatifloxacin*	10 mg/kg/day	1	o/i.v.	5–7	10–14	
Ceftriaxone	50–80 mg/kg/day	1–2	i.m./i.v.	7–10	10–14	
Cefotaxime	100–150 mg/kg/day	3–4	i.m./i.v.	7–10	10–	
Cefixime	20–30 mg/kg/day	2	o	7–10	Not recommended	
Azithromycin	20 mg/kg/day	1	o	5–7	Not recommended	

i.m., intramuscularly; i.v., intravenously; o, orally.
*Nalidixic acid-resistant isolates may not respond.

the Indian subcontinent, countries of South East Asia and some countries in Africa.

The fluoroquinolone antibiotics, third-generation cephalosporins and azithromycin have proved effective alternatives for treating MDR infections. Unfortunately, these antibiotics are expensive, in particular the cephalosporins. Widespread use of fluoroquinolones has led to the emergence of strains with low-level and full resistance to these antibiotics. In some countries in Asia (Indonesia, Papua New Guinea), Africa (except Kenya and some countries in West Africa) and South and Central America, many strains remain susceptible to chloramphenicol.

Relapses after chemotherapy occur in a variable proportion of patients (2–10%), are usually rather less severe than the initial illness and respond to the same chemotherapy.

Fluoroquinolones

A 5–7-day course of a fluoroquinolone such as ciprofloxacin (Table 39.1) has proved extremely effective for the treatment of fully susceptible isolates, with rapid resolution of fever and symptoms. There have been concerns about the use of fluoroquinolones in children, because of evidence of damage to the cartilage in the growing joints of animals. However, compassionate use of short courses of fluoroquinolones in children with multiresistant Gram-negative infections, where alternatives were unavailable, has proved safe.

Strains with decreased susceptibility to fluoroquinolones have appeared, in the Indian subcontinent and South East Asia. Infections with these strains may fail to respond to ciprofloxacin or ofloxacin therapy. There is evidence that the newer fluoquinolone gatifloxacin is better for treating such infections. Microbiology laboratories can have difficulty in detecting these strains with the currently recommended methods. Resistance to the related antibiotic nalidixic acid, however, is a useful marker. Patients with enteric fever who are still sick after 5-7 days of an adequate dose of fluoroquinolone are likely to be infected with a resistant strain and should be changed to an alternative antibiotic. Fully fluoroquinolone-resistant strains are now appearing in the major cities in India.

Third-generation cephalosporins

Third-generation cephalosporins such as ceftriaxone, cefotaxime and cefixime are effective in treating MDR strains. The response to treatment may be slow, with the fever and symptoms taking 7–10 days to resolve. There are sporadic reports of ESBL producing strains resistant to this class of drug.

Azithromycin

Azithromycin is another effective oral alternative for MDR typhoid in adults and children. It has not been used yet in severe disease.

Chloramphenicol

A fairly prolonged course must be given to prevent relapse, such as a total of 14 days, or 12 days after fever has abated. It commonly takes 48 h before the fever shows a response, and 5 days or more until the patient becomes completely afebrile in severe cases. A Herxheimer-type reaction is sometimes seen early in treatment, and should be treated with steroids.

Amoxicillin

This is at least as effective as chloramphenicol if given in high doses. Ampicillin is inferior to chloramphenicol.

Co-trimoxazole

The clinical response is at least as rapid as with chloramphenicol.

Steroids

Adults and children with severe typhoid characterized by delerium, obtundation, coma or shock were shown to benefit in a small study from Indonesia from the prompt administration of dexamethasone. The dosage given was 3 mg/kg by slow intravenous infusion over a period of 30 min followed by 1 mg/kg given at the same rate every 6 h for eight additional doses. Hydrocortisone given at a lower dose was not effective.

Carrier state

This commonly persists for some months into convalescence, and when it terminates spontaneously such patients are called convalescent carriers. They are an obvious source of infection to others, but even more important are chronic carriers (1–3% of cases) in which a persisting focus of infection smoulders on in the gallbladder (faecal carriers) or urinary tract (urinary carriers) for more than 1 year. In most endemic areas, few carriers are identified because culture facilities do not exist. Persistent elevation of Vi antibodies often accompanies the carrier state.

The excretion of organisms by carriers is variable and erratic. Chronic faecal carriers may have chronic cholecystitis with or without gallstones, or pathological abnormalities in the urinary tract, including *Schistosoma haematobium* infection in chronic urinary carriers. *Schistosoma mansoni* may be associated with a relapsing non-typhoid *Salmonella* septicaemia.

Treatment of chronic carriers

Antimicrobial therapy should be guided by the susceptibility of the isolated bacteria. Ciprofloxacin 750 mg twice daily for 28 days has proved effective. If ciprofloxacin is unavailable and the strains are susceptible, two tablets of co-trimoxazole twice a day for 3 months, or 100 mg/kg/day amoxicillin combined with 30 mg/kg/day probenecid, both for 3 months, may also be effective. Faecal carriers with gallstones only respond temporarily to chemotherapy and cholecystectomy is needed to terminate the carrier state in such cases.

If the patient is intelligent and conscientious, and not a food-handler, the carrier state need not be treated at all, for the fastidious maintenance of high standards of environmental and personal hygiene will prevent transmission of the infection to others.

Typhoid vaccine

Two vaccines are currently available. The live attenuated oral vaccine (Ty21a) requires three doses over 5 days with a booster recommended every 5 years. This vaccine is not recommended for children under the age of 6 years. The second, a purified Vi antigen vaccine, is given as a single dose intramuscularly; boosters are recommended every 3 years. It is not recommended for children under the age of 2 years. A new modified conjugate Vi vaccine and single dose attenuated oral vaccines are in development. These vaccines aim to be effective in very young children. The disadvantage of all these vaccines is their cost.

The use of vaccination as a public health tool is now recommended by WHO in highly endemic areas where there are high rates of resistance to available antimicrobials.

If typhoid does develop in a vaccinated subject, it is no less severe than in the unvaccinated.

Paratyphoid A and B

These usually infect via contaminated foods in which the organisms have multiplied. For this reason, diarrhoea and vomiting may precede septicaemia. Many mild cases occur. Treatment is as for typhoid. Drug resistant strains have become common in some areas of the Indian subcontinent.

Paratyphoid C

This commonly produces septicaemia without involvement of the gut, and abscess formation is common.

 Visit www.lecturenoteseries.com/tropicalmed to test yourself on this chapter using interactive MCQs.

 FURTHER READING

Bhan MK, Bahl R, Bhatnager S (2005) Typhoid and paratyphoid fever. *Lancet* **366**: 749–62.

Bhutta ZA (2006) Current concepts in the diagnosis and treatment of typhoid fever. BMJ **333**: 78–82.

 SUMMARY

- Enteric fever (typhoid and paratyphoid) is acquired from contaminated water and food.
- Mild infections are under-reported and can be managed in the community.
- Most of the complications of severe typhoid become apparent in the third week of illness.
- Multidrug resistance is common, especially in Asia, where *S. enterica* var. typhi and *S. enterica* var. paratyphi A are often resistant to fluoroquinolones as well as 'first-line drugs' such as amoxicillin, chloramphenicol and co-trimoxazole.
- Alternative treatments include third generation cephalosporins or azithromycin.
- Mass immunization against typhoid is recommended by the WHO as a control measure in settings where disease transmission is common, especially if multidrug resistance is also a problem.

40

Arboviruses

Tom Solomon
University of Liverpool

Arbovirus (short for arthropod-borne virus) is an ecological description for viruses that are transmitted between vertebrate hosts by insects – principally mosquitoes, ticks, sandflies or midges. There are more than 500 arboviruses, in four viral families, but only a small number are medically important (Fig. 40.1). Some arboviruses are named after the disease they cause (e.g. Yellow fever, or O'nyong nyong – 'joint weakening' in a Ugandan dialect), some after their insect vector (e.g. phleboviruses after 'phlebotomus' – sandflies) and some after the geographical area where the disease first occurred (e.g. Japanese encephalitis).

Vectors and hosts

Following infection with an arbovirus, most animals develop life-long immunity to that virus. An arbovirus therefore needs a ready supply of immunologically naïve hosts. A few arboviruses (notably dengue) have evolved to use humans as the 'natural host'; however, most use small mammals or birds because of their high reproductive rate. For these 'enzootic' viruses, humans are coincidentally infected 'dead-end hosts' and do not transmit the disease. In some situations an 'amplifying host' increases the amount of circulating virus and acts as a link to human infection.

Clinical syndromes

The majority of human infections with arboviruses are asymptomatic or cause a mild non-specific febrile illness. When an arbovirus causes disease, it usually leads to one of three clinical syndromes.

1 Fever–arthralgia–rash (FAR).
2 Viral haemorrhagic fever.
3 Central nervous system (CNS) infection.

Most viruses cause a single syndrome, but there can be overlap; e.g. dengue viruses can present with a FAR syndrome (dengue fever), a haemorrhagic syndrome (dengue haemorrhagic fever) and even, occasionally, CNS disease. The most important haemorrhagic fevers are considered in Chapter 41, and CNS arboviruses are discussed in Chapter 33. FAR arboviruses are summarized below.

Fever–arthralgia–rash arboviruses

Chikungunya

Chikungunya ('that which bends you over' in Makonde dialect) occurs in Africa, India and South-East Asia. Humans and primates are the natural hosts and both *Aedes* and *Culex* mosquitoes can transmit the disease. Since March 2005 the virus has caused large outbreaks in the Pacific islands, and Asia, and has even reached southern Europe. It is often present in the same areas as, and confused with, dengue. The main clinical distinguishing feature of chikungunya is frequent multiple joint pain, which may persist for some months. Haemorrhagic complications are rare and thrombocytopenia and neutropenia are much less common than in dengue.

Tropical Medicine Lecture Notes, Seventh edition. Edited by Nick Beeching and Geoff Gill. © 2014 John Wiley & Sons, Ltd. Published 2014 by John Wiley & Sons, Ltd.

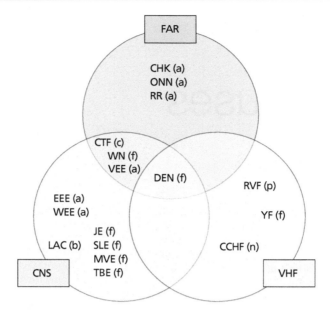

Key

(a) Alphavirus genus [Togaviridae]
- CHK = Chikungunya
- ONN = O'nyong nyong
- RR = Ross River
- VEE = Venezuelan equine encephalitis
- EEE = Eastern equine encephalitis
- WEE = Western equine encephalitis

(f) Flavivirus genus [Flaviviridae]
- JE = Japanese encephalitis
- SLE = St Louis encephalitis
- MVE = Murray valley encephalitis
- TBE = Tick borne encephalitis
- WN = West Nile
- DEN = Dengue
- YF = Yellow fever
- ZV = Zika virus

(b) Bunyavirus genus [Bunyaviridae]
- LAC = La Crosse

(n) Nairovirus genus [Bunyaviridae]
- CCHF = Crimean–Congo haemorrhagic fever

(c) Coltivirus genus [Rheoviridae]
- CTF = Colorado tick fever

(p) Phlebovirus genus [Bunyaviridae]
- RVF = Rift Valley fever

Figure 40.1 Medically important arboviruses grouped according to disease syndrome (top), and listed by genus (bottom). CNS, central nervous system; FAR, fever–arthralgia–rash; VHF, viral haemorrhagic fever. Viral families are indicated by [ ].

O'nyong nyong

O'nyong nyong occurs in Africa and is the only arbovirus transmitted by *Anopheles* mosquitoes. Humans are the only hosts and a common clinical feature is conjunctivitis.

Ross River

This occurs in Australia and is transmitted by *Aedes* and *Culex* mosquitoes. It can cause 'epidemic polyarthritis'.

Colorado tick fever

This is found in the Rocky Mountain states of the USA and is transmitted among small mammals by *Dermacentor* ticks. It causes CNS disease in 10% of children; haemorrhagic disease is rarer. It is easily confused with the rickettsial disease, Rocky Mountain spotted fever.

Dengue virus

This is the most common FAR arbovirus and is discussed more fully in Chapter 41.

SUMMARY

- Arbovirus (short for arthropod-borne virus) is an ecological description for viruses that are transmitted between vertebrate hosts by insects – principally mosquitoes, ticks, sandflies or midges.

- The majority of human infections with arboviruses are asymptomatic or cause a mild non-specific febrile illness.

- When an arbovirus causes disease, it usually leads to one of three clinical syndromes: Fever–arthralgia–rash (FAR); viral haemorrhagic fever (VHF); central nervous system (CNS) infection.

- Relatively common arboviruses include mosquito-borne chikungunya (Africa and Asia), O'nyong nyong (Africa), Ross River virus (Australia) and tick-borne Colorado tick fever (USA).

- The most important FAR viruses, dengue and yellow fever, and the VHF group are considered in separate chapters.

Visit **www.lecturenoteseries.com/tropicalmed** to test yourself on this chapter using interactive MCQs.

FURTHER READING

Chen LH, Wilson ME (2012) Dengue and chikungunya in travelers: recent updates. *Curr Opin Infect Dis* **25**: 523–9. doi: 10.1097/QCO.0b013e328356ffd5 [Update on epidemiology and clinical issues – common problems in returned travelers.]

Randolph SE, Rogers DJ (2010) The arrival, establishment and spread of exotic diseases: patterns and predictions. *Nat Rev Microbiol* **8**: 361–71.

Weaver SC, Reisen WK (2010) Present and future arboviral threats. *Antiviral Res* **85**: 328–45. [Review.]

41

Viral haemorrhagic fevers

Tom Solomon[1] and Nick Beeching[2]
[1]University of Liverpool; [2]Liverpool School of Tropical Medicine

Few diseases cause as much terror as the viral haemorrhagic fevers (VHFs), but this is often out of proportion to the actual harm they do. VHFs are caused by a diverse group of viruses from four viral families: the Arenaviridae, Filoviridae, Bunyaviridae and Flaviviridae (Table 41.1).

Epidemiology

The epidemiology can be simplified by considering three questions (Figure 41.1).

1 How is the virus transmitted in its natural cycle – via arthropods, directly or unknown?
2 How do human index cases become infected – via insects, directly or unknown?
3 Is there direct transmission between humans to cause nosocomial spread?

Pathogenesis

The pathogenesis varies according to virus, but usually includes a combination of vascular damage, coagulopathy, immunological impairment and end-organ damage. These lead to:

- increased vascular permeability – the major pathophysiological process for most VHFs, which allows plasma to leak from the vessels into the tissue and causes shock, oedema and effusions;
- haemorrhagic manifestations, which are sometimes relatively minor (e.g. petechiae) or can be major (e.g. gastrointestinal bleeding in Crimean–Congo haemorrhagic fever [CCHF]);
- hepatic and renal failure;
- encephalopathy.

Management

The management of VHFs includes the identification and treatment of suspected cases, limiting further spread (for the directly transmissible VHFs) and identifying others who may have been infected.

Identifying VHF in the febrile patient

Most patients with suspected VHF turn out to have malaria, typhoid or another non-transmissible disease. Unnecessary alarm can be avoided, and attention focused on likely cases of VHF, by considering the following (Figure 41.2).

- Most VHFs are acquired in rural rather than urban areas.
- Travel history should include details of activities that may have caused exposure.
- An interval of 3 weeks between possible exposure and onset rules out VHF.
- Most early symptoms are non-specific but certain features should ring alarm bells; for example pharyngitis with ulcers or causing difficulty swallowing, retrosternal chest pain, conjunctival injection and prostration.
- Haemorrhagic manifestations may not be obvious – look for petechiae in the skin folds and axillae, gum bleeding and microscopic haematuria and perform a tourniquet test (see Chapter 42).
- Look, repeatedly if necessary, for a rising haematocrit (caused by plasma leakage), pleural effusions on decubitus chest X-ray, leucopenia, thrombocytopenia and proteinuria.

Tropical Medicine Lecture Notes, Seventh edition. Edited by Nick Beeching and Geoff Gill. © 2014 John Wiley & Sons, Ltd. Published 2014 by John Wiley & Sons, Ltd.

Table 41.1 Overview of the major viral haemorrhagic fevers

Virus	Genus, family	Geographical area	Natural cycle	Human disease
Lassa	*Arenavirus*, Arenaviridae	Western Africa	*Mastomys* rodent	Human–human spread occurs. 2–15% mortality. Treat with ribavirin
Lujo	*Arenavirus*, Arenaviridae	Zambia; uncertain range	Unknown	Human–human and nosocomial spread occurs. 80% mortality in 5 cases
Ebola and Marburg	*Filovirus*, Filoviridae	Sub-Saharan Africa	(Unknown) Bats implicated	Nosocomial spread common. 25–90% mortality. No antiviral treatment
Hantaan and others (Haemorrhagic fever with renal syndrome)	*Hantavirus*, Bunyaviridae	Far East, Europe	Various rural rodents	No human–human spread. 1–15% mortality depending on virus. Treat severe disease with ribavirin
Crimean–Congo haemorrhagic fever	*Nairovirus*, Bunyaviridae	Eastern Europe, Asia, Africa	*Hyalomma* ticks and livestock	Human–human spread. 15–30% mortality. Treat with ribavirin
Rift Valley fever	*Phlebovirus*, Bunyaviridae	Africa, Middle East	*Aedes* and other mosquitoes and livestock	Human–human spread not documented, but possible. Most infections asymptomatic. 50% mortality for VHF. Treat with ribavirin
Dengue	*Flavivirus*, Flaviviridae	Tropics and subtropics worldwide	*Aedes* mosquitoes and humans	No human–human spread. Mortality, 1% with adequate fluid treatment. No antivirals
Yellow fever	*Flavivirus*, Flaviviridae	Africa, South America	Various mosquitoes and monkeys	No human–human spread. 20–50% mortality. No antivirals

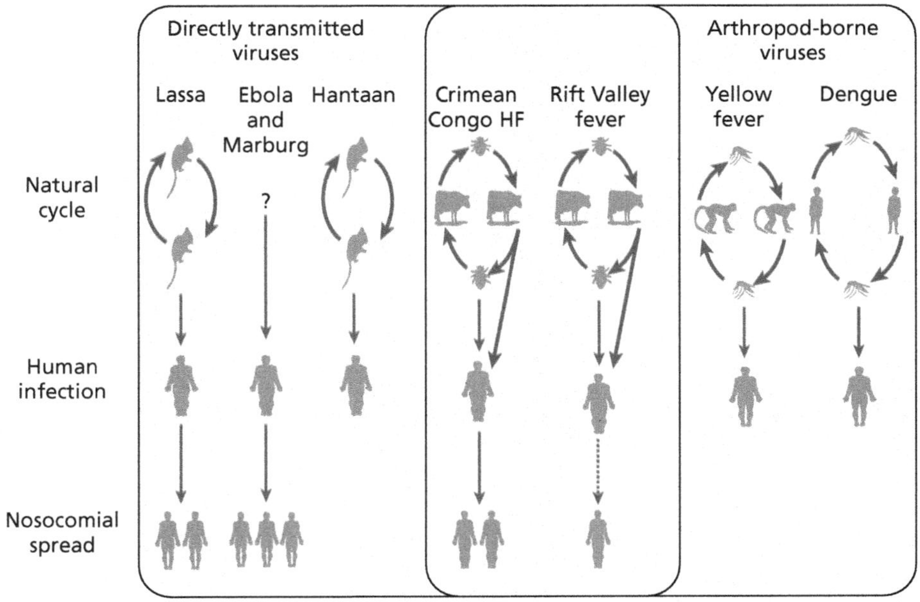

Figure 41.1 Ecological overview of viral haemorrhagic fevers showing natural cycle, transmission to humans and potential for nosocomial spread. Note the distinction between directly transmissible viruses (Lassa, Ebola, Marburg and Hantaan), arboviruses (yellow fever and dengue), and those transmitted by both routes (Crimean–Congo haemorrhagic fever and Rift Valley fever). *Source:* Modified from Solomon (2002).

	Directly transmissible VHF *					Non-directly transmissible VHF		
	Ebola/ Marburg	Lassa	South American VHFs	CCHF	RVF	HFRS	DHF	Yellow fever

1. Obtain a travel history:

	Ebola/ Marburg	Lassa	South American VHFs	CCHF	RVF	HFRS	DHF	Yellow fever
Africa	+	+		+	+		+	+
Middle East				+	+		+	
Asian subcontinent				+			+	
Europe				+		+		
Far East						+	+	
Americas			+				+	+

2. Ask about activities that may have caused exposure to virus:

	Directly transmissible VHF					Non-directly transmissible VHF		
Exposure to human cases	Recent contact (<3 weeks) with any sick individual with unexplained fever and bleeding					–	–	–
Exposure to animal reservoir	?Monkeys ?Bats	Rodent excreta (urban)	Rodent excreta (rural)	Livestock	Livestock	Rodent excreta	–	Monkeys
Activities undertaken	Jungle visits, caving	Cleaning basements, etc.	Farming, harvesting	Farming, abattoir work, rural activities	Farming, abattoir work, rural activities	Rural, agricultural work	Urban mosquito exposure	Jungle mosquito exposure

3. Look for suggestive clinical features:

Early features	Pharyngitis	Rash	Facial oedema
	Conjunctival injection	Venepuncture oozing	Small pleural effusions
	Retrosternal chest pain	Petechial haemorrhages	Abdominal pain
	Prostration	Mucosal bleeding	Tender hepatomegaly

Late features	Shock	Haematemesis	Renal failure
	Pleural effusions	DIC	Encephalopathy
	Ascites	Hepatic failure	Acidosis
	Pericardial effusions		

4. Consider investigative findings common in VHFs:

Leucopenia	Proteinuria	Prolonged TT, APTT
Thrombocytopenia	Haematuria	Elevated transaminases
Rising haematocrit	Renal impairment	

5. If malaria film and other tests negative, and patient deteriorating despite presumptive treatment, suspect VHF:

For a directly transmissible VHF, begin isolation procedure; alert medical, nursing, laboratory, cleaning and laundry staff, public health officials	For non-transmissible VHF, ensure standard safe practices are being followed. Inform public health authorities

6. Start intravenous ribavirin if one of the following suspected:

–	+	+	+	+	+	–	–
Ebola/ Marburg	Lassa	South American VHFs	CCHF	RVF	HFRS	DHF	YF

Directly transmissible VHF   Non-directly transmissible VHF

Figure 41.2 Algorithm for identifying VHF patients. *Directly transmissible between humans. †Patients with VHF caused by RVF should be treated as infectious, although direct transmission between humans has not yet been shown. CCHF, Crimean Congo haemorrhagic fever; DHF, dengue haemorrhagic fever; HFRS, haemorrhagic fever with renal syndrome; RVF, Rift Valley fever; YF, yellow fever. *Source:* Modified from Solomon (2002).

Table 41.2 **Differential diagnosis of viral haemorrhagic fevers**

Viral haemorrhagic fevers (in order of incidence)
Dengue haemorrhagic fever
Haemorrhagic fever with renal syndrome
Yellow fever
Lassa fever
Crimean–Congo haemorrhagic fever
Argentine, Bolivian and Venezuelan haemorrhagic
  fevers
Rift Valley fever
Omsk haemorrhagic fever, Kyasanur Forest
  disease and Al Khurma virus
Ebola and Marburg haemorrhagic fevers
Lujo virus

Treatable causes of fever with rash/haemorrhage
Parasites
  Malaria (rash/haemorrhage rare)
Bacteria
  Meningococcal
  Typhoid
  Septicaemic plague
  Shigellosis
  Any severe sepsis with DIC

Rickettsia
  Tick and epidemic typhus
  Rocky Mountain spotted fever
Spirochaetes
  Leptospirosis
  Borreliosis

Causes of fulminant hepatic failure
Hepatitis viruses A–E
Paracetamol and other drugs
Reye's syndrome
Alcohol

Arboviral causes of fever with rash
Alphaviruses
  Chikungunya
  O'nyong nyong
  Sindbis
Bunyaviruses
  Oropouche
Phleboviruses
  Sandfly fever
Coltiviruses
  Colorado tick fever
Flaviviruses
  Zika virus

Non-arboviral causes of fever with rash
Enteroviruses
  Coxsackie viruses
  Echoviruses
  Enteroviruses 68–71
Paramyxoviruses
  Measles
Herpes viruses
  Herpes zoster virus
  Human herpes virus 6 and 7
Orthomyxoviruses
  Influenza A and B
Rubiviruses
  Rubella

Miscellaneous

Drug reactions
Toxins
Acute surgical emergencies (upper gastrointestinal
  bleeding)

DIC, disseminated intravascular coagulation.

Diagnosis

The differential diagnosis of VHFs includes many causes of fever in the tropics (Table 41.2). Early laboratory diagnosis of the illness is by virus isolation, reverse transcriptase PCR or antigen capture ELISAs. Subsequently, IgM and IgG ELISAs are used. Because of the infectious nature of the directly transmissible VHFs, these tests must be carried out in biosafety level-4 facilities (high levels of staff protection only available in specialist centres).

Management

Encourage oral fluid intake with oral rehydration solution, and a straw if the patient cannot sit up. For patients with suspected Lassa fever, CCHF, Rift Valley fever (RVF) and haemorrhagic fever with renal syndrome (HFRS), ribavirin should be started as soon as possible (30 mg/kg loading dose, then 16 mg/kg q.d.s. for 4 days, then 8 mg/kg t.d.s. for 6 days). However, the evidence to support the use of ribavirin is poor for most VHFs except for Lassa and possibly CCHF. Hypovolaemic shock should be treated with crystalloids and colloids, and inotropes may be needed. Pulmonary oedema and effusions are common because of the increased capillary permeability. Blood transfusions are not required in most patients, but fresh frozen plasma may be needed.

Nosocomial spread is limited by isolating the patient, strict barrier nursing (with goggles and mask), proper decontamination and disposal of clinical waste and sharps and prompt disposal of bodies by specialized burial teams. Laboratory staff must be warned about possible hazardous specimens. The risks of respiratory spread are probably negligible. Negative pressure isolation units are used in the West, but not in the African countries where most cases occur. Here implementation of the measures outlined above has dramatically reduced nosocomial transmission. 'High risk' contacts who were exposed to blood, secretions or body fluids (usually before the diagnosis is suspected) should have their temperature checked twice daily for 3 weeks. Casual contacts at low risk should be told to report if they have fever. Survivors can suffer severe psychological damage, and support is needed.

Lassa fever

Lassa fever is the directly transmissible VHF most often seen in returning travellers, because of its wide distribution and long incubation period (5 days to 3 weeks). Lassa virus (genus Arenavirus, family *Arenaviridae*) is found across West Africa and is transmitted naturally between *Mastomys* rodents via their urine and faeces. Humans are infected by contact with these secretions, possibly by inhalation of aerosolized virus or by ingestion of food contaminated by rodents. Secondary human cases may occur by nosocomial spread. It is estimated that there are 100 000 cases and 5000 deaths annually, plus many unapparent infections.

Clinically, Lassa fever usually presents as a non-specific febrile illness, followed by conjunctival injection, sore throat with a pharyngeal exudate, retrosternal chest pain, vomiting and diarrhoea. Some patients progress to facial and laryngeal oedema, a mild bleeding diathesis and shock. Sensorineural deafness is a late complication in 30% of patients. The disease should be treated with ribavirin. Control measures include rodent control.

South American haemorrhagic fevers

Related arenaviruses with epidemiological and clinical similarities to Lassa are found in South America: Junin, Machupo and Guanarito viruses cause Argentine, Bolivian and Venezuelan haemorrhagic fever respectively. Whitewater Arroyo virus is a recently identified rare cause of VHF in southern United States.

Ebola and Marburg haemorrhagic fevers

These are caused by Ebola and Marburg viruses (genus *Filovirus*, family Filoviridae), which are presumed to be zoonotic. The natural reservoir remains unconfirmed but evidence is accumulating to implicate bats in transmission, especially for Marburg virus. Marburg virus first caused human disease in 1967 in laboratory workers in Marburg, Germany, who were handling tissue from African green monkeys imported from Uganda. Occasional cases followed in Africa, then a large outbreak in the Democratic Republic of Congo in 1999, with subsequent similar outbreaks. The first outbreak of Ebola occurred in 1976 in southern Sudan and the Democratic Republic of Congo (formerly Zaire). Subsequent outbreaks occurred in 1979, 1995 (Congo), 2000 (Uganda) and 2001–03 (Gabon and Congo) and more recently in Uganda. Five biotypes have been identified: Ebola-Zaire, Ebola-Sudan, Ebola-Côte d'Ivoire, Ebola-Bundibugyo (in Uganda) and Ebola Reston (which originated in the Philippines).

Naturally acquired human index cases of Ebola and Marburg always occur in rural areas, sometimes in association with bat-infested caves or mines, and sometimes following contact with diseased primates. Secondary cases are infected by contact with blood or other fluids from primary cases and hence are mostly carers. The route of virus entry is uncertain, but is possibly via small cuts in the skin or conjunctivae. Reuse of unsterile needles and lack of barrier nursing were important factors in early nosocomial outbreaks.

Clinically, the incubation period is 4–10 days. Patients present with a febrile illness with myalgia, abdominal pain (which may be severe enough to mimic peritonitis), sore throat, herpetic lesions in the mouth and pharynx, conjunctival injection, diarrhoea and a maculopapular rash. Prostration is a characteristic feature of Ebola. There is sometimes bleeding from the gastrointestinal tract, nose or injection sites. Petechiae, shock and neurological manifestations can occur. The case fatality rate is 30% (Marburg) and 60–90% (Ebola). Supportive treatment only can be given. Convalescent serum from survivors may help, and barrier nursing is essential. A range of experimental treatments are in development.

Haemorrhagic fever with renal syndrome

This is caused by four viruses (all members of the genus *Hantavirus*, family Bunyaviridae), which are transmitted naturally between various rural rodents in their excreta.

- Hantaan virus causes epidemic HFRS in the Far East.
- Seoul virus causes a milder syndrome in the same geographical area and in Europe.
- Dobrova virus causes severe HFRS in the Balkans (Europe).
- Puumula virus causes a milder variant across Scandinavia and northern Europe, with renal predominance (also called nephropathia epidemica).

Hantavirus pulmonary syndrome (a related condition with non-cardiogenic pulmonary oedema and shock) occurs in the Americas and is caused by Sin Nombre and other 'new world' hantaviruses. Humans are infected with hantaviruses by contact with rodent excreta. There is no evidence of human–human spread. Classically, HFRS patients have five phases: febrile, hypotensive phase (with haemorrhage), oliguric, diuretic and then convalescent. Severe illness should be treated with ribavirin. Prevention and control measures include minimizing human exposure to rodent excreta; for example, by rodent-proofing homes. Formalin-inactivated vaccines are used in Asia.

Crimean–Congo haemorrhagic fever

This virus is transmitted naturally between animals (small mammals and livestock) by ixodid ticks, especially of the *Hyalomma* genus. It is endemic throughout Africa, Asia, the former USSR, eastern Europe and the Middle East. There have been recent outbreaks in Afghanistan, Pakistan, the Russian Federation and South Africa. Humans are infected after being bitten by, or crushing, an infected tick; or by contact with blood from infected livestock or patients (hence barrier nursing is necessary). Unlike other VHFs, major haemorrhage is more important than vascular leakage in the pathophysiology and clinical presentation of CCHF. The mortality associated with different regional strains varies, and can be reduced considerably by full supportive care including adequate blood and fluid replacement. The role of ribavirin therapy is controversial. Prevention is by minimizing tick exposure.

Rift Valley fever

RVF is endemic in the African Rift Valley and much of sub-Saharan Africa and Egypt and has spread to Saudi Arabia and Yemen. It is transmitted naturally between livestock by many mosquito species, especially *Aedes* and *Culex*. Epidemics are associated with increases in mosquito populations following heavy rains, or irrigation projects. Humans are infected by mosquitoes and by contact with animal products. Direct transmission between humans has not been documented, but barrier nursing is advisable. RVF also causes disease in sheep and cattle (abortions). Clinically, it usually presents as a mild febrile illness in humans; 5% have haemorrhagic manifestations, meningoencephalitis or retinitis. Ribavirin treatment is probably effective, and control measures include livestock vaccination, personal protection of workers in the livestock industry and mosquito control.

Emerging viruses

Over the past decade, Al-Khurma virus, a new tick-borne flavivirus, has been shown to cause a VHF syndrome similar to Kyasanur Forest disease (to which it is related) in Saudi Arabia, and cases have also been reported in Egypt. The true clinical spectrum and geographical range of this infection remain to be determined. In 2008, a novel arenavirus called Lujo virus (after Lusaka and Johannesburg) was described in 5 patients. The index case, who was evacuated from Zambia to South Africa, died along with 3 of the 4 contacts, mostly health care workers. These infections remind us of the need to keep an open mind about the possibility of novel as well as known VHFs in the tropics and in returning travellers.

Dengue haemorrhagic fever and yellow fever

These are discussed in Chapter 42.

SUMMARY

- Viral haemorrhagic fevers (VHF) are caused by a diverse group of zoonotic viruses from four viral families: the Arenaviridae, Filoviridae, Bunyaviridae and Flaviviridae.

- The management of VHFs includes the identification and treatment of suspected cases, limiting further spread (for the directly transmissible VHFs) and identifying others who may have been infected.

- The greatest risk of healthcare associated transmission is posed by Crimean Congo haemorrhagic fever, which has a wide distribution from Africa across to Asia but is rarely imported by travellers returning from these areas.

- Healthcare associated transmission is limited by isolating the patient, strict barrier nursing (with goggles and mask), proper decontamination and disposal of clinical waste and sharps and prompt disposal of bodies by specialized burial teams. Laboratory staff must be warned about possible hazardous specimens.

- Early administration of ribavirin is effective in Lassa fever and is often used in Congo Crimean haemorrhagic fever, although the evidence base for this is less secure.

- Most returning travellers suspected to have a VHF turn out to have malaria or an arboviral infection.

Visit www.lecturenoteseries.com/tropicalmed to test yourself on this chapter using interactive MCQs.

FURTHER READING

Advisory Committee on Dangerous Pathogens (2012) *Management of Hazard Group 4 viral haemorrhagic fevers and similar human infectious diseases of high consequence.* Department of Health. http://www.hpa.org.uk/webc/HPAwebFile/HPAweb_C/1194947382005 [Revised British guidelines and algorithm for assessing returned travellers with possible VHF. Other documents also available from same HPA website.]

Beeching NJ, Fletcher T, Hill DR, Thomson GL (2010) Travellers and viral haemorrhagic fevers – what are the risks? *Int J Antimicrob Agents* **36**(Suppl): S26–S39. [Summary of VHF cases imported to industrialised countries, emphasising their rarity and very low risk of onward transmission in those settings.]

Centers for Disease Control and Prevention and World Health Organization (1998) *Infection Control for Viral Haemorrhagic Fevers in the African Health Care Setting.* Atlanta: Centers for Disease Control and Prevention. http://www.cdc.gov/ncidod/dvrd/spb [Very helpful manual for use in the field. Any other useful materials and updates on this site.]

Memish ZA, Fagbo SF, Assiri AM, *et al.* (2012) Alkhurma viral hemorrhagic fever virus: proposed guidelines for detection, prevention, and control in Saudi Arabia. *PLoS Negl Trop Dis* **6**(7): e1604. doi:10.1371/journal.pntd.0001604 [Summary of new virus and control methodology.]

ProMED-mail http://www.promedmail.org/aboutus/ [A very good source of current and archived information about outbreaks and isolated cases of VHFs and all emerging or unusual infections.]

Solomon T (2000) Viral haemorrhagic fevers. In G Cook, A Zumla (eds), *Manson's Tropical Diseases*, 21st edn. London: Saunders, pp. 773–93. [Detailed discussion of the ecology, pathophysiology and clinical aspects of viral haemorrhagic fevers.]

42

Dengue and yellow fever

Tom Solomon
University of Liverpool

While the most important viral haemorrhagic fevers numerically (dengue and yellow fever) are transmitted exclusively by arthropods, other arboviral haemorrhagic fevers (Crimean–Congo and Rift Valley fevers) can also be transmitted directly by body fluids. A third group of haemorrhagic fever viruses (Lassa, Ebola, Marburg) are only transmitted directly, and are not transmitted by arthropods at all. The directly transmissible viral haemorrhagic fevers are discussed in Chapter 41.

Dengue

Dengue virus is numerically the most important arbovirus infecting humans, with an estimated 100 million cases per year and 2.5 billion people at risk. There are four serotypes of dengue virus, transmitted by *Aedes* mosquitoes, and it is unusual among arboviruses in that humans are the natural hosts. Dengue fever ('breakbone fever') has been around for many hundreds of years; dengue haemorrhagic fever (DHF) emerged as an apparently new disease in South East Asia in the 1950s.

Epidemiology

Dengue has spread dramatically since the end of World War II, in what has been described as a global pandemic. Virtually every country between the tropics of Capricorn and Cancer is now affected (Fig. 42.1). Epidemics occur when the virus is introduced to new areas and there are susceptible hosts and mosquitoes; hyperendemic transmission refers to continuous transmission of multiple dengue virus serotypes. In addition to the annual large outbreaks across South East Asia, and in South America, in recent years there has been increasing disease in India.

Factors implicated in the spread of dengue viruses include poor control of its principal vector (*Aedes aegypti*) as well as reintroduction of this insect into Central and South America (it was largely eradicated in the 1960s), and expansion of the range of the other main vector *Aedes albopictus*. Other factors include intercontinental transport of car tyres containing *Aedes albopictus* eggs, overcrowding of refugee and urban populations and increasing human travel. In hyperendemic areas of Asia, disease is seen mainly in children (because adults are immune from prior exposure). However, the disease is being seen increasingly in non-immune adults travelling to endemic regions, and in adults when the disease arrives in new areas.

Aedes mosquitoes are 'peri-domestic': they breed in collections of fresh water around the house (e.g. water storage jars). They feed on humans (anthrophilic), mainly by day, and feed repeatedly on different hosts (enhancing their role as vectors).

Clinical features

Dengue virus may cause a non-specific febrile illness or asymptomatic infection, especially in young children, or more severe disease

Traditionally, two main clinical dengue syndromes: have been described dengue fever (DF) and dengue haemorrhagic fever (DHF). For many years, a WHO classification system for distinguishing DF from DHF, and classifying four severity grades of DHF has been used. Although it is being superceded by a newer classification, the older terms are still widely used, and so both are described here.

Tropical Medicine Lecture Notes, Seventh edition. Edited by Nick Beeching and Geoff Gill. © 2014 John Wiley & Sons, Ltd. Published 2014 by John Wiley & Sons, Ltd.

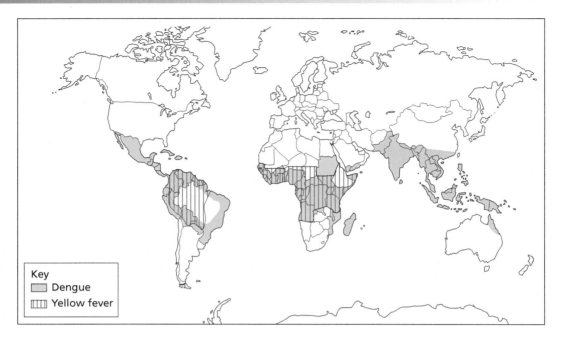

Figure 42.1 Map showing the approximate distribution of dengue and yellow fever viruses (see further reading for revised local maps).

Dengue fever

This is a classical fever–arthralgia–rash syndrome (Chapter 40), with retro-orbital pain, photophobia, lymphadenopathy and, in about 50% of patients, a rash. This is usually maculopapular, but may be mottling or flushing. In addition, there may be petechiae and other bleeding manifestations including gum, nose or gastrointestinal haemorrhage; according to the previous WHO classification of dengue, these features would not define it as DHF – see below (Table 42.1). About one-third of patients have a positive tourniquet test (a blood pressure cuff inflated to half way between systolic and diastolic pressure for 5min produces 20 or more petechiae in a 2.5-cm square on the forearm).

Dengue hemorrhagic fever

Initially, patients have a non-specific febrile illness, which may include a petechial rash. Then on the third to seventh day of illness, as the fever subsides, there is a massive increase in vascular permeability (this is the major pathophysiological process). This leads to plasma leakage from the blood vessels into the tissue, causing an elevated haematocrit, oedema and effusions. In addition,

there is thrombocytopenia and haemorrhagic manifestations.

If a positive tourniquet test is the only such manifestation, then this was defined as DHF grade I according to the previous classification system (Table 42.1). If there is spontaneous bleeding this is grade II. In grade III, the plasma leakage is sufficient to cause shock (defined in children as a pulse pressure <20 mmHg). In grade IV, the blood pressure is unrecordable. Collectively, grades III and IV are known as dengue shock syndrome (DSS). Patients with DHF are restless or lethargic, and often have tender hepatomegaly or abdominal pain.

In adults, especially the elderly, fever, abdominal pain and rash are less often seen. In this group gastrointestinal bleeding, bacteraemia, and acute renal failure are more common, and may be associated with a poor outcome

New WHO classifications of dengue infections

The previous WHO classification system had several limitations: the implication was that haemorrhage is the cardinal manifestation of disease, whereas plasma leakage into the interstitia is more

Table 42.1 Traditional World Health Organization criteria for distinguishing dengue fever (DF) and dengue haemorrhagic fever (DHF) grades I–IV. DHF grades III and IV are collectively known as dengue shock syndrome (DSS)

	Plasma leakage*	Platelets (/µL)	Circulatory collapse	Haemorrhagic manifestations
DF	No	Variable	Absent	Variable
DHF I	Present	<100 000	Absent	Positive tourniquet test (or easy bruising)
DHF II	Present	<100 000	Absent	Spontaneous bleeding[†] with or without positive tourniquet test
DHF III	Present	<100 000	PP<20 mmHg[‡]	Spontaneous bleeding and/or positive tourniquet test
DHF IV	Present	<100 000	Pulse and BP undetectable	Spontaneous bleeding and/or positive tourniquet test

BP, blood pressure; DF, dengue fever; DHF, dengue haemorrhagic fever; PP, pulse pressure.
*Identified by haematocrit 20% above normal, or clinical signs of plasma leakage.
[†]Skin petechiae, mucosal or gastrointestinal bleeding.
[‡]Pulse pressure less than 20 mmHg, or hypotension for age.

important; many patients with severe disease did not meet all the criteria required for DHF; the classification required regular platelet and haematocrit measurements, which are not possible in many areas where dengue occurs; finally, it ignores other important manifestations such as neurological dengue disease.

For this reason, a newer classification has been adopted which describes patients as having dengue with or without warning signs (of more severe disease), and severe dengue (Fig. 42.2). Warning signs of severe disease include abdominal pain or tenderness, persistent vomiting, clinical fluid accumulation, mucosal bleeding, lethargy or restlessness, liver enlargement >2 cm, or increase in hematocrit concurrent with rapid decrease in platelet count). Patients with 'severe dengue' have signs of severe plasma leakage (i.e. leading to shock or fluid accumulation with respiratory distress), severe haemorrhage (as defined by the treating physician), or severe organ impairment (defined as liver transaminase level ≥1000 iu/L, impaired consciousness, or severe involvement of the heart or other organs).

Investigations

Leucopenia and thrombocytopenia are common. In the first few days of illness dengue virus can be isolated from plasma or detected by polymerase chain reaction (PCR). After the fever subsides, IgM and then IgG antibodies can be detected by ELISA. New enzyme immunoassay kits allow rapid diagnosis in the field. Rapid assays for measuring the viral antigens are also available. Lateral chest X-ray may show a pleural effusion in DHF. See Box 42.1.

Box 42.1 Differential diagnosis of dengue

Fever with arthralgia or rash

- *Arboviruses:* Chikungunya, O'nyong nyong, sindbis, West Nile, Ross River, Oropouche, sandfly fevers, Colorado tick fever, Zika virus
- *Other viruses:* rubella, measles, herpes, enteroviruses
- *Bacteria:* meningococcus, typhoid
- *Spirochaetes:* leptospirosis, Lyme disease, relapsing fevers
- *Rickettsiae:* tick and endemic typhus, Rocky Mountain spotted fever
- *Parasites:* malaria

Fever with haemorrhage

- *Arboviruses:* yellow fever, Crimean–Congo haemorrhagic fever, Rift Valley fever, Omsk haemorrhagic fever
- *Other viruses:* hantaviruses, fulminant hepatitis (A–E); Lassa; South American haemorrhagic fevers, Ebola, Marburg
- Any severe sepsis with disseminated intravascular coagulation (DIC)
- Drug reactions

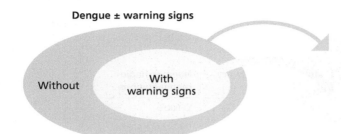

Dengue ± warning signs

Without | With warning signs

Severe dengue

1. Severe plasma leakage
2. Severe haemorrhage
3. Severe organ impairment

Criteria for dengue ± warning signs		Criteria for severe dengue
Probable dengue Live in/travel to dengue endemic area. Fever and two of the following criteria: • Nausea, vomitng • Rash • Aches and pains • Tourniquet test positive • Leucopenia • Any warning sign **Laboratory confirmed dengue** (Important when no sign of plasma leakage)	**Warning signs*** • Abdominal pain or tenderness • Persistent vomiting • Clinical fluid accumulation • Mucosal bleed • Lethargy, restlessness • Liver enlargement >2 cm • *Laboratory:* Increase in HCT concurrent with rapid decrease in platelet count **Requiring strict observation and medical intervention*	**1. Severe plasma leakage** leading to: • Shock (DSS) • Fluid accumulation with respiratory distress **2. Severe bleeding** as evaluated by clinician **3. Severe organ involvement** • Liver: AST or ALT>=1000 • CNS: Impaired consciousness • Heart and other organs

Figure. 42.2 The revised dengue case classification. *Source:* WHO (2009).

Management

Dengue fever

Most cases are self-limiting. Oral fluids should be encouraged, and paracetamol given. Patients may have a maculopapular recovery rash and prolonged lethargy and depression after recovery are common. Aspirin should be avoided.

Dengue haemorrhagic fever

For grades I and II DHF, oral fluids should be encouraged, vital signs closely monitored, as well as haematocrit and platelet count, which may warn of deterioration to grades III and IV. For grades III and IV (dengue shock syndrome), central venous pressure (CVP) should be monitored if possible. Intravenous crystalloid (10–20 mL/kg/h) should be given, followed by intravenous colloid if shock persists. Patients should be watched carefully for fluid overload, and infusions reduced accordingly.

Other severe manifestations of dengue infection

These include hepatitis, or fulminant hepatic failure (Reye-like syndrome) as well as neurological complications (metabolic encephalopathy, cerebral oedema or, occasionally, viral encephalitis).

Pathogenesis of dengue haemorrhagic fever

Current evidence suggests two mechanisms may be important:

1 *Antibody-dependent enhancement* – antibodies against one dengue virus serotype (from a previous infection) enhance the entry of a second dengue virus into macrophages, leading to a more severe infection.
2 Viral strain differences – e.g. increased virulence of South East Asian strains of dengue-2 virus.

Prevention

Prevention is by control of *Aedes* mosquitoes. Methods include treating stored water with larvicides (e.g. temephos), educating people to remove collections of water around the house (e.g. in rubbish), and spraying with insecticide during epidemics.

Future developments include tetravalent vaccines (effective against all four dengue serotypes), which are in development, for example, live attenuated vaccines and recombinant copy DNA infectious clone vaccines. However, no vaccine is currently licensed.

Yellow fever

Epidemiology

Yellow fever virus is naturally transmitted between primates by various mosquitoes in jungle cycles in Central America and Africa (Fig. 41.1 and Fig. 42.1). *Aedes aegypti* transmits the virus to humans in urban cycles. The disease has reemerged in South America since the 1970s, when the Aedes eradication programme was relaxed. There are an estimated 200 000 cases, with 30 000 deaths annually. Declining population immunity to infection, deforestation, urbanization, population movements and climate change are all thought to have contributed to the increased number of yellow fever cases over the past two decades.

Clinical features

The illness is biphasic and often mild. Severe disease is characterized by jaundice, fulminant hepatic failure and gastrointestinal bleeding. Faget's sign is the failure of the heart rate to increase with a rising temperature and is indicative of cardiac damage. Elevated liver function tests, leucopenia, thrombocytopenia and clotting abnormalities may occur. Liver histology reveals Councilman bodies, which also occur in Crimean–Congo haemorrhagic fever and Rift Valley fever.

Control

Yellow fever control consists of use of the highly effective 17D live attenuated vaccine. This vaccine is safe, affordable and highly effective, and appears to provide protection for 30–35 years or more. The vaccine provides effective immunity within one week for 95% of persons vaccinated. In recent years there have been increasing reports of adverse events, particularly in older adults receiving immunization for the first time. The risk of death from yellow fever far outweighs the risk of adverse events for those living in endemic or epidemic settings. However, vaccine is not recommended for:

- children aged less than 9 months for routine immunization (or less than 6 months during an epidemic);
- pregnant women – **except** during a yellow fever outbreak when the risk of infection is high;
- people with severe allergies to egg protein;
- people with severe immunodeficiency due to symptomatic HIV/AIDS or other causes, or in the presence of a thymus disorder;
- older travellers visiting low-risk areas in a country where yellow fever transmission occurs (detailed individual risk assessment required).

Vector control is as for dengue fever.

SUMMARY

- Dengue virus is numerically the most important arbovirus infecting humans, with an estimated 100 million cases per year and 2.5 billion people at risk.

- Factors implicated in the spread of dengue viruses include poor control of its principal vector, *Aedes aegypti* as well as reintroduction of this insect into Central and South America and expansion of the range of the other main vector *Aedes albopictus*.

- Symptoms of dengue include retro-orbital pain, photophobia, severe muscle pain, lymphadenopathy and in about 50% of patients, a rash. In addition, there may be petechiae and other bleeding manifestations including gum, nose or gastrointestinal haemorrhage.

- More severe bleeding manifestations occur mostly in children exposed to repeated infection, but stroke and other major bleeds may complicate infection in adults.

- Yellow fever virus is naturally transmitted between primates by various mosquitoes in jungle cycles in Central America and Africa. *Aedes aegypti* transmits the virus to humans in urban cycles.

- Yellow fever illness is biphasic and often mild. Severe disease is characterized by jaundice, fulminant hepatic failure and gastrointestinal bleeding.

- Effective vaccines exist to prevent yellow fever, with rare viscerotropic and neurotropic side effects in the elderly, pregnant women and severe immunosuppression.

 Visit www.lecturenoteseries.com/tropicalmed to test yourself on this chapter using interactive MCQs.

📖 FURTHER READING

Anon (2012) The safety of yellow fever vaccine 17D or 17DD in children, pregnant women, HIV+ individuals, and older persons: systematic review. *Am J Trop Med Hyg* **86**: 359–72. [Review.]

DengueMap: a website produced by HealthMap in collaboration with the CDC which has up to date information on dengue disease. http://www.healthmap.org/dengue/index.php

Jentes ES, Poumerol G, Gershman MD, *et al.* (2011) The revised global yellow fever risk map and recommendations for vaccination, 2010: consensus of the Informal WHO Working Group on Geographic Risk for Yellow Fever. *Lancet Infect Dis* **11**(8): 622–32. Erratum in: *Lancet Infect Dis* 2012; **12**: 98. [Important update of maps, to assist risk assessment as part of revised International Health Regulations.]

Lee IK, Liu JW, Yang KD (2012) Fatal dengue hemorrhagic fever in adults: emphasizing the evolutionary pre-fatal clinical and laboratory manifestations. *PLoS Negl Trop Dis* **6**(2): e1532.

National Travel Health Network and Centre (NaTHNaC) website http://www.nathnac.org/pro/factsheets/yellow.htm [Updated information on outbreaks and travel-related issues including yellow fever.]

Simmons CP, Farrar JJ, Nguyen van Vinh Chau N, Wills B (2012) Dengue. *N Engl J Med* **66**: 1423–32. [Recent comprehensive review.]

Thomas RE, Lorenzetti DL, Spragins W, Jackson D, Williamson T (2012) The safety of yellow fever vaccine 17D or 17DD in children, pregnant women, HIV+ individuals, and older persons: systematic review. *Am J Trop Med Hyg*; **86**: 359–72. doi: 10.4269/ajtmh.2012.11-0525. [Free on-line review]

World Health Organization (2009) *Dengue: Guidelines for Diagnosis, Treatment, Prevention and Control – New Edition.* Geneva: WHO.

43

Relapsing fevers

Tim O'Dempsey
Liverpool School of Tropical Medicine

Relapsing fevers are caused by various species of *Borrelia*. They fall into two main categories: epidemic or louse-borne relapsing fever (LBRF) caused by *Borrelia recurrentis*; and endemic or tick-borne relapsing fever (TBRF) caused by numerous other species of *Borrelia*, depending on the geographical location. Untreated, these infections are characterized by a series of febrile episodes, often associated with systemic symptoms, separated by periods of relative well-being. TBRF is usually clinically milder and may be associated with up to 11 relapses, whereas LBRF is more severe but seldom gives rise to more than three relapses.

Epidemiology

Louse-borne relapsing fever, in common with many louse-borne infections, tends to occur in epidemics in situations of poor hygiene and overcrowding, such as in prisons and among refugee, displaced and homeless populations. The disease is most common in the highland regions of Ethiopia and Burundi and, to a lesser extent, in other highland areas of Africa, India and the Andes. Humans are the reservoir host. The louse, most commonly the human body louse (*Pediculus humanus*) but also occasionally the head louse (*P. capitis*) and, possibly, the crab louse (*Phthirus pubis*), becomes infected following a blood meal and remains infected for life. The louse provokes itching and is crushed when the host scratches, releasing *Borrelia* which enter the new host via abrasions and mucous membranes. Blood-borne and congenital infections may also occur.

TBRF occurs in geographically widespread endemic foci: central, eastern and southern Africa (*B. duttonii*); North-Western Africa and the Iberian peninsula (*B. hispanica*); central Asia and parts of the Middle East, India and China (*B. persica*); and various regions of the Americas (*B. hermsii*, *B. turicatae*, *B. venezuelensis*). Animal reservoirs include wild rodents, lizards, toads and owls. Recently *Borrelia* species have been identified in pigs and chickens in East Africa, raising the possibility that domestic animals also may be implicated as reservoir hosts. Transmission to humans occurs following the bite of an infected argasid (soft) tick of the genus *Ornithodorus* via tick saliva or coxal fluid. Soft ticks favour cool, relatively humid environments such as caves or the mud walls or thatch of huts. They exhibit 'transovarial transmission': vertical transmission of *Borrelia* from one tick generation to the next without further exposure to a reservoir host. Human congenital infections may also occur.

A recent study in rural Senegal concluded that the incidence of TBRF was higher than that of any other bacterial disease and that TBRF was likely to be a common cause of disease in similar rural communities elsewhere in West Africa.

Pathology

Borreliae multiply in blood by simple fission and are taken up by the reticuloendothelial system. They have a predisposition for the liver (sometimes resulting in intrahepatic biliary obstruction), spleen and the central nervous system (CNS). Widespread vascular endothelial damage and platelet sequestration in the bone marrow occur. Myocardial and pulmonary damage are also common. Clinical severity tends to correlate with the level of spirochaetaemia. Relapses result from antigenic variation.

Tropical Medicine Lecture Notes, Seventh edition. Edited by Nick Beeching and Geoff Gill. © 2014 John Wiley & Sons, Ltd. Published 2014 by John Wiley & Sons, Ltd.

Clinical features

The incubation period is usually 4–8 days (range 2–15). Typically, there is a sudden onset of high fever accompanied by headache, confusion, meningism, myalgia, arthralgia, nausea, vomiting and, sometimes, dysphagia.

Dyspnoea and cough may be severe and, if productive, sputum may contain *Borrelia*. Hepatomegaly is common and is associated with jaundice in 50% of patients with LBRF and in less than 10% of those with TBRF. Splenomegaly is common and may be associated with an increased risk of rupture. Petechiae, erythematous rashes, epistaxis, conjunctival injection and haemorrhages are more common in LBRF. Complications include pneumonia, nephritis, parotitis, arthritis, cranial and peripheral neuropathies, meningoencephalitis, meningitis, acute ophthalmitis and iritis. Myocarditis may give rise to sudden and fatal arrhythmias. Most complications are more common and more severe in LBRF. Case fatality rates may reach 70% in epidemics of LBRF. In contrast, with the exception of children and pregnant women, case fatality rates rarely exceed 10% in untreated cases of TBRF.

Differential diagnosis

The differential diagnosis is wide and includes malaria, typhus, typhoid, meningococcal septicaemia/meningitis, dengue, hepatitis, leptospirosis, yellow fever and other viral haemorrhagic fevers.

Diagnosis

Borrelia are large spirochaetes measuring 10–30 × 0.2–0.5 µm. They are visible in Giemsa or Field stained blood films, and may be a surprise finding in a patient with suspected malaria. Dual infections of with malaria and *Borrelia* may occur and, usually the latter, may be overlooked. The spirochaetes are also visible unstained using darkfield or phase-contrast microscopy. They may be concentrated above the buffy coat following centrifugation of anticoagulated whole blood. The acridine orange-coated quantitative buffy coat (QBC) technique is also useful. Infected blood or cerebrospinal fluid (CSF) inoculated into mice or rats yields borreliae in the peripheral blood after 2–3 days. Serology is unreliable. Examination of the vector may also be useful. PCR assays are becoming available for diagnosis and speciation. In a recent study, PCR was shown to be at least twice as sensitive as microscopy for detecting *Borrelia* infections among children in Tanzania and led to the discovery of a new species of *Borrelia*.

Treatment

A single dose of antibiotic is effective in about 95% of cases of LBRF and in up to 80% of those with TBRF. However, the usual practice is to give a 5-10-day course to minimize the likelihood of relapses. Effective antibiotics include tetracycline, doxycycline, penicillin, erythromycin, chloramphenicol and ciprofloxacin. Ceftriaxone is recommended for patients presenting with meningitis or encephalitis. The choice will depend on drug availability, age, allergies, whether the patient is pregnant and one's confidence in the diagnosis.

A potentially fatal Jarisch–Herxheimer reaction (JHR) has been reported in up to 80–90% of patients treated for LBRF and in up to 50% of those treated for TBRF. A JHR is more likely to occur in patients treated with bactericidal antibiotics (e.g. penicillins and cephalosporins). The JHR usually follows within two hours of the first dose of antibiotic and is characterized by intense rigors, restlessness and anxiety. The temperature rises sharply accompanied by an initial rise in pulse rate and blood pressure. This is followed by marked vasodilation and sweating, sometimes resulting in collapse and shock. Patients must be closely monitored for this complication and may require intravenous fluids to maintain blood pressure. If available, meptazinol, an opioid antagonist, should be given to reduce the severity of the reaction. Anti-tumour necrosis factor alpha antibiodies may also be effective. Steroids are of no benefit.

Prevention and control

Prevention of LBRF is largely a matter of improving hygiene, reducing crowding and delousing. Post-exposure antibiotic prophylaxis with tetracycline or doxycycline may be recommended in high-risk situations. TBRF is best prevented by avoiding tick habitats.

SUMMARY

- Louse-borne relapsing fever (LBRF) is caused by *Borrelia recurrentis* and tick-borne relapsing fever (TBRF) by various other *Borrelia* species. LBRF is often described as 'epidemic', and TBRF as 'endemic'.

- Relapsing fevers remain common infections in some tropical areas. The condition causes a septicaemia-like illness, but a variety of complications can occur.

- Complications are more common with LBRF, and include meningitis, neuropathies, arthritis, parotitis, iritis and myocarditis.

- Antibiotic treatment (e.g. doxycycline or penicillin) is effective, but a Jarisch-Herxheimer reaction (JHR) can occur.

 Visit www.lecturenoteseries.com/tropicalmed to test yourself on this chapter using interactive MCQs.

📖 FURTHER READING

Guerrier G, Doherty T (2011) Comparison of antibiotic regimens for treating louse-borne relapsing fever: a meta-analysis. *Trans Roy Soc Trop Med Hyg* **105**:483–90. [Recent meta-analysis with recommendations for antibiotic treatment of LBRF based on best, albeit limited, available evidence.]

Parola P, Raoult D (2001) Ticks and tickborne bacterial diseases in humans: an emerging infectious threat. *Clin Infect Dis* **32**: 897–928. [This article reviews and illustrates various aspects of the biology of ticks and the tickborne bacterial diseases – rickettsioses, ehrlichioses, Lyme disease, relapsing fever borrelioses, tularaemia and Q fever – particularly those regarded as emerging diseases.]

Raoult D, Ndihokubwayo JB, Tissot-Dupont H *et al.* (1998) Outbreak of epidemic typhus associated with trench fever in Burundi. *Lancet* **352**: 353–8. [This epidemic highlights the appalling conditions in central African refugee camps and the failure of public health programmes to serve their inhabitants.]

Kisinza WN. McCall PJ. Mitani H. Talbert A, Fukunaga M (2003) A newly identified tick-borne *Borrelia* species and relapsing fever in Tanzania. *Lancet* **362**: 1283–4. [Illustrates how advances in molecular techniques are leading to some interesting new discoveries concerning the epidemiology and clinical importance of *Borrelia* infections.]

McCall PJ, Hume J, Motshegwa K, *et al.* (2007) Does tick-borne relapsing fever have an animal reservoir in East Africa? *Vector-Borne and Zoonotic Diseases* **7**: 1–8. [Reports interesting epidemiological findings on TBRF in East Africa.]

Vial L, Diatta G, Tall A, *et al.* (2006) Incidence of tick-borne relapsing fever in West Africa: longitudinal study. *Lancet* **368**: 37–43. [Highlights the importance of TBRF as a common cause of fever in parts of rural West Africa.]

44

Rickettsial infections

Geoff Gill
Liverpool School of Tropical Medicine

There are many species and subspecies of *Rickettsiae* that can infect humans. They may also infect rodents, and are transmitted to humans by the bites, body fluids or faeces of a variety of arthropods. The illness is very variable in intensity, but is characterized by fever and rash. There is therefore often a wide differential diagnosis. In this chapter only the three main types of typhus seen worldwide are considered: louse-borne typhus, scrub typhus and African tick typhus.

Louse-borne typhus

This is caused by *Rickettsia prowazekii*, which is transmitted to humans from the infected faeces of the human body louse, *Pediculus humanus*, usually by being scratched into the skin. Louse-borne typhus may be epidemic, and occurs particularly in malnourished migrant populations with poor hygiene (e.g. in refugee camps). The disease can occur in wide geographical areas; indeed it was common in Europe in the 19th century and was a frequent cause of death in concentration camps in World War II.

Clinical features

The disease incubates for about 12 days following which there is high fever, myalgia, headache and prostration. The conjunctivae may be suffused and delirium is common. A rash appears on about the third or fourth day – it is central and macular, although the lesions may later become petechial or purpuric. Pneumonia and/or meningoencephalitis frequently occur later, as can sometimes myocarditis. Untreated, the disease has a high mortality. Diagnosis is usually made clinically, especially in epidemic situations. The Weil–Felix serological test can still be useful, but modern, specific serological and polymerase chain reaction (PCR) techniques are better.

Treatment

As well as full supportive medical and nursing care, the disease usually responds well and rapidly to either tetracycline or chloramphenicol as below.

- Tetracycline 500 mg four times daily (adult dose) orally or intravenously for 1 week.
- Chloramphenicol 500 mg four times daily (adult dose) orally or intravenously for 1 week.
- Doxycycline 200 mg daily (or 100 mg b.d.) for 7 days.

Preventive measures are important in epidemics; as well as delousing procedures, 200 mg doxycycline as a single dose to all those at risk may be useful.

Scrub typhus

This is also known as mite typhus or Tsutsugamushi fever. It is caused by *Orientia tsutsugamushi* (previously known as *Rickettsia orientalis* or *R tsutsugamushi*). It is a zoonosis of rodents, and humans are infected by the bites of infected larval mites. Scrub typhus occurs in wide parts of South East Asia, Oceania and northern parts of Australia.

Clinical features

The incubation period is 5–10 days, and a small eschar may be noted at the site of the mite bite. There is an abrupt fever, as well as headache, myalgia and prostration, as in louse-borne typhus. The rash is also similar. Lymphadenopathy may be generalized or local (related to the eschar). Hepatosplenomegaly

Tropical Medicine Lecture Notes, Seventh edition. Edited by Nick Beeching and Geoff Gill. © 2014 John Wiley & Sons, Ltd. Published 2014 by John Wiley & Sons, Ltd.

may also occur, as may pneumonia and myocarditis. Delirium is frequently marked, although neuropsychiatric features are not as prominent as in louse-borne typhus and the overall mortality is lower. Hearing loss is under-recognized. Diagnosis is usually clinically based. The Weil–Felix test is insensitive in this form of typhus.

Treatment

Tetracycline and chloramphenicol are effective, in regimens as in other forms of typhus (see above). However, the simplest and most optimal treatment is doxycycline 200 mg orally once daily for 3–7 days.

Resistance to both tetracycline and chloramphenicol has been reported in northern Thailand, and here rifampicin or ciprofloxacin may have to be used. Preventive measures include avoidance of mite-infested areas, impregnation of clothing with permethrin and prophylactic doxycycline (200 mg weekly while in high-risk areas).

African tick typhus

There are various forms of tick typhus (e.g. Rocky Mountain spotted fever, Siberian tick typhus, Queensland tick typhus, etc.). African tick typhus occurs in wide areas of Africa, but particularly central and southern parts. The causative organism is usually *R. africae*, which has a reservoir in cattle, domestic cattle and even in the hippopotamus and rhinoceros. A variety of tick species are involved as both vectors and reservoirs. The infection is usually caught by hikers and campers in veld areas or grasslands. The disease may present as an 'imported' tropical infection when travellers and holidaymakers return home.

Clinical features

The illness mimics a mild attack of scrub typhus. There is usually a noticeable eschar with local lymphadenopathy, and a mild fever with toxaemic symptoms. A central maculopapular rash later spreads to the limbs. The disease is brief and complications are rare. There is almost no mortality. Diagnosis is usually clinically based.

Treatment

Mild cases may not require treatment. If necessary, tetracycline or chloramphenicol can be used as above, or doxycycline 200 mg for 3–7 days. Azithromycin is also effective, but less widely available. Preventive measures include tick-avoidance strategies such as appropriate clothing and insect repellents.

> **SUMMARY**
>
> - There are various forms of typhus, transmitted by different insects.
> - Fever and rash are the commonest features. Some types (e.g. louse-borne) can cause serious illness.
> - African tick typhus is very common in sub-Saharan Africa, and usually causes a mild illness.
> - Tetracycline drugs are the most useful anti-rickettsial agents (usually doxycycline).

 Visit www.lecturenoteseries.com/tropicalmed to test yourself on this chapter using interactive MCQs.

📖 FURTHER READING

Bechah Y, Capo C, Mege J-L, Raoult D (2008) Epidemic typhus. *Lancet Infect Dis* **8**: 417–26. [Useful review of louse-borne typhus.]

Oostvagel PM, van Doornum GJ, Ferreira R, *et al.* (2007) African tickbite fever in travelers to Swaziland. *Emerg Infect Dis* **13**: 353–5. [One of a number of reports in recent years emphasizing the increasing problem of African tick typhus presenting after travellers and holidaymakers have returned to their home countries, including Europe.]

Renvoise A, Mediannikor O, Raoult D (2009) Old and new tick-borne rickettsioses. *Int Health* **1**: 17–25. [Good review of tick-borne typhus.]

45

Leptospirosis

Alastair Miller
Liverpool School of Tropical Medicine

Introduction

Leptospirosis is a zoonotic infection that can cause a variety of clinical pictures in man ranging from asymptomatic infection to fulminant hepato-renal failure (Weil's disease). It has a worldwide distribution (except for the Polar regions) but can cause particular problems in the tropics.

Microbiology

The causative organism belongs to the genus *Leptospira* which is part of the Spirochaete family (that also includes *Treponema* and *Borrelia*). The nomenclature of the leptospires is complex and undergoes frequent change. Historically there were two species (*L. interrogans* and *L. bireflexa* – not known to be related to human disease) but these have recently been reclassified. There are about 250 serovars that are potentially pathogenic and there is some evidence that certain serovars may be more associated with severe disease.

Epidemiology

Rodents and other small mammals are the most important animal reservoirs. They are usually infected during infancy and continue with chronic renal infection for life. They excrete the organism in the urine to infect other mammals or humans. Larger mammals such as dogs and cattle may become chronic carriers or they may develop symptomatic infection that may be fatal. Excreted organisms may remain viable in soil or water for weeks and the incidence of infection is of-ten higher after heavy rainfall and flooding. Over 3000 cases were reported in the Philippine floods of 2009. Those most at risk have direct contact with soil, water or animals. Therefore, at particular risk are farmers, veterinary workers, sewage workers and the military. In a Western setting, infection is frequently acquired recreationally by canoeists or triathletes. In one of the most well know outbreaks in Sabah (Borneo) in 2000, 42% of competitors in an adventure race met the case definition for clinical leptospirosis.

Pathogenesis

Infection is produced by leptospirae penetrating the skin through minor cuts and abrasions or by penetrating mucous membranes. It is not established whether they can penetrate intact skin. The bacteria are disseminated via the bloodstream and are therefore widely distributed through the body where they produce a vasculitis, the exact mechanism of which remains obscure.

Clinical features

This is incredibly variable. Many of those infected will have an asymptomatic seroconversion. Others may have a mild non-specific febrile illness and others may have one of the more easily appreciated syndromes. The average incubation period seems to be about 10 days although it is usually difficult to establish exactly when infection occurred and a range of incubations from 2 to 26 days has been reported. The majority of symptomatic cases then present with sudden onset of fever, rigors, myalgia and headache. Nausea, vomiting, diarrhoea and cough are also common

Tropical Medicine Lecture Notes, Seventh edition. Edited by Nick Beeching and Geoff Gill. © 2014 John Wiley & Sons, Ltd. Published 2014 by John Wiley & Sons, Ltd.

features. On examination, the most characteristic findings are conjunctival suffusion and muscle tenderness but these probably only occur in a minority of cases. Physical findings described more rarely include lymphadenopathy, hepatosplenomegaly, chest signs and a rash. Clinical features of meningitis may also be present. Although the illness is classically described as 'biphasic', in practice such a pattern is rarely recognized. However, as the immune response appears the patient may deteriorate and develop one of the more specific syndromes associated with leptospira infection.

These include the following.

- Aseptic meningitis – this may occur in up to 50–80% of cases and is difficult to distinguish from other causes of aseptic meningitis.
- Weil's disease – this is the classical presentation of jaundice, thrombocytopenia and renal failure. Despite the jaundice, liver function is usually relatively well preserved.
- Pulmonary syndrome – this has been described especially in South America and may vary from mild respiratory symptoms and signs to severe pulmonary haemorrhage and adult respiratory distress syndrome. A recent study in Peru suggested that nearly 4% of patients with serologically confirmed *Leptospira* infection had severe pulmonary manifestations and would not have been diagnosed had they not been part of the study.
- Cardiac syndrome – recently severe cardiac involvement has been described in India and Sri Lanka, with myocarditis leading to cardiac failure.

Several of these syndromes may coexist.

Diagnosis

The differential diagnosis during the non-specific febrile phase is wide and includes malaria, typhoid, influenza, rickettsial infection (especially scrub typhus) and arbovirus infections (including dengue). Routine laboratory investigations are similarly non-specific – white cell count may be elevated or lowered (usual range 3000 to 25 000 × 10^9/L) often with a left shift. About half the patients have elevations of liver transaminases (fairly mild) and creatine kinase. The urine is often abnormal with proteinuria, white cells, casts and occasionally microscopic haematuria. In Weil's disease, the renal function deteriorates and the serum bilirubin may be very high. Chest X-ray may show non-specific shadowing. The platelet count is sometimes be reduced. The CSF may show an elevated white cell count with neutrophils or lymphocytes, minimal to moderately elevated protein concentrations and normal glucose.

Because of the non-specific nature of the clinical picture and the laboratory findings, a high index of suspicion must be maintained if the diagnosis is not to be missed.

Leptospirae can be seen microscopically in blood or urine but sensitivity and specificity is low and these techniques are rarely used in practice. The organism can also be isolated in blood cultures from specimens taken from the patient in the first 10 days of illness and before antibiotics have been administered. Urine cultures may become positive a week into the illness and remain positive for some time afterwards. A urinary antigen test was described but does not seem to have been developed further.

Most patients have their infection identified serologically. The traditional gold standard test has been the microscopic agglutination (MAT) test that uses live organisms and can be technically difficult to perform. Therefore, most laboratories would use a screening test first such as an ELISA for IgM antibodies – these are usually detectable on day 5 of illness. Polymerase chain reaction (PCR) methods are in development but are not yet widely used.

Treatment

Leptospirosis is sensitive to many antibiotics and many have been used to treat it (eg ceftriaxone, penicillin, doxycycline and azithromycin). There is dispute over how effective antibiotics are, unless they are given very early in the natural history of the condition and there is similar doubt about the need to treat mild disease. In endemic areas it is common for leptospirosis to be misdiagnosed as a rickettsial infection or vice versa, therefore oral doxycycline 100 mg b.d. is a sensible empirical option effective against both conditions while awaiting serological confirmation. If the patient is very unwell, intravenous penicillin 1.2 G 6 hourly or ceftriaxone 1 gm once daily should be used. There are no trials on duration of therapy but 10 days is usually recommended, although a recent trial in Thailand suggested that 3 days of azithromycin is as effective as 7 days of doxycycline.

Prevention

The risk of infection can be reduced by avoiding high risk exposure. A human vaccine has been used but is not widely available. A vaccine is used in veterinary practice. A study from 1984 showed significant benefit of weekly doxycycline 200 mg amongst US troops in the jungles of Panama.

SUMMARY

- Leptospirosis is a zoonoses with a worldwide distribution, spread to humans via contamination of the environment by infected animal urine.
- Rodents are the most important animal reservoirs.
- Excreted organisms may remain viable in water or soil for weeks; flooding is commonly followed by an increase in local cases.
- Clinical features vary from minor fever to severe hepatorenal failure, often accompanied by conjunctival haemorrhages. Other severe complications include pulmonary disease, myocarditis and and meningoencephalitis.
- Although the evidence base for effectiveness of antibiotic therapy is poor, most patients are treated with penicillin, doxycycline, ceftriaxone or azithromycin.

Visit www.lecturenoteseries.com/tropicalmed to test yourself on this chapter using interactive MCQs.

FURTHER READING

Brett-Major DM, Coldren R (2012) Antibiotics for leptospirosis. *Cochrane Database Syst Rev* **15**(2): CD008264. doi: 10.1002/14651858.CD008264.pub2. [Comprehensive review.]

Helmerhorst HJ, van Tol EN, Tuinman PR, *et al.* (2012) Severe pulmonary manifestation of leptospirosis. *Neth J Med* **70**(5): 215–21. [Report of travel related case and detailed review of under-recognised syndrome. Free download.]

Navinan MR, Rajapakse S (2012) Cardiac involvement in leptospirosis. *Trans R Soc Trop Med Hyg* **106**: 515–20. [Useful review.] http://www.hpa.org.uk/Topics/InfectiousDiseases/InfectionsAZ/Leptospirosis [Useful links to wide variety of helpful websites.]

46

Melioidosis

David Lalloo
Liverpool School of Tropical Medicine

Epidemiology

Melioidosis is caused by the Gram-negative bacillus, *Burkholderia pseudomallei*. In endemic areas, the organism can be easily found in the soil and surface water such as in rice paddies, but only certain strains are pathogenic to humans. Melioidosis was initially recognized as a serious problem during the Vietnam war and now causes clinical disease in a relatively geographical constrained area of South East Asia. In Thailand, the most affected country, 3000–5000 new cases are diagnosed annually. Clinical cases are also regularly reported from Vietnam, Malaysia, Singapore and northern Australia, although sporadic cases occur over a far greater geographical area including India, China, the Caribbean and Brazil.

Pathogenesis

Infection is acquired primarily by inoculation of contaminated soil or water, but may also be acquired by inhalation. Most infection is asymptomatic; organisms may remain latent within macrophages and can cause disease many years after infection. Localized abscesses may develop at the site of inoculation which can lead to bacteraemia and dissemination of the organism. Up to 70% of patients have predisposing diseases. Diabetes mellitus is the most common, but chronic renal impairment, cirrhosis, steroid therapy and malignancy are also important. There is no association with HIV infection.

Clinical features

Many individuals are found to have positive serology without having had obvious clinical symptoms. Acute presentations can be with localized or septicaemic disease. The most common form of localized disease is pneumonia, but abscesses may also be found in the skin and soft tissue or organs such as the spleen and liver. Localized disease may lead to subsequent bacteraemia. Septicaemic disease is associated with a poor prognosis: an obvious focus of disease cannot always be found. If patients survive the initial stages of septicaemic disease, dissemination can occur to cause abscesses in a number of different sites.

Diagnosis

Definitive diagnosis of melioidosis is by culture of the organism from blood or pus. Molecular techniques are available but are of limited utility in routine diagnosis. Serological tests can detect rising titres of IgG or a raised specific IgM in acute infections, but are far less sensitive than culture in endemic areas.

Treatment

Melioidosis is both difficult and expensive to treat. *Burkholderia pseudomallei* is intrinsically resistant to a large number of antibiotics. Initial treatment should be with parenteral ceftazidime or a carbopenem for a minimum of 10 days. Ceftazidime or meropenem are sometimes combined with co-trimoxazole (trimethoprim/sulfamethoxazole), although the value of this is uncertain. Amoxicillin-clavulanate may also be used but has higher treatment failure rates. Several weeks of intravenous therapy may be needed to produce clinical improvement in patients with visceral abscesses. The response of symptoms to treatment is slow: fever may often persist for over a week and does not imply failure of antibiotic therapy.

Oral maintenance therapy is required following completion of parenteral therapy to prevent relapse: relapse rates may reach 25% in severe disease. The combination of doxycycline and co-trimoxazole is cheap and effective if compliance can be maintained. Amoxicillin-clavulanate is less effective and more expensive. 20 weeks' therapy is advocated to reduce the relapse rate to less than 10%. Aggressive supportive therapy is required for individuals with septicaemic disease: the use of granulocyte colony stimulating factor along with meropenem appears to have reduced mortality in Australia. Abscesses should be surgically drained when feasible.

Prognosis

There is a very high mortality rate (up to 50%) in septicaemic melioidosis, even with adequate treatment. Long-term follow-up is necessary to detect relapse.

 SUMMARY

- Meliodosis is caused by the Gram-negative bacillus *Burkholderia pseudomallei*. Infections occur mainly in South East Asia and northern Australia.
- Clinically, patients present with a septicaemic illness or focal infection causing pneumonia or abscesses (both superficial and deep).
- Treatment is difficult, and relapses are common. Initial treatment may be with intravenous ceftazidime (there are other regimens), followed by a combination of doxycycline and co-trimoxazole for 20 weeks.
- Despite adequate treatment, septicaemic meliodosis has a high mortality rate (up to 50%).

 Visit www.lecturenoteseries.com/tropicalmed **to test yourself on this chapter using interactive MCQs.**

FURTHER READING

Wiersinga WJ, Currie BJ, Peacock SJ (2012) Melioidosis. *N Engl J Med* **367**: 1035–44. [Comprehensive review.]

47

Tropical ulcer

Geoff Gill
Liverpool School of Tropical Medicine

Tropical ulcer is a term used to describe ulcers of the ankle and lower leg occurring in the tropics and subtropics that are not typical of other leg ulcers of more definitive aetiology (e.g. Buruli ulcers, diabetes, leprosy).

Clinical features

The vast majority of tropical ulcers occur below the knee, usually around the ankle. They are often initiated by minor trauma, and subjects with poor nutrition are at increased risk (Fig. 47.1). Once developed, the ulcer may become chronic and stable, but also it can run a destructive course with deep tissue invasion, osteitis and risk of amputation. Unlike Buruli ulcer (Chapter 48), tropical ulcers are typically painful.

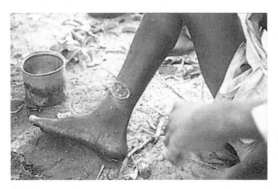

Figure 47.1 A chronic tropical ulcer in a poor and malnourished young Nigerian patient.

Microbiology

There is no single agreed causative organism for tropical ulcers, although early lesions may be colonized or infected by *Bacillus fusiformis*, anaerobes and spirochaetes. Later, tropical ulcers may become infected with a wide variety of organisms, notably staphylococci and/or streptococci.

Epidemiology

Tropical ulcer is seen throughout the tropics and subtropics. Prevalence rates of up to 7% were reported from rural Ethiopia in the early 1990s, but frequency has generally declined since then. Tropical ulcer has been described as a disease of the 'poor and hungry', and it may be that slowly improving socioeconomic conditions and nutrition account for its decline. Urbanization of populations is another factor, as tropical ulcer is usually a rural problem. More widespread use of shoes and socks also provides protection from initiating trauma. Despite this, susceptible individuals still develop tropical ulcers. Sometimes 'outbreaks' can occur; one was recorded in Tanzania in sugar cane workers (cutting the crop in bare feet). The disease was very common amongst Allied prisoners of war working on the Thai–Burma railway in the early 1940s. The men often suffered very severe ulcers which frequently required amputation.

Tropical Medicine Lecture Notes, Seventh edition. Edited by Nick Beeching and Geoff Gill. © 2014 John Wiley & Sons, Ltd. Published 2014 by John Wiley & Sons, Ltd.

Treatment

Antibiotics should be given in adequate dosages. For early ulcers, penicillin is usually sufficient, although later broad-spectrum antibiotics are likely to be needed. Improved nutrition and vitamin supplementation is helpful. The important principle of dressings is that they must be non-adherent (e.g. saline soaks, petroleum jelly impregnated gauze), otherwise they will stick to the ulcer surface and when removed they will disrupt granulation tissue. For sloughy ulcers, honey, sugar paste or paw paw (papaya) are useful inexpensive dressings. Large infected ulcers may require curettage and débridement under anaesthetic. Skin grafting can occasionally be helpful. In extreme cases, amputation may be inevitable.

Prevention

Trauma avoidance is important – in particular wearing adequate footwear. General good health and nutrition also reduce ulcer risk. Adequate and prompt treatment of ankle and leg skin breaks is also important.

Complications

- *Chronic ulceration* – particularly if poorly treated, tropical ulcers may rarely become chronic. In former Far East prisoners of war of World War II, they have been recorded for over 50 years since original development of the ulcer.
- *Deep tissue invasion* – often with bone involvement, and potentially leading to amputation.
- *Recurrent ulceration* – in the same site may occur when a 'paper-thin' scar forms over the ulcer.

- *Squamous cell carcinoma* – may occasionally develop, usually in very chronic cases, and at the edge of the ulcer.
- *Tetanus* – by entry of tetanus bacilli through the ulcer.

SUMMARY

- Tropical ulcers usually affect the lower leg and may run a destructive course with deep tissue invasion.
- Tropical ulcers are usually painful.
- The incidence of tropical ulcer is decreasing.
- The main principle of treatment is adequate debridement of necrotic tissue and covering the wound with non-adherent dressings to allow healing by secondary intention.
- Penicillin is often given as an adjunct and other antibiotics will be needed if the ulcer becomes secondarily infected.

Visit www.lecturenoteseries.com/tropicalmed to test yourself on this chapter using interactive MCQs.

FURTHER READING

Naafs B (2009) Rural dermatology in the tropics. *Clin Dermatol* **27**: 252–70. [A useful review of dermatological disease in the rural tropics, including a section on tropical ulcer.]

Robson D, Welch E, Beeching NJ, Gill GV (2008) Consequences of captivity: health effects of Far East imprisonment in World War II. *Quart J Med* **102**: 87–96. [A summary of tropical disease in captivity amongst 2nd World War Far East POWs, including a description of severe and debilitating tropical ulcer.]

48

Buruli ulcer

Tim O'Dempsey
Liverpool School of Tropical Medicine

Buruli ulcer is a highly destructive ulcerating condition caused by *Mycobacterium ulcerans*. Any part of the body may be affected, particularly areas exposed to minor trauma such as the limbs. *Mycobacterium ulcerans* ranks third among mycobacterial infections affecting immunocompetent humans.

Microbiology

Mycobacterium ulcerans, a slowly growing acid- and alcohol-fast organism, belongs to a large group of environmental mycobacteria. Three different genetic strains have been identified but their relationship to virulence remains uncertain. Local immunosuppression, ulceration and necrosis are caused by mycolactones, soluble polyketide toxins that also appear to be responsible for the painlessness that is characteristic of uncomplicated lesions. There is some evidence that intercurrent helminthic infections may also predispose to ulceration.

Background and epidemiology

Buruli ulcer has been reported from several parts of Africa, notably the Buruli region of Uganda, Ghana, Papua New Guinea, the Americas, South East Asia and China. Buruli ulcer (or Bairnsdale ulcer as it is known 'down under') has also been described among koala bears, possums and Australian golfers.

Predominantly a disease of children, infection is thought to occur following a penetrating injury – usually minor – resulting in inoculation of the organism, which is found naturally in soil or stagnant water. It has been postulated that transmission may also follow the bite of an infected water bug. *Mycobacterium ulcerans* has also been identified in mosquitoes captured during an outbreak in Australia. Whether this is of any epidemiological or clinical significance is unclear. Person–person transmission is very rare.

Clinical features

A non-ulcerative lesion usually precedes ulceration. Four non-ulcerative presentations are recognized.

1 *Papule* – painless, sometimes itchy, non-tender palpable intradermal lesion (seen in Australia but rare in Africa).
2 *Nodule* – painless palpable firm lesion, 1–2 cm in diameter, situated in the subcutaneous tissue and usually attached to the skin (uncommon in Australia).
3 *Plaque* – painless well-demarcated elevated dry indurated lesion more than 2 cm.
4 *Oedematous* – diffuse extensive non-pitting swelling, ill-defined margin, firm, usually painful, with or without colour change over the affected skin.

In due course, the overlying skin breaks down and an ulcer forms with a necrotic centre, often spreading very rapidly in all directions. The following features are clinically very characteristic.

- The ulcer is usually painless, a factor contributing to the delay in health care seeking behaviour.
- The skin at the edge of the ulcer is deeply undermined.
- Satellite ulcers often communicate with the original ulcer by a subcutaneous tunnel, so the skin between adjacent ulcers is often unattached to the underlying tissues. The extent of the damage is always much greater than it looks from the surface.

Tropical Medicine Lecture Notes, Seventh edition. Edited by Nick Beeching and Geoff Gill. © 2014 John Wiley & Sons, Ltd. Published 2014 by John Wiley & Sons, Ltd.

Table 48.1 **Differential diagnosis of Buruli ulcer**

Papule	Nodule	Plaque	Oedema	Ulcer
Granuloma annulare	Boil	Cellulitis	Actinomycosis	Cutaneous diphtheria
Herpes	Cyst	Haematoma	Cellulitis	Guinea worm
Insect bites	Leishmaniasis	Insect bites	Elephantiasis	Leishmaniasis
Leishmaniasis	Lipoma	Leishmaniasis	Necrotizing fasciitis	Necrotizing fasciitis
Pimple	Lymphadenitis	Leprosy	Onchocercoma	Neurogenic ulcer
Pityriasis	Mycosis	Mycosis	Osteomyelitis	Tropical ulcer
Psoriasis	Onchocercoma	Psoriasis		Tuberculosis
				Sickle cell disease
				Squamous cell carcinoma
				Syphilis
				Venous ulcer
				Yaws

Source: Modified from *Diagnosis of* Mycobacterium ulcerans *disease* (Buruli ulcer). WHO/CDS/CPE/GBUI/2001.4.

Regional adenitis and systemic symptoms are unusual and, if present, are suggestive of primary or secondary bacterial infection. Erosion of underlying tissue may involve nerves, blood vessels and bone (in up to 15%). Complications such as tetanus and primary or secondary osteomyelitis may occur. Eventually, after months or years, healing may result in scarring, ankylosis and contractures. Currently, 25% of those affected develop long-term complications that may include amputation or loss of sight. HIV infection, and other immunodeficiency states, can exacerbate Buruli ulcer and lead to severe complications.

Differential diagnosis

Differential diagnosis is shown in Table 48.1.

Investigations

The slough from the ulcer usually contains numerous acid-fast bacilli on Ziehl–Neelsen stain, but may be negative. Culture is time-consuming, expensive and too frequently gives rise to false-positive results to make it worthwhile. Polymerase chain reaction (PCR) has been used as an epidemiological tool and is now increasingly used in diagnosis with sensitivity of > 90%. Recently, a highly sensitive dry reagent–based PCR assay has been developed that is better suited for use in most endemic countries.

Management

Significant progress in management has been made since the WHO began its Global Buruli Ulcer Initiative in 1998. Current strategies involve a combined medical and surgical approach. The combination of rifampicin with streptomycin or amikacin for 8 weeks is the preferred WHO antimicrobial regimen.

Small early lesion (eg, nodules, papules, plaques, ulcers < 5 cm in diameter): For papules and nodules, if immediate excision and suturing is possible, start antibiotics at least 24 hours before surgery and continue for 4 weeks. Otherwise, treat all lesions in this category with antibiotics for 8 weeks.

Non-ulcerative and ulcerative plaque and oedematous forms; Large ulcerative lesions (>5 cm in diameter); Lesions in the head and neck region, particularly the face: Treat with antibiotics for at least 4 weeks, then surgery (if necessary), followed by another 4 weeks of antibiotics.

Disseminated/mixed forms (e.g. osteitis, osteomyelitis, joint involvement): Treat with antibiotics for at least 1 week before surgery and continue for a total of 8 weeks.

Supervised combination therapy using oral rifampicin (10 mg/kg) plus intramuscular streptomycin (15 mg/kg) daily for eight weeks was shown to be highly effective in Benin when used in conjunction with surgery depending on the size of the ulcer at presentation, with an overall treatment success rate of 96%. Antibiotic combination treatment without surgery achieved a cure rate of 47% and was most successful in patients with nodules, papules, plaques and ulcers < 5 cm. Recurrence occurred in less than

2% overall. Antibiotic combination treatment, by reducing ulcer size, also makes larger ulcers more amenable to surgery and grafting.

Recently, an open-label, randomized trial in Ghana evaluating antibiotic treatment of early (< 6 months) limited (< 10 cm) ulcers, demonstrated that 4 weeks of streptomycin and rifampicin followed by 4 weeks of rifampicin and clarithromycin was as effective as 8 weeks of streptomycin and rifampicin and had the advantage of halving the number of injections of streptomycin required.

In Australia, a combination of rifampicin (10 mg/kg per day up to 600 mg daily) plus one other oral antibiotic (either clarithromycin 500 mg twice daily, or ciprofloxacin 500–750 mg twice daily, or moxifloxacin 400 mg once daily) is recommended for a total of 3 months (a) when the histology of resection margins shows either necrosis or acid fast bacilli or granulomata, or (b) when the initial lesion was large enough to require grafting, or (c) for complex, recurrent disease. Intravenous amikacin is recommended where surgical resection is necessarily incomplete. Recommended antibiotics and doses for children are rifampicin 10–20 mg/kg once daily not to exceed adult dose; Clarithromycin 15–30 mg/kg/day in two divided doses if < 12 years; dose as for adults if > 12 years, not to exceed adult doses; ciprofloxacin 20 mg/kg/day in two divided dose, not to exceed adult dose. Moxifloxacin is not recommended for children.

Necrotic ulcers should be excised with care to remove all affected tissue by extending the margin into healthy tissue. Excision is followed by primary closure or split-skin grafting. Surgery and physiotherapy may be required for patients with contractures. The need for surgery, and the risks of permanent deformity and disability, could be considerably reduced in the future through greater public awareness, earlier diagnosis and wider availability of effective combination treatment with oral antibiotics.

Prevention and public health aspects

Long trousers and other mechanical barriers reduce the likelihood of infection. There is no specific vaccine available at present, although bacille Calmette–Guérin (BCG) offers some protection. A prospective vaccine candidate is the environmental mycobacterium *M. vaccae*.

The Global Buruli Ulcer Initiative, launched by the World Health Organization (WHO) in 1998 is an important initiative targeting this neglected disease. The following control strategies are being promoted.

- Health education and staff training in the communities most affected.
- Development of educational materials adapted to the needs of the countries.
- Community-based surveillance system to increase early detection and referral for treatment in collaboration with diseases such as leprosy and Guinea worm.
- Assessment of local health services and resources currently available for the diagnosis and treatment of Buruli ulcer in endemic areas.
- Strengthening of the capacity of health systems in endemic areas by upgrading surgical facilities and improving laboratories.
- Rehabilitation of those already deformed by the disease.

 SUMMARY

- Buruli ulcer is a destructive ulcer caused by *Mycobacterium ulcerans*, occurring in wide areas of the tropics.
- The ulcer is characteristically painless, but is often deeply undermined.
- Surgical excision of the ulcer is needed in most cases.
- Prolonged antibiotic treatment is important (e.g. a combination of rifampicin and streptomycin), and should be started prior to surgery.

 Visit www.lecturenoteseries.com/tropicalmed to test yourself on this chapter using interactive MCQs.

 FURTHER READING

Anonymous (2008) Buruli ulcer: progress report, 2004–2008. *Wkly Epidemiol Rec* **83**: 145–54. [Review summarizing some of the key developments made in recent years.]

Boyd SC *et al.* (2012) Epidemiology, clinical features and diagnosis of *Mycobacterium ulcerans* in an Australian population. *Medical Journal of Australia* **196**: 341–4.

Converse PJ, Nuermberger EL, Almeida DV, Grosset JH (2011) Treating Mycobacterium ulcerans disease (Buruli ulcer): from surgery to antibiotics, is the pill mightier than the knife? *Future Microbiol* **6**: 1185–98. [Comprehensive review and horizon gazing.]

Johnson PDR *et al.* (2007) Consensus recommendations for the diagnosis, treatment and control of Mycobacterium ulcerans infection (Bairnsdale or Buruli ulcer) in Victoria, Australia. *MJA* **186**: 64–8. [Way to go? Heads up from down under.]

van der Werf TS, van der Graaf WT, Tappero JW, Asiedu K (1999) *Mycobacterium ulcerans* infection. *Lancet* **354**: 1013–18. [Highly recommended, this concise review includes some good clinical photographs and an excellent figure illustrating pathogenesis.]

Wansbrough-Jones M, Phillips R (2006) Buruli ulcer: emerging from obscurity. *Lancet* **367**: 1849–58.

[Comprehensive review explaining the current understanding of *M ulcerans* and its relations with human beings.]

World Health Organization. *Provisional Guidance on the Role of Specific Antibiotics in the Management of Mycobacterium Ulcerans Disease (Buruli Ulcer).* http://www.who.int/buruli/information/antibiotics/en/index.html [Extensive information is also available from the WHO at http://www.who.int/gtb-buruli/ Click on 'information resources'. This will lead you to further links providing a wealth of useful information.]

49

Myiasis

Geoff Gill
Liverpool School of Tropical Medicine

The term myiasis refers to a variety of conditions characterized by insect larvae invading the subcutaneous tissues or body cavities. There are only three common syndromes: the Tumbu fly, the Bot fly and Chiggers.

Tumbu fly

This is also sometimes known as the 'Putzi fly' in central and southern Africa. It is caused by the larvae of *Cordylobia anthropophaga*, which mostly inhabits sub-Saharan Africa. The fly lays its eggs on clothing (often on a washing line) and these hatch with body warmth when the clothes are worn. The larvae invade the skin and develop over the next 2 weeks, causing a 'blind boil'. The lesion is painful and often 'prickles' as a result of larval movement. The small dark 'head' of the boil is actually the respiratory spiracles of the larva. Multiple lesions may be present.

Treatment is to partly suffocate the larva by putting petroleum jelly or other oil or grease over the spiracles. The larva will become activated, and will partly extrude from the lesion when it can be grasped with forceps and removed intact. Care must be taken as maceration of the larva causes a severe inflammatory reaction. A novel described treatment is 'bacon therapy' – putting strips of bacon over the lesion to lure the larva out! Prevention is by hot-ironing all clean clothes after drying.

Bot fly

This is *Dermatobia hominis*, and is found in Central and South America. The Bot fly deposits eggs directly on the skin, rather than via clothes as does the Tumbu fly. The lesion that develops is similar; however, removal is more difficult. Occasionally, mechanical extraction of the larva can be done, but its shape often makes this difficult and incision under local anaesthetic is often needed. After infiltration of lidocaine, a cruciate incision should be made over the lesion, taking care not to incise the larva itself. Following this, extraction with forceps is usually easy. The lesions of both the Bot and Tumbu flies are usually microbiologically sterile, but sometimes secondary infection can occur, and antibiotics may be required.

Chiggers

Chiggers (or 'jiggers') are caused by *Tunga penetrans*, a flea that is widely distributed around the tropics – including much of Central and South America, Africa and the Asian Subcontinent. The gravid jigger flea invades exposed human skin – almost always the feet, and usually the interdigital clefts or the base of the toes. The flea encapsulates itself and produces eggs about 10 days later. A papular – and often later pustular – lesion develops which is painful and itchy. Excoriation helps to expel the eggs. Secondary infection and even ulceration can occur and multiple 'jigger' lesions may be present.

The flea should be carefully removed with a sterile needle, following which the lesion usually heals. Late ulcerative lesions will require antibiotics. The main aspect of prevention is good foot care and wearing shoes.

Body cavity myiasis

A variety of syndromes of myiasis exist in which various larvae invade body cavities – including wounds, urethra, vagina, anus, eye and ear. Nasal myiasis is

Tropical Medicine Lecture Notes, Seventh edition. Edited by Nick Beeching and Geoff Gill. © 2014 John Wiley & Sons, Ltd. Published 2014 by John Wiley & Sons, Ltd.

the most common, caused usually (but not always) by maggots of the so-called screw-worm flies *Chrysomia bezziana* (Old World) or *Cochliomyia hominivorax* (New World). Cold-like symptoms develop, followed by nasal obstruction and epistaxis. The fly maggots can usually be seen with a nasal speculum. Application of 15% chloroform in vegetable oil to the nasal cavity causes the larva to appear, when it can be removed with forceps. In occasional advanced cases, invasions of the nasal sinuses and even the brain can occur.

SUMMARY

- Myiasis is the invasion of insect larvae into the subcutaneous tissues, or sometimes body cavities.
- Specific conditions are Tumbu Fly (in Africa), Bot Fly (in Central and South America), and Chiggers (widely distributed).
- Myiasis is usually a nuisance rather than a danger, but removal techniques for the larvae are specific and must be done carefully.

 Visit www.lecturenoteseries.com/tropicalmed **to test yourself on this chapter using interactive MCQs.**

FURTHER READING

Francesconi F, Lupi O (2012) Myiasis. *Clin Microbiol Rev* **25**: 179–205. [Useful up to date review.]

50

Cutaneous larva migrans

Geoff Gill
Liverpool School of Tropical Medicine

Cutaneous larva migrans is an intensely itchy and slowly moving linear rash under the skin of the foot and ankle. It represents the subcutaneous meanderings of invading dog hookworms, and is one of the most common exotic diseases imported to Western countries (usually after tropical beach holidays).

Parasitology

The disease is caused by the larvae of animal hookworms – most commonly the dog hookworm *Ancylostoma braziliense*. Eggs are shed in the faeces of canine hosts to the soil or sand. Humans walking barefoot, or lying on the soil or sand, can become infected by larval invasion through intact skin. Sometimes infection can arise from towels or clothes which have been in contact with infected sand. Humans are an incidental host, and infection represents a cul-de-sac of the lifecycle. The larvae therefore travel aimlessly under the skin, causing the typical clinical eruption, until they eventually die.

Clinical features

A typical cutaneous larva migrans rash is shown in Fig. 50.1. The rash is a very itchy serpiginous red track, which is often excoriated. The larva advances by only a few millimetres a day, so the rash is relatively static. This is in contrast to the very rapidly moving linear rash of larva currens caused by *Strongyloides stercoralis* (Chapter 52). Although the foot and ankle are by far the most common sites for cutaneous larva migrans, it can occur on other parts of the body in contact with the ground. 'Hookworm folliculitis' is an uncommon form of the disease characterized by pustular folliculitis of the buttocks.

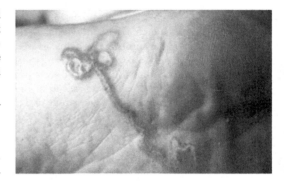

Figure 50.1 Typical rash of cutaneous larva migrans in a holidaymaker returned from a beach holiday in the Caribbean.

Treatment

There is no constitutional disturbance and the rash will heal spontaneously within a few weeks. However, it is aesthetically unpleasant and the severe itch can be debilitating. Also, some larvae can survive for several months. Older treatments included local freezing of the head of the larval track with an ethyl chloride spray, or occlusive application of 10% or 15% tiabendazole in emulsifying ointment. Neither were highly effective, and oral treatments are better. Current options are as follows.

- *Albendazole* – a single dose of 400 mg is usually completely effective, and if available this is the drug of choice.
- *Ivermectin* – is also highly effective in a single dose (12 mg for adults).
- *Tiabendazole* – is less effective than albendazole and ivermectin, and also more prone to

Tropical Medicine Lecture Notes, Seventh edition. Edited by Nick Beeching and Geoff Gill. © 2014 John Wiley & Sons, Ltd. Published 2014 by John Wiley & Sons, Ltd.

side-effects (e.g. dizziness, nausea and vomiting). It should only be used if albendazole or ivermectin are not available. The dose is 25 mg/kg twice a day for 3 days.

Prevention

Contamination of soil and sand by dog faeces is the cause of the disease. Beaches are a particular hazard, so banning dogs from beaches is an effective option (widely practised in Australia, but difficult to enforce in most developing countries). Programmes to de-worm dogs regularly will also be effective, provided the uptake is high. On an individual basis, wearing shoes or sandals on beaches helps, as well as avoiding lying on dry sand (preferably using sand that has been washed by the tide). It can be seen that both these practices significantly detract from the pleasures of a tropical beach, and many may prefer to risk infection from these annoying but benign parasites!

 SUMMARY

- Cutaneous larva migrans (CLM) is an itchy slowly moving linear rash, usually on the feet or ankles.
- CLM is due to subcutaneous invasion by animal hookworms. The condition is self-limiting.
- If treatment is needed, single dose albendazole or ivermectin is effective.

 Visit www.lecturenoteseries.com/tropicalmed **to test yourself on this chapter using interactive MCQs.**

FURTHER READING

Heukelbach J, Feldmeir H (2008) Epidemiological and clinical characteristics of cutaneous larva migrans. *Lancet Infect Dis* **8**: 302–9. [Useful and up-to-date review.]

51

Scabies and lice

Geoff Gill
Liverpool School of Tropical Medicine

Scabies

Scabies is a common skin condition globally, but it is seen particularly frequently and severely in tropical countries. Infection rates of 10% overall, and up to 50% in children, have been reported from some areas. It is caused by infestation with the mite *Sarcoptes scabiei*. Infection occurs by direct skin contact, and there is often then a 4–6-week period before clinical symptoms occur. The mite burrows beneath the skin, causing an inflammatory reaction and an intensely itchy generalized rash ensues. The itchy rash can disturb sleep and significantly reduce life quality. The classical diagnostic lesion is the interdigital burrow, from which the mite can be sometimes extracted with a sterile needle. In practice, however, the diagnosis is frequently made clinically and empirical treatment given.

The classical eruption is not always seen in tropical countries. Secondary infection and/or allergic hypersensitivity to the mite can alter the rash significantly. Thus, infected papules, widespread vesicles and papular urticaria may occur. In all types of rash, excoriation often alters its appearance. The important clinical principle is to *always* think of scabies when presented with an intensely itchy generalized rash in the tropics (especially in a child). A history of nocturnal itch in other family members is good supportive evidence.

'Norwegian scabies' or 'crusted scabies' occurs sometimes in immunologically compromised patients (e.g. HIV or lepromatous leprosy), and represents a massive proliferation of infecting mites (perhaps analogous to the hyperinfection syndrome of *Strongyloides stercoralis*). The skin becomes scaly or 'crusted' and is frequently not as itchy as classical scabies. Crusted scabies also occurs sporadically for no obvious reason, and is relatively common in Australian aborigines.

Scabies treatment is usually topical and is applied from the neck down to all parts of the skin, with particular attention to crevices and the genitalia. For severe cases, a second treatment 5–7 days later should be given. All household contacts must be treated at the same time. The preparations available are as follows.

- *Benzyl benzoate 25%* – old-fashioned but still effective and cheap; however, best avoided in children under 4 years of age.
- *Sulphur 6% ointment* – a better alternative for young children (<4 years).
- *Permethrin 5% cream* – more effective than benzyl benzoate and the treatment of choice, if available.
- *Ivermectin 200 µg/kg* – a single oral dose is effective in severe cases (including the 'Norwegian' variant).

The itch may continue for some weeks after effective treatment, and can be controlled with calamine lotion. Preventive measures for scabies include general principles of hygiene, and also the use of Tetmosol (5% tetraethylthiuram monosulphide) soap or rubbing oils.

Lice

Lice infestations of humans include *Pediculus humanus* (the body louse), *Phthirus pubis* (the pubic or crab louse) and *Pediculus capitis* (the head louse). Transmission is by close contact (usually head–head for head louse).

Pediculus humanus can transmit louse-borne relapsing fever, louse-borne typhus and trench fever, but only the local effects are considered here. Body lice cause generalized itch and often a maculopapular

Tropical Medicine Lecture Notes, Seventh edition. Edited by Nick Beeching and Geoff Gill. © 2014 John Wiley & Sons, Ltd. Published 2014 by John Wiley & Sons, Ltd.

rash which may become secondarily infected. Pubic and head lice cause local itch and sometimes excoriation, but their importance is frequently more aesthetic than medically important.

A variety of insecticidal preparations are available for treatment. These include lotions, dusting powders or shampoos of malathion, permethrin and dichlorodiphenyl-trichloroethane (DDT). Head lice can sometimes be managed physically with a 'lice comb' (a fine-toothed comb that removes the eggs or 'nits' from the shaft of the hair). This process can be aided by the use of hair conditioner.

Body lice will recur if clothing is not treated by heating to about 70 °C for 30 min. It should also be remembered that there are wide geographical variations in the susceptibility of lice to drug treatment, and local information on resistance patterns should be sought.

 Visit www.lecturenoteseries.com/tropicalmed to test yourself on this chapter using interactive MCQs.

FURTHER READING

Clarke JM, Lee SH, Yoon KS, Strycharz JP, Kwon DH (2009) Human head lice: status, control and resistance. In: *Advances in Human Vector Control*. Washington: American Chemical Society, pp. 73–88. [An up-to-date general review, including discussion of drug resistance.]

Hengge UR, Currie BJ, Jager G, Lupi O, Schwartz RA (2006) Scabies: a ubiquitous neglected skin disease. *Lancet Infectious Diseases* **6**: 769–79. [Review including Norwegian scabies.]

Heukelbach J, Feldmeier H (2006) Scabies. *Lancet* **367**: 1767–74. [A comprehensive review, including a section on developing world aspects.]

Moss PJ, Beeching NJ (2010) Arthropods and ectoparasites. In Cohen J, Powderly WG, Opal SM (eds), *Infectious Diseases*, 3rd edn, London: Elsevier Science, Chapter 11, pp. 128–39. [Illustrated summary of scabies, lice and other ectoparasites.]

🔑 SUMMARY

- Scabies is a global skin infection, but in the tropics is often extensive and sometimes bacterially infected.

- Particularly extensive scabies ('Norwegian scabies') is sometimes seen in immunocompromised patients (e.g. with HIV), and may need treatment with oral ivermectin.

- Body lice are very common. They are usually easily eradicated, but there may be local variations in drug sensitivity.

52

Strongyloidiasis

Geoff Gill
Liverpool School of Tropical Medicine

Strongyloides stercoralis is a highly advanced nematode worm that inhabits the small bowel of human hosts. It occurs in widespread areas of the tropics and subtropics and has also been reported in more temperate climates (e.g. southern parts of North America, southern Europe and even the UK).

Most infections cause minor symptoms or none at all. However, because of its 'autoinfective' life-cycle, strongyloidiasis can become permanently established in human hosts without the need for reinfection. In this situation, a more chronic clinical syndrome may occur. Of particular importance in such cases is the potential for fatal 'hyperinfection' if host immunity is reduced. Strongyloidiasis has been recorded in patients with HIV infection, but the association appears weak or absent, and the condition is not generally regarded as a classical HIV-associated infection. There is, however, a well established association with HTLV-1 infection.

A related worm *S fülleborni* has been reported to infect children, and to be associated with a condition known as 'swollen belly syndrome' in young children in Papua New Guinea.

Usual life-cycle

Adults live in the small intestine of humans only. The females, 2 mm long and very slender, live in the mucosa. They lay eggs that soon release microscopic larvae which usually escape at the non-infective (rhabditiform) stage in the faeces. Adult male worms are rapidly expelled and reproduction is probably usually parthenogenetic.

In the hospitable environment of warm moist soil, the larvae develop into free-living male and female worms within a week. The free-living females produce another generation of rhabditiform larvae, which develop into infective filariform larvae under certain environmental conditions. Humans are infected by penetration of the intact skin. Larvae may persist in the soil for many weeks, and the free-living cycle may be repeated many times. *Stercoralis stercoralis* is the only common soil-transmitted helminth infecting humans in which the worms can multiply in the free-living stage. After penetrating the skin, the larvae are carried to the lungs, migrate through the alveoli to reach the bronchial tree, and are swallowed to reach their normal habitat. From initial infection to maturity probably takes less than 4 weeks.

Autoinfection cycle

The rhabditiform larvae, after their release into the bowel lumen, sometimes change into the infective filariform stage. They may then reinfect the same host by either penetrating the perianal skin or the bowel wall. They then migrate through the tissues and the lungs and re-establish themselves in the intestine as new adult worms. This is how infection can persist for more than 40 years, even in the absence of external reinfection, such as in about 1 in 5 of ex-prisoners of war of the Japanese who worked on the infamous Thai–Burma railway during World War II.

Clinical features

Many infections are asymptomatic. However, both acute and chronic stages of infection can have symptoms that are quite distinct from each other. Untreated

Tropical Medicine Lecture Notes, Seventh edition. Edited by Nick Beeching and Geoff Gill. © 2014 John Wiley & Sons, Ltd. Published 2014 by John Wiley & Sons, Ltd.

acute infections may resolve spontaneously, or become chronic because of the autoinfective cycle. Immunologically, acute strongyloidiasis is characterized by a marked IgE and blood eosinophil response, but these are less constant in the chronic form of the disease, presumably because of the host becoming immunologically tolerant.

Acute infection

1 An itchy eruption at the site of larval penetration (patients seldom recollect this).
2 Cough and wheeze because of larvae in the lungs (also uncommon).
3 Abdominal pain and diarrhoea. Pain is usually vague and ill-defined. Diarrhoea can be marked. Occasionally, steatorrhoea and even bloody diarrhoea occurs.
4 Weight loss (usually associated with diarrhoea).

Chronic strongyloidiasis

1 *Larva currens* ('creeping eruption'). This is a characteristic, virtually pathognomonic skin eruption (Fig. 52.1). It is caused by the migration of larvae through the skin during autoinfection. The eruption is typically:
    - a serpiginous wheal (a raised line) surrounded by a flare;
    - evanescent (comes and goes in a few hours);
    - very itchy;
    - confined to the trunk between the neck and the knees; and
    - tends to appear in crops at irregular and unpredictable intervals.

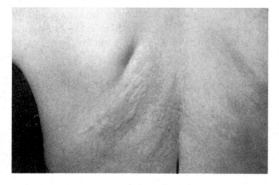

Figure 52.1 The 'larva currens' rash of strongyloidiasis in a former prisoner of World War II of the Japanese. The serpiginous wheals come and go in a few hours and travel rapidly over the central body areas. The rash is due to tissue larval migration of *Strongyloides stercoralis*.

2 *Intestinal symptoms.* These are usually vague, taking the form of irregular bouts of looseness of the stools. Diarrhoea is not constant, and the patient may only recognize that his or her bowels were abnormal in retrospect, when the infection has been eliminated. Bloody diarrhoea is not a feature of uncomplicated chronic strongyloidiasis. Very occasionally, a 'sprue-like' syndrome of diarrhoea and weight loss occurs.

Hyperinfection syndrome

Hyperinfection syndrome is a rare complication of *Strongyloides stercoralis* infection – usually the chronic form of disease. It occurs when host immunity is significantly and usually abruptly reduced, allowing rapid and disseminated migration of filariform larvae into tissues not involved in the normal human life-cycle. Conditions reported to be associated with hyperinfection include the following:

- diabetic ketoacidosis;
- lepromatous leprosy.
- leukaemia and lymphoma;
- immunosuppressive therapy;
- post-irradiation treatment;
- severe malnutrition;
- systemic steroid treatment.

Of all the causes, corticosteroid treatment is the most common. A well-reported scenario for hyperinfection is postrenal transplant (resulting from steroid and other immunosuppressant therapy).

Features of the hyperinfection syndrome are as follows:

1 severe and often bloody diarrhoea;
2 bowel inflammation with multiple microperforations;
3 bacterial peritonitis and paralytic ileus;
4 Gram-negative septicaemia;
5 pulmonary exudates, haemoptysis, pleural effusions and hypoxia;
6 encephalitis and bacterial meningitis.

The diagnosis of hyperinfection is essentially clinical and a high index of suspicion is needed. Eosinophilia is usually absent, but larvae are generally easy to find in stool and other body fluids (e.g. peritoneal and/or pleural exudates, bronchoalveolar lavage samples). Treatment is with standard antihelmintic drugs (see below) as well as full supportive therapy (e.g. fluids, antibiotics); however, the outcome is poor. For patients in endemic areas who are likely to need steroid treatment (e.g. severe asthmatics), there is a case for regular diagnostic screening for strongyloidiasis, with appropriate eradication if the disease is found.

Diagnosis

Diagnosis of strongyloidiasis is notoriously difficult. The following strategies may be useful:

- clinical suspicion;
- direct stool microscopy;
- duodenal biopsy;
- microscopy of duodenal juice;
- serological tests (e.g. ELISA);
- stool culture (charcoal culture or agar culture methods);
- stool microscopy after concentration;
- therapeutic trials.

Except in hyperinfection, larvae in the stool are frequently scant and appear intermittently. This is especially true with chronic *Strongyloides* infections. Even with concentration techniques, there are well-documented cases of patients with up to 12 consecutive negative stool samples although subsequently shown to have strongyloidiasis. Stool culture with charcoal may be helpful, but duodenal aspirates can be especially helpful, although difficult to obtain. Flexible gastroduodenoscopy is an option (as well as an aspirate for microscopy, a duodenal biopsy for histological examination should be taken). However, such techniques are frequently not available in tropical countries, although an option is the Enterotest capsule (sometimes known as the 'hairy string' test). This is a small, weighted capsule containing a hairy nylon thread, the end of which is taped to the cheek while the capsule is swallowed. The capsule dissolves in the stomach, releasing the thread, which is carried through to the duodenum, usually in 2–3 h. The string is withdrawn and the part which has entered the duodenum is stained yellow with bile. The duodenal juices are squeezed into a Petri dish between the thumb and forefinger of a gloved hand, and the fluid is then examined microscopically. Finally, a variety of serological tests have been developed, the best of which is probably the ELISA method, which is highly sensitive and specific.

Despite all these techniques, diagnosis may remain in doubt, and clinical features should remain part of the diagnostic process. High eosinophilia, unexplained diarrhoea and a typical larva currens rash are all highly suggestive evidence of *Strongyloides* infection in at-risk subjects. In such cases, and even in the absence of supportive parasitology, a therapeutic trial may be worthwhile, and is often rewarding.

Treatment

There are three possible therapeutic agents. If available, ivermectin is now generally regarded as the most effective therapy.

- *Ivermectin.* The dose is 200 µg/kg/day for 3 days, although single doses of 6 mg (again, daily for 3 days) have been effective. A single one-day dose may be as effective. A veterinary parenteral preparation of ivermectin is available, and cases of *Strongyloides* hyperinfection syndrome have been reported to have been successfully treated with 12 mg of subcutaneous ivermectin given as single or repeated doses.
- *Albendazole.* The usual dose is 400 mg/day for 3 days, but there is evidence that 400 mg twice daily is more effective. A 7-day course should be given in chronic cases.
- *Tiabendazole.* This is a more traditional treatment, but it is less effective than albendazole or ivermectin and prone to side-effects (nausea, vomiting, dizziness and occasional neuropsychiatric problems). However, it may be the only drug available in some developing countries. The dose is 25 mg/kg twice daily for 3 days (usually 1.5 g twice daily). It should be given as syrup, or tablets which are chewed before swallowing.

Epidemiology and control

The occurrence of strongyloidiasis in the tropics is variable – with intense infection in some parts and apparent absence in others. The variability is partly climatic – prevalence is increased in wetter and humid areas. The free-living cycle of *Strongyloides* does better in such conditions than, for example, hookworm. Diagnostic problems may account for the apparent absence or rarity in some areas.

Because infection enters the human host by larval soil transmission through intact skin, encouragement to wear footwear is the mainstay of control strategies. The only case of strongyloidiasis recorded in Britain was in a young woman who was in the habit of walking barefoot in the local park! The major control method for prevention of the hyperinfection syndrome is to screen people who need, or are likely to need, steroid or immunosuppressive therapy. Asthmatics are the most common group, but others include those with ulcerative colitis, collagen vascular disease, leukaemias, lymphomas, other malignancies and those on transplant waiting lists. Amoebiasis and tuberculosis should also be screened for in such individuals. Like strongyloidiasis, these conditions also may be seriously exacerbated by immunosuppressive therapy.

SUMMARY

* *Strongyloides stercoralis* is an advanced nematode with a complex life cycle. It occurs widely in the tropics and subtropics.

* Once infection is established, the disease can continue indefinitely through the autoinfective part of the life-cycle.

* Infections may be asymptomatic, but can also cause diarrhoea, cough and wheeze. A common feature – particularly of chronic infection – is the larva currens rash, due to larval migration.

* A rare but potentially fatal manifestation is hyperinfection, due to massive larval migration in immunocompromised hosts.

Visit www.lecturenoteseries.com/tropicalmed to test yourself on this chapter using interactive MCQs.

FURTHER READING

Gill GV, Welch E, Bailey JW, Bell DR, Beeching NJ (2004) Chronic *Strongyloides stercoralis* infection in former British Far-East prisoners of war. *Quart J Med* **97**: 789–95. [Analysis of a large number of UK ex-World War II Far East prisoners with chronic strongyloidiasis, emphasizing diagnostic delays and difficulties, and the small but important occurrence of fatal hyperinfection.]

Lewthwaite P, Gill GV, Hart CA, Beeching NJ (2005) Gastrointestinal parasites in the immunocompromised. *Curr Opinion Infect Dis* **18**: 427–35. [Good review of immunosuppression and gastrointestinal parasite infection in general, including strongyloidiasis and its relationship with steroid treatment, HIV and HTLV-l infection.]

Olsen A, van Lieshout L, Marti H, *et al.* (2009) Strongyloidiasis – the most neglected of the neglected tropical diseases? *Trans Roy Soc Trop Med & Hyg* **103**: 967–72. [Useful up-to-date review emphasizing the problem of under-diagnosis, and need for greater awareness of *Strongyloides* infection.]

Suputtamongkol Y, Kungpanichkul N, Silpasakorn S, Beeching NJ (2008) Efficacy and safety of a single-dose veterinary preparation of ivermectin versus 7-day high-dose albendazole for chronic strongyloidiasis. *Int J Antimicrob Agents* **1**: 46–9. [Recent clinical trial of single dose ivermectin versus prolonged albendazole, showing superiority of ivermectin with an approximate 90% cure rate.]

53

Guinea worm infection (dracunculiasis)

Nick Beeching
Liverpool School of Tropical Medicine

Guinea worm infection, a subcutaneous parasitic disease caused by *Dracunculus medinensis*, was a major cause of disability in Asia and Africa but is now confined to a few African countries and is expected to become the second disease after smallpox to be eradicated by public health efforts (Fig. 53.1).

Life-cycle

Larvae of guinea worm are drunk in water containing their intermediate host, the freshwater copepod (water flea) *Cyclops*. The larvae then penetrate the gut wall and develop within subcutaneous tissue into adults over about 3 months. Adult female worms grow to about 50–100 cm long and, as they become distended with millions of larvae, they migrate to dependent parts of the body after about 1 year. Here they secrete enzymes that allow them to emerge through the skin and discharge huge numbers of larvae once the skin is immersed in water. The active larvae that emerge swim for 2–3 days and must be ingested by a suitable *Cyclops*, within which they develop for a further 2 weeks before they become infective to humans.

Clinical features

Patent human infections are usually highly seasonal and are often most frequent in the height of the dry season when water is scarce. Developing worms do not usually cause symptoms, but as guinea worms emerge, they cause burning pain that motivates patients to immerse the limb in water, thus encouraging transmission. Sometimes, emerging worms provoke allergic responses including urticaria or even asthma. A blister forms at the point of emergence; this is usually on the foot or lower leg but sometimes the arm, scrotum or indeed any part of the body. After discharging larvae, the worm dies and may gradually extrude or become absorbed. However, the process often takes many weeks and local ulceration with spreading secondary bacterial infection can cause disability for months, especially if there are multiple worms. Abscess formation is common. Worms migrating near a joint sometimes cause arthritis with effusion and, rarely, aberrant migration of a worm to the spinal cord causes paraplegia. The prolonged disability caused by guinea worm disrupts childrens' schooling and agricultural work.

Diagnosis

This is clinical. The white cloud of larvae extruded from a female worm immersed in water is characteristic. Dead calcified worms are sometimes seen on X-rays.

Treatment

There is no specific drug treatment. Courses of albendazole or metronidazole have been recommended as a means of reducing the inflammatory response, but they are of marginal benefit. If the uterus has emerged, discharge the larvae by immersion in water and take

Tropical Medicine Lecture Notes, Seventh edition. Edited by Nick Beeching and Geoff Gill. © 2014 John Wiley & Sons, Ltd. Published 2014 by John Wiley & Sons, Ltd.

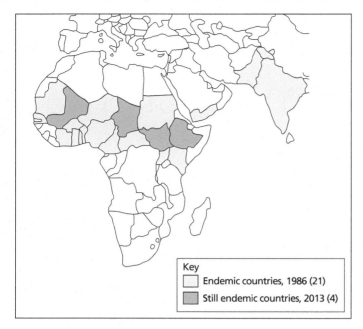

Key
☐ Endemic countries, 1986 (21)
▨ Still endemic countries, 2013 (4)

Figure 53.1 Distribution of guinea worm infection – endemic in 21 countries in 1986 (light colour) and only 4 countries (dark colour) in 2013. *Source:* Carter Center: www.cartercenter.org

care to dispose of the water hygienically. The traditional method is to tie the end of the emerging worm to a small stick and wind the worm out slowly over many days, taking care not to rupture the worm as this can cause severe allergic responses. Ulceration requires antiseptic dressings. Tetanus immunization should be checked and updated if necessary. Surgical removal of the worm before it emerges, by extraction through small transverse incisions, reduces the risk of infection and disability. However, surgical facilities are usually lacking in the poor villages where the disease occurs.

Control

Provision of a safe drinking water supply is the key to control. Wells must be protected to prevent contamination by people bathing infected limbs. Even straining water through cloth or unglazed pottery will filter out *Cyclops* and prevent infection. Filters made of monofilament nylon cloth for individuals, or within oil drums for a community, have proved useful in eradication projects. Efforts at prevention have been highly successful; from a peak of perhaps 50 million infections annually in the 1950s there were about 10 000 infections in 2007 and just 148 cases in 2013. The disease has been eradicated from Asia and transmission is now concentrated in 4 countries in Africa, particularly in South Sudan. The WHO is hoping for global disease eradication in the near future.

 SUMMARY

- Previously a major problem, Guinea worm has almost been eradicated.
- Disease is caused by the nematode worm *Dracunculus medinensis*, the larvae of which are drunk in water containing the intermediate host, the freshwater copepod (water flea) *Cyclops*.
- Disability is caused by local ulceration and abscess formation at the site of release of larvae from the adult worm, usually on the lower leg.
- Transmission can be interrupted by provision of a protected water supply and by filtering water through gauze to remove the *Cyclops* intermediate host.

 Visit www.lecturenoteseries.com/tropicalmed **to test yourself on this chapter using interactive MCQs.**

FURTHER READING

Barry M (2007) The tail end of guinea worm – global eradication without a drug or vaccine. *New Engl J Med* **356**: 2561–4. [Nice illustrated editorial with key refs. Free.]

Website of the Carter Center www.cartercenter.org/health/guinea_worm/index.html [Useful resource from this centre which has taken the lead in final eradication efforts.]

54

Histoplasmosis

Geoff Gill
Liverpool School of Tropical Medicine

There are two main types of histoplasmosis. 'Classical' histoplasmosis is caused by the dimorphic fungus *Histoplasma capsulatum* var. *capsulatum*, and occurs in many parts of the world outside Europe. Central and South America are areas of particularly high occurrence, although it also occurs in the USA, the Asian Subcontinent and the Far East. Cases imported to temperate countries have been recorded. African histoplasmosis is classically caused by *Histoplasma capsulatum* var. *duboisii*, which is usually confined to Central and West Africa. However *Histoplasma capsulatum capsulatum* is found in southern Africa.

Classical histoplasmosis

Clinical features

The fungus is present in bat and bird excreta, and is a particular hazard for cave explorers in endemic areas. Infection is by inhalation, following which a number of clinical syndromes can result.

- *Asymptomatic.* Many infected individuals develop no illness, but may have serological evidence of past exposure.
- *Acute pulmonary histoplasmosis.* This is a febrile bronchitic illness occurring 10–14 days after exposure. There is usually systemic malaise and myalgia, and the chest X-ray shows generalized diffuse pulmonary shadows and sometimes hilar lymphadenopathy. The illness may resolve spontaneously with no treatment.
- *Chronic pulmonary histoplasmosis.* Sometimes the disease can cause asymptomatic single or multiple pulmonary nodules, often found on routine chest radiography. More importantly, and usually in patients with underlying chronic lung damage, focal consolidation and cavitation can occur, often in the lung apices, and this can mimic pulmonary tuberculosis (cough and haemoptysis may occur).
- *Acute disseminated histoplasmosis.* In this form of the disease liver, spleen, bone marrow and lymph glands are infected. Patients are usually ill and febrile, with weight loss, lymphadenopathy and/or hepatosplenomegaly. This form of the disease is often associated with AIDS. Fever may be accompanied by small umbilicated skin lesions resembling those of cutaneous cryptospococcosis or penicilliosis, but oral ulceration in such patients is more common in histoplasmosis.
- *Chronic disseminated histoplasmosis.* Sometimes, years after exposure, various organ-specific syndromes resulting from histoplasmosis can present. These include oral ulceration, hypoadrenalism, meningitis and endocarditis.
- *Atypical presentations.* These include polyarthritis or polyarthralgia, erythema multiforme, eruythema nodosum, and hypoadrenalism.

Diagnosis

This is ideally made by finding the fungus in body secretions or tissues (e.g. sputum, buffy coat layer, lymph node aspirates, bone marrow samples and biopsies of liver or pulmonary nodules). If culture facilities are available, the yeast can be grown from sputum or blood. There are a variety of serological tests available, as well as an intradermal histoplasmin skin test.

Treatment

Treatment should be reserved for severe cases or immunocompromised patients. Ideally, 200–400 mg/day itraconazole should be given. Fluconazole is

Tropical Medicine Lecture Notes, Seventh edition. Edited by Nick Beeching and Geoff Gill. © 2014 John Wiley & Sons, Ltd. Published 2014 by John Wiley & Sons, Ltd.

probably also effective, but there is less experience. Amphotericin B is more difficult and toxic to use, but it is widely available. The dosage is 0.6–1.0 mg/kg/day by slow intravenous infusion. In advanced HIV infection, relapses are inevitable and, if possible, patients should receive long-term itraconazole or fluconazole as secondary prophylaxis.

African histoplasmosis

The portal of entry and source of the fungus is poorly understood. The most common presentation is with skin nodules or ulcers, enlarged lymph nodes or lytic lesions in bones. Disseminated disease (sometimes known as 'progressive disseminated histoplasmosis' or PDH) can occur with lung and gastrointestinal involvement. Diagnosis can be made histologically from biopsy specimens, and treatment is as for classical histoplasmosis. Though there has been some doubt in the past, it is now generally accepted that African histoplasmosis is more severe in HIV-infected patients, who often also have tuberculosis, leading sometimes to diagnostic delays.

SUMMARY

- Two main types of histoplasmosis occur – 'classical' (occurring widely and due to *Histoplasma capsulatum* var *capsulatum*), and 'African' (found only in Africa, and due to *Histoplasma capsulatum* var *duboisii*).

- Immunocompromised patients (e.g. with HIV) are particularly at risk from histoplasmosis, which can be clinically severe.

- The drug of choice is itraconazole, though fluconazole and amphotericin B can also be used.

 Visit www.lecturenoteseries.com/tropicalmed to test yourself on this chapter using interactive MCQs.

FURTHER READING

Alonso D, Munoz J, Letang E, *et al.* (2007) Imported acute histoplasmosis with rheumatologic manifestations in Spanish travelers. *J Travel Med* **14**: 338–42. [Report of both imported cases to temperate climates, and also atypical clinical presentations.]

Govender NP, Chiller TM, Poonsamy B, Frean JA (2011) Neglected fungal diseases in sub-Saharan Africa: a call to action. *Curr Fungal Infect Rep* **5**: 224–32. [Review of fungal disease in general in Africa, including a section on African histoplasmosis.]

Kauffman CA (2007) Histoplasmosis: a clinical and laboratory update. *Clin Microbiol Rev* **20**: 115–32. [Useful and comprehensive review of histoplasmosis in general.]

55

Other fungal infections

David Lalloo
Liverpool School of Tropical Medicine

Mycetoma (Madura foot)

Mycetoma is defined as chronic swelling, induration and sinus formation with the discharge of fungal grains, involving the skin, subcutaneous tissue and bone, usually of the foot. The clinical syndrome is caused by a variety of different fungi (Eumycetes) and also by aerobic *actinomycete* bacteria. Differentiation is important because of the differing response to treatment. Actinomycetes are Gram-positive organisms with branching filaments whose width is generally less than 1 mm. Fungal hyphae stain with special fungal stains (periodic acid–Schiff (PAS) or methenamine silver) and are usually more than 2 mm in diameter; chlamydospores may also be seen.

Epidemiology

These are saprophytic organisms introduced through the skin by a thorn prick. They are not contagious and can also occur in animals. The diseases are widely distributed in tropical areas from 18°N–18°S, commonly among barefoot farmers. Some areas, particularly in the Sudan and India, have a high incidence. The chief agents of mycetoma differ in different areas (e.g. Mexico 80% *Nocardia brasiliensis*, India chiefly *Madurella mycetomatis* and *Streptomyces somaliensis*).

Clinical features

Mycetoma presents with painless (80%) swelling usually involving the foot, less commonly the hands, back or head. After several years, nodules form in the skin and break down to form discharging sinuses from which pus and coloured fungal grains emerge. There are no systemic effects unless secondary infection occurs. The condition progresses slowly and

relentlessly but lymphatic spread is late and is more likely in actinomycotic infection. Eumycetomas are better circumscribed with a palpable edge, while actinomyectomas are more diffuse.

Diagnosis

The colour, size and consistency of grains obtained from deep within a sinus together with microscopy after they are crushed in 10% sodium hydroxide gives a provisional diagnosis. Cultures are necessary and are best obtained by deep biopsy and the material also sent for histology. Antibiotic sensitivities should be obtained for actinomycotic infections. Use of serological techniques has generally been disappointing but may occasionally be used to follow the effects of treatment in actinomycetoma. Radiological examination may show large erosions of bone, especially in eumycotic infections, while many small cavities and extensive bone sclerosis is more likely to be caused by actinomycotic disease.

Treatment

Drug treatment is often only partially effective in true fungal infections despite organisms that are sensitive to antifungal drugs in vitro. However, successful treatment of *Madurella mycetomatis* infections with prolonged (over a year) use of itraconazole or ketoconazole has been recorded, particularly if disease is limited. Many actinomycotic infections respond to treatment with antibiotics. Co-trimoxazole (trimethoprim/sulfamethoxazole) alone or in combination with an aminoglycoside (amikacin or streptomycin) is most commonly used. Amoxycillin-clavulanate may also be effective. Treatment may need to be continued for many months until clinical improvement occurs and repeat biopsies are culture negative.

Tropical Medicine Lecture Notes, Seventh edition. Edited by Nick Beeching and Geoff Gill. © 2014 John Wiley & Sons, Ltd. Published 2014 by John Wiley & Sons, Ltd.

Surgery may be useful, particularly in eumycetoma. Ideally, the affected area should be completely excised, with care taken not to rupture the 'capsule' that often surrounds the infection. Small nodules are often successfully treated in this way. Below-knee amputation may be needed, but sometimes the heel can be conserved. In poor farmers, amputation is often best left until the limb has become useless. Recurrences are quite common after surgery and so surgery should be both preceded and followed by chemotherapy.

Chromoblastomycosis

These are warty violaceous, often ulcerated, chronic skin lesions usually involving the leg and causing itching. Further spread is by scratching or via lymphatics. The condition is usually found in Latin America or Africa. Several different fungi are responsible (e.g. *Fonsecaea pedrosoi*). They are saprophytes of wood and transmitted by skin trauma.

Diagnosis

Diagnosis is by finding the chestnut brown thick-walled fungal cells, often in a wall-like pattern, or branching hyphae in skin smears or histological sections.

Treatment

Treatment is unsatisfactory. Itraconazole and terbinafine in combination may be effective: 5-flucytosine may also be used. Surgical treatment tends to spread infection but cryosurgery is useful for small lesions and long-term use of local heat packs has been successful.

Sporotrichosis

This infection is caused by *Sporothrix schenckii*, a worldwide saprophyte of decaying vegetation, sphagnum moss and soil. It typically affects farmers and florists. Cats and other animals can inoculate the organism by scratching. An epidemic in South African miners was caused by infected wooden pit props.

Clinical features

Infection manifests as a pustule or nodule typically on a finger or hand, often followed by spread along lymphatics causing nodular ulcerating lesions. Osteoarticular, disseminated and pulmonary forms are uncommon except in the immunosuppressed.

Diagnosis

Diagnosis is by microscopy and culture of material from pus, crusts or biopsies. Yeast forms, hyphae or asteroid bodies (from antigen–antibody complexes on the fungal surface) can be demonstrated, often with a background of polymorph leucocytes. The differential diagnosis of the 'sporotrichoid' lesions along lymphatics includes cutaneous leishmaniasis, nocardiosis, tuberculosis and atypical mycobacterial infection, especially *Mycobacterium marinum* (fish tank granuloma).

Treatment

Itraconazole (100–200 mg daily) is the treatment of choice. Saturated potassium iodide orally is also effective, starting with 1mL three times daily and rising to 15 mL/day as tolerated. Treatment should be continued for at least 3 months.

 SUMMARY

- Mycetoma ('Madura foot') is a chronic infection of the skin, subcutaneous tissues and sometimes bones of the foot.
- Treatment is difficult and may involve both drugs and surgery. Various fungi or bacteria may be involved, and identification is important as it will affect drug treatment.
- Sporotrichosis usually causes a nodule or pustule on the hand. It usually responds to itraconazole.

 Visit www.lecturenoteseries.com/tropicalmed **to test yourself on this chapter using interactive MCQs.**

FURTHER READING

Hay RJ (ed.) (1989) Tropical fungal infections. In *Ballière's Clinical Tropical Medicine and Communicable Diseases*. London: Baillière Tindall. [An older but still useful review that includes the fungal infections mentioned above.]

Kauffman CA, Bustamante B, Chapman SW, Pappas PG (2007) Clinical practice guidelines for the management of sporotrichosis: 2007 update by the Infectious Diseases Society of America. *Clin Infect Dis* **45**: 1255–65.

Welsh O, Vera-Cabrera L, Salinas MC (2007) Mycetoma. *Clin Dermatol* **25**: 47–71. [Review of the disease and current treatment.]

56

Haemoglobinopathies and red cell enzymopathies

Jecko Thachil[1] and Imelda Bates[2]

[1]Manchester Royal Infirmary; [2]Liverpool School of Tropical Medicine

Defects in the haemoglobin or enzymes within red cells interfere with red cell function and cause a range of clinical features depending on the type and degree of abnormality.

Haemoglobinopathies

Sickle cell anaemia

Sickle cell anaemia was the first condition for which a molecular basis was identified and is the result of a β-globin chain mutation that alters the structure and function of haemoglobin. When the circulating red cells containing sickle haemoglobin encounter conditions of low oxygen tension the haemoglobin polymerizes and deforms the cells which eventually take up a sickle shape (Fig. 56.1). Polymerization, and therefore the clinical features of sickle cell anaemia, can be affected by many factors including temperature and hydrodynamics. Although normal red cells have a diameter of 7 μm they are very flexible and able to squeeze through small capillaries such as those in the spleen, which are only 3 μm wide. Sickled red cells get stuck in these small vessels, and also become more adhesive to vascular endothelium. These factors in combination with the platelet aggregation, vasoconstriction and coagulation acti-

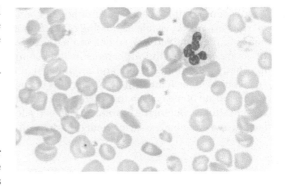

Figure 56.1 Sickle cells. *Source:* From B. Bain (2002) *Blood Cells: A Practical Guide*, 3rd edn. Oxford: Blackwell Science.

vation cause microthrombi and ischaemia of the tissues. These pathological events precipitate the anaemia, chronic organ damage, pain crises and consequent organ failure and chronic bony deformities which are so characteristic of sickle cell anaemia. In an individual with sickle cell anaemia, 80–95% of the haemoglobin is sickle haemoglobin (HbS) with the remainder being made up of HbF. In carriers of the sickle cell gene (sickle cell trait; HbAS) only about 30% of haemoglobin is HbS and the rest is predominantly HbA.

Tropical Medicine Lecture Notes, Seventh edition. Edited by Nick Beeching and Geoff Gill. © 2014 John Wiley & Sons, Ltd. Published 2014 by John Wiley & Sons, Ltd.

Epidemiology and protection against malaria

The geographical distribution of sickle cell disease follows that of malaria transmission. Carriers of the sickle cell gene have up to 10 times better protection against severe malaria than those with normal haemoglobin. This protection is in part due to accelerated acquisition of malaria immunity. The highest frequencies of the carrier state are generally found in Africa (e.g. up to 30% of all births are HbAS in parts of Nigeria, Ghana and central Africa) but the sickle gene is also common in parts of eastern Saudi Arabia and east central India.

Clinical features (Fig. 56.2)

At all ages, chronic haemolysis of abnormal red cells means that sickle cell anaemia is associated with steady state haemoglobin levels of 60–80 g/L. The response to this anaemia is pronounced bone marrow expansion visible as bossing of the frontal bones in the skull and overgrowth of the maxillae. In young children, clinical features include stunting, bony deformities, pain and swelling of the small bones in the hands and feet (dactylitis), acute sequestration of red cells in the spleen, aplastic crises and strokes. Before the introduction of early detection and systematic care for young children with

sickle cell anaemia, the mortality in under-fives exceeded 95%. Much of this mortality can be prevented by neonatal screening programmes which provide close monitoring of infants and young children during the critical first few years of life. The lives of older children and adults are punctuated by acute severe episodes of pain in the bones of the trunk and limbs, as well as organ-related complications such as sickle chest syndrome. Splenic atrophy due to microthrombi results in increased risk of infection particularly by encapsulated organisms. The chronic and unpredictable nature of sickle cell anaemia can make it difficult for patients to achieve adequate schooling and to sustain regular employment. The carrier state, HbAS, is not normally associated with any clinical problems. However, an increased incidence of renal problems including haematuria, urine concentrating problems, medullary carcinoma and rare reports of exercise-induced sudden death have been observed. Conditions that are clinically similar to sickle cell anaemia can result from a combination of HbS with other haemoglobin variants (e.g. HbSC, HbS thalassaemia and HbSD).

Diagnosis

Often the family history and clinical findings clearly point towards a diagnosis of sickle cell disease and during an acute crisis abundant sickled red cells

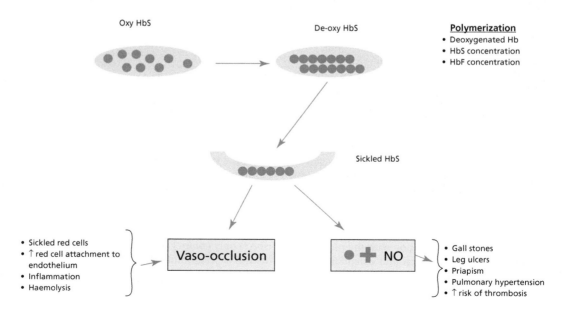

Figure 56.2 Complications of sickle cell disease (NO; nitric oxide.)

can be seen on a blood film. The presence of sickle haemoglobin (e.g. HbAS, HbSS, HbSC) can be confirmed by a simple sickle slide or solubility test. Haemoglobin electrophoresis will distinguish between HbAS and HbSS. High performance liquid chromatography and iso-electric focusing may be available in specialist centres.

Management

Individuals with sickle cell anaemia are best managed by a multidisciplinary team as they may require a variety of specialist inputs including haematology, ophthalmology, nephrology, obstetrics, orthopaedics and physiotherapy. In steady state it is usual practice to give sickle cell patients folate supplements (5 mg/day) because their high rates of haemopoiesis put them at risk of deficiency. They should also receive prophylactic oral penicillin (250 mg twice a day) and be monitored closely for signs of infection. Management can be broadly divided into acute and chronic care.

Acute care: Severe pain crises are generally managed in hospital with intravenous fluids and adequate, often opiate, analgesia. If the crisis was precipitated by an infection this should also be treated. Because of the increased risk of thrombosis in sickle cell disease, blood transfusions should only be given for emergencies such as sequestration or aplastic crises and should not aim to increase the haemoglobin above steady state levels. Manual or automated replacement of the patient's blood with normal blood from donors to reduce the level of HbS to 30% (exchange transfusion) is only beneficial for specific clinical indications such as respiratory distress syndrome or incipient stroke.

Chronic care: This is based on increasing HbF levels which can reduce the frequency of painful episodes, the need for blood transfusion, and admission to hospital. Hydroxycarbamide is the main agent used for this purpose, starting at a small dose (500 mg daily in adults) and gradually increasing the dose while monitoring the white cell and platelet counts. Regular transfusions have been tried in countries where this is possible aiming at reducing HbS levels to less than 30%. This has been successful to reduce the incidence of stroke, recurrence of acute chest syndrome and preventing long-term organ complications.

β Thalassaemia

β Thalassaemia is a genetic defect that results in insufficient production of the β-globin chains which are needed to form HbA ($\alpha\alpha\beta\beta$) which makes up 97%

of normal adult haemoglobin. The amount of β chain produced can vary from none ($\beta0$) to almost normal levels ($\beta+$) and the degree of anaemia and compensatory bone marrow overactivity determines the clinical severity.

Epidemiology

β Thalassaemia is present in all ethnic groups but has the highest incidence in the Mediterranean basin (15–20%) and South East Asia and Africa (5–10%).

Clinical features (Fig. 56.3)

Classification of β thalassaemias is based on clinical criteria.

- *β Thalassaemia trait* – clinically well with normal haemoglobin in steady state.
- *β Thalassaemia intermedia* – symptoms of anaemia (Hb 70–80 g/L) but not completely transfusion dependent.
- *β Thalassaemia major* – dysmorphic and transfusion dependent (Hb 20–30 g/L). The presentation is usually in the first year of life with severe anaemia, jaundice and hepato-splenomegaly due to extramedullary haemopoesis. Marked erythroid hyperplasia in the bones can cause the typical thalassaemic facies with expansion of the skull and maxillary bones.

Diagnosis

Clinical features and family history should indicate the diagnosis but definitive investigations require demonstration of increased HbA2 levels or molecular studies. The blood film shows hypochromic microcytic red cells with more target cells than are seen in iron deficiency. Basophilic stippling is common and the reticulocyte count is high but not in keeping with the severity of anaemia because erythropoeisis is ineffective. A diagnostic clue for thalassaemia trait is an inappropriately low mean corpuscular haemoglobin (MCH) compared to the degree of anaemia. If there is severe anaemia then marked bone marrow overactivity may be evident by the presence of many polychromatic red cells (seen as reticulocytes if a special staining technique is used) or even nucleated red cells.

Management

Management varies with the severity of the anaemia. To prevent death in β thalassaemia major in the first few years of life regular transfusions must be given.

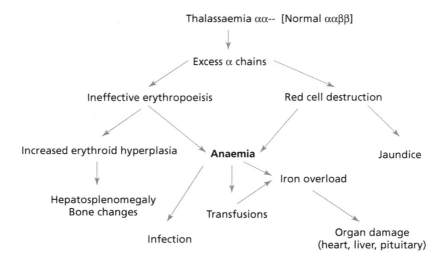

Thalassaemia αα-- [Normal ααββ]

Excess α chains

Ineffective erythropoeisis   Red cell destruction

Increased erythroid hyperplasia   **Anaemia**   Jaundice

Iron overload

Hepatosplenomegaly
Bone changes   Transfusions

Infection   Organ damage
(heart, liver, pituitary)

Figure 56.3 Complications of thalassaemia.

This will lead to iron overload and death in the second decade unless an iron chelation programme is initiated. This involves overnight subcutaneous infusions of desferrioxamine, which may not be affordable for poorer patients. Alternatively deferiprone, an oral iron chelator can be used either alone or in combination with desferrioxamine. Long-term follow-up of individuals with thalassaemia is important to monitor the growth and bone changes (osteopenia), and for early identification of endocrine disturbances and cardiac or liver damage from iron overload. Follow-up reviews should include assessment for complications of chronic blood transfusions (e.g. viral hepatitides, blood group antibodies) and iron chelating therapies (e.g. auditory and visual disturbance)

Enzymopathies

Glucose-6-phosphate dehydrogenase deficiency

Epidemiology

The enzyme glucose-6-phosphate dehydrogenase (G6PD) is present in red cells and protects them from oxidant damage (e.g. infection, drugs, fava beans). G6PD deficiency is common and associated with many different X-linked genetic defects which alter enzyme stability and therefore its half life. Early red cells have higher levels of enzyme than older cells. The degree of haemolysis, and hence clinical severity,

is dependent on the quantity and half-life of the abnormal enzyme. Like sickle haemoglobin, G6PD deficiency has a protective effect against malaria and has its highest prevalence in the Mediterranean basin (35–40%) and Africa (25%).

Clinical features

G6PD deficiency is X-linked and therefore manifests predominantly in males. It can cause neonatal anaemia and jaundice with a risk of kernicterus. In older children and adults, oxidant stress caused by drugs (e.g. primaquine, sulfonamides, nitrofurantoin), infections or fava beans (Mediterranean variety of G6PD deficiency) cause sudden haemolysis. The severity is dependent on the levels of G6PD, which are genetically determined. The African type (G6PD A–) tends to be mild and self-limiting whereas the Mediterranean variety can cause life-threatening haemolysis.

Diagnosis

During an acute haemolytic episode caused by G6PD deficiency, the blood film appearances are very characteristic. The haemoglobin in the red cells appears to be pushed into the middle or to one side of the cell ('bite' and 'helmet' cells (Fig. 56.4)). Screening tests such as the methaemoglobin reduction test can detect an 80% reduction in G6PD levels and can be performed by district hospitals in resource-poor countries where G6PD is common. Enzyme assays and genetic analyses are the definitive investigations but need a specialist laboratory. Enzyme assays for

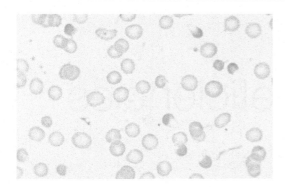

Figure 56.4 Red cell appearances during acute haemolytic crisis caused by G6PD deficiency. *Source:* From B. Bain (2002) *Blood Cells: A Practical Guide*, 3rd edn. Oxford: Blackwell Science.

SUMMARY

- The major tropical haemoglobinopathies are sickle cell anaemia (SCS) and thalassaemia.
- SCS is characterized by chronic ill health and acute crises. Long-term treatments include folic acid, prophylactic penicillin and hydroxycarbamide.
- Beta thalassaemia requires regular blood transfusion, and associated iron overload is a problem. Ideally chelation treatment should also be given.
- Glucose-6-phosphate dehydrogenase (G6PD) deficiency can lead to haemolytic episodes often precipitated by specific drugs.

G6PD deficiency should be carried out 6–8 weeks after an acute attack because the cells that are deficient in G6PD are destroyed during the haemolytic episode leaving only cells with normal levels of enzyme. An enzyme assay carried out during acute haemolysis will therefore not detect a deficiency.

Management

As many episodes of G6PD haemolysis are self-limiting, particularly in Africa, transfusions are rarely required. In very severe cases, such as those associated with fava bean ingestion, acute renal failure necessitating dialysis may supervene. Once a patient has been identified as G6PD deficient they should be advised to avoid drugs that may precipitate a haemolytic episode (Box 56.1).

Box 56.1 **Common drugs that can cause haemolysis in G6PD-deficient individuals**

Analgesics – acetylsalicylic acid
Antimalarials – primaquine, pamoquine, dapsone
Antimicrobials – sulfonamides, nitrofurantoin
Others – vitamin K analogues, probenecid, PAS

Visit www.lecturenoteseries.com/tropicalmed to test yourself on this chapter using interactive MCQs.

FURTHER READING

Bain B (2006) *Haemoglobinopathy Diagnosis* (2e). Oxford: Blackwell Publishing Ltd. [Details and rationale of standard methods for laboratory diagnosis of haemoglobinopathies, covering a range of tests; includes a self assessment exercise.]

Key NS, Derebail VK (2010) Sickle-cell trait: novel clinical significance. *Hematology Am Soc Hematol Educ Program*: **2010**: 418–22.

Kwiatkowski DP (2005) How malaria has affected the human genome and what human genetics can teach us about malaria. *Am J Hum Genet* **77**(2): 171–92. [>200 references relating to malaria and red cell abnormalities.]

Mason PJ, Bautista JM, Gilsanz F (2007) G6PD deficiency: the genotype-phenotype association. *Blood Reviews* **21**(5): 267–83. [Good overview of complex relationship between genetic mutations and resultant clinical picture.]

Platt OS (2008) Hydroxyurea for the treatment of sickle cell anemia. *N Engl J Med* **27**: 358(13): 1362–9. [Rationale, benefits and complications of hydroxycarbamide use for sickle cell disease.]

Rees DC, Williams TN, Gladwin MT (2010) Sickle-cell disease. *Lancet* **11**: 376(9757): 2018–31. [Overview of sickle cell disease with focus on children in Africa.]

Roberts DJ, Brunskill SJ, Doree C, Williams S, Howard J, Hyde CJ (2007) Oral deferiprone for iron chelation in people with thalassaemia *Cochrane Database of Systematic Reviews* **3**: CD004839. [Systematic review of use of oral chelator.]

57

Haematinic deficiencies

Jecko Thachil[1] and Imelda Bates[2]

[1]Manchester Royal Infirmary; [2]Liverpool School of Tropical Medicine

Haemopoiesis can be reduced by lack of many micronutrients including vitamin A and zinc, but this chapter will focus on the more common iron, folate and cobalamin deficiencies.

Iron deficiency

Iron deficiency is the most common cause of anaemia and affects 20–50% of the world's population. The WHO has ranked iron deficiency anaemia as the third leading cause of morbidity for females of childbearing age, and among the top 10 disease burdens for men aged 15–44 years. In developing countries, about half of all cases of anaemia in women and children are the result of iron deficiency. In regions where infections and inflammatory conditions are prevalent, ferritin levels are difficult to interpret because ferritin is an acute phase protein and can be raised even in the presence of iron deficiency. Prevalence studies about iron deficiency therefore need to be interpreted with caution unless the authors rigorously evaluated iron status. Iron deficiency can be caused by excessive loss of red cell iron from the body but may also be caused by insufficient intake or poor absorption. Iron deficiency is a particular problem in childhood and pregnancy when physiological requirements are high. The body has very little capacity to regulate either iron absorption or iron loss. The maximum absorptive capacity of the gut for iron is about 3.5 mg/day and iron requirements in pregnancy are approximately 2.0 mg/day. Other factors that commonly coexist with iron deficiency and can contribute to anaemia include gastrointestinal infections (e.g. hookworm infestation, Shigellosis or entero-invasive *Escherichia coli* dysentery), HIV infection, tuberculosis, folate deficiency, infections, cow-milk intolerance and anaemia of chronic disease. Chronic intravascular haemolysis which can occur in red cell membrane or enzyme abnormalities can also lead to urinary iron loss. Anaemia is one of the later manifestations of iron deficiency and tissue function can be impaired even before there is a detectable reduction in haemoglobin level. This can lead to subtle changes in behaviour, cognition and psychomotor development in children, and preterm delivery in pregnant women.

Clinical features

The symptoms of iron deficiency may be due to (1) the primary disorder which led to the deficiency; (2) symptoms related to the degree and rapidity of development of anaemia; and (3) impaired function of tissues or organs which require iron proteins for their normal function. If iron deficiency develops slowly, as in chronic hookworm infestation, physiological compensation mechanisms ensure that symptoms do not become significant until the haemoglobin has reached very low levels. Physical signs specifically associated with iron-deficiency anaemia include spoon-shaped nails (koilonychia) and angular stomatitis. Clinical examination is not a reliable method for diagnosing anaemia but is helpful to indicate some of the causes of iron deficiency. Common causes of excessive iron loss include menorrhagia, haemorrhoids, hookworm, bowel carcinoma, hiatus hernia and treatment with aspirin or non-steroidal anti-inflammatory drugs. The best dietary source of iron is red meat so reduced iron intake is commonly associated with a vegetarian diet and can be exacerbated by phytates and tannates in cereals and tea, which inhibit iron absorption.

Investigations

In rural health facilities where specific tests to measure iron status may not be available, a reasonably firm

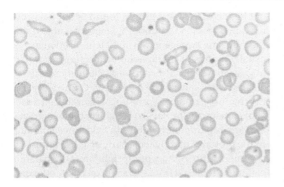

Figure 57.1 Iron-deficient red cells. The cells are paler and more irregular in shape than normal red cells. *Source:* B. Bain (2002) *Blood Cells: A Practical Guide*, 3rd edn. Oxford: Blackwell Science.

diagnosis can be made from a well-prepared blood film. In iron deficiency the red cells appear hypochromic (over half of the diameter of the cell is pale rather than only one-third as in normal cells) and microcytic (significantly smaller than a small lymphocyte) (Fig. 57.1). The red cells may also appear flattened ('pencil cells'). If an automated blood count is available the mean corpuscular volume (MCV), mean corpuscular haemoglobin concentration (MCHC) and mean corpuscular haemoglobin (MCH) will all be reduced. Iron deficiency is often associated with a mildly raised platelet count which resolves as the anaemia improves. Thalassaemia can also produce hypochromic, microcytic anaemia.

If iron studies are available they will demonstrate low serum iron with raised total iron-binding capacity and a low ferritin. In pregnancy, the haemoglobin is affected by the physiological changes in plasma volume and red cell mass and the use of a low MCV may be misleading because of the higher proportion of larger younger red cells. The 'gold standard' investigation for iron deficiency is demonstration of a lack of iron stores in aspirated bone marrow. A dietary history should be obtained and tests to determine the cause of the iron deficiency should be performed and may include stool examination for hookworm ova or blood, and endoscopy or radiography of the gastrointestinal tract.

Management

Treatment of the iron deficiency itself comprises iron sulphate 200 mg three times a day; absorption can be enhanced by ascorbic acid. Compliance can be a major issue with iron tablets since they often cause gastrointestinal upsets. Unfortunately intake with food delays its absorption. Altering the formulation to ferrous fumarate or gluconate or liquid preparation or starting on a lower dose may help to avoid gastrointestinal symptoms. In true iron deficiency early red cells should appear in the peripheral blood within 4–5 days of starting iron therapy. Early red cells are slightly larger and bluer (polychromatic) than normal red cells and can be specifically visualized using a reticulocyte stain. Iron supplementation should be continued for at least 3 months after a normal haemoglobin is achieved to replenish body stores. The cause of the iron deficiency should also be rectified to prevent recurrence of the anaemia. This may involve encouraging inclusion of locally available iron-rich foods in the diet, or explaining the need for farmers to wear shoes when working in their fields to prevent hookworm infestations. Iron supplementation can reverse some developmental delays in anaemic children, even in the absence of an overall increase in haemoglobin. A negative association between iron deficiency and severe infection has been found in Malawian children suggesting a protective effect for iron deficiency on bacteraemia. There is some evidence suggesting iron replacement may exacerbate infections in children in malarious areas and consideration should be given to prescribing antimalarial treatment prior to iron therapy.

Folate deficiency

Folate deficiency is more often caused by insufficient intake than by malabsorption. It can be exacerbated or precipitated by the excessive physiological demands for folate that occur in pregnancy and childhood, and in chronic haemolytic states. Folate is widely available in liver, yeast, spinach, green leafy vegetables and nuts but it is easily destroyed by boiling. Bone marrow stores only last a few months. Alcohol abuse can cause a rapid drop in serum folate by impairing the enterohepatic cycle and interfering with gut absorption. Other causes of folate deficiency include chronic hemolytic anemias, exfoliative skin diseases and some drugs which can affect folate metabolism including trimethoprim and pyrimethamine. Mixed iron and folate deficiencies are not uncommon and may indicate poor diet. The clinical and laboratory features that result from combined deficiency are a mixture of those occurring in isolated iron and folate deficiencies.

Clinical features

In addition to general symptoms of anaemia, folate deficiency can cause anorexia, change in bowel habit, glossitis and a mild haemolytic anaemia.

Investigations

Folate and cobalamin deficiency both cause enlarged, slightly oval red cells and hypersegmented neutrophils (six or more nuclear lobes) on the peripheral blood film (Fig. 57.2) and a bone marrow examination will show typical changes of megaloblastic anaemia. On automated blood counts, an MCV over 100 fL indicates macrocytosis. Serum and red cell folate assays can provide a definitive diagnosis but are not always available in poorer countries. As folate is required for DNA synthesis, severe chronic deficiency can eventually cause a reduction in white cells and platelets as well as red cells (pancytopenia).

Management

Treatment comprises folic acid 5 mg/day but, as with all anaemias, the underlying cause should be corrected. Appropriate advice should be given to maximize dietary folate intake.

Cobalamin (vitamin B$_{12}$) deficiency

Deficiency of cobalamin was thought to be much less common than folate deficiency in resource-poor countries but resent research suggests that this may

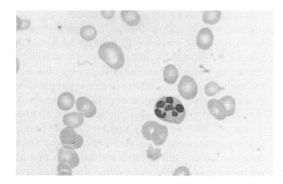

Figure 57.2 Oval macrocytes and hypersegmented neutrophils in folate deficiency. *Source:* B. Bain (2002) *Blood Cells: A Practical Guide*, 3rd edn. Oxford: Blackwell Science.

not be the case. Cobalamin is found in animal products. Body stores last about 2 years and absorption mechanisms are generally efficient. Deficiency is usually the result of impaired absorption secondary to gastrointestinal disorders, especially those that affect the small bowel and ileum (e.g. Crohn's disease, tuberculosis, tropical sprue). Cobalamin deficiency can occasionally be caused by lack of dietary cobalamin and is particularly common in lacto-vegetarians. In the presence of reduced gastric acid secretion (e.g. treatment with proton pump inhibitors) cobalamin cannot be released from dietary proteins. Metformin, an oral anti-diabetic drug, can also lead to cobalamin deficiency through a calcium-dependent abnormality of absorption in the ileum. Low serum levels of cobalamin can be seen in up to 40% of patients infected with HIV. Several reasons contribute including poor nutritional status, diarrhoea, and exudative enteropathy. Tropical sprue is a cause of combined cobalamin and folate deficiency. Pernicious anaemia is a specific failure of B$_{12}$ absorption because of a lack of intrinsic factor production by gastric parietal cells. It can be associated with antibodies to gastric parietal cells or intrinsic factor. Pernicious anaemia occurs in all races and up to 30% of patients have relatives with the same disorder.

Clinical features

The typical neurological symptoms of cobalamin deficiency – posterolateral column degeneration, peripheral neuropathy and optic atrophy – can occur in the absence of anaemia. Subtle neuropsychiatric changes like memory loss, personality changes and paraesthesias can also occur. In severe cases, profound life-threatening anaemia may develop. As with folate deficiency, a reduction in platelets and white cells can occur. These abnormalities are generally mild so severe infections or bleeding episodes are unusual. Features that may indicate an underlying cause of small bowel dysfunction, such as diarrhoea or abdominal pain, should be sought. Pernicious anaemia may be associated with thyroid disease, vitiligo, Addison's disease and other auto-immune disorders, and clinical evidence of these may be apparent.

Investigations

The peripheral blood film is indistinguishable from that seen in folate deficiency and the combination of macrocytosis and hypersegmented neutrophils is virtually pathognomonic of cobalamin or folate deficiency. Assays of cobalamin levels will provide a definitive diagnosis but it is also important to determine any underlying cause.

Management

Treatment is with hydroxycobalamin injections 1 mg every 3 months after an initial loading dose (e.g. 1 mg three times a week for 2 weeks). Oral cobalamin (1 to 2 mg *daily*) may be used once cobalamin levels have normalized. Any underlying condition should be treated appropriately and unless the cause of the deficiency can be eliminated, treatment will be needed for life.

If the patient is anaemic, a reticulocyte response will be noted within a week of starting treatment, disappearance of hypersegmented neutrophils and a rise in haemoglobin in about two weeks and normalization of haemoglobin within two months depending on the severity of anaemia. Neurological abnormalities take longer (up to 3 to 6 months) to resolve although a complete recovery may be depend on the extent and duration of the abnormality.

SUMMARY

- Deficiency of haematinics (iron, folate and B$_{12}$) are common causes of anaemia.
- Iron deficiency is the commonest type, and is particularly common in children and women of child-bearing age.
- Simple haematological tests such as the mean corpuscular volume (MCV) and blood film can be diagnostically useful.

 Visit **www.lecturenoteseries.com/tropicalmed** **to test yourself on this chapter using interactive MCQs.**

📖 FURTHER READING

Bain B (2006) *Blood Cells: A Practical Guide*, 4th edn. Oxford: Blackwell Science. [Atlas of haematological morphology with clear illustrations and accompanying text. Good guide to the use of the diagnostic laboratory.]

Balarajan Y (2011) Anaemia in low and middle income countries. *Lancet* **378**: 2123–35. doi:10.1016/S0140-6736(10)62304-5. [Comprehensive overview of haematinics and other causes of anaemia.]

Boele M, Calis J, Phiri K *et al.* (2010) Pathophysiological mechanisms of severe anaemia in Malawian children. *PLOS One* **5**(9): e12589. [Review of interdependency of haematinics and other factors causing anaemia.]

Hall A (2007) Micronutrient supplements for children after deworming. *Lancet Infect Dis* **7**(4): 297–302. [Review of complexities surrounding haematinic supplementation and de-worming programmes.]

Phiri K, Calis JCJ, Siyasiya A *et al.* (2009) New cut off levels for ferritin and soluble transferring receptor for the assessment of iron deficiency in children in a high infection pressure area. *J Clin Path* **62**: 1103–6. [Usefulness of various methods for measuring iron deficiency in tropical settings.]

58

Bites and stings

David Lalloo
Liverpool School of Tropical Medicine

Snakebite

Clinical features

There are a large number of species of venomous snakes throughout the world. These can be divided into three main categories: vipers, elapids and sea snakes. The pattern of envenoming depends upon the biting species. Only 50–70% of patients bitten by venomous snakes develop signs of envenoming.

The major clinical effects following snakebite can be divided as follows.

1 *Local effects.* Pain, swelling or blistering of the bitten limb. Necrosis at the site of the wound can sometimes develop.
2 *Systemic effects.*
   - Non-specific symptoms: vomiting, headache, collapse.
   - Painful regional lymph node enlargement, indicating absorption of venom.
   - Specific signs:
     (a) non-clotting blood;
     (b) bleeding from gums, old wounds, sores;
     (c) neurotoxicity: ptosis, bulbar palsy and respiratory paralysis;
     (d) rhabdomyolysis; muscle pains and black urine;
     (e) shock; hypotension, usually resulting from hypovolaemia.

Vipers most commonly cause local swelling, shock, bleeding and non-clotting blood. Elapids cause neurotoxicity and usually minimal signs at the bite site (with the exception of some cobras which also cause necrosis). Sea snakes cause myotoxicity and subsequent paresis. There are exceptions to this general rule, some vipers cause neurotoxicity and Australian elapids also cause non-clotting blood and haemorrhage.

First aid for snakebites

1 Reassure the patient. Many symptoms following snakebite are caused by anxiety.
2 Immobilize the limb. Moving the limb may increase systemic absorption of venom. Splinting is especially helpful in children.
3 Avoid harmful manoeuvres such as cutting, suction or tourniquets.
4 Consider a pressure bandage in regions where snakebite does not cause tissue necrosis, particularly if rapid transport to hospital is not possible. This is especially important for snakes that cause neurotoxicity. A firm crêpe bandage should be applied over the bite site and wound up the limb.
5 Transport the patient to hospital as soon as possible.
6 If the snake has been killed, take it to hospital with the patient.

Diagnosis and initial assessment

Think of envenoming in unusual cases.

1 Carefully examine bitten limb for local signs.
2 Measure the pulse, respiration rate, blood pressure and urine output. The blood pressure must be watched if patients are unwell, are bleeding or have significant swelling; shock is common in viper bites.
3 Look for non-clotting blood. This may be the only sign of envenoming in some viper bites. The 20-min whole blood clotting test (WBCT20; Box 58.1) is an extremely easy and useful test. This should be performed on admission and repeated 6h later.

Tropical Medicine Lecture Notes, Seventh edition. Edited by Nick Beeching and Geoff Gill. © 2014 John Wiley & Sons, Ltd. Published 2014 by John Wiley & Sons, Ltd.

4 Look carefully for signs of bleeding, which may be subtle (gums/old wounds/sores). Bleeding internally (most often intracranial) may cause clinical signs.
5 Look for early signs of neurotoxicity; ptosis (this may be interpreted as feeling sleepy), limb weakness, or difficulties in talking, swallowing or breathing.
6 Check for muscle tenderness and myoglobinuria in sea-snake bites.
7 Take blood for:
   - haemoglobin, white cell count and platelet count;
   - prothrombin time, activated partial thromboplastin time and fibrinogen levels if available;
   - serum urea and creatinine; and
   - creatine phosphokinase, reflecting skeletal muscle damage.
8 ECG if available.

Management

General management

All patients should be observed in hospital for 12–24 h, even if there are no signs of envenoming initially. They should be regularly reviewed; envenoming can develop quite rapidly. Nurse patients on their side with a slight head down tilt to prevent aspiration of blood or secretions. Avoid intramuscular injections and invasive procedures in patients with incoagulable blood. Tetanus prophylaxis should be given, but routine antibiotic prophylaxis is not required unless necrosis is present.

Antivenom

Antivenom is indicated for signs of systemic envenoming. Evidence for its efficacy in severe local envenoming is poor, but it is usually indicated if swelling extends over more than half the bitten limb. Mono-specific (monovalent) antivenom can be used for a single species of snake; polyspecific (polyvalent) for a number of different species. The choice and dose of antivenom depends upon manufacturers' recommendations and local experience (see Theakston & Warrell 1991 for a list of available antivenoms; reference details in Further reading). Children require exactly the same dose as adults as the dose is dependent upon amount of venom injected, *not* bodyweight.

- Antivenom should be diluted in 2–3 volumes of dextrose/saline and infused over an hour or so. The infusion rate should be slow initially and gradually increased.
- Adrenaline (epinephrine) should be drawn up in a syringe ready for use. Routine prophylaxis with adrenaline against antivenom may be effective but should not generally be used:
- Patients should be observed closely during antivenom administration. Common early signs of an antivenom reaction are urticaria and itching, restlessness, fever, cough or feeling of constriction in the throat.
- Patients with these signs should be treated with adrenaline (0.01 mg/kg) intramuscularly. An antihistamine, e.g. chlorphenamine (0.2 mg/kg i.m. or i.v.) should also be given.
- Unless life-threatening anaphylaxis has occurred, antivenom can cautiously be restarted after this treatment.

The response to antivenom should be monitored. In the presence of a coagulopathy, restoration of clotting depends upon hepatic resynthesis of clotting factors. The WBCT20 should be repeated 6 h after antivenom; if blood is still non-clotting, further antivenom is indicated. After restoration of coagulation, measurement of the WBCT20 should be repeated every 6–12 h as a coagulopathy may recur because of late absorption of venom from the bite site.

The response of neurotoxicity to antivenom is less predictable. In species with predominantly postsynaptically acting toxins, antivenom may reverse neurotoxicity; failure to do so is an indication for further doses. However, response to antivenom is poor in species with presynaptically acting toxins.

Other therapy

- Sloughs from necrotic wounds should be excised. Skin grafting may be necessary. Severe swelling may lead to a suspicion of compartment syndromes. Fasciotomy should *not* be performed unless there is definite evidence of raised intracompartmental pressure (>45 mmHg) and any coagulopathy has been corrected.

- Blood products are not necessary to treat a coagulopathy if adequate antivenom has been given.
- Endotracheal intubation should be performed to prevent aspiration if bulbar palsy develops, often obvious when difficulty in swallowing leads to pooling of secretions.
- Paralysis of intercostal muscles and diaphragm requires artificial ventilation. This can be performed by manual bagging and may need to be maintained for days, using relays of relatives if necessary.
- Anticholinesterases may reverse neurotoxicity following envenoming by some species with postsynaptic toxins.
- Careful fluid balance should be maintained to treat shock and prevent renal failure.
- Some cobras spit venom into the eyes of their victims. Rapid irrigation with water will prevent severe inflammation. 0.5% adrenaline drops may help to reduce pain and inflammation.

Epidemiology and prevention

Snakebite is mainly a rural and occupational hazard: farmers, plantation workers, herdsmen and hunter-gatherers are at greatest risk. Children also are frequently bitten as a result of their inquisitive nature. Most bites occur in the daytime and involve the foot, toe or lower leg as a result of accidentally disturbing a snake. However, some species of snake (e.g. kraits) may bite sleeping victims at night. In some areas of the world, snakebite is one of the most common causes of death and severe morbidity can result from snakebite. Sensible footwear, discouraging handling of potentially venomous animals and keeping the grass short around dwellings can all reduce the chance of snakebite.

Scorpion stings

In some areas of the world, scorpion stings are more common than snakebites and cause significant mortality. The stinging scorpion is often not seen. A number of different species have broadly similar clinical effects. The major feature of envenoming is severe pain around the bite site, which may last for many hours or even days. Systemic envenoming is more common in children and may occur within minutes of a bite. Major clinical features are caused by activation of the autonomic nervous system (Table 58.1). Severe hypertension, myocardial failure and pulmonary oedema are particularly prominent in severe envenoming.

Table 58.1 **Clinical features of scorpion stings**	
Tachypnoea	Muscle twitches and
Excessive salivation	spasms
Nausea and vomiting	Hypertension
Lachrymation	Pulmonary oedema
Sweating	Cardiac arrhythmias
Abdominal pain	Hypotension
	Respiratory failure

Management

Patients should be taken to hospital immediately; delay is a frequent cause of death. Control pain with infiltration of lidocaine around the wound or systemic opiates (with care). Scorpion antivenom is available for some species. It should be given intravenously in systemic envenoming, but intramuscular injection has been used with good effect. Prazosin is particularly effective for treating hypertension and cardiac failure. Severe pulmonary oedema requires aggressive treatment with diuretics and vasodilators.

Spider bites

Many species of spiders cause significant envenoming in the tropics. Fatal envenoming is rare.

Widow spiders

Widow spiders (*Latrodectus* spp.) are found throughout the world. Severe pain at the bite site is common. Rare cases develop systemic envenoming with abdominal and generalized pain and other features resulting from transmitter release from autonomic nerves. Hypertension is characteristic of severe envenoming. Antivenom is available in some regions and is effective for relief of pain and systemic symptoms. Opiates and diazepam are also useful for treatment of pain.

Recluse spiders

Recluse spiders (*Loxosceles* sp.) have a wide distribution and cause bites in which pain develops over a number of hours. A white ischaemic area gradually breaks down to form a black eschar over 7 days or so. Healing can be prolonged and occasionally causes severe scarring. The efficacy of antivenom and other advocated treatment (dapsone, steroids, hyperbaric oxygen) remains uncertain.

Banana (Brazilian wandering) spiders

Phoneutria spp. occur only in South America. They usually cause severe burning pain at the site of the bite, but in severe cases can cause systemic envenoming with tachycardia, hypertension, sweating and priapism. A polyspecific antivenom is available in some regions.

Funnel-web spider

Bites by funnel web spiders in Australia may cause systemic envenoming with autonomic effects on the cardiovascular system and neurological symptoms. Antivenom is available and has helped to reduce fatalities.

Marine envenoming

Venomous fish

Many different venomous fish, for example stonefish, can sting patients if they are stood on or touched. Systemic envenoming is rare. Excruciating pain at the site of the sting is the major effect. Regional nerve blocks and local infiltration of lidocaine may be effective, but most marine venoms are heat labile. Immersing the stung part into hot water is extremely effective in relieving pain. Care should be taken to avoid scalding; the envenomed limb may have abnormal sensation. Clinicians should check the water temperature with their own hand. Asking the patient to also immerse the non-bitten limb may help to avoid scalding.

Jellyfish

Venomous jellyfish have a large number of stinging capsules (nematocysts) on their tentacles that inject venom when tentacles contact skin. Pain and wheals are the usual effects but, rarely, systemic envenoming can be life-threatening. Many of the nematocysts remain undischarged on tentacles that adhere to the victim and rubbing the area of the sting causes further discharge and worsens envenoming. In box jellyfish stings, pouring vinegar over the sting prevents the discharge of nematocysts. For most other jellyfish, seawater should be poured over the stings and adherent tentacles gently removed. Ice may be useful for pain relief and hot water is effective in reducing pain for some species. Box jellyfish stings can occasionally be rapidly life-threatening. Antivenom is available and can be administered intramuscularly. The Irukandji syndrome may occur in Info-Pacific regions when patients develop systemic envenoming shortly after a minor or sometimes unnoticed sting in deep waters. Muscle pains, spasms and hypertension with cardiac failure may occur. Treatment is supportive; i.v. magnesium has been used to reduce pain and hypertension.

SUMMARY

* As well as snakebite, venomous animals include some fish (e.g. stonefish), jellyfish, spiders (e.g. widow, recluse), and scorpions.
* Snakebite is a major problem, particularly in the rural tropics, with significant morbidity and mortality.
* The major types of venomous snakes are vipers, elapids and sea snakes. Effects of envenomation can be both local and systemic.
* First-aid measures for snakebite are important. Antivenom is normally only indicated in cases of systemic envenomation.
* Anaphylaxis is a continuing potential problem with antivenom treatment. When used, adrenaline should be immediately available.

 Visit **www.lecturenoteseries.com/tropicalmed** to test yourself on this chapter using interactive MCQs.

 ## FURTHER READING

Isbister GK, Fan HW (2011) Spider bite. *Lancet* **378**: 2039–47. doi: 10.1016/S0140-6736(10)62230-1. [Practical spider bite management.]

Meier J, White J (1995) *Handbook of Clinical Toxicology of Animal Venoms and Poisons*. Florida: CRC Press. [A comprehensive summary of venomous animals and the effects of their bites.]

Theakston RDG, Lalloo DG (2013) Venomous bites and stings. In J Zuckerman (ed.), *Principles and Practice of Travel Medicine*. Chichester: John Wiley and Sons Ltd, 2013. [A practical approach to venomous bites and stings.]

Theakston RD, Warrell DA (1991) Antivenoms: a list of hyperimmune sera currently available for the treatment of envenoming by bites and stings. *Toxicon* **29**(12): 1419–70.

Warrell DA (2005) Treatment of bites by adders and exotic venomous snakes. *BMJ* **331**: 1244–7. [Summary of snakebite management.]

http://apps.who.int/bloodproducts/snakeantivenoms/database/ [A useful website with details of distribution of venomous snakes and antivenoms.]

59

Non-communicable diseases

Geoff Gill,[1] Maureen Wilkinson[2] and Kevin Mortimer[1]
[1]Liverpool School of Tropical Medicine; [2]Cheshire and Wirral Partnership NHS Foundation Trust

Introduction

Disease spectrum

Non-communicable diseases (NCDs) are of increasing importance all over the world, but particularly in developing countries. NCDs include all chronic disease processes, which may be treatable but are frequently not curable. By definition, they are not caused by infectious agents. Common NCDs are as follows.

- Hypertension
- Cardiovascular disease
- Diabetes
- Asthma
- Epilepsy
- Sychiatric disease
- Stroke
- Trauma
- Cancer
- Arthritis

The pattern of NCDs encountered in tropical countries is often different from that seen in the Western world. Thus, coronary artery disease is the most important form of cardiac disease in developed countries, but in many areas of the tropics the most important is rheumatic heart disease. Cardiomyopathy and hypertensive heart disease are also frequent. Similarly, although chronic obstructive pulmonary disease (COPD) is seen in the tropics, asthma is usually the most common respiratory problem encountered. Road traffic accidents (RTAs) are a particularly problematic form of trauma in developing countries, as well as the effects of war and civil unrest. Malignancy patterns vary: hepatoma, Burkitt's lymphoma, Kaposi's sarcoma, nasopharyngeal carcinoma and bladder cancer are particular tropical problems.

Mortality patterns

These are often difficult to determine in tropical countries because of diagnostic difficulties, problems of enumerating deaths outside hospital, and variable and mobile populations. In general, NCDs are globally the major cause of death, although in tropical countries infectious disease remains the major killer, as shown in Table 59.1. However, there is good evidence that the proportion of deaths caused by NCDs in developing countries is steadily increasing. Thus, in the Gambia, NCDs made up about 32% of total deaths in the 1970s but in the 1990s the proportion had risen to 49%. General projections are that, despite the HIV/AIDS epidemic, proportionate NCD mortality will overtake that caused by communicable diseases in most developing countries in the next 10–20 years.

Epidemiological transition

The reasons for the rising mortality from NCDs in tropical countries are various. Overall mortality caused by infectious disease is falling; and even in poor countries life expectancy is slowly increasing. As many NCDs increase in prevalence with rising age (e.g. diabetes and hypertension), extended life expectancy necessarily increases the rates of such diseases. Increased vehicle use and social unrest are also

Tropical Medicine Lecture Notes, Seventh edition. Edited by Nick Beeching and Geoff Gill. © 2014 John Wiley & Sons, Ltd. Published 2014 by John Wiley & Sons, Ltd.

Table 59.1 World patterns of proportionate mortality (communicable and non-communicable disease)

Population	Communicable disease (%)	Non-communicable disease (%)
Total world	35	65
Poorest countries	60	40
Richest countries	10	90

leading to more traumatic deaths. A further problem is that of 'epidemiological transition'. This term refers broadly to sociocultural population changes that can have profound effects on disease patterns. Population transition is a complex process, but approximately equates to what is often referred to as 'Westernization' or sometimes, more light-heartedly, as 'Coca-colonization' (Box 59.1).

Box 59.1 Features of epidemiological or demographic transition

- Urban–rural migration
- Adoption of 'Western' lifestyles
- Increased food intake
- Reduced dietary quality
- Reduced exercise
- Increased alcohol intake
- Smoking
- Higher salt intake
- Pollution
- Family and social breakdown

These processes are best seen at work in the effect on tropical populations migrating to urban environments from the country. Many studies have shown that dramatic increases in NCD prevalence occur following rural–urban migration, as shown by the figures from East Africa in Table 59.2. Obesity is a major

Table 59.2 Non-communicable diseases and rural–urban migration in East Africa

	Rural (%)	Urban (%)
Hypertension	13	23
Diabetes	1	6
Childhood asthma	11	26

effect of rural–urban migration, and is a major risk factor for several important NCDs (in particular, accidents, hypertension and diabetes). In Africa, obesity is an especial problem in women, and in some areas up to 40% of adult urban women are significantly obese, compared with less than 5% in rural environments. Tackling this problem is especially difficult as in a number of areas of Africa, it is regarded as culturally advantageous to be overweight or obese.

Diabetes mellitus

Epidemiology

Diabetes is an especially important NCD in the tropics as it is common, rapidly increasing, is difficult to manage adequately, and is associated with morbidity and mortality from specific acute and chronic complications. The latter two factors in particular make it different from and more problematic than other NCDs. Not surprisingly, its mortality is high: 20 years ago a study from Zimbabwe showed that 6 years after diagnosis, nearly 50% of diabetic patients had died – predominantly from metabolic problems (hypoglycaemia, ketoacidosis and other glycaemic states) or infections. There have been relatively few studies since, but what information there is suggests that there have been only modest improvements. However, in some communities renal failure (as a result of diabetic nephropathy) and cardiovascular disease are emerging causes of mortality. Diabetes outcome everywhere is highly dependent on local medical services, patient education and the availability of insulin and other appropriate medication.

Diagnosis

All type 1 diabetes, and much type 2 diabetes, present no diagnostic challenges, as patients present with classical symptoms (thirst, polyuria, weight loss, etc.) and obviously raised blood glucose levels. Some type 2 diabetic patients, however, have borderline values (particularly those who may be found accidentally). The World Health Organization (WHO) diagnostic criteria are shown in Box 59.2. Note that glycated haemoglobin (HbA_{1c}) has recently been accepted for diagnostic purposes in type 2 diabetes (cut off >6.5%). HbA_{1c} as a diagnostic test for type 2 diabetes is unlikely at present to become widely used in the tropics, as it is an expensive test and not widely available.

A glucose tolerance test (GTT) should be rarely needed, but if so a 75-g glucose load should be used, and tests performed at 0 and 2 h only. The basal and 2-h cut-off levels are the same as for the fasting and random levels above. It should be remembered that although most European and North American laboratories have standardized to *plasma* glucose levels, many tropical laboratories still measure *blood* glucose. The values are not the same: a plasma glucose of 7.0 is equivalent to a blood glucose of 6.1 mmol/L; and a plasma glucose of 11.1 mmol/L equivalent to a blood glucose of 10.0 mmol/L.

Prevalence

Fifty years ago diabetes was thought to be rare or even non-existent in tropical countries. It was probably genuinely less common than in Western countries, but high mortality prior to presentation at hospital may well have accounted for much of this 'rarity' (this remains a problem). In the last decade, type 2 diabetes in particular has reached epidemic rates all over the world, and the rate of expansion appears to be faster in developing as compared to developed countries. The total world number of people with diabetes will double in the next 10–15 years, and by 2020 diabetes will (in terms of mortality) almost certainly be the most important NCD. Actual prevalence rates of type 2 diabetes vary enormously. Global world prevalence was estimated as 6% in 2007, but some areas of the Caribbean have rates of 10–15%, and of the Middle East over 20%. Particularly high rates are seen in the elderly, and also in Asian migrants. In the tropics, urbanization and Westernization are particular risk factors. These lead to increased body weight and reduced exercise, both of which are potent causes of insulin resistance, which is the hallmark of type 2 diabetes.

Type 1 diabetes appears less common than in Western countries, and contributes usually less than 10% of the total diabetic population. The incidence in Africa is about 3–5 per 100 000 per year (compared to about 15–20 per 100 000 per year in Europe).

Enumeration difficulties, as referred to previously, may partly account for this difference. Type 1 diabetes in sub-Saharan Africa also appears to have a later age of onset than in Western countries (early twenties, rather than early teens).

Causes

The causes of diabetes in tropical countries are essentially similar to elsewhere. Type 2 diabetes can be seen as a 'lifestyle' disease, rapidly increasing as a result of excessive eating and a sedentary lifestyle. The tropical townships in particular are highly 'diabetogenic'. One popular explanation for this is the thrifty genotype theory. This theory suggests that genetically predisposed individuals may have reduced insulin secretory capacity or insulin resistance, which can be beneficial in a 'subsistence' or 'hunter-gatherer' situation, as ingested carbohydrate tends to be stored as fuel rather than rapidly burnt off. This 'thrifty' genotype loses its advantage when food supplies increase and exercise reduces (the urbanization situation). Here the reduced insulin reserves are overwhelmed and type 2 diabetes results. Although still theoretical, possible examples of the 'thrifty genotype' in action can be seen. Thus, in the late 1980s, a group of Africans from a famine area in northern Ethiopia were moved to Israel and within 4 years type 2 diabetes prevalence had risen from 0.1 to 8.9%.

There are certain diabetes syndromes seen particularly in the tropics with unusual causes, as follows:

- **Malnutrition-related diabetes mellitus (MRDM).** This was described many years ago, and has had a controversial history. It is seen in certain geographical areas of the tropics, and its exact cause is unknown though it appears related to past or present malnutrition. Patients present at a young age, and there is a male excess. They have low body weight and are hyperglycaemic but not ketotic. Sometimes there is obvious generalized pancreatic destruction, with fibrosis or calcification, and steatorrhoea. Treatment of MRDM depends on the degree of pancreatic damage – some may be controllable with sulphonylureas, but some will need insulin.
- **Atypical ketosis-prone type 2 diabetes.** This has been described particularly in West Africans, or migrants from this area. Patients are typically young and present acutely with marked hyperglycaemia or even ketoacidosis (DKA). After appropriate insulin treatment, however, the disease often remits, and patients can be controlled on oral agents or even diet. An association has been described with the herpes virus HHV-8.

- **ART-related diabetes**. Antiretroviral treatment (particularly with protease inhibitors or nucleoside reverse transcriptase inhibitors) can cause central obesity, with insulin resistance, glucose intolerance and potentially type 2 diabetes. With the widespread and increasing use of ART in the tropics, this cause of diabetes is likely to markedly increase in the next few years.

Complications

Acute complications

These are hypoglycaemia, ketoacidosis (DKA) and hyperosmolar hyperglycaemic states (HHS). They are seen more frequently in the tropics and carry a higher mortality. DKA mortality is now below 5% in Europe, but ranges from 10 to 30% or more in developing countries. Hypoglycaemia is not infrequently caused by sulphonylurea drugs; the commonly used glibenclamide is long-acting and may cause severe and prolonged hypoglycaemia.

Chronic complications

These include the classic specific complications of retinopathy, neuropathy and nephropathy, as well as the non-specific large vessel complications caused by atherosclerosis of the lower limb, coronary and cerebral arteries. Other complications include cataracts and erectile dysfunction. Diabetic complications – in particular those caused by small vessel disease – are strongly related to the degree of glycaemic control and the duration of disease. In some poorly resourced areas, the occurrence of diabetic complications may appear low; however, this may be because of inadequate surveillance or patients simply dying prematurely before complications have time to appear.

Infection

Infections are more common and more severe in diabetic patients, particularly those with poor control. Infective complications can be dramatic in the tropics – caused both by high blood glucose levels and delayed presentation. As well as standard infections involving, e.g. the chest, urinary tract and foot, some particularly dramatic and specific diabetic infections can be seen in the tropics. These include severe deep sepsis of the hand and orofacial mucormycosis.

Management

Diet

Diet and exercise are the prime treatments for type 2 diabetes, particularly when associated with obesity.

Unfortunately, even with good provision of expert dietetic and patient educational support, lifestyle change rarely controls diabetes adequately. Nevertheless, even in resource-poor situations, simple but firm advice should be offered.

Oral agents

Metformin should be used for obese and overweight patients inadequately controlled on diet alone, and sulphonylureas for the non-obese with similarly inadequate control. A body mass index (BMI) of 27.0 can be used for the obese/non-obese cut-off. This standard practice may be giving way to a 'metformin-for-all' policy in the future, with sulphonylureas as 'add-on' treatment.

All sulphonylurea drugs can cause hypoglycaemia, but glibenclamide and chlorpropamide are the most problematic. Oral hypoglycaemic agents should be started in low doses, and then increased as necessary. Combination treatment (metformin plus sulphonylureas) can be used if control is poor on maximal doses of one drug, but beyond this insulin may be needed.

Insulin

All type 1 diabetic patients obviously require insulin for survival, but many type 2 patients ideally require insulin for control. If insulin is in short supply, it may need to be reserved for type 1 patients only. The potential benefits of insulin in type 2 diabetes also need to be weighed against hypoglycaemic risks (especially if patient self blood glucose monitoring is not available). When insulin is given, as simple and safe a system as possible should be used. A twice-daily intermediate-acting insulin system (e.g. lente or isophane) is often successful and safe. A common misconception is that patients need a refrigerator to store their insulin. Insulin is relatively stable in all but the hottest conditions, and storage in a cool and shady area of the home is sufficient.

Ketoacidosis treatment

Successful and standard protocols are widely available for the management of DKA with intravenous insulin and fluids. However, such systems often require equipment not available in developing countries. A simple system requiring no special technology is shown in Box 59.3, which assumes that only bedside reagent-strip monitoring is available. In all cases of DKA it is also important to consider an infective precipitant, such as pneumonia, urinary infection, skin sepsis (e.g. foot or hand) or malaria.

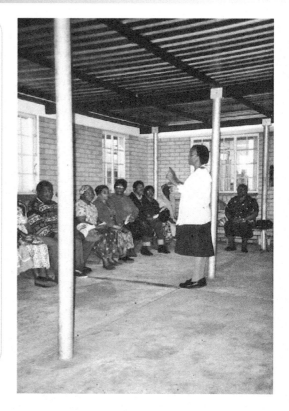

Box 59.3 Treatment of ketoacidosis in resource-poor settings

Fluids	Give 500 mL 0.9% saline quickly, then 500 mL hourly for 4–6 h
Potassium	Give none for the first hour, then 20 mmol KCl hourly for 3 h, then 10 mmol hourly for 2 h (diluted in the saline infusion)
Insulin	Give any soluble insulin 20 units i.m. stat, then 10 units i.m. hourly. If no soluble is available, give lente or isophane i.m. similarly
Bicarbonate	Give only if the patient is very ill and not improving. Give 50 mmol $NaHCO_3$ slowly i.v.
Monitoring	Blood glucose (BG) hourly by reagent strip
Later	When BG = 15 mmol/L, convert intravenous saline to 5% dextrose. Continue i.m. insulin, and change to a subcutaneous regimen when the patient can eat

Figure 59.1 Diabetes education at a primary health clinic in rural South Africa.

Education

An inexpensive but highly effective treatment modality is patient education. This should be delivered to patients by local nurses or other health workers, often at primary health centre level. A simple 'syllabus' should be agreed, incorporating for example an explanation of what diabetes is and why treatment is important, tablet and insulin treatment, diet, foot care, monitoring control, social aspects etc. Simple visual aids (eg flip charts) can be helpful. This type of education has been shown to be beneficial in rural African settings (see Figure 59.1).

Monitoring

Ideal diabetes monitoring is with self-glucose testing (for those on insulin), and regular HbA1c tests in clinic. Both techniques are expensive and rarely affordable in resource-limited settings. Urine glucose testing is often used as an alternative, but it is insensitive and of doubtful value. Symptom surveillance can be surprisingly effective – for example, in type 2 diabetes nocturia is a sensitive indicator of glycaemic status. Body weight should be monitored and hypoglycaemia always enquired about.

Organization of care

Although the skilled use of individual drugs and insulin is important, the real challenge of diabetes management in the tropics is of delivery of care in difficult circumstances. Particular problems are:

- late presentation;
- low and irregular food supply;
- lack of insulin and oral agents;
- absence of dietitians and podiatrists;
- lack of monitoring equipment;
- poor laboratory support.

Insulin shortage is a particular problem. It is an expensive drug in developing countries, and supplies are often poor and erratic. With all these problems, the aims of treatment may need to be compromised, with relief of symptoms and avoidance of hypoglycaemia the main aims. Diabetes is an NCD ideally suited to nurse-led and community-delivered care. The major factors in setting up a district diabetic service in

- Organization and delegation
- Central hospital referral clinic
- Decentralized peripheral clinic care
- Nurse-led protocols for type 2 diabetes
- Patient and staff education system
- Medical protocols for diabetic ketoacidosis treatment
- Simple dietetic and foot care
- Sensible use of drugs and insulin
- Hypertension management
- Complication surveillance
- Gestational diabetic care
- Diabetic retinopathy screening

a tropical country are shown in Box 59.4. Obviously, the list will need to be adapted to the geographical situation, resources available and particular clinical problems present.

Nurse-led care of type 2 diabetic patients in primary health care units is especially appropriate, and has been shown to be highly successful. Figure 59.2 shows an algorithm that has been used successfully. It assumes metformin and glibenclamide are the available drugs, but obviously must be adapted to local conditions.

Hypertension

Epidemiology

Hypertension is globally by far the most common NCD, and in the tropics it makes up approximately 40% of the total NCD burden. Globally, at least 25% of the world's population have hypertension. The major importance of hypertension is that it is a potent risk factor for stroke and, because of the frequency of raised blood pressure (BP), it leads to a very high population stroke risk. Effective treatment of hypertension lowers risk by at least 40%, and such treatment can involve relatively simple and inexpensive drugs. Sadly, however, much hypertension remains undiagnosed, and of those cases diagnosed many are inadequately controlled.

Diagnosis

Population BP levels are continuously distributed, and there is therefore no clear dividing line between hypertensive and non-hypertensive levels. Diagnostic

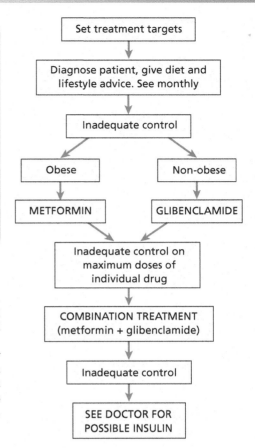

Figure 59.2 Nurse-led algorithm for treating patients with type 2 diabetes. Note: (1) The treatment target must be set locally depending on resources. Without laboratory support it should be 'absence from hyperglycaemic symptoms, and drug-induced hypoglycaemia'. Laboratory targets may be a fasting blood glucose, 8.0 mmol/L, or an HbA_{1c}, 8.0%. (2) Ideally, patients should see a doctor at diagnosis for complication screening. (3) Obesity can be defined as a body mass index 27.0. (4) The drugs are given in stepwise increments increasing each month as follows: metformin 500 mg/day and then 500 mg b.d., then 500 mg t.d.s., then 1 g b.d., then 1 g t.d.s. For glibenclamide, give 2.5 mg/day, then 5 mg/day, then 5 mg b.d., then t.d.s. (5) When using combination treatment, use the second drug according to the dose regimen mentioned earlier. (6) At each visit reinforce lifestyle advice, check for diabetic symptoms and possible drug side effects (hypoglycaemia with glibenclamide, and dyspepsia or diarrhoea with metformin). (7) Weigh patient and check urine at clinic visits. Always check BP and, if constantly > 140/80 mmHg, treat vigorously.

cut-off levels are therefore decided on the basis of risk, and these levels have been progressively decreasing. WHO currently recommends a diagnostic cut-off of 140/90 mmHg. There is, however, evidence that in certain high-risk groups (notably those with diabetes) the cut-off level should be lower – probably 130/80 mmHg.

Accurate measurement is important in diagnosing hypertension. A good quality mercury sphygmomanometer, with an adequate-sized and well-fitting cuff, remains the 'gold standard' system. However, the use of such equipment is declining, as a number of countries are restricting their use because of concerns over mercury toxicity. The alternative electronic machines are expensive and difficult to maintain. Aneroid models are a reasonable compromise, although they can read slightly lower than other systems. Overall, the major problem in accurate BP measurement is failure to use a large-sized cuff in an obese patient.

Prevalence

As may be expected, prevalence rates vary widely geographically. In some poor rural areas of the tropics, where obesity is rare, rates of well below 5% are found. Conversely, in many urban areas of sub-Saharan Africa, where obesity is very common, hypertension may be found in 40–50% of the population or more. Most tropical doctors will find themselves working in areas with hypertension prevalence rates of 10–20% at least. It should always be remembered that the prevalence of known hypertension (those on antihypertensive medication) always considerably underestimates the total hypertension prevalence – often by about one-half. In view of this, and the essentially asymptomatic nature of the disease, opportunist hypertension screening should be undertaken whenever possible (e.g. at inpatient or outpatient hospital attendances, regardless of the reason for the consultation).

Causes and risk factors

About 95% of cases of hypertension are 'essential' (with no definable underlying cause). Secondary hypertension is always rare. Causes include Cushing's syndrome, Conn's syndrome, phaeochromacytoma and a variety of renal disorders. A number of aetiological factors have been suggested for essential hypertension, including genetic factors, fetal malnutrition (the 'fetal origins' hypothesis), salt retention (in West Africa and North American Afro-Caribbeans, sometimes known as the 'Slave Hypothesis') and subtle abnormalities of the renin–aldosterone system. It is more useful to think in terms of risk factors for

essential hypertension, rather than actual causes. In the tropics, the main risk factors are as follows:

- obesity (especially central);
- high salt intake;
- urbanization;
- excess alcohol intake;
- reduced activity.

It can be seen that these make up a 'package' of adverse lifestyle factors similar to those predisposing to urban diabetes. Reduced activity and central obesity leads to insulin resistance, and this is strongly associated with hypertension, as well as diabetes. Increased salt intake is probably a major feature of tropical urbanization, and some individuals may be particularly prone to the potential hypertensive effect of increased dietary salt.

Complications

The long-term result of uncontrolled hypertension can be a variety of complications resulting from end-organ damage. These are as follows:

- stroke;
- left ventricular hypertrophy;
- renal failure;
- coronary artery disease;
- hypertensive retinopathy.

Of these, stroke is by far the most important, with hypertension leading to an excess risk of up to 10 times that in non-hypertensive subjects. Stroke in hypertensive patients can be caused by cerebral thrombosis as well as cerebral haemorrhage. Left ventricular hypertrophy is also a serious complication, which may lead to hypertensive heart failure. Hypertensive renal disease is one of the most common causes of chronic renal failure.

A rare acute complication is the 'hypertensive crisis' that occurs in severe and accelerated disease. Patients usually have a diastolic BP in excess of 140 mmHg, encephalopathy and hypertensive retinopathy (often with papilloedema).

Management
Principles of treatment

Treatment of hypertension should follow a logical pathway, bearing in mind the important basic principles of management below.

- *Education* is vital; patients must understand what the disease is, and how treatment will help them.
- *Non-drug treatment* includes weight reduction, reduced salt intake, reduced alcohol, avoidance of smoking, and increased exercise.

- *Compliance* is a major barrier to good BP control. Try to use once daily drug systems and be sensitive to possible side-effects.
- *Side-effects* can be minimized by using low doses of more than one drug, rather than very high doses of a single drug.
- *Organization* of hypertension care is very important, as the number of patients involved is likely to be high.

Drug treatment

Popular antihypertensive drugs in developed countries include angiotensin-converting enzyme (ACE) inhibitors or ARBs (angiotensin receptor blockers) if ACE drugs cause side effects, and calcium channel blockers. All these drugs are relatively expensive and often unavailable in resource-limited tropical countries. There are important ethnic factors in drug effectiveness; thus, ACE inhibitors, ARBs and beta-blockers work less well in black compared with white subjects. However, the addition of a thiazide diuretic to ACE or ARB treatment appears to restore most of their effectiveness.

In developing countries, the choice will usually be dependent on cost and availability. Simple and cheap drugs such as thiazides and methyldopa may be appropriate and effective. Side effects are rarely a problem. Thiazide doses should be low (e.g. hydrochlorothiazide 12.5 mg or bendrofluazide 2.5 mg) – at these levels adverse effects on blood glucose do not occur, and antihypertensive effect is as good as at higher doses. More expensive drugs such as ACE inhibitors or calcium blockers should (if available) be reserved for more difficult cases.

It has already been mentioned that only about half of hypertensive patients are detected. In addition, it is known that of those detected cases, only about one-half are treated; and of those treated, only about half reach treatment targets (this is the so-called 'Rule of Halves'). Detection and treatment therefore needs to be improved, and patients should be 'treated to targets' (usually below 140/90, though this may be lower in some situations, e.g. diabetes).

Special situations

There are specific clinical situations where the standard progression of treatment (first-line, second-line, etc.) should not be followed, as specific drugs may be indicated or contraindicated. Beta-blockers should be avoided in asthma, but they are good first-line drugs in the presence of angina. Similarly, ACE inhibitors (if available) are ideally suited to patients with heart failure, or diabetes with renal complications (nephropathy or microalbuminaemia).

Hypertensive crisis

Patients should be bed-rested and observed closely, with hourly BP measurements. A simple, but often surprisingly effective treatment is simply to give methyldopa orally, 1 gm stat and then 500 mg 4-hourly. Otherwise, hydralazine 10 mg i.m. every 2–4 h is usually effective.

Organization of care

As with type 2 diabetes, routine hypertension management is ideally suited to primary health clinic care by suitably trained nurses. In most areas, there are large numbers of hypertensive patients, and such a system will allow medical staff to concentrate on more difficult cases. Again, as with diabetes, the protocol needs to be adapted to local needs and drug supplies. Figure 59.3 assumes that a thiazide drug and methyldopa are the main available, cheap and effective medications in use.

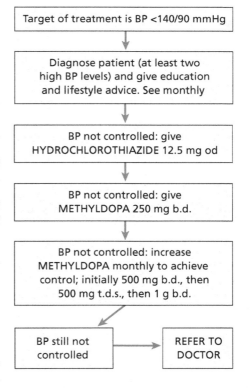

Figure 59.3 Nurse-led algorithm for treating patients with hypertension. Note: (1) Any low-dose thiazide can be used. (2) Make sure BP is measured carefully and correctly. (3) At each visit, reinforce lifestyle advice and check compliance.

Initial patient education is important, and should carry two messages. First, advice should be given on non-drug aspects of treatment. Secondly, the nature and importance of hypertension should be carefully explained. In most cases hypertension is asymptomatic, and patients will not comply with long-term treatment unless they understand the benefits.

Asthma

Epidemiology

Asthma is a chronic clinical syndrome of reversible airways obstruction, characterized by wheeze and shortness of breath. Airways obstruction is caused by inflammation, resulting in bronchial oedema, mucus production and smooth muscle contraction. Asthma particularly affects younger age groups and, if poorly controlled, is likely to interfere with school or work attendance. A significant amount of asthma is undiagnosed and misdiagnosed. In the tropics, asthma is increasing and becoming a major problem in urban environments. Effective drugs are expensive and often poorly available. The death rate is unknown, but is certainly higher than in developed countries.

Diagnosis

The hallmark of asthma is reversible airways obstruction, and the key features in the history are wheeze, cough and breathlessness. Wheezes may be present on chest auscultation, but their absence does not exclude the diagnosis, which is essentially made on the history. Asthma symptoms are often worse at night, or in the early morning and may be provoked by trigger factors (e.g. allergens, cold, exercise). Sometimes, particularly in children, a dry (and often nocturnal) cough may be the only feature. In adults, breathlessness without wheeze may indicate asthma. If available, patient records of peak flow (PF) measurements are useful in making the diagnosis. PF readings will usually be variable, often low, but in particular show classical 'early morning dipping'. In doubtful cases spirometry with and without bronchodilation may be useful diagnostically: the FEV1 is reduced (to below 80% of the predicted value), as is the FEV1:FVC ratio (to below 70%). Without this equipment a simple clinic PF measurement, repeated 20 min after two puffs of a salbutamol inhaler, can give similar information.

Frequently in developing countries, the diagnosis is made on history, perhaps confirmed by a trial of bronchodilator treatment. The diagnosis of asthma is summarized in Box 59.5.

Box 59.5 **Diagnosis of asthma**

- History
- Patient peak flow (PF) charts
- Spirometry with bronchodilation
- PF with bronchodilation
- Response to treatment

Some care must be taken with the differential diagnosis. In children, simple wheezy bronchitis may be mistaken for asthma. In adults, chronic obstructive pulmonary disease (COPD) is the main alternative diagnosis. Tropical pulmonary eosinophilia should also be considered.

Prevalence

Studies of prevalence of asthma in the tropics vary widely. This is partly a result of diagnostic difficulties. Other factors affecting prevalence results include patient age (rates will be higher in younger age groups) and whether the environment is rural or urban. Rates are generally low in rural areas (usually below 5%), but in towns can rise to 10–15% or more. In Western countries asthma prevalence has greatly increased in recent decades, and asthma is now rapidly increasing also in the developing world.

Causes

General

There are several factors related to the causation of asthma, although the overall explanation for individual disease (and indeed increasing population trends) is often uncertain.

- *Allergens* – allergy is very important in many cases. The most important allergen is the house dust mite, but in tropical countries cockroaches and bed bugs can also be important. Other allergens include pollens, animal dander and fungal spores.
- *Genetic factors* – there is familial clustering of atopy and allergy in general, and asthma in particular.
- *'Hygiene hypothesis'* – this hypothesis is based on the observation that children who have relatively little infection or vaccination exposure early in life have a greater risk of later asthma.
- *Obesity* – the reason for this association is uncertain but asthma is certainly more common in the obese.

In addition to the above, there are a number of environmental precipitants or triggers to asthma.

These include some drugs (e.g. non-steroidal anti-inflammatory drugs, beta-blockers), and active or passive smoking. Atmospheric pollution in general is not thought nowadays to be a true cause of asthma. Asthma rates are rising in Europe while the air gets cleaner.

Urban asthma

There are several potential causes of the marked rise in asthma prevalence seen in tropical urban, compared with rural, environments. The major reason is probably increased exposure to house dust mites, and this is supported from studies in Ethiopia. Rural dwellings tend to be spacious and well ventilated, and have rudimentary furniture. In towns, houses are smaller, and have doors and windows that reduce ventilation. There may also be curtains, carpets, easy chairs, etc. Overall, the environment is ideal for house dust mites! A further interesting factor may be the reduced childhood intestinal parasite load found in urban areas. There is evidence that increased parasite exposure in childhood reduces the risk of later asthma. Obesity increases with urbanization. Finally, the urban environment has more 'triggers' to asthma for those with a predisposition to the disease (e.g. smoking, household fires, occupational irritants).

Complications

The main complication of asthma is sudden and severe decompensation to acute severe asthma (status asthmaticus). This is usually brought on by infection and is heralded by increasing need for reliever (bronchodilator) aerosols, reduced effect of such treatment, and severe nocturnal breathlessness. Patients at presentation usually have tachypnoea, distress and marked airways obstruction. There is often tachycardia and sometimes pulsus paradoxus. Blood gas levels are initially well-preserved, but a rising pCO_2 is a dangerous sign. Cyanosis and a 'silent chest' are similarly serious signs suggesting the likely impending need for ventilatory assistance. Status asthmaticus is a serious complication of asthma with a small but significant mortality.

Management
Routine treatment

The most effective treatment is based on beta-2 agonist and steroid aerosols. Beta-2 agonists can be considered to be 'relievers'. The most commonly used is salbutamol (Ventolin) although there are several others (e.g. terbutaline). Steroid inhalers

can be considered to be 'preventers', and again there are several, although the most common is beclometasone. Reliever treatment gives rapid improvement and can be given either as needed or, if necessary, on a regular basis. Preventer aerosols are given regularly, regardless of current symptoms. They are now regarded as primary asthma treatment in all but the mildest cases. Asthma can be managed in a simple drug cascade system, adding in further treatment if initial management fails to control the disease or trialling reduced therapy if symptom relief is good and stable ('step up' and 'step down' treatment).

Tropical adaptations to treatment

Asthma inhalers are expensive and often difficult to obtain in developing countries. Simple identification and removal of precipitants can be helpful. Oral bronchodilators may have to be the mainstay of treatment. These are difficult drugs to use, with a narrow therapeutic window and relatively weak bronchodilator activity. Cromoglycate (Intal) is now rarely used in modern asthma practice, but if available (and steroid inhalers are not) it is worth using as a preventor inhaler.

Treatment of exacerbations

Infective exacerbations should be treated with antibiotics and a brief course of steroids (e.g. prednisone or prednisolone 40 mg/day for 5–10 days). Assuming the patient is on a beta-2 agonist inhaler (e.g. salbutamol), this should be given in a high dose (e.g. 4–8 puffs q.d.s.) via a spacer inhaler (which can, if necessary, be home made – see below). Antibiotics may be needed but most underlying infections are viral.

Treatment of acute severe asthma (status asthmaticus)

If asthmatic exacerbations are treated promptly and adequately, this is an avoidable complication. Nevertheless, when it does occur, it must be treated vigorously. The principles of management are shown in Box 59.6.

If nebulized salbutamol is not available, high-dose inhalers with a spacer device should be used. If available intravenous magnesium (1.2–2.0 g by single i.v. infusion over 20 minutes) can be helpful. The dose in children over 2 years is 40 mg/kg i.v. up to a maximum of 2 g. Aminophylline can also be used (250–500 mg or 5 mg/kg by slow i.v. infusion). If

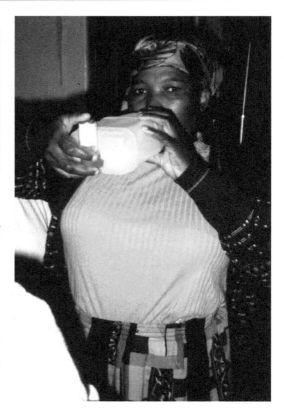

Figure 59.4 A makeshift bronchodilator aerosol spacer device. This woman from rural South Africa is using an adapted plastic milk container to effectively inhale salbutamol. *Source:* Parry *et al.* (2004); reproduced with permission.

nothing else is available, adrenaline (epinephrine) can be life-saving, used in a subcutaneous dose of 0.1 mL of 1/1000 solution per 10 kg body weight (give 0.75 mL if the patient is too ill to be weighed).

Organization of care

Patient education

Patient education is especially important if asthma treatment is to be successful, and all newly diagnosed patients should be given simple advice and training as follows:

- understanding asthma;
- avoiding allergic triggers;
- importance of regular treatment;
- correct use of inhalers;
- concept of reliever and preventer treatment;
- recognizing deterioration and seeking help.

Particularly in younger asthmatic patients, attention to allergic triggers can be helpful. This includes avoiding domestic pets, good home ventilation, and regular beating and cleaning of bedclothes, mattresses and settees. Inhaler technique is vitally important – many patients find these difficult to use, and without training they will be ineffective and a waste of resources. Spacer devices are very effective, and these can be homemade. An empty plastic milk or fruit juice container is ideal – a hole is cut at or near the bottom to fit the mouthpiece of the inhaler, the required dose is delivered into the container, and then rebreathed through the top. These systems have been shown to be as effective as expensive proprietary spacers (see Figure 59.4).

Doctor education

Doctor education is also important. Protocols of routine and emergency management should be widely displayed and distributed. Many patients develop acute severe asthma because of inadequate preceding medical treatment. In particular, steroids are widely underused – a course of prednisolone 40 mg/day for 5–7 days given on an outpatient basis frequently resolves significantly deteriorating asthma. There are few acute dangers with such short courses and, in particular, adrenal suppression does not occur. In areas where *Entamoeba histolytica* and/or *Strongyloides stercoralis* are found, asthmatic patients should be regularly screened for these infections, as steroids may cause serious deterioration of amoebic dysentery, or the hyperinfection syndrome of strongyloidiasis.

Nurse-led treatment protocols

As with other NCDs, basic asthma treatment is well-suited to protocol-based stepwise care, delivered by nurses (Fig. 59.5). Although PF measurements can

Aim of treatment is freedom from asthma symptoms

↓

Diagnose patient, give education, and train in inhaler technique

↓

Give 'RELIEVER' inhaler (e.g. salbutamol) to take as required

↓

If not controlled, take reliever inhaler regularly

↓

If still not controlled, add 'PREVENTOR' inhaler (e.g. beclometasone) regularly

↓

If still not controlled

↓

REFER TO DOCTOR

Figure 59.5 Nurse-led algorithm for treating patients with asthma. Note: (1) At each clinic visit record symptoms, measure peak flow and check inhaler technique. (2) Beyond currently taken reliever and preventor aerosols, medical staff may have to consider oral theophylline or aminophylline preparations, or even sometimes low-dose maintenance steroids.

be useful to detect` improvement and deterioration, the basic aim of treatment should be freedom from significant asthmatic symptoms.

Epilepsy

Epidemiology

Although epilepsy is much less common than hypertension or asthma, it is an important NCD for several reasons. Diagnosis is often difficult, and there are many with undiagnosed epilepsy. Those with known disease are frequently poorly controlled, and their continuing seizures carry a significant social stigma and life burden. The condition also carries an excess mortality of 2–5 times that of non-epileptic people. Treatment is often made difficult by a lack of modern drugs, and many doctors do not understand the basic principles of anticonvulsant therapy. There are also cultural problems affecting the person with epilepsy

in the tropics. It is not always seen as a disease at all in some cultures (it may be considered a form of bewitching or possession by demons). In other societies it may be thought to be contagious.

Diagnosis

The diagnosis rests on a history of at least two typical attacks, preferably witnessed, and with the history obtained from the witness. A good description of typical grand mal (tonic–clonic) seizures should lead to a firm diagnosis, but it must be remembered that there are other less obvious types of seizure: absence attacks (or petit mal – usually in childhood); and a variety of partial seizures, with or without impairment of consciousness (e.g. focal motor epilepsy, temporal lobe epilepsy). A simple and useful modern classification of seizures is as shown in Box 59.7.

Box 59.7 Classification of epilepsy

- Grand mal (tonic–clonic)
- Absence attacks (petit mal)
- Simple partial seizures (patient conscious), for example focal motor or temporal lobe
- Complex partial seizures (as above, but with loss of consciousness)
- Myoclonic epilepsy (rare)

Note: Partial seizures may sometimes progress to grand mal attacks.

When attacks are atypical, and especially where they are not witnessed, diagnosis may be difficult. Electroencephalography (EEG) is rarely available in tropical countries, and is anyway often unreliable. A trial of anticonvulsant therapy is sometimes a reasonable option, with the patient keeping a close record of attacks.

Prevalence

Rates of reported epilepsy in developing countries greatly underestimate the extent of the problem. Their variability also reflects diagnostic difficulties, which may alter geographically, and also local causative factors (e.g. prevalence of neurocysticercosis). Overall prevalence rates are probably around 2%. Reported studies have demonstrated prevalences of 0.5% in Ethiopia, 1.0% in Uganda, 3.0% in Tanzania and 5.0% in India.

Causes

Most epilepsy in developed countries is idiopathic, but in developing countries proportionally more cases have a definable cause. Tropical causes of epilepsy include the following:

- birth hypoxia/injury;
- past head injury;
- past meningitis/encephalitis (e.g. cerebral malaria, bacterial meningitis, sleeping sickness);
- HIV infection (usually caused by an associated opportunist infection or tumour, such as toxoplasmosis, cryptococcosis, tuberculoma or lymphoma);
- brain tumours, cysts (e.g. hydatid);
- neurocysticercosis (*Taenia solium*);
- past stroke.

Complications

Burns and other trauma occurring during seizures are the most common complications of epilepsy. Sudden death may occur during fits. Status epilepticus is a serious complication. It normally occurs in pre-existing epilepsy and can be provoked by infection or alcohol excess. It carries significant mortality and must be treated vigorously.

Management

Drug treatment

Infections leading to epilepsy should always be treated. It has been shown that albendazole or praziquantel treatment for neurocysticercosis reduces seizure frequency, though long-term anticonvulsant treatment is still often necessary. Anticonvulsants commonly used in Western countries are rarely affordable in the tropics, but phenobarbitol (and sometimes phenytoin) are usually available, and if used properly can be very effective. Side-effects can sometimes be problematic. Phenobarbital can cause drowsiness, and sometimes behaviour change in children. Phenytoin may lead to gum hypertrophy, acne and hirsutism; as well as sedation and, in excessive doses, vertigo and incoordination. Like other anticonvulsants, phenytoin and phenobarbital are potentially difficult drugs to use as they have a 'therapeutic window' of blood levels. Below this window they are ineffective, but above it they are toxic. In the absence of drug level estimations in the blood, the drugs should be started at a low dose and gradually titrated up until seizure control is obtained. Experience from India suggests that adult doses of phenobarbital should start at 30 mg/day, and be slowly titrated up to 90 mg/day (in 30 mg increments). For phenytoin the range is 100–300 mg (in 50 mg increments). Both drugs should be given once daily at night. Effective seizure control can often be obtained using either of these drugs in this way.

Patients, with family members, should be seen monthly with a record of epileptic attack, and enquiries made regarding possible side effects.

Status epilepticus

If available, intravenous or rectal diazepam is ideal, but if not intravenous phenytoin can be used (this can also be given if diazepam has failed). The dose schedules are as follows:

- *Diazepam* – 2 mg slow i.v. per minute (up to 20 mg);
- *Phenytoin* – 18 mg/kg by slow i.v. infusion, usually 750–1500 mg over 30–60 minutes.

Old-fashioned paraldehyde (5 mL deep i.m. in each buttock) can still be effective (remember to use a glass syringe!). In severe refractory cases, general anaesthesia with muscle relaxation and anaesthesia may be needed.

Organization of care

Education

Successful epilepsy management programmes in the tropics involve education of patients, carers and the community. As with other NCDs, patients need to understand the nature of their disease and the importance of regular treatment, particularly as most fits in established epileptic patients result from poor compliance. Other precipitants are infections, alcohol excess and some drugs which lower seizure threshold. Patients may recognize their own triggers (e.g. excessive fatigue, psychological stress and, in women, prior to menstruation). Carers should if possible be involved to provide support and sometimes to supervise medication. Attempts should be made at a community level to increase understanding of epilepsy, and to prevent distrust of or discrimination against the epileptic patient.

Drug treatment

Although there is less experience with nurse-led epilepsy care than with other NCDs, once the diagnosis is made and treatment initiated by medical staff, there is no reason why nursing staff cannot supervise the dose increases of phenobarbital or phenytoin mentioned above. Figure 59.6 illustrates a suggested protocol using phenobarbital, although a similar one could be produced with phenytoin.

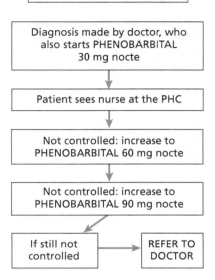

Figure 59.6 Nurse-led algorithm for treating patients with epilepsy. Note: (1) At each visit check compliance, disease understanding and any side effects of treatment. (2) Patients are asked to keep a diary of fits. PHC, primary health clinic.

Mental illness

WHO recognizes that mental disease is an important cause of disability throughout the world but in most developing countries it has received little attention and few resources. Much mental illness presents to traditional healers, and people with serious disease such as schizophrenia may be tied up or chained for many years without effective treatment (see Fig. 59.7). Those with depression and anxiety are more likely to present in general medical clinics and if the diagnosis is missed an opportunity to provide cheap and effective treatment is lost. The patient is then likely to keep on returning, his or her symptoms unresolved.

Assessment of acute mental disturbance

There are three important questions to ask when examining the acutely disturbed patient:

1 **Is this person physically ill?** Acute infections, metabolic disturbance, epilepsy or trauma may all cause confusion and sometimes frank delirium.

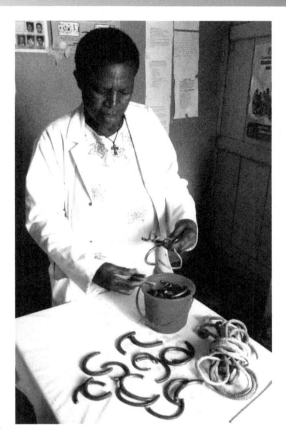

Figure 59.7 A psychiatric clinical officer with shackles removed from mentally ill patients at a hospital in Uganda.

Eliminate physical causes before assuming that the patient is mentally ill. Check especially for cognitive impairment. Impaired concentration, attention, orientation and memory characteristically suggest organic disorders. Be careful when administering sedative drugs to patients who may be physically ill. Give only what is needed to allow safe examination and establishment of diagnosis. Benzodiazepines may be used provided the patient's conscious level is normal and there are no respiratory problems. A combination of antipsychotic such as haloperidol with lorazepam is usually effective.

2 **Is this person under the influence of drugs or alcohol?** Use of illicit drugs and alcohol are common; ask the patient and their relative for details. Patients who appear to be simply drunk and confused may also have a head injury or metabolic disturbance: check for dehydration, hypoglycaemia and hepatic dysfunction.

3 **Is this person mentally ill?** If physical illness and drug-related problems have been eliminated examine the patient's mental state in more detail to establish the diagnosis. Remember the patient is likely to be frightened so needs care and kindness as well as a safe environment.

Schizophrenia

Schizophrenia is a common and serious mental disorder affecting every part of a patient's mental state. Key features are:

- **hallucinations:** the patient commonly hears people talking about him or her, often to each other and usually with an unpleasant or frightening content; there may also be disturbed perception in any other sensory modality, e.g. tingling or burning of limbs or body, abnormal tastes or smells;
- **delusions:** often as a result of hallucinations the person begins to believe things which are not true, e.g. that people are out to kill them or that they are being subject to mysterious forces;
- **affective (mood) changes:** unexpected aggression, inappropriate laughter or social withdrawal may occur, again often in response to the hallucinations or delusions;
- **disturbed behaviour:** as a result the patient in a frightened or defensive state may hide away, run off, or express aggression to others.

Treatment

Treatment of schizophrenia is cheap, and in the setting of a primary care programme is usually very effective.

Be sure to eliminate physical causes for the psychotic symptoms (especially illicit drugs or epilepsy). Once the diagnosis is made, the key is maintenance treatment with **antipsychotics**. If the patient has a supportive family these may be given orally, e.g. chlorpromazine 100 mgs t.d.s. or haloperidol 5 mgs t.d.s. initially. Reduce the dose once the acute phase is over, but maintain treatment to keep the patient well.

If atypical antipsychotics are available, use olanzapine for more aggressive patients. Dosage should be titrated against symptoms: check with the family as well as the patient to judge whether the psychotic symptoms are improving.

Treat side effects such as muscle stiffness and tremor with an antiparkinsonian agent, e.g. benzhexol 5 mg or procyclidine 5 mg two or three times a day.

If depot antipsychotics are available these are ideal in a primary care mental health programme. Give the patient a monthly injection of fluphenazine 25 mgs or flupenthixol 20–40 mgs, again titrating against symptoms. Regular treatment and family and community support can transform a patient's mental health so that he or she can become happy and productive again.

Depression

WHO figures suggest that depressive disorder is the 4th leading cause of disease burden worldwide, and the burden of disability caused by depression comes into the same range as ischaemic heart disease, diarrhoeal disease, or asthma and COPD. It is a relapsing and remitting disorder, often closely linked to events or relationships in the person's life, so a careful history is needed. In developing countries the presenting symptoms are likely to be:

- low mood;
- physical symptoms, e.g. headache, backache, general body pains, palpitations; it is helpful to learn the local language of emotional distress in order to identify the real cause of vague physical symptoms which appear to have no organic cause;
- anxiety and fearfulness;
- insomnia, especially with early waking;
- change in appetite, usually eating less with weight loss;
- poor concentration and memory;
- loss of energy and motivation, withdrawal;
- loss of hope and optimism.

If depression is suspected, discuss the patient's life circumstances to check for an obvious cause. Often talking over problems with a sympathetic health worker will be helpful in itself. If the patient appears to be becoming more severely ill, the options are:

- **antidepressants,** e.g. amitriptyline or imipramine in gradually increasing doses up to 150 mg at night or fluoxetine 20–40 mgs daily;
- **cognitive behaviour therapy (CBT)** either alone or with antidepressants; patients with very low mood cannot concentrate well enough for psychotherapy so will need pharmacological treatment first;
- **electroconvulsive therapy:** a specialist treatment, which may be highly effective in severe cases.

Be sure to check for suicidal ideas in any patient with depression. If the patient has clear plans and intention to harm or kill himself seek specialist help. A pathway of care for suicidal patients is shown in Figure 59.8.

Bipolar affective disorder

When the patient experiences discrete episodes of high mood as well as depression, they

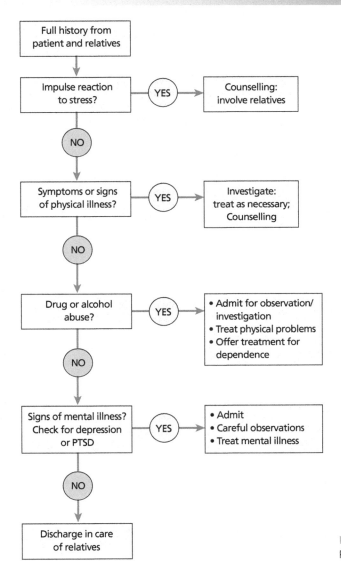

Figure 59.8 Management of suicidal patients.
PTSD: Post-traumatic stress disorder.

may have bipolar disorder. This may be treated symptomatically – antipsychotics for the high or manic mood, and antidepressants for depression.

If there is access to specialist support, better still is a mood stabilizer, eg lithium. This is excellent but needs careful monitoring including regular checks on serum levels of lithium, renal function and thyroid function. Alternative mood stabilizers are carbamazepine and sodium valproate. Do not use lithium and anticonvulsants in women of childbearing age in view of the risk of teratogenesis, instead, use maintenance antipsychotics.

Post-traumatic stress disorder (PTSD)

People who have been subject to life-threatening situations over which they have no control may develop PTSD, a disabling condition. Check for this in any person who has been subject to trauma, especially in war or refugee situations. Symptoms are as follows:

- high anxiety with high vigilance;
- insomnia with nightmares;
- day time 'flashbacks' (seeing images of the original trauma);
- depression and suicidal ideas;

Be alert for sexual trauma in women and girls especially. The effects are profound and long-lasting, but difficult to disclose, and the patient will need careful and sympathetic management. Treatment for PTSD is with antidepressants such as fluoxetine 20–60 mgs daily, and cognitive behaviour therapy.

Organization of care

Most mental illnesses can be effectively treated in primary care.

- Include mental illness in the list of conditions managed in primary care clinics.
- Train general health workers in common signs and symptoms.
- Maintain people with schizophrenia on oral or depot antipsychotics.
- Maintain people with recurrent depression on antidepressants.
- Work with community volunteers or health workers to identify mental illness and signs of relapse in known patients.
- Work with local leaders, traditional healers and communities to reduce stigma and ensure that patients receive effective treatment.

🔑 SUMMARY

- Non-communicable diseases (NCDs) are rapidly increasing in prevalence in tropical countries.
- The adoption of Western lifestyles ('epidemiological transition') is increasing the prevalence of many NCDs – notably diabetes.
- NCD-associated mortality is now approaching that related to infective disease.
- Important NCDs in tropical countries include diabetes, asthma, hypertension, epilepsy, cardiovascular disease, stroke and mental health disorders.
- Models of NCD care delivery in the tropics differ from those used in developed countries. Nurse-led, community-based systems are often successful.

 Visit www.lecturenoteseries.com/tropicalmed to test yourself on this chapter using interactive MCQs.

📖 FURTHER READING

Bhugra D, Bhui K (eds) (2007) *Textbook of Cultural Psychiatry.* Cambridge: Cambridge University Press. [A very helpful perspective on practicing psychiatry in difficult cultures.]

Gill GV, Mbanya J-C, Ramaiya KL, Tesfaye S (2009) A sub-Saharan African perspective of diabetes. *Diabetologia* **52**: 8–16. [A comprehensive update of diabetes in sub-Saharan Africa, including epidemiology, complications and management.]

Mabey D, Parry E, Gill G, *et al.* (2013) *Principles of Medicine in Africa.* 4th ed. Cambridge: Cambridge University Press. [Contains several useful chapters on NCDs, relevant to Africa and elsewhere in the tropics. These include 'Diabetes' (Gill GV, Mbanya JC, pp. 498–509), 'Asthma' (Fullerton DG *et al.*, pp. 566–577), 'Hypertension' (Walker RW, Edwards R, pp. 510–524), 'Epilepsy' (Prevelt MC, Newton CR, pp. 531–542), and 'Mental Health' (Gureje O, Oladeji B, pp. 543–565).]

Mani KS *et al.* (2001) Epilepsy control with phenobarbitol or phenytoin in rural south India: the Yelandur study. *Lancet* **357**: 1316–20. [An excellent report showing successful epilepsy control with appropriately delivered monotherapy.]

Meyer A-C, Dua T, Ma J, Saxena S, Birbeck G (2010) Global disparities in the epilepsy treatment gap: a systemic review. *Bull Wld Hlth Org* **88**: 260–6. [A literature review demonstrating a significant 'treatment gap' amongst epileptic patients in tropical compared with non-tropical countries.]

Patel V (2001) *Where There Is No Psychiatrist.* Gaskell. [An excellent and user-friendly manual of practical psychiatry in resource-limited areas.]

Price C, Shandu D, Dedicoat M, Wilkinson D. Gill GV (2011) Long-term glycaemic outcome of structured nurse-led diabetes care in rural Africa. **104**: 571–4. [This paper describes the outcome of structured nurse-led diabetes care in rural South Africa, using clinical algorithms and patient education.]

Prince M *et al.* (2007) Global Mental Health I. No health without mental health. *Lancet* **370**: 859–77. [A good overview of the world impact of mental health – 14% of the global burden of disease, and a particular problem in the developing world.]

Wjst M, Boakye D (2007) Asthma in Africa. *PLOS Medicine* **4**: e72. [An open access article reviewing asthma in Africa, particularly aetiology and epidemiology.]

World Health Organization (2010) *mhGAP Intervention Guide for Mental Neurological and Substance Use Disorders in Non-specialized Health Settings.* Geneva: WHO. [A WHO-developed technical tool for managing common mental health disorders in resource-poor areas.]

World Health Organization/WONCA (2008) *Integrating Mental Health into Primary Care – A Global Perspective.* Geneva: WHO/WONCA. [A publication giving management models from around the world.]

60

Refugee health

Tim O'Dempsey
Liverpool School of Tropical Medicine

Humanitarian emergencies in resource poor countries

Most refugees/internally displaced persons (IDPs) are displaced because of Complex Humanitarian Emergencies (CHEs) or natural disasters. CHEs are primarily internal wars in which conflicting groups compete for limited resources. CHEs are characterized by administrative, economic, political and social disruption, usually accompanied by high levels of violence. Major violations of the Geneva Conventions and Universal Declaration of Human Rights are common and cultural, religious and ethnic groups may be at risk of extinction. CHEs frequently result in catastrophic public health emergencies as coping capacities are exceeded by need, placing vulnerable populations at greatest risk of epidemic diseases and malnutrition. CHEs may smoulder on for many years as 'chronic emergencies' with fluctuating levels of violence, displacement and disease.

Natural disasters (floods, earthquakes, famine) may also become complex humanitarian emergencies, particularly when they affect vulnerable populations in weakened or disrupted states.

Global Climate Change is affecting the frequency and magnitude of natural disasters, aggravating the burden of malnutrition and communicable diseases, intensifying competition for scarce resources, and increasing the likelihood of conflict and population displacement.

Responding to humanitarian emergencies

Emergency phase

The initial phase of an emergency is characterized by need overwhelming available resources and resulting in increased mortality rates. Crude Mortality Rate (CMR) is generally used as an indicator of the severity of an emergency. Under Fives Mortality (UFM) may also be used (see Table 60.1).

The emergency phase of an intervention can be regarded as over when the CMR is < 1 per 10 000/day and basic needs have been met. The figures quoted above refer to current recommendations particularly applicable to countries in sub-Saharan Africa. Thresholds for most countries in other regions are significantly lower.

Effective action in response to a humanitarian emergency depends on individuals, governmental and non-governmental organizations (NGOs), working in a coordinated and complementary manner. Intersectoral collaboration is the key to success in emergency interventions. *Médecins Sans Frontières* (MSF) emphasize ten priorities in an emergency response:

1 Initial assessment

The initial assessment is usually conducted in two phases.

Tropical Medicine Lecture Notes, Seventh edition. Edited by Nick Beeching and Geoff Gill. © 2014 John Wiley & Sons, Ltd. Published 2014 by John Wiley & Sons, Ltd.

Table 60.1 **Levels of Crude Mortality Rate (CMR) or Under Fives Mortality (UFM) that indicate levels of severity of an emergency**

	CMR	UFM
	(per 10 000/day)	
Major catastrophe	> 5	> 10
Emergency: out of control	> 2	> 4
Emergency/relief programme: situation serious	> 1	> 2
Emergency/relief programme: under control	< 1	< 2
Normal rate for stable developing country	0.5	1.0

Phase I:

- Objective to enable rapid decision regarding the need for and scale of an intervention
- Completed within three days
- Focus
  - (a) Geo-political context, including the background to the displacement
  - (b) Demographic description of the population and map of site
  - (c) Characteristics of the environment in which refugees have settled
  - (d) Availability of water, food and shelter
  - (e) Major health problems, epidemic diseases and mortality rates
  - (f) Human and material resources required
  - (g) Operating partners (eg. local and national authorities, local and international organizations)

Phase II:

- Conducted simultaneously with the implementation of relief actions
- Allows more detailed programme planning and wider dissemination of information.
- Similar range of issues to Phase I, but with greater depth and emphasis.

2 Measles immunization

Measles can be a devastating illness in refugee populations, particularly if there is also a high level of malnutrition and vitamin A deficiency. Herd immunity is only achieved when over 90% of those susceptible have been immunized, a figure rarely achieved in any country in the world. Therefore, all children aged between six months and fifteen years should be immunized against measles and given vitamin A.

3 Water and sanitation

Access to adequate supplies of water is critical in reducing the likelihood of diarrhoeal diseases. Quantity is more important than quality. A minimum of five litres per person per day is required for essential needs such as drinking and cooking in the acute stages of an emergency. This should be increased to at least 15–20 litres per person per day as soon as possible to reduce the risk of water-borne and water-washed diseases. Having sourced a sufficient quantity of water, attention can be given to assessing quality by determining the level of faecal coliforms using a field testing kit such as the Del Agua/Oxfam kit. Chlorination is the most effective way of treating water in emergencies.

During the initial stages of an emergency, it may be necessary to identify defecation areas or fields for excreta disposal. However, construction of shallow trenches or collective latrines is preferable. The target should be one latrine or trench per 50–100 people. As the situation stabilizes, the aim is for one latrine per 20 people, or, ideally, one latrine per family.

4 Food and nutrition (see also Chapter 61)

Existing malnutrition in a population is exacerbated by circumstances giving rise to humanitarian emergencies. Establishing and maintaining food security (access by all people at all times to enough food for an active, healthy life) can present an enormous logistical challenge. The minimum mean population requirement is 2100 kcals per person per day. Attention must be given to ensuring that the basic food ration includes an appropriate mix of vitamins and other micronutrients. The prevalence of malnutrition among children aged less than five years is usually an indication of the level of malnutrition in the entire population. Therefore, the initial health assessment should include a nutritional survey of a sample of these children by measuring the weight-for-height (W/H) index and identifying children with bilateral pedal oedema.

Prevalence rates can be calculated for:

- global malnutrition (% children with moderate or severe malnutrition);
- severe malnutrition (% children with W/H Z-Scores < – 3 and/or oedema);
- moderate malnutrition (% children with W/H Z-Scores < – 2 but > – 3 Z-Scores)

where 'Z-Scores' refer to the number of standard deviations above (+) or below (-) the median in the reference population;

Mid-upper arm circumference (MUAC) is less accurate but is sometimes used for rapid screening in children aged 6–59 months if a W/H survey is impossible.

MUAC < 125 mm indicates global acute malnutrition; MUAC < 110 mm indicates severe malnutrition. Bilateral pedal oedema is used as an indicator of severe malnutrition.

The results of the survey can then be used to guide the level of intervention.

In addition to ensuring that general food distributions provide adequate food rations for all, there is often need for selective feeding programmes (SFPs). Blanket SFPs provide food supplements to vulnerable groups (e.g. pregnant women). Targeted SFPs provide food supplements and medical follow-up for the moderately malnourished. Therapeutic feeding programmes are used in the management of severely malnourished children and include an initial 'intensive care' phase for careful resuscitation, management of medical problems and initiation of nutritional treatment. Once complications have been brought under control and feeding has been established, the child can be transferred to a day-care unit for on-going nutritional and medical management and follow-up.

Routine inpatient management of severe malnutrition is now being questioned. It has become evident that the traditional therapeutic feeding centre (TFC) may be suboptimal. Access to TFC's may be difficult in complex emergencies and concentration of vulnerable individuals in centres increases risk of exposure to infectious diseases, such as measles, and may also result in greater vulnerability to security threats. Carers are often dislocated from their families and communities and are unable to work or fulfil domestic responsibilities. Recently, Community-based Therapeutic Care (CTC) has been developed as an innovative approach to management of severe malnutrition that addresses many of these issues.

The core operating principles of CTC are as follows.

- Maximum coverage and access – ideally, reach the entire severely malnourished population.
- Timeliness – begin case-finding and treatment before the prevalence of malnutrition escalates and additional medical complications occur.
- Appropriate care – Provide simple, effective outpatient care for those who can be treated at home and clinical care for those requiring inpatient treatment.

- Care for as long as it is needed – by improving access to treatment, ensure that children remain in the programme until they have recovered. By building local capacity and integrating the programme within existing structures and services.
- CTC also aims to ensure that effective treatment is available for as long as acute malnutrition is present in the population.

Acutely malnourished children are identified through population screening or by community/self-referral. Three forms of treatment are provided according to the severity of malnutrition as follows.

- Moderate acute malnutrition without medical complications. Support in a SFP providing dry take-home rations and basic medicines.
- Severe acute malnutrition (SAM) without medical complications. Treat in an Outpatient Therapeutic Programme (OTP), which provides ready-to-use therapeutic food (RUTF) and medicines for simple medical conditions. Children are managed at home with weekly OTP attendance for check ups and supplies of RUTF.
- Acutely malnourished with medical complications. Treat in an inpatient stabilization centre until well enough to continue on OTP.

The CTC approach is proving effective in a wide range of contexts with outcomes equivalent to or better than those achieved in TFCs.

5 Shelter and site planning

Overcrowding and lack of hygiene and sanitation are major factors in the spread of communicable diseases among large populations of refugees in 'camps'. In some situations, it may be possible and preferable for refugees to be integrated among the host population.

In planning a refugee camp site, attention must be given to security, access, protection from environmental health risks and provision of essential services (reception, administration, storage, distribution, water, sanitation, cemetery, health facilities, nutrition centre(s), places for social, commercial, educational and religious activities). Careful consideration should also be given to the social, economic, health and environmental impact that refugees may have on the host population and services.

Small camps, accommodating up to about 10 000 persons, are preferable to larger camps and should be organized according to social and cultural norms, shelter and accommodation being provided on the basis of family groupings.

6 Health care in the emergency phase

Whenever possible, health care should be planned and implemented in consultation with national and local health authorities. Responding to the essential health care needs of refugees in camps usually requires the establishment of specific services for this population focussing on basic curative care. Having established a central health facility, priority should be given to providing a network of peripheral health centres and health posts and developing outreach activities. There should be standardized systems for data collection and surveillance, clear management protocols appropriate to different levels of health facility, and clear guidelines for referral. Contingency plans should be developed so that appropriate action can be taken as circumstances change, for example, in response to an epidemic, or in managing a sudden influx of new arrivals.

7 Control of communicable diseases and epidemics

Diarrhoeal diseases especially cholera and *Shigella dysenteriae* type 1, acute respiratory infections, measles, meningitis and, in many regions, malaria are among the leading infectious causes of excess mortality in refugee populations. There may also be a risk of epidemic louse borne typhus or relapsing fever, and a variety of other infections depending on the region or circumstances.

The emphasis should be on prevention, epidemic surveillance using agreed case definitions, contingency planning and epidemic response appropriate to the specific disease and circumstances of the outbreak. The number of clinical cases may overwhelm existing facilities and specific treatment centres may have to be set up and staffed.

Sexually transmitted infections (STIs) including HIV may be a serious problem in refugee populations, as a result of sexual violence or social disruption. Their long-term impact may be as devastating as any of the diseases mentioned above. Therefore, implementation of measures to prevent and treat STIs should be an early consideration following the initial emergency response.

The risk of reactivation and transmission of tuberculosis is increased in refugee populations. However, WHO recommend that a TB control programme should not be initiated until the following criteria have been fulfilled: data indicate that TB is an important health problem; the emergency phase is over;

basic needs of water, adequate food, shelter and sanitation are available; essential clinical services and basic drugs are available; security in, and stability of, the camp are envisaged for at least 6 months; sufficient funding is available for at least 12 months; laboratory services for sputum smear microscopy are available. Similar, though even more complex, issues require consideration with regard to provision of antiretroviral treatment for people with HIV/AIDS. Difficult ethical dilemmas face health care providers in emergency settings who must reconcile an individual's 'right to life with dignity' with the need to adopt a Public Health approach for the 'greater common good'.

8 Public health surveillance

Effective programme planning, implementation, monitoring and evaluation depends on a system for the collection of data on demography, morbidity, mortality, basic needs and programme activities. Simple, standardized indicators should be used. A minimum data set in the initial emergency phase should include CMR, cause-specific mortality and morbidity using simple case definitions, malnutrition rate among under-fives, and indicators of access to water and sanitation facilities.

9 Human resources and training

Recruitment, training and management of staff are critical to the success of an intervention. It is important to determine appropriate staffing levels for a given task, prepare specific job descriptions, and establish lines of management and communication. Consideration should be given to contracts, legal status and salaries. Local services can be severely disrupted when their staff are lured by superior salaries and conditions offered by refugee agencies.

10 Coordination

A reliable coordination mechanism and leadership should be established early in the initial phase of an emergency. Coordination requires regular meetings involving representatives from key ministries in the host government, the host community, the refugee population, and the agencies involved in the response. Common objectives should be agreed and tasks determined and formally allocated. Technical guidelines and standardized policies should be introduced from the outset, and procedures agreed for reporting and dissemination of data.

Post-emergency phase

The post-emergency phase commences when basic needs have been met and excess mortality has been controlled (CMR < 1/10 000/day). Continued attention is given to the 'top ten' priorities indicated in the emergency phase, whilst adapting health programmes to address additional issues that may not have been received particular attention, for example reproductive and mental health. The post-emergency phase may end with repatriation and resettlement, or, if a population faces long-term displacement, there may be a gradual process of adaptation of services according to need, or integration into mainstream services for the host population.

The Sphere Project and Humanitarian Reform

The need for greater accountability and professional standards in humanitarian interventions received critical attention in the evaluation of the international response to the 1994 Rwandan genocide. Three years later a multi-agency initiative, the Sphere Project, was launched. Sphere defined minimum standards in core sectors of humanitarian assistance and advocated a universal humanitarian charter. Sphere is based on two core beliefs: first, that all possible steps should be taken to alleviate human suffering arising out of calamity and conflict, and second, that those affected by disaster have a right to life with dignity and therefore a right to assistance.

Over the past decade the frequency, magnitude, complexity and cost of humanitarian emergencies have continued to escalate. Following the Humanitarian Response Review in 2005, the international humanitarian community developed the Humanitarian Reform Agenda which aims to enhance the timeliness and effectiveness of humanitarian responses, prioritize the allocation of resources and offer more comprehensive needs-based relief and protection. The bed-rock of humanitarian reform is increased capacity, predictability, accountability, and partnership among humanitarian actors. This forms the foundation for the three 'pillars' of reform.

1 Improving the predictability of funding through the Central Emergency Response Fund.
2 Strengthening the Humanitarian Coordinator System.
3 The Cluster Approach coordinating effective responses through global and country cluster lead organizations addressing gaps in activities such as health, water/sanitation, logistics, nutrition, emergency shelter, camp coordination and management, emergency telecommunications, protection, education, agriculture and early recovery.

Health issues among asylum seekers in developed countries

There is a common perception in industrialized countries that asylum seekers are a threat to the health of the host population. Asylum seekers may be at risk of certain infectious diseases because of possible exposure either in their country of origin or during their migration in search of asylum, however the risk posed by members of the host population who travel abroad on holiday or business in numbers far exceeding those of asylum seekers entering industrialized countries receives comparatively little attention. Mandatory 'screening' for infectious diseases may be perceived as stigmatizing and may deter individuals from seeking health care. It is in everyone's best interest to keep a sense of proportion and encourage asylum seekers to regard access to health care as an opportunity rather than as a threat.

Health assessment of asylum seekers

In considering the health needs of asylum seekers it is important to consider the person and their predicament. Health care providers should be aware of issues related to language, communication, culture, religion, gender, family, community and social circumstances. Social, economic, physical, psychological and emotional needs may greatly outweigh medical needs.

The 'health assessment' approach is preferable to 'screening' as the latter is often narrowly focussed and may have negative connotations from viewpoint of the asylum seeker.

The key elements in a programme for health care of asylum seekers and refugees include:

- close liaison with other services;
- communication and continuity of care;
- continuing access to specialist services;
- early initial health assessment;
- information and encouragement;

- integration into mainstream services;
- specialist follow-up according to need.

The history and examination should include assessment of:

- evidence of substance misuse;
- evidence of torture;
- infectious diseases;
- mental health status;
- non-infectious diseases (e.g. haematological – sickle cell, thalassaemia, G6PD; cardiac – rheumatic heart disease, endomyocardial fibrosis [EMF]);
- nutritional status;
- obstetric and gynaecological problems;
- presence and level of disability;
- risk of exposure to toxins (e.g. lead);
- vaccination status;
- vision, hearing and dental problems.

The choice of laboratory investigations will depend on the findings of the health assessment, and whether specific 'screening' programmes are to be followed.

Assessment of children should also include: whether the child is accompanied or unaccompanied, growth and development (including language, hearing, vision) and the possibility of congenital diseases routinely screened for in neonates in the UK (e.g. hypothyroidism, phenylketonuria). Another important issue to consider in children is that of child protection, for example, certain cultural practices, notably female genital mutilation (FGM), may be traditional in the child's country of origin but illegal in the country of asylum.

Infectious diseases

Infectious diseases that are likely to be more prevalent among refugees and asylum seekers include tuberculosis, hepatitis B and C, HIV, STIs, gastrointestinal infections (bacterial/parasitic), malaria, typhoid and other tropical diseases, infestations (lice, scabies) and multidrug resistant bacterial infections. In most cases, these infections are likely to be asymptomatic. Therefore, 'screening' programmes may be recommended for specific infections, particularly those of greatest public health interest (eg. tuberculosis, hepatitis B/C, HIV, STIs). Issues concerning ethics, consent, confidentiality, cost effectiveness and continuity of care deserve consideration.

Decisions regarding routine screening for intestinal helminths should be made on the basis of risk assessment. Empirical treatment with albendazole has been shown to be more cost effective than routine screening of immigrants in the USA.

Many latent imported infections may cause clinical disease following immunosuppression, including tuberculosis, leprosy, amoebiasis, strongyloidiasis, visceral leishmaniasis, histoplasmosis, malaria, filariasis, and American trypanosomiasis.

Some imported infections, if untreated, may persist for years, for example strongyloidiasis (> 60 yrs), schistosomiasis (> 30 yrs), melioidosis (> 25 yrs), hydatid (> 20 yrs), and trichinella, cysticercosis, onchocerciasis (all > 15 yrs).

Torture and other traumatic experiences

It is estimated that 10–30% of asylum seekers will have survived torture, sexual violence or other seriously traumatizing experiences. Many will experience on-going psychological problems including nightmares, hallucinations, flash-backs, panic attacks, sexual problems, phobias, difficulty trusting people or forming relationships, depressive illness and anxiety. The medical documentation and reporting of such experiences may be a critical factor in the asylum determination process.

Reactions to trauma and loss may include poor concentration, memory impairment, day-dreaming, intrusive thoughts and images, irritability, confusion, tiredness, lethargy, sleep difficulties and loss of motivation. Sufferers may become withdrawn and isolated and may self harm. It is often very difficult for a person to articulate these experiences. Somatization is common and unexplained backache, headache, stomach ache or other body pains should prompt further careful enquiry. Children may, in addition, experience interrupted or uneven emotional development, or failure to thrive.

 SUMMARY

- Natural disasters, wars and political upheaval continue to lead to humanitarian emergencies and problems of refugee health.

- Initial assessment and intervention involves provision of water, food and shelter. The sociocultural characteristics of the displaced population must also be assessed.

- Diarrhoeal diseases, in particular cholera and bacillary dysentery, can cause major epidemics. Other epidemic-prone diseases in refugee camps include measles, meningitis, malaria and other vector-borne infections.

- A significant proportion of refugees and asylum seekers may have survived torture or sexual violence and have associated psychological problems.

Visit www.lecturenoteseries.com/tropicalmed to test yourself on this chapter using interactive MCQs.

FURTHER READING

Burkle FM (1999) Lessons learnt and future expectations of complex emergencies. *BMJ* **319**: 422–6.

Checchi F *et al.* (2009) Public health in crisis affected populations: A practical guide for decision-makers. http://www.odihpn.org/report.asp?id=2902 [A great overview and friendly introduction for non-specialists.]

Coker R, Lambregts van Weezenbeek K (2001) Mandatory screening and treatment of immigrants for latent tuberculosis in the USA: just restraint? *Lancet Infect Dis* **1**: 270–6.

Collins S, *et al.* (2006) Management of severe acute malnutrition in children. *Lancet* **368**: 1996–2000.

Connolly M, *et al.* (2004) Communicable diseases in complex emergencies: impact and challenges. *Lancet* **364**: 1974–83.

Goma Epidemiology Group (1995) Public health impact of Rwandan refugee crisis: what happened in Goma, Zaire, in July 1994. *Lancet* **345**: 339–44.

Lifson AR, Thai D, O'Fallon A, Mills WA, Hang K (2002) Prevalence of tuberculosis, hepatitis B virus, and intestinal parasitic infections among refugees to Minnesota. *Public Health Rep* **117**: 69–77.

Médecins Sans Frontières (1997) *Refugee Health: An Approach to Emergency Situations*. London: Macmillan. [This is essential reading for anyone involved in humanitarian emergencies in developing countries. Refugee Health and other key MSF books are also available on CD-ROM, and online at: http://www.msf.org/source/refbooks/E_MSF-docmenu.htm]

Muennig P, Pallin A, Sell RL, Chan M-S (1999) The cost effectiveness of strategies for the treatment of intestinal parasites in immigrants. *N Engl J Med* **340**: 773–9.

Perrin P (1996) *War and Public Health*. Geneva: ICRC. [Clear and systematic text with the added bonus of chapters on international humanitarian law and ethics. Also available online at WHO/PAHO Health Library for Disasters.]

World Health Organization (2005) *Communicable Disease Control in Emergencies. A Field Manual*. Connolly MA (ed.). WHO 2005.

Websites

Female Genital Mutilation: BMA guidelines revised July 2011: http://www.bma.org.uk/ethics/human_rights/femalegenitalmutilation.jsp

Humanitarian Reform: http://www.humanitarian-reform.org/

Freedom from Torture (previously known as The Medical Foundation for the Care of Victims of Torture) is a registered charity that provides care and rehabilitation to survivors of torture and other forms of organised violence. http://www.freedomfromtorture.org/

Physicians for Human Rights website provides access to reports and training materials, including the 'Istanbul Protocol' (Manual on the effective investigation and documentation of torture and other cruel, inhuman or degrading treatment or punishment). http://www.phrusa.org

Sphere Project: Humanitarian Charter and Minimum Standards in Disaster Response. http://www.sphereproject.org/

WHO Emergency Humanitarian Action website has excellent links including access to a huge range of electronic handbooks, manuals and emergency bibliography, many of which are also available on CD ROM. http://www.who.int/disasters/

The WHO/PAHO 'Health Library for Disasters' is also outstanding. http://helid.desastres.net/

61

Syndromes of malnutrition

Rebecca Sinfield[1] and Tom Doherty[2]
[1]Edge Hill University; [2] The Hospital for Tropical Diseases

Malnutrition in children

Malnutrition in all its forms remains a major public health problem throughout the developing world and is an underlying factor in over 50% of the 10–11 million deaths in children under 5 years of age who die each year from preventable causes. Worldwide approximately 60 million children are suffering from moderate acute malnutrition and 13 million from severe acute malnutrition at any one time.

Definition

Severe acute malnutrition is defined as a weight-for-height measurement of <70% of the median or ≥ 3 SD below the mean National Centre for Health Statistics reference values (termed wasting/marasmus); the presence of bilateral pitting oedema of nutritional origin (termed oedematous malnutrition/kwashiorkor); or a mid upper arm circumference (MUAC) of <110 mm in a child between 1 and 5 years of age. By contrast, chronic malnutrition (termed stunting) is identified using a height-for-age indicator (Table 61.1).

Aetiology

There are many factors involved in the aetiology of malnutrition, varying between geographical regions, including famine, drought, war, poverty/social disadvantage, lack of food, infections and neglect. The principal pattern is of a child who is underweight due to poor nutrition and recurrent infections, who then develops a severe infection e.g. diarrhoea or measles, which precipitates severe acute malnutrition. The varied presentations are determined by the severity, duration and complexity of interactions of specific macro- and micronutrient deficiencies, yet despite much research there is as yet no clear explanation as to why children present with such differing clinical features.

Oedematous malnutrition is commonly seen in areas where high energy – low protein foods are the staple diet; however the concept that protein deficiency causes this form of malnutrition has now been refuted. It is thought that oedematous malnutrition is precipitated by a variety of environmental insults, termed noxae. The child's protective mechanisms are compromised by a whole range of dietary deficiencies or depletions. Oedematous malnutrition results from an imbalance between the production of toxic radicals by the noxae and their safe disposal. The important noxae are infections, but other possible noxae are exogenous toxins such as aflatoxin and its metabolites. Oedema, aside from a low intravascular protein, is caused by leaking membranes which have lost their integrity through oxidative stress.

Clinical Features

The principal clinical feature in children with severe wasting is wasting of muscle and fat (Fig. 61.1). This can be particularly marked around the ribs, long bones and buttocks (resulting in so called 'baggy

Tropical Medicine Lecture Notes, Seventh edition. Edited by Nick Beeching and Geoff Gill. © 2014 John Wiley & Sons, Ltd. Published 2014 by John Wiley & Sons, Ltd.

Table 61.1 Classification of childhood malnutrition. Weight-for-height 'Z-score' is defined as standard deviation (SD) below the mean for that population.

	Classification	
	Moderate malnutrition	Severe malnutrition
Symmetrical oedema	No	Yes (oedematous malnutrition or kwashiorkor) 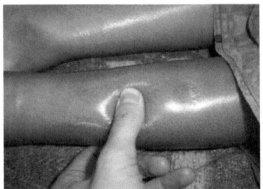
Weight-for-height Z-score	–3 SD to –2 SD (70–79%)	< –3 SD (<70%) (wasting or marasmus)
Height-for-age	–3 SD to –2 SD (85–89%)	< –3 SD (<85%) (stunting)

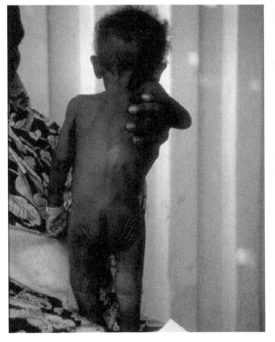

Figure 61.1 Severe visible wasting. (Source: IMCI teaching material).

pants'). There may be hair changes in long-standing cases. Oedematous malnutrition is characterized by:

- Oedema of a type and distribution similar to that in nephrotic syndrome, however without proteinuria. Ascites is rare (Fig. 61.2).
- Enlarged fatty liver: 20–40% wet liver weight is triglyceride

Figure 61.2 Oedematous malnutrition or kwashiorkor.

- Progressive skin changes: hyperpigmented and dry skin is followed by flaking, peeling and hypopigmentation ('flakey paint dermatitis' – Fig. 61.3).
- Straightened and bleached hair which is sparse and easily pluckable (Fig. 61.4).
- Mental changes ranging from irritability and apathy to semi consciousness.
- Eye changes of vitamin A deficiency affecting particularly the cornea (see Chapter 62).
- Anorexia.
- Moderate anaemia which is commonly due to a mixed deficiency of iron, folic acid, riboflavin and other haematinics, along with general depression of bone marrow production.

Clinical features of common infections (e.g. pneumonia, urinary tract infection, gastroenteritis) may complicate all types of severe acute malnutrition, although typically clinical signs may be subtle or absent.

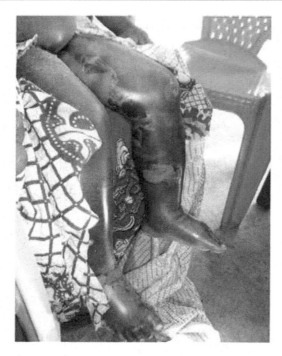

Figure 61.3 Oedematous malnutrition demonstrating hypo-hyper-hyperpigmented areas and flaking skin.

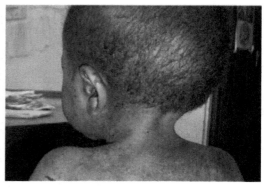

Figure 61.4 Straightened, sparse hair that is easily pluckable (in oedematous malnutrition).

Investigations

Malnourished children have marked derangement of serum electrolytes. Typical changes include hypokalaemia (due to GI losses and dietary deficiency), hypocalcaemia and hypomagnesaemia. There is an increase in total body sodium although paradoxically this may be accompanied by hyponatraemia.

Cell mediated immunity is compromised; B lymphocytes and immunoglobulins are usually normal or raised, although the immune response to bacterial infections may be suboptimal. Complement levels are reduced alongside the activity of polymorphs. Thus ensues a vicious cycle where infection results in malnutrition which in turn depresses the activity of the immune system which further leads to anorexia, weight loss and malnutrition. Serum albumin is low as amino acids are diverted away from albumin production for synthesis of acute phase proteins and immunoglobulins.

Management

For all cases of severe acute malnutrition the WHO management protocol has recommended medical and nutritional treatment regimes that are inpatient based and administered by trained health care professionals in ten steps in two phases, termed **resuscitation/stabilization** and **rehabilitation**.

The principal tasks during **initial resuscitation/ stabilization** are as follows.

1 *To prevent hypoglycaemia* by initiating frequent small feeds as soon as possible and continuing these throughout the day and night. Where hypoglycaemia is established it should be treated with 5 ml/kg of 10% dextrose given orally/NGT/i.v., and followed up with frequent small feeds.

2 *To treat or prevent hypothermia* by covering the child, including the head, reducing draughts and initiating 'kangaroo care' where possible.

3 *To treat or prevent dehydration and shock.* Dehydration can be very difficult to recognize in a wasted child because many of the signs of dehydration will be present by virtue of the malnutrition (e.g. sunken eyes, slow skin pinch). Therefore any child with watery diarrhoea or vomiting should be assumed to have dehydration. ReSoMal (**Re**hydration **So**lution for the **Mal**nourished – a modified ORS) should be commenced slowly, at an approximate rate of 5 ml/kg every 30 minutes for the first 2 hours followed by 5–10 ml/kg every hour, until signs of improvement or a maximum of 10 hours. i.v. fluids should not be used for the treatment of dehydration in malnourished children, due to the risk of fluid overload and cardiac failure.

In malnourished children, some of the signs of shock can also be present all the time. Therefore shock is defined as:

Lethargy/unconsciousness <u>and</u> cold hands, <u>plus either</u> slow capillary refill <u>or</u> weak or fast pulse

When shock is identified it should be treated with:

- oxygen;
- 5 ml/kg of intravenous 10% glucose or 1 ml/kg of 50% glucose;
- warmth;
- intravenous fluids: 15 ml/kg of fluid over 1 hour. The fluid of choice is half-strength Darrows with 5% glucose.

4 *To correct electrolyte imbalance.* Malnourished children require extra potassium (3–4 mmol/kg/day) and extra magnesium (0.4–0.6 mmol/kg/day). If using F75 (see below) these supplements will not be necessary as the milk has a combined mineral and vitamin mix added already. Malnourished children should also receive a low sodium diet.

5 *To treat or prevent infection.* All severely malnourished children should be treated for infection even if there are no signs. If no complications are present, an oral antibiotic such as co-trimoxazole can be used. If complications (e.g. shock, hypoglycaemia, dermatosis with raw skin/fissures, pneumonia, UTI) are present, parenteral antibtioics e.g. chloramphenicol and gentamicin should be used. Antibiotic choices will depend upon local microbiology knowledge and sensitivity patterns.

6 *To correct micronutrient deficiencies.* All children should receive a multivitamin supplement, folic acid 1 mg/day, zinc 2 mg/kg/day and copper 0.3 mg/kg/day. All of these are provided within F75 (see below). In addition, malnourished children will require prophylactic vitamin A. Iron (3mg/kg/day) should only be given once the child has a good appetite and has started gaining weight. Single doses of vitamin A are: age <6 months, 50 000 IU; age 6–12 months, 100 000 IU; age >12 months, 200 000 IU.

7 *To start to feed the child.* During the resuscitation phase of treatment, a low protein milk formula feed should be commenced, with small volumes given 2 or 3 hourly. The recommended WHO feed is F75 (Formula 75, i.e. 75 kcal/100 ml of milk; Table 61.2). Unless the child is able to take the required volume by cup, it should be given wholly or partly by nasogastric tube.

During the **Rehabilitation phases**

8 *This is the phase of rapid catch-up growth, when the child is encouraged to eat as much as possible* (e.g. 130–200 kcal/kg/day). WHO recommend F100 (Formula 100, i.e. 100 kcal/100 ml of milk) in addition to a normal diet and breast milk where appropriate.

Table 61.2 Constituents of F75 and F100 feeds

Constituents	Amount per 100 mL	
	F75	F100
Energy	75 kcal (316 kJ)	100 kcal (420 kJ)
Protein	0.9 g	2.9 g
Lactose	1.3 g	4.2 g
Potassium	3.6 mmol	5.9 mmol
Sodium	0.6 mmol	1.9 mmol
Magnesium	0.4 mmol	0.7 mmol
Zinc	2.0 mg	2.3 mg
Copper	0.25 mg	0.25 mg
Osmolarity	333 mOsmol/L	419 mOsmol/L

9 *As the child improves, sensory stimulation and emotional support* become essential.

10 *Discharge and follow-up should be planned.* The time of discharge will vary from unit to unit; certainly the child should have regained their appetite and have achieved a weight-for-height (WFH) measurement of 80% of the median. Recovery can take 4–6 weeks. Follow-up after recovery is essential to reduce the risk of relapse or recurrence.

Community-based therapeutic care (see also Chapter 60)

Despite the success of these protocols when implemented in selected units, their publication has not led to a widespread decrease in case fatality rates in most hospitals in the developing world (which remain at 20–30% for marasmus and up to 50–60% for kwashiorkor). There are often insufficient skilled staff and limited inpatient capacity. The centralized nature of hospitals also promotes late presentation, high opportunity costs for carers and risks of cross infection. Therefore an increasing number of countries have adopted a community-based model for the management of acute malnutrition, called community-based therapeutic care (CTC). CTC consists of four elements:

1 measures to mobilize the community in order to encourage early presentation and compliance;

2 outpatient supplementary feeding protocols for those with moderate acute malnutrition and no serious medical complications;

3 outpatient therapeutic protocols for those with severe acute malnutrition and no serious medical complications;

4 inpatient therapeutic protocols for those with acute malnutrition also suffering from serious medical complications.

Experience over the past 10 years indicates that many cases of acute malnutrition can be successfully treated solely as outpatients, enabling resource intensive inpatient care to be reserved for the minority suffering from malnutrition with complications. CTC complements the existing WHO inpatient protocols, using ready-to-use therapeutic foods for most children. This new approach has dramatically reduced case fatality rates and increased coverage rates. Initial data indicate that it has improved the cost-effectiveness of treating severe acute malnutrition.

Effect of HIV and tuberculosis

In sub-Saharan Africa, a high proportion of severely malnourished children admitted to nutritional rehabilitation units are now HIV-positive, particularly those with severe wasting. HIV and tuberculosis are increasing the workload of units treating severe acute malnutrition through both the direct effects of infection and the indirect negative effects on livelihoods and food security. HIV not only raises the prevalence of severe acute malnutrition, but also increases the complication and case-fatality rates. Experience has shown that whilst such children can achieve a full recovery using standard protocols, they recover more slowly than HIV-uninfected children.

Malnutrition in adults

Severe malnutrition among an adult population is unusual, but does occur predominantly in the context of a famine or as a consequence of late stage HIV infection. The same principles apply to the classification of severe malnutrition among children – severe wasting, represented by a significant reduction in Body Mass Index (BMI) and oedematous malnutrition presenting as kwashiorkor. The use of the Mid Upper Arm Circumference (MUAC) has not yet been formally validated in adults.

Managing severe malnutrition among adults should follow the same principles as those outlined for children above – cautious introduction of food in the acute stage, liberal use of multivitamins and antibiotics and more aggressive rehabilitation during the 'catch-up' phase. As with children, community based therapy may be the most appropriate for most people, particularly in the context of a famine.

Specific deficiencies of one or more micro-nutrients may be more commonly seen in an adult as opposed to a paediatric population and are occasionally a reflection of the staple elements of the diet consumed by the local population. This varies across different parts of the tropics, from predominantly rice based in most of Asia, to cassava and maize in parts of Africa. The clinical features of specific vitamin deficiencies are listed below:

Vitamin A

Vitamin A is found predominantly in green leafy vegetables. In the early stages of deficiency there may be no clinical signs but patients may report an impairment in their night vision. The first sign of vitamin A deficiency is a dryness of the eyes, which may feel gritty, and can be clinically apparent. This is known as xerophthalmia. Bitot's spots are grey or white plaques of damaged epithelium usually seen on the lateral aspect of the conjunctiva. They may be present with normal serum retinol levels, ie they indicate vitamin A deficiency at some time. They do not represent a stage of progression of the disease. As the deficiency worsens, keratomalacia may occur where the whole structure of the eye breaks down, leading to irreversible blindness (see Chapter 62 on eye disease).

Vitamin B1 (thiamine)

Thiamine deficiency is classically associated with a diet consisting of polished rice – or alcohol – and ultimately results in the condition 'beriberi', a word probably derived from *beri*, the word for 'weak' in one of the Malay dialects. Two forms are described, 'wet' and 'dry'. Wet beriberi presents as a form of cardiomyopathy in which peripheral oedema is prominent. Dry beriberi is characterized by a painful polyneuropathy. Thiamine deficiency is also the cause of the Wernicke-Korsakoff syndrome, or alcoholic psychosis, which is seen sporadically throughout the world. The diagnosis is usually made clinically, but in a research setting, a reduction in the red blood cell transketolase enzyme is diagnostic.

Vitamin B6 (niacin or nicotinic acid)

Niacin deficiency is primarily associated with a diet based on maize and is seen most commonly in southern Africa. Ultimately, niacin deficiency results in pellagra, a disease characterized by diarrhoea, dermatitis that predominantly affects sun exposed skin,

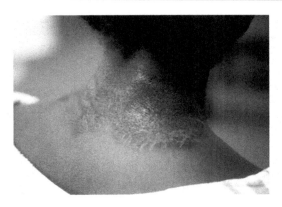

Figure 61.5 African adult with pellagra, showing the typical 'Casal's necklace'.

and dementia. A hyperpigmented rash affecting the neck and known as 'Casal's necklace' is characteristic (Fig. 61.5) and is not uncommon in southern Africa among marginalized adults whose diet comprises little more than maize meal porridge – 'sadza' as it is known in Zimbabwe, for example.

Vitamin C (ascorbic acid)

Vitamin C deficiency, or scurvy, occurs among those whose diet is deficient in any form of fruit or vegetable. Classically it produces gingivitis and ultimately bleeding – both from the gums and into the skin, often around the base of the hair follicles. In practice, scurvy is very rarely seen any longer.

Vitamin D

Rickets is usually seen in young children, but may occasionally present in young adults whose bones are still growing. Bony changes include the 'rickety rosary' caused by widening of the costophrenic junctions and a recognized association of severe protein-energy malnutrition. The radiological signs are often seen in X-rays of the wrists and forearms and comprise 'cupping, splaying and fraying' – in other words the joint spaces become wider in both longitudial ('cupping') and transverse ('splying') sections while the joint margins become irregular ('fraying'). Involvement of the femur may result in either 'bowlegs' or 'knock knees'. Although sunlight is an important cofactor in the metabolism of dietary vitamin D to its active metabolite, rickets is still seen occasionally in parts of the tropics where, either for cultural or religious reasons, children are kept covered from the sun.

Other manifestations of vitamin deficiencies

Glossitis, angular stomatitis and a range of dermatoses are all features of protein energy malnutrition in children and are occasionally seen in adults. They are a manifestation of a range of vitamin deficiencies rather than attributable to the lack of a specific vitamin. All will respond to multivitamin replacement therapy.

 SUMMARY

- Severe acute malnutrition in children is defined as low weight-for-height, bilateral pitting oedema of nutritional origin, or low mid-arm circumference.
- Chronic malnutrition (stunting) is defined as low height-for-age.
- The aetiology of childhood malnutrition is multifactorial and includes famine, drought, war, poverty/social disadvantage, lack of food, neglect and infections.
- Infections that have been implicated include measles, gastroenteritis, TB and HIV; the latter also increases the complication and case-fatality rate.
- The management of severe acute malnutrition incorporates a 10-step protocol of inpatient management, divided into a resuscitation/stabilization phase followed by a rehabilitation phase.
- Introduction of community-based therapeutic care protocols for prevention, early detection and management in the community has improved outcomes for children.

 Visit www.lecturenoteseries.com/tropicalmed to test yourself on this chapter using interactive MCQs.

FURTHER READING

Collins S, Dent N, Binns P, *et al.* (2006). Management of severe acute malnutrition in children. *Lancet* **368**:1992-2000. [Good review]

Manary MJ, Sandige HL (2008). Management of acute metabolic and severe childhood malnutrition. *BMJ* **337**: 1227–30. [Useful recent review]

WHO (1999). *Management of severe malnutrition: a manual for physicians and other senior health workers.* Geneva: WHO. [http://whqlibdoc.who.int/hq/1999/a57361.pdf.]

62

Eye disease in the tropics

Malcolm Kerr-Muir
Liverpool School of Tropical Medicine

About 161 million people worldwide have visual impairment, of whom 37 million are blind and 124 million have low vision (<6/18 to 3/60). Thus globally, 1 in 36 people have significant visual impairment. Ninety per cent of the world's blind live in developing countries. 80% of blindness is avoidable, either treatable such as cataract, or preventable such as trachoma, onchocerciasis and vitamin A deficiency. Fifty per cent of blindness is due to cataract. This chapter includes a short section on eye disease in leprosy (see also Chapter 18). Onchocerciasis is covered in Chapter 14.

A country's economic status and availability of health care determine the prevalence of blindness. In most resource poor countries in the tropics the number of blind is 10 per 1000 (1%), compared to prevalence in industrialized economies of 2 per 1000 (0.2%). Blindness in poorer socioeconomic communities aggravates the reduction in an individual's independence, his/her contribution to the family and society and leads to social disintegration.

Blindness, as defined by the WHO, is a level of vision that prevents a person walking alone unaided. This functional definition translates to an objective measure of Snellen acuity <3/60 in the better eye with best correction. A visual acuity of <6/60 to 3/60 is defined as severe visual impairment (Table 62.1).

Examination of the eye

For the majority of ocular diagnoses in primary care, the only equipment required is a form of magnification and good focal illumination.

The red eye

Redness, due to dilated conjunctival blood vessels, is a common manifestation of most inflammatory eye disease. It is important to distinguish the 'safe' from the 'serious' red eye which is a potential threat to vision. Diffuse (safe) redness of the eye without a change in vision is due to surface inflammation (conjunctivitis) and is likely to be microbial or allergic in origin (Fig. 62.1). Redness concentrated at the junction of the sclera and cornea (limbus), usually accompanied by an impairment of vision and/or pain indicates serious intraocular inflammation and needs specialist referral (Fig. 62.2, Table 62.2).

Pathways to blindness

The principal pathways to blindness in the tropics and low income economies are diseases of the lens and cornea. The uvea (iris, choroid and ciliary body), retina and optic nerve make up the remainder.

Cataract

Cataract is an opacification of the lens and accounts for 50% of world blindness and is readily treatable (Fig. 62.3). 15% of childhood blindness (1.5 million age 0–16) is due to cataract. Adult cataract is predominantly age-related (80%). Recurrent dehydrational illness, ultraviolet B exposure, smoking, diabetes and intraocular inflammation are contributory factors.

Tropical Medicine Lecture Notes, Seventh edition. Edited by Nick Beeching and Geoff Gill. © 2014 John Wiley & Sons, Ltd. Published 2014 by John Wiley & Sons, Ltd.

Table 62.1 Categories of visual impairment. Visual acuity in better eye with best correction (WHO, 1993)

From	To	Category
6/6	6/18	Normal
<6/18	6/60	Visual impairment
<6/60	3/60	Severe visual impairment
<3/60	No perception of light	Blind

<10 degrees central visual field is equivalent to blindness.

Table 62.2 The red eye

Diffuse – safe	Limbal – serious
Microbial conjunctivitis	Acute corneal inflammation (keratitis)
Allergic conjunctivitis	Acute elevation of intra-ocular pressure (glaucoma)
Chemical conjunctivitis	Acute inflammation of the iris/ciliary body (iritis/uveitis)

The treatment is surgical removal of the opaque lens which is replaced with a prosthetic intra-ocular lens to restore optical normality. There may be poor uptake of surgery which may relate to poor access to services, cost, and fear.

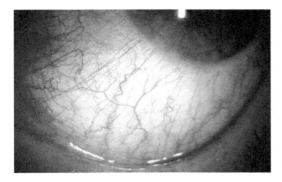

Figure 62.1 Diffuse redness – usually safe.

Microbial keratitis

Keratitis (inflammation of the cornea) is an ocular emergency, which needs early intervention in primary care (Fig. 62.4). It is a major cause of blindness, due to scarring and/or loss of the hitherto transparent corneal collagen. A prerequisite for infection is corneal trauma to allow ingress of microorganisms which can be bacterial, fungal, viral or acanthamoeba. This trauma is either a direct injury (common in agricultural workers) or the result of a loss of integrity of the ocular surface, for example when the cornea is exposed (lagophthalmos or trachomatous trichiasis) or anaesthetic (leprosy, herpes simplex and herpes zoster). The eye becomes intensely inflamed and painful with impaired vision, light sensitivity and excess watering or discharge. Suppurative corneal infection proceeds to scarring or perforation (Fig. 62.5). It may be compounded by delayed presentation and by traditional medicines.

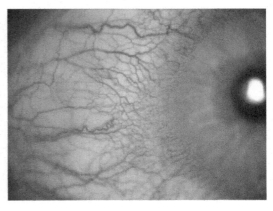

Figure 62.2 Limbal inflammation – potentially serious.

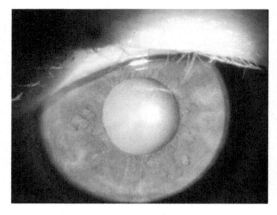
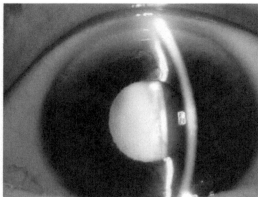

Figure 62.3 Cataract.

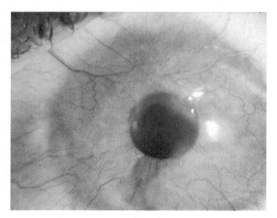

Figure 62.4 Keratitis with fibrovascular ingrowth into cornea.

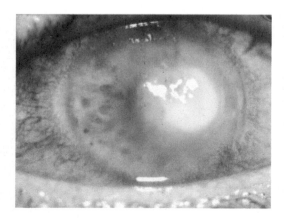

Figure 62.5 Acute suppurative keratitis with corneal ulcer and stromal disorganization.

Ideally, microbiological assessment would dictate appropriate antimicrobial treatment. Primary care involves frequent administration of a topical antibiotic e.g cefazolin 5% or ofloxacin 0.3% hourly and an antifungal agent e.g. natamycin 5% together with twice daily atropine 1% drops. Steroid drops and padding of the eye are contraindicated. Systemic analgesia and vitamin A should also be given.

Vitamin A deficiency disorders

500 000 children are blinded each year from vitamin A deficiency. The infant and pre-school child are preferentially affected when demands for this essential vitamin are greater. It is always associated with malnutrition. There can be lifelong morbidity and considerable mortality. This blindness is entirely preventable.

Vitamin A is needed for maturation of all epithelial cells, for a normal interactive immune system and for the rod photoreceptor pigment rhodopsin. The source of vitamin A (retinol) includes both animal products such as liver, meat, poultry and dairy products and vegetable products (provitamin A) such as dark green leafy vegetables, yellow and red fruits and palm oil. It is absorbed in the small intestine and the sole storage site is the liver. It is protein-bound for transport to the target tissues. The daily requirement is greater in the young, during intercurrent illness (notably infection) and in pregnancy.

It is possible, therefore, that despite a reasonable vitamin A intake, tissue levels may be compromised by malabsorption, failure of liver storage and failure to elaborate retinol transport proteins.

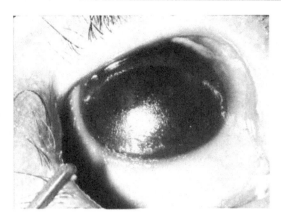

Figure 62.6 Corneal xerosis. Abnormal pre-corneal tear film, no stromal change. Reversible. © HKI.

In the eye a deficiency of vitamin A results in impaired differentiation of the conjunctival and corneal epithelium which become lacklustre and stippled due to squamous metaplasia and keratinization (Fig. 62.6). Specific mucus secreting cells (goblet cells) become depleted and the ocular surface becomes non-wetting (xerophthalmia) and therefore loses its protective mechanisms. Bitot's spots represent focal areas of conjunctival epithelial dysplasia which become colonized by resident conjunctival bacteria and can have a foamy, cheesy, or pigmented appearance. They indicate vitamin A deficiency at some time but do not represent a stage of disease and can persist indefinitely even with a normal serum retinol (Fig. 62.7).

Chronic vitamin A deficiency causes mild ocular discomfort and night blindness. Once there is a break in the surface corneal epithelium it should be regarded as a medical emergency. The blinding process is often rapid, over hours. This is due to a sudden demand on already diminished vitamin A stores. This demand accompanies acute events such as measles, respiratory tract infection or diarrhoeal disease. Corneal ulceration proceeds to liquefaction (keratomalacia) of the corneal stroma, without significant inflammation (Fig. 62.8). The inevitable result is corneal scarring, but if the eye perforates the vision may be irretrievably lost.

Malnourished children with acute pyrexial illness, particularly measles and diarrhoea, must have vitamin A as part of the treatment regimen. The objectives of management are to halt active disease and to replenish the stores of vitamin A, summarized as:

- identify children with active disease;
- immediate massive dose of vitamin A (Table 62.3);
- treat underlying/provoking condition;
- prevent recurrence.

In the presence of concurrent intestinal malabsorption/diarrhoea, the oral preparation (which is oil based) should be substituted with intramuscular (water based) vitamin A, 200 000 IU. If corneal ulceration

Table 62.3 **Vitamin A treatment regimens for active disease**

Age	Oral Treatment	Frequency
< 6 months	50 000 IU	Day 1, 2 and 14
6–12 months	100 000 IU	Day 1, 2 and 14
> 1 year	200 000 IU	Day 1, 2 and 14

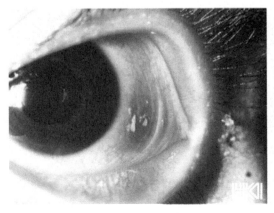

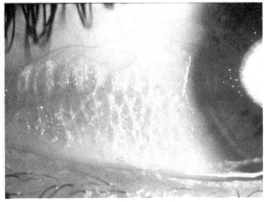

Figure 62.7 Bitot's spot. © HKI.

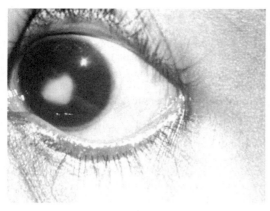

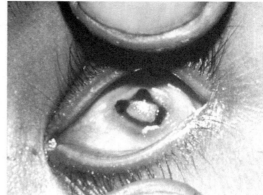

Figure 62.8 Keratomalacia outcome. © HKI.

Table 62.4 **Prevention of vitamin A deficiency**

Age	Oral treatment	Frequency
< 6 months	50 000 IU	3 times one month apart
6–12 months	100 000 IU	Every 6 months
> 1 year	200 000 IU	Every 6 months
Women	200 000 IU	Day 1 and 2 after delivery

is present, prophylactic topical antibiotics (tetracycline of chloramphenicol) and an antiviral (aciclovir) should be given. Topical steroids and padding of the eye are contraindicated.

Prevention of vitamin A deficiency demands regular surveillance of affected or at risk communities. Strategies depend on the severity of vitamin A deficiency and include:

- massive dose regimens (Table 62.4);
- food fortification;
- health and dietary education;
- encouraging use of local vegetable and animal vitamin A sources.

Trachoma

Once a debilitating condition throughout the world, trachoma is now largely confined to tropical regions. It is the prime cause of blindness due to infection. 150 million children have active infection and 5 million people are bilaterally blind from corneal scarring.

The reservoir for this chlamydial eye disease is the copious discharge from eyes with active disease. Eye to eye transmission of *Chlamydia trachomatis* (an obligate intracellular organism) occurs through direct contact with fingers and clothes and especially the mixing of ocular discharges by eye-seeking flies (*Musca domestica* and *M. sorbens*).

Trachoma is a chronic recurring keratoconjunctivitis. As there is no protective immunity, repeated infection leads to diffuse conjunctival scarring. Subsequent scar contraction of the conjunctiva of the posterior surface of the lids turns the lid margin inwards (entropion) and the lashes abrade the globe (trichiasis) (Fig. 62.9). This continuous trauma causes chronic keratitis. This together with incomplete lid closure and corneal exposure, increases the risk of acute microbial infections with bacteria and/or viruses, with eventual irreversible and potentially blinding corneal scars.

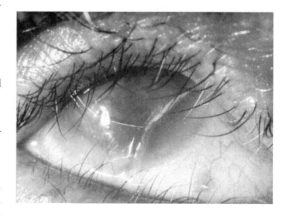

Figure 62.9 Late effects of trachoma. Retracted and inturned lid with lash abrasion of the cornea.

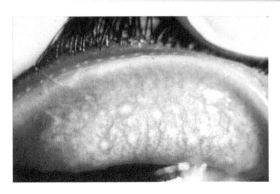

Figure 62.10 Trachoma. Upper tarsal follicles.

Acute inflammation occurs mainly in children and women, whilst trichiasis and corneal scarring occur in adults. Acute keratitis affects the limbus and with recurrent inflammation leads to neovascularization (pannus) of the peripheral and then central cornea. The tarsal conjunctivitis is manifest as aggregations of white cells (follicles Fig. 62.10), vascular proliferation (papillae Fig. 62.11) and cellular infiltrate followed by scarring (Fig. 62.12) which form the basis for the WHO classification of disease (Table 62.5).

Management of trachoma

The objectives are to identify and decrease the reservoir of active disease, to reduce eye to eye

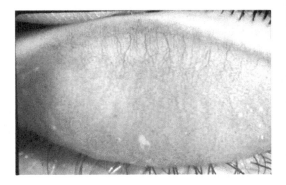

Figure 62.11 Trachoma. Upper tarsal papillae.

Table 62.5 Simplified WHO grading system for trachoma

Stage	Clinical features
Trachomatous inflammation, follicular (TF)	Five or more follicles of >0.5 mm on the upper tarsal conjunctiva
Trachomatous inflammation, intense (TI)	Papillary hypertrophy and inflammatory thickening of the upper tarsal conjunctiva obscuring more than half the deep tarsal vessels
Trachomatous scarring (TS)	Presence of scarring in tarsal conjunctiva.
Trachomatous trichiasis (TT)	At least one ingrown eyelash touching the globe, or evidence of epilation (eyelash removal)
Corneal opacity (CO)	Corneal opacity blurring part of the pupil margin

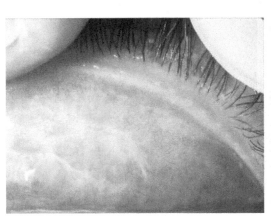

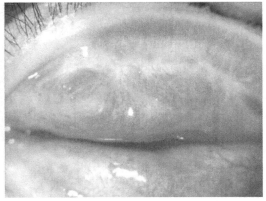

Figure 62.12 Trachoma. Upper tarsal scarring due to fibrosis.

Table 62.6 The SAFE strategy for management of trachoma

S	Surgery for in-turned lashes
A	Antibiotics: azithromycin (20 mg/kg) single dose or tetracycline ointment 1% twice daily for 6 weeks
F	Face washing
E	Environmental improvement

transmission and to protect the cornea from continuous lash induced abrasion.

The WHO has developed the SAFE strategy (Table 62.6)

Surgery to rotate the lashes away from the globe is simple and effective. The antibiotic of choice is a single dose of azithromycin, which is concentrated in macrophages and tears and is highly effective in clearing ocular and non-ocular sources of chlamydia. The simple measure of face washing is an effective way to reduce transmission. It reduces the attraction for flies by decreasing the volume of ocular discharges.

In terms of prevention, environmental improvements will eventually eliminate the blinding forms of trachoma. Improved water supply, decrease in population density and better hygiene will all contribute to reducing transmission of chlamydia.

Leprosy

The prevalence of leprosy is 12 million, with at least 250 000 new cases per year. Sight threatening lesions occur in 15–20% and there are 200 000 blind, mainly due to cataract. Most of these cases are from the pre-multidrug therapy (MDT) era (see Chapter 18).

Patients with complications due to leprosy need to know where they are placing their feet, to see to handle work tools, and to be able to dress ulcers with confidence. Living with peripheral neuropathy and damaged limbs is severely compromised if there is accompanying impairment of vision.

Eye involvement in leprosy occurs in several ways:

- direct invasion of the anterior one third of the eye (cornea, sclera, iris);
- as part of leprosy reactions;
- from massive mycobacterial invasion and secondary atrophy.

Primary ocular infection causes a fleeting neurokeratitis and invasion of the iris, ciliary body and sclera (these sites are cooler than core body temperature).

Type 1 leprosy reactions (reversal reactions) involve tissues already infiltrated with mycobacteria. They can occur in paucibacillary (PB) or multibacillary (MB) leprosy. Thus acute inflammation in relation to the facial (VII) or trigeminal (V) nerves may lead to irreversible facial palsy and an anaesthetic cornea/conjunctiva (Fig. 62.13). Early treatment lessens the completeness of the paresis (Chapter 18).

Type 2 leprosy reaction (erythema nodosum leprosum-ENL) is an immune-complex mediated multisystem disease occurring in MB patients only. The ocular sequelae are recurrent acute irits or scleritis, which may lead to acute glaucoma and cataract. Urgent treatment is with topical steroids and atropine (Fig. 62.14).

Massive bacillary invasion may affect the cornea and sclera as a discrete mass at the limbus (leproma). Invasion of the iris may produce discrete white

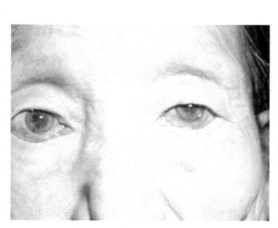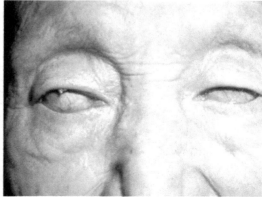

Figure 62.13 End-stage multibacillary leprosy with bilateral facial palsy, lagophthalmos and exposure keratitis.

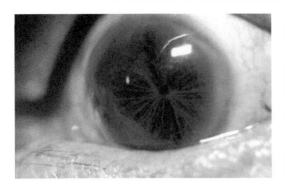

Figure 62.14 Neuroparalytic iritis with small pupil and dilator muscle atrophy.

 SUMMARY

- About 161 million people worldwide have visual impairment, of whom 37 million are blind.
- 80% of blindness is avoidable, either treatable such as cataract or preventable such as trachoma, onchocerciasis and vitamin A deficiency.
- Vitamin A deficiency blinds 500 000 children.
- Trachoma is the leading infectious cause of blindness.
- In addition to case detection and management, environmental improvements are essential to eliminate the blinding forms of trachoma.

particles which extrude and fall from the iris surface (iris pearls). Massive skin invasion causes bilateral facial palsy with incomplete closure of the lids (lagophthalmos) and exposure of the anesthetic cornea leads to acute on chronic keratitis and scarring (Fig. 62.13).

Chronic infiltration of the iris, particularly the dilator muscle, results in a very small non-dilatable pupil due to the unopposed action of the constrictor. This can cause night blindness or severe loss of vision due to even mild cataract in the visual axis.

Early MDT markedly reduces the risk of complications. Treatment of lagophthalmos is a combination of protective measures including lid exercises (forced blinking) to maintain regular corneal coverage and lid surgery. As patients may not feel pain, daily self (or relative or carer) examination for redness of the eye is essential to prompt early attendance for diagnosis and treatment.

A summary of management of ocular leprosy is given in Table 62.7.

 Visit **www.lecturenoteseries.com/tropicalmed** **to test yourself on this chapter using interactive MCQs.**

📖 FURTHER READING

World Health Organization (1993) *International Statistical Classification of Diseases, Injuries and Causes of Death,* Tenth Revision. Geneva: WHO.

World Health Organization (1997) *Vitamin A Supplements: A Guide to Their Use in the Treatment and Prevention of Vitamin A Deficiency and Xerophthalmia,* 2nd edn. WHO/UNICEF/IVACG Task Force. Geneva: WHO.

World Health Organization. *Causes of blindness* site at http://www.who.int/blindness/en/ including downloadable cards for classification of trachoma at http://www.who.int/blindness/causes/trachoma_documents/en/index.html

Table 62.7 **Management of ocular leprosy**

Early diagnosis and MDT
Recognize and treat leprosy reactions
Regular eye examination
Lagophthalmos surgery
Cataract extraction

63

Neglected tropical diseases

David Molyneux
Liverpool School of Tropical Medicine

Introduction

Since 2004 many of the individual diseases mentioned in the chapters of this book have been categorized as' Neglected Tropical Diseases' or NTDs. These diseases have become of increased interest and priority in Global Health as they are now recognized as important causes of poverty as well as being characteristic of conditions of poverty. Indeed, the prevalence of NTDs has been suggested as one of the indicators of poverty. The WHO categorizes 17 infections as NTDs (Table 63.1), although there are many other infections which have an almost equal right to be included in the list. Some of these are zoonotic infections, adding to the difficulties of control. The WHO definition of NTDs excludes HIV/AIDS, TB and malaria, often called the 'big three'. These are no longer felt to be neglected problems in terms of the resources which are flowing into research and because of the creation of the Global Fund for AIDS TB and malaria (GFATM), which provides huge financial support to help countries control of these infections.

Strategic approaches

The WHO recommends five strategies for the control or elimination of the NTDs. These are:

- the expansion and up-scaling of preventive chemotherapy;
- intensification of case detection and management;
- improved vector control or intermediate host control where feasible and cost effective;
- implementation of appropriate veterinary public health measures for control of the zoonotic diseases;
- the provision of safe water, sanitation and hygiene.

'Tool-ready diseases'

The particular strategy for the treatment or control of any disease is dependent on several factors. Some diseases have been selected for elimination because there are tools available, which can have a significant or even permanent impact on both the prevalence and incidence of diseases such as leprosy, onchocerciasis, lymphatic filariasis and schistosomiasis. Ultimately this should lead to elimination of transmission, greatly reduced morbidity and reduction of the disease incidence to a level at which it is no longer a public health issue. These diseases are referred to as 'tool-ready diseases'. In the case of dracunculiasis (Guinea worm) it is expected that eradication can be achieved despite there being no drug or vaccine available. Eradication is defined as the reduction of incidence to zero on a global scale. To date this has only been achieved for smallpox. The eradication strategy for Guinea worm is based on simple public health approaches-surveillance for cases, case containment, intermediate host control (using temephos), provision of safe/protected drinking water or provision of cloth filters, health education and instigation of a

Tropical Medicine Lecture Notes, Seventh edition. Edited by Nick Beeching and Geoff Gill. © 2014 John Wiley & Sons, Ltd. Published 2014 by John Wiley & Sons, Ltd.

Table 63.1 List of diseases included by the WHO in list of Neglected Tropical Diseases (in alphabetical order)

Buruli ulcer
Chagas' disease (American trypanosomiasis)
Cysticercosis
Dengue
Dracunculiasis (Guinea worm disease)
Echinococcosis
Endemic treponematoses
Foodborne trematode infections
Human African trypanosomiasis (sleeping sickness)
Leishmaniasis
Leprosy
Lymphatic filariasis
Onchocerciasis (river blindness)
Rabies
Schistosomiasis (bilharzia)
Soil-transmitted helminthiases
Trachoma

rumour register and reward system to encourage reporting of suspect cases.

In many diseases, however, the provision of safe drinking water and sanitation as well as health education can have a permanent impact on transmission and exposure to the sources of infection, particularly the soil-transmitted helminth diseases and schistosomiasis. Health education messages are important in transmitting information on the biology of transmission of the cestode diseases, cysticercosis and echinococcosis and food borne trematodes. Reducing transmission through behaviour change is a particular challenge when there is a need to change deeply entrenched cultural practices.

'Tool-deficient diseases'

A group of NTDs have been described as 'tool deficient' as there are currently inadequate curative treatments and diagnostics. This includes visceral and mucocutaneous leishmaniasis, human African trypanosomiasis and Chagas' disease, and Buruli ulcer. The drugs available are toxic, expensive for poor people (if not donated or subsidized by government) and hence not readily accessed. Drug administration requires skilled medical care and requires the follow-up of patients. Diagnosis, particularly in the early stages, is difficult or invasive and late diagnosis when the disease has progressed makes treatment more complex and difficult. Early

diagnosis of these diseases is important and requires awareness of the problem as well as the necessary skill such as microscopy, as many present clinically with fever that may be mistaken for malaria. This group of diseases needs improved drugs which have a profile of low toxicity, are affordable (or donated) and can be given orally, preferably over short periods of time. Most of the currently available drugs do not match this profile and progress has been slow in introducing new products, despite intensive research efforts.

The zoonotic NTDs

The WHO have included in the list of NTDs a group of infections which are zoonoses such as rabies, cysticercosis, echinococcosis, trypanosomiasis and some forms of leishmaniasis. These diseases pose particular problems for their control as interventions often have to be targeted at infections in both animals and humans. For example, rabies control is most effective if dog vaccination is introduced, whilst zoonotic human trypanosomiasis in Uganda can be controlled by treatment of the cattle reservoir with trypanocidal drugs and by spraying the legs of cattle with insecticide to kill the vector tsetse fly, *Glossina*. Control of cysticercosis (*Taenia solium*) is best achieved by measures which involve the veterinary public health sector. These include improved and more rigorous meat inspection of pigs to reduce the consumption of larval tapeworms in pig muscle and reducing access of pigs to human faeces. For hydatid disease (*Echinococcus granulosus*), the most successful approaches have been to regulate sheep slaughtering practices to prevent dogs accessing offal containing cysts of *Echinococcus*, as well as reducing human exposure to tapeworm eggs by treating the adult phase in dogs with praziquantel. Control of zoonotic diseases requires close cooperation between human health and other national ministries such as those responsible for livestock, agriculture and water and sanitation. Control and elimination of some neglected zoonotic diseases, with wild reservoir hosts such as rodents which are reservoirs of cutaneous leishmaniasis, plague, and leptospirosis, is extremely challenging. There are many different rodent reservoir species which act as hosts and these may have high infection rates. Further, they are abundant in a variety of environments such tropical forests, urban slums and arid desert, where targeted control is challenging.

Vector control and NTDs

The WHO has promoted the concept of integrated vector management (IVM) as one approach to reducing the transmission of some diseases and to improve the cost effectiveness of vector control operations. The key elements to the IVM strategy are to:

1 promote an integrated approach to ensure rational use of resources to target multiple diseases through use of both non-chemical and chemical methods of vector control;
2 adopt strategies and interventions relevant to the ecology of the vector and the epidemiology of the disease;
3 develop collaboration with other sectors for planning purposes;
4 develop capacity and infrastructure to manage IVM dependent on the local situation;
5 promote the principles of integrated vector management. through advocacy, social mobilization and appropriate legislation.

Examples are vector control through impregnated/long lasting bednets on malaria and lymphatic filariasis for which *Anopheles* mosquitos are the vectors in Africa, and in Asia and the Pacific where *Aedes* mosquitoes are responsible for transmission of both lymphatic filariasis and dengue. However, challenges include the limited resources and expertise available in vector control and the reality of operationalizing the IVM concept in the face of other priorities.

Common features of neglected tropical diseases

The impact and the burden

Neglected Tropical Diseases afflict at least one billion people, hence the poorest people on the planet are disproportionately affected – 'the bottom billion'. These diseases have a serious impact of individuals, families (as carers) and communities. They impact on the quality of life and cause loss of productivity and hence family income, inflicting a burden of cost on poor families for long-term care. This can drive people who are already poor into the medical poverty trap, as the family incurs direct and indirect medical costs which are often inappropriate. NTDs have a physical impact on individual health through the symptoms/ pathology of the infection as well as a burden of stigma and social exclusion from disfiguring conditions, causing mental health problems. Females are often disproportionately affected by NTDs; anaemia and other problems contribute to higher risks in pregnancy and pregnancy outcome, while stigmatizing/ disfiguring infections such as cutaneous leishmaniasis or lymphatic filariasis may reduce their marital prospects, thus exposing them to abuse and vulnerability. Intestinal worm infections have been shown to have a direct impact on growth and are a cause of stunting, and worm infections retard educational performance through impaired cognitive development and physical performance, whilst reducing school attendance as measured by absenteeism. The overall burden of these diseases when aggregated, because people are commonly infected with more than one of these infections ('polyparasitism'), is at least equivalent to that of malaria and tuberculosis. These diseases are characteristic of marginalized populations with limited political voice, who often have limited or no access to government health or education services, and may live in remote rural areas as well as the expanding urban areas where services are minimal.

The costs and benefits in development terms

Only 0.6% of Overseas Development Assistance for health is directed towards the control of NTDs, which is an inequitable distribution of resources, given the high burden and the numbers of people affected (over 1 billion). Neglect of these diseases can be attributed to their long names, the lack of familiarity with the diseases in the developed world and the low risk of their spread to afflict populations outside the tropics. This is because conditions for transmission are based on determinants such as the ecology of vectors and reservoir hosts, which are confined to tropical environments. However, the costs to both individuals and their societies and the savings that can be made if the diseases are controlled, are dramatic. Recent estimates of productivity losses have demonstrated that the cost of all NTDs when aggregated is in the billions of dollars, whereas economic rates of return on investment in their control range from 15–30%.

Studies on the lymphatic filariasis programme show that cost savings of its activities over 8 years (2000–08) are of the order of US$ 24 billion. In the Onchocerciasis Control Programme, economic gains included the agricultural benefits derived from freeing up river valleys previously not habitable due to the high risk of blindness, with an estimated 25 million hectares of land becoming available for cultivation. Independent assessment of those NTD programmes which use mass chemotherapy, such as lymphatic filariasis, soil-transmitted helminth, schistosomiasis and onchocerciasis has also shown that these programmes are amongst the best buys of all public heath interventions, with estimated cost per DALY averted being US$2–22. The unit costs of delivery of donated drugs for these programmes are recognized as being around US$ 0.03–0.60 per treatment per year, depending on the setting. The unit costs depend on several factors, including the availability of donated drugs and the willingness of volunteers to play a key role in their distribution. However, where NTDs require treatment through intensified case management, costs are higher not only because of the costs of hospital facilities but because of the costs of the drugs themselves

Drug donation programmes

Several major pharmaceutical companies provide donated products for the control or treatment of the Neglected Tropical Diseases; these donations are long-term and some are for as long as required until the public health goals are reached. Many of the control or elimination programmes depend on this generosity. Drug donations are available for onchocerciasis, lymphatic filariasis, trachoma, leprosy, fascioliasis, soil-transmitted helminths, schistosomiasis, and curative drugs are provided for sleeping sickness. These donation programmes are managed in collaboration with the WHO by the pharmaceutical companies who are committed to making quality controlled drugs available. Well- defined application processes are in place, together with monitoring and feedback, ensuring accountability of the use of the drugs through the complex route from manufacture, delivery and importation to their entry into the supply chain in the endemic country. This involves duty free importation, storage, distribution from the centre to communities including training needs at each level of the system and the need to monitor any adverse events.

Examples of successful NTD control and elimination and the wider benefits

Historically, there are several examples of successful control or elimination of NTDs (see below). These are the result of well-defined strategies, sustained country commitment to financing and the demonstration that rapid scaling up is possible following the establishment of proof of principle of the strategy. In addition, several of the products donated for mass drug administration for control of specific diseases such as lymphatic

filariasis and onchocerciasis have broad spectrum efficacy impacting on other infections including the soil-transmitted helminths – hookworm, *Trichuris* and *Ascaris* – and ectoparasites such as lice and scabies. School-based deworming treatment also results in educational benefits including improved school attendance and improved physical growth and cognition. HIV prevention could be assisted by treatment with the drug praziquantel if given to prevent urogenital schistosomal lesions. In addition, community-based interventions have been demonstrated to provide a platform for other health interventions such as vitamin A supplementation, provision of insecticide treated bednets and home-based management of malaria.

Interventions through school-based delivery provide access to the school age population, notwithstanding the need to reach those who are of school age but do not attend school.

The wider dimension social dimensions of NTD control

Freedom from preventable diseases including NTDs has a human rights dimension given the availability of affordable, donated medicines for some conditions. This raises issues of equity as mass drug distribution of safe and effective drugs covers large numbers of individuals who benefit directly and who would otherwise have no access to them. Such programmes often deliver drugs to populations who are beyond the reach of health services – for example 50% of treatments for river blindness through the African Programme for Onchocerciasis Control are provided to communities more than 20 km from the nearest health centre. The effectiveness of interventions for elimination or control is demonstrated by historical success and in the progress of ongoing programmes, but also because communities have sustained their commitment to delivery without remuneration. The arguments of equitable access to health are enshrined in several UN charters including the WHO Charter. The ability of the WHO strategy of preventive chemotherapy not only reduces the morbidity and transmission of disease, but prevents future generations from acquiring conditions which blight lives and communities.

Additional needs through research

Research needs are well defined-in particular the need for better drugs for some diseases such the human trypanosomiases and leishmaniases, as existing drugs are toxic, expensive, and difficult to transport and administer. These need to be given parentally but drugs which can be given orally are a pre-requisite for more effective treatment and control. Programmes should also monitor drug efficacy as there is always a risk of resistance which becomes particularly important when few (if any) alternatives are available. Diagnostic and monitoring tools are also required as some diseases are difficult to diagnose clinically and need invasive procedures.

Policy considerations

NTDs form a diverse group of infections, caused by the range of infectious agents from viruses such as dengue to guinea worm, hence control strategies differ. As the diseases are often found in particular geographic regions there is a need to address them in a regional context due to the different epidemiology, diversity of health systems and health financing mechanisms. The NTDs are characterized as infections of poverty and their prevalence has been used as an indicator of poverty. They were however, 'lumped' by policy-makers within the 'other diseases' of Millennium Development Goal 6, which only mentions HIV and malaria. Tuberculosis was ignored but was later included in the Global Fund, the major financing mechanism for control of the big three diseases – AIDS, TB and malaria. This has led to the NTDs being ignored as health problems for many years. Recently, NTDs have been included with HIV, TB and malaria in the post-2015 health development targets. The situation has changed due to advocacy efforts and the realization that successful programmes can be implemented at low cost, the interventions are highly cost-effective. Many are based on the availability of donated drugs which are largely safe for mass drug distribution. The impact of control can be monitored and assessed by various surveillance methods providing evidence of progress towards end points established by the WHO. It is also essential that there is a continuing commitment for health systems to conduct post intervention or control surveillance for several years to detect and prevent resurgence of disease.

Successes in the control of Neglected Tropical Diseases

Lymphatic filariasis has been successfully controlled in China in a population of 350 million people and in the Republic of Korea (South Korea); transmission has also been arrested in several countries where it is no longer a public health problem in – Thailand, Sri Lanka (*Brugia*), Suriname, the Solomon Islands, Togo Trinidad and Tobago and Costa Rica. The Global Programme for the Elimination of Lymphatic Filariasis (GPELF) has reported that over 500 million treatments are being distributed each year in over 50 countries with savings of US$ 24 billion between 2000–08 through prevention of loss of labour. Annual treatments of ivermectin and albendazole are given in Africa where onchocerciasis is coendemic. In the rest of the world, the drugs used are diethylcarbamazine (DEC) and albendazole. As a result of the GPELF to date, 66 million newborns have been prevented from becoming infected, 2.2 million protected from developing clinical disease and 28.7 million who have problems of existing infection have seen their clinical symptoms diminish and not progress to further disability.

River blindness (onchocerciasis) has been eliminated as a public health problem and as a disease of socioeconomic importance in ten West Africa countries, the original area of the Onchocerciasis Control Programme (OCP), protecting a population of some 50 million people. The benefits of the OCP have been quantified as 600 000 cases of blindness prevented, 18 million born free of the risk of blindness, 25 million hectares of arable land reclaimed for settlement and agricultural production. Control of blindness and skin disease via the donated drug ivermectin (Mectizan; donated by Merck & Co. Inc) is now reaching some 90 million people each year in 19 countries by the Africa Programme for Onchocerciasis Control (APOC). This is supported by national governments and NGDOs through over 748 000 community workers trained in 120 000 communities. Onchocerciasis is also endemic in 6 countries in Latin America where twice yearly distribution of ivermectin has resulted in the elimination of transmission in several foci. In Africa there is evidence that annual distribution may also eliminate transmission if sustained for 15 years at 70% coverage.

Domestic transmission of **Chagas' disease** due to *Trypanosoma cruzi* has been controlled in five South American countries by domestic spraying of insecticide against the vector *Triatoma infestans,* providing economic rates of return of around 30% on the investment in vector control. In Central America there is similar progress through control of *Rhodnius prolixus.* Transmission by blood transfusion has been substantially reduced throughout Latin America. Sustaining the advances made and maintaining an effective surveillance system are necessary whilst research for new and effective drugs continues to be a high priority to treat those infected.

Leprosy has been reduced as a public health problem as a result of the use of multidrug therapy of three donated drugs-rifampicin, dapsone and clofazimine. Of the 122 countries considered endemic for leprosy, the WHO states that 119 have eliminated the disease as a public health problem (defined as 1 case per/ 10 000). The 213 000 cases reported are confined to 17 countries reporting more than a 1000 cases/year. The figures suggest a prevalence reduction of 90% in endemic countries through case finding and multidrug therapy, which have prevented disabilities in between 1 and 2 million people. Since 1985 some 14.5 million people have been cured through multidrug therapy. The numbers of new cases per year have fallen dramatically. The drugs for the cure of leprosy are donated by Novartis.

Guinea worm is moving towards eradication. The number of cases has been dramatically reduced from over 3.5 million in 1986 to 542 in 2012; the disease remains endemic in four countries – Chad, Ethiopia, Mali and South Sudan. There are several countries which have not reported cases during the previous year (Burkina Faso, Côte d'Ivoire, Ghana, Kenya, Niger, Nigeria, Togo) and are considered to be in a precertification phase awaiting formal certification as being free of transmission. Post certification there is a continued need for surveillance until global certification is achieved.

Schistosomiasis affects 200 million people. Intensive control in Egypt has reduced prevalence from around 20% to less than 1–2% using the drug praziquantel (now 0.32 US$/treatment) over the last two decades. Transmission in Egypt has been largely eliminated over the last five years and control focuses on hotspots of transmission – the result has been a massive reduction in incidence of bladder cancer. China continues to make considerable progress and now there are less than 1 million people infected and a national programme continues. Programmes in Africa are now reaching school age children in 17 countries in Africa and initial results show dramatic reductions in prevalence over a period of 4 years of annual treatment.

Trachoma A trachoma programme has been established to eliminate blinding trachoma by 2020 through a SAFE strategy (S=surgery; A=antibiotics; F=facial cleanliness through washing; E=environmental control). Trachoma is endemic in 57 countries and the cost of in terms of lost productivity is estimated at US$2.9–5.3 billion/annum. The antibiotic azithromycin has been donated by Pfizer. Three countries have reported reaching their elimination targets (Iran, Morocco and Oman) but there is a need for further up-scaling in the highest burden countries such as Ethiopia, Nigeria and Sudan.

Human African trypanosomiasis Over recent years the numbers of reported new cases of sleeping sickness has been declining between 1999 and 2008 and the number of new cases reported has fallen by 62% from over 27 000 to 10 372. However, these figures are likely to be underestimates because of the remoteness of many endemic areas that may not be covered by regular surveillance. There is evidence that the disease is no longer present in many West African countries probably due to climate change and population pressure on habitat of the tsetse fly vector. The problem remains focussed on Angola, the Democratic Republic of Congo and Sudan who report over 1000 cases of chronic *T. gambiense* annually. More extensive surveillance and the availability of treatment provided through WHO of donated drugs is the likely cause of the reduction in reported incidence. There has also been a 58% decline in reported cases of acute *T. rhodesiense* in East and Southern Africa whilst the adoption of cattle treatment and spraying of cattle the reservoir in Uganda has had a major impact on transmission of *T. rhodesiense* to humans.

Soil-transmitted helminth infections targets three important worms which inhabit the gut-hookworm (*Necator* and *Ancylostoma*), whipworm (*Trichuris*) and roundworm (*Ascaris*), the combined global prevalence of which is probably greater than all the other NTDs combined. Mass drug distribution annually of mebendazole or albendazole through deworming programmes, usually by school based health delivery programmes, has had a significant impact on educational achievement, increased growth and weight gain, cognitive and physical performance. Deworming of pregnant women in the second and third trimester of pregnancy increased child survival at the age of 6 months by over 40% in areas of hookworm endemicity. The cost per person of these deworming programmes in South East Asia is of the order of 2 US cents/year. The onchocerciasis and lymphatic filariasis programmes also act as deworming programmes as the drugs used have powerful effects on the worms of the gut.

Health systems and partnerships

The control of NTDs, achieved in many different settings, also has benefits for the health system. Experience over the last three decades demonstrates contributions in the areas of:

- improving national surveillance and monitoring systems;
- institutional capacity development;
- strengthening laboratory services;
- enhanced operational research capacity;
- improved drug distribution systems;
- development of drug storage, quality control and supply chains;
- extensive inter-country interactions at various levels;
- development of community networks of volunteers able to collect, manage and distribute drugs, undertake monitoring of adverse events, submit reports, provide census data;
- community directed approaches which are catalytic, enabling expansion of delivery channels for other interventions (e.g. mosquito bed nets, vitamin A and condoms).

However, there have been criticisms that, if NTD-specific interventions are implemented in parallel with ongoing health services, this can disrupt routine health provision, especially if such health systems are weak. One of the characteristics of NTD control based around the drug donation programmes has been the development of supportive partnership and alliances, whose function is to provide advocacy support and mobilize resources for the implementation and to raise the profile of the problem within the global health community (Table 63.2). These partnerships are also designed to reflect the mandate of the WHO to support countries in implementing the World Health Assembly Resolutions, which are focused on specific diseases (Table 63.3).

Table 63.2 List of some Neglected Tropical Disease partnerships

APOC	African Programme for Onchocerciasis Control; hosted by World Bank/WHO/UNDP MOU with World Bank and WHO, endemic countries, international organizations, NGOs, private sector
GAELF	Global Alliance for the Elimination of Lymphatic Filariasis; hosted by academic institution; countries, international organizations, NGOs, private sector, academia
GWEP	Guinea Worm Eradication Programme; hosted by NGO; international organizations, endemic countries, NGOs, private sector; certification by WHO Commission
ILEP	International Federation of Anti-Leprosy Associations; hosted by NGOs; coordination/advocacy
INCOSUR	Southern Cone Initiative to Control/Eliminate Chagas' Disease. Hosted by PAHO countries, international organizations
ITI	International Trachoma Initiative; countries, international organizations, NGOs, private sector
OEPA	Onchocerciasis Elimination Programme for the Americas; hosted by an NGDO; endemic countries, international organizations, NGOs, private sector
SCI	Schistosomiasis Control Initiative; hosted by NGOs, private sector academia; financing/technical assistance

Table 63.3 Selected World Health Assembly resolutions pertaining to Neglected Tropical Disease control programmes which specify targets for control, elimination or eradication

Leprosy – elimination as a public health problem in all countries (i.e. prevalence of 1 case per 10 000 population in each country)

Buruli ulcer – surveillance and control of *Mycobacterium ulcerans* disease

Dracunculiasis (guinea worm) – eradication; country-by-country certification of elimination of transmission; certificated by the International Commission

Chagas' disease – interruption of vector and serological (transfusion) transmission in all endemic countries in Latin America

Lymphatic filariasis – elimination as a public health problem and the interruption of transmission

Onchocerciasis – in the Americas (OEPA), elimination as a public health problem, defined as elimination of morbidity in the six countries in the Americas. Eliminate parasite transmission in those countries or foci where feasible. In Africa (APOC), onchocerciasis control through ivermectin distribution

Trachoma – elimination of trachoma as a blinding disease by 2020

SUMMARY

- The WHO currently identifies 17 diseases as 'Neglected Tropical Diseases' (NTD).

- These are important causes of poverty as well as being characteristic of conditions of poverty.

- As the NTDs form a diverse group of infections caused by a range of pathogens, from dengue virus to guinea worm, details of emphasis in control strategies differ.

- Five overall strategies are recommended for NTD control: expansion of access to chemotherapy; intensified case detection and management; improved vector or intermediate host control; improved veterinary/joint public health measures to control zoonotic diseases; provision of safe water, sanitation and hygiene.

 Visit www.lecturenoteseries.com/tropicalmed to test yourself on this chapter using interactive MCQs.

FURTHER READING

Hotez PJ, Fenwick A, Savioli L, Molyneux DH (2009) Rescuing the bottom billion through control of neglected tropical diseases. *Lancet* **373**: 1570–5. [Free download from http://thelancet.com]

Lancet Neglected Tropical Diseases Series (2010) http://www.thelancet.com/series/neglected-tropical-diseases. [Reviews elimination and control programmes for lymphatic filariasis, onchocerciasis, schistosomiasis, and soil-transmitted helminthiasis, and describes the effect, governance arrangements, and financing mechanisms of selected international control initiatives. Free downloads.]

World Health Organization (2010) *Working to Overcome the Global Impact of Neglected Tropical Diseases*. Geneva: WHO.

World Health Organization (2011) Working to overcome the global impact of neglected tropical diseases-summary. *Weekly Epidemiological Record* **86**: 113–28.

Useful websites

www.who.int/neglected_diseases
www.filariasis.org
www.trachoma.org
www.who.int/blindness/partnerships/APOC
www.cartercenter.org/health/river_blindness/oepa.html
www.who.int/topics/leprosy

Index

A

abacavir (ABC), 110–11
abdominal pain, 3–4
achalasia, 3
acute dermatolympangioadenitis (ADLA), 135
acute filarial lymphangitis (AFL), 135
acute flaccid paralysis, 248
  nerve conduction studies, 250
  pathophysiology and clinical presentations, 248
    acute motor axonal neuropathy (AMAN), 249–50
    eneterovirus, 71, 249
    Guillain–Barré syndrome, 249
    Japanese encephalitis, 249
    polio, 248
acute HIV seroconversion illness, 101–2
acute motor axonal neuropathy (AMAN)
  pathophysiology and presentation, 249–50
acute papular onchodermatitis (APOD), 127
adequate clinical and parasitological response (ACPR) rate, 60
African histoplasmosis, 318
African Programme for Onchocerciasis Control (APOC), 132
African tick typhus, 293
  clinical features, 293
  treatment, 293
African trypanosomiasis, 141
  clinical picture
    early stage, 142–3
    late stage symptoms and signs, 143
  control and surveillance, 146
  diagnosis
    early stage, 143–4
    immunological diagnostic methods, 144
    late stage (CNS involvement), 144
  disease
    immune response and pathogenesis, 142
    local effects, 141
    systemic effects, 141–2
  epidemiology, 145–6
  life-cycle, 141
  parasites, 141

  treatment, 144
    early stage, 144
    late stage, 144–5
    relapse, 145
AIDS, 102
albendazole, 9, 106, 133, 136
  ascariasis, 201
  hookworm, 202
  strongyloidiasis, 313
aminosidine (paromomycin), 74
amodiaquine (AQ), 62
  pregnancy, 65
amoebiasis, 106
  clinical features, 178
    amoebic liver abscess (ALA), 179–80
    intestinal amoebiasis, 178–9
  epidemiology, 177
  investigations
    antigen detection, 180
    endoscopy, 180
    imaging, 180–81
    microscopy, 180
    serology, 180
  management
    cyst eradication, 181
    invasive amoebiasis, 181
    practical aspects, 181
  parasite and life-cycle, 177–8
  pathogenesis, 178
  prevention and public health aspects, 182
  recent developments, 182
amoxicillin, 271
amphotericin B, 73–4
  liposomal, 74
anaemia, 33
  blood transfusion in developing countries, 36–7
  causes, 33
  clinical diagnosis, 33
  laboratory investigations, 33–4
    haemoglobin measurement, 34
    macrocytic anaemia, 35–6
    microcytic anaemia, 34–5
    normocytic anaemia, 36
    peripheral blood film, 34
  management without laboratory investigations, 36
  patient management algorithm, 35
antibiotics for malaria, 63

antifolate drugs, 63
antiretroviral therapy (ART), 94
  4-S guide, 112
    starting ART, 113–14
    stopping treatment, 114
    substituting drugs, 114
    switching regimen, 114
  adult prescription flowchart, 125
  boosted protease inhibitors, 111
  common drugs and regimens, 110
  delivery, 115
  follow-up visit format, 113
  Immune Reconstitution Inflammatory Sysndrome (IRIS), 114–15
  non-nucleoside reverse transcriptase inhibitors (NNRTIs), 111
  nucleoside reverse transcriptase inhibitors (NRTIs), 110–11
  public health approach, 110
  screening tests, 112
  special population regimens, 112
arboviral encephalitis, 243
arboviruses, 273
  clinical syndromes, 273
    fever-arthralgia-rash arboviruses (FAR), 273–4
  vectors and hosts, 273
artemisinin combination therapy (ACT), 61, 64, 66–7
artemisinin derivatives, 60–61
  pregnancy, 65
artesunate, 61
ARV-related diabetes, 337
ascariasis
  clinical features, 200
  investigations, 200
  management, 201
  parasite and life-cycle, 200
  prevention and public health aspects, 201
asthma, 14
  care organization
    doctor education, 344
    nurse-led treatment protocols, 344–5
    patient education, 344
  causes
    general, 342–3
    urban asthma, 343
  complications, 343
  diagnosis, 342

asthma, *(cont'd)*
  epidemiology, 342
  management
    acute severe asthma, 343–4
    exacerbations, 343
    routine treatment, 343
    tropical adaptations, 343
  prevalence, 342
asylum seekers, 355
  health assessment, 355–6
  infectious diseases, 356
  torture and traumatic experiences, 356
atazanavir (ATZ), 111
atovaquone, 63
azithromycin, 106, 271

B

bacillary dysentery, 183
  clinical features, 183–4
  investigation, 184
  management, 184
  microbiology and epidemiology, 183
  prevention and public health aspects, 184–5
Balantidium coli, 192
bancroftian filariasis
  clinical effects, 134–5
  life-cycle, 134
BCG vaccination, 92, 109
bilharzia, 151
bipolar affective disorder, 348–9
bithionol, 215
Bitot's spots, 363, 367
Blantyre coma scale, 19
Blastocystis hominis, 192
blindness, 364
  cataracts, 364–5
  microbial keratitis, 365–6
blood transfusion in developing
    countires, 36–7
blood, vomiting, 3
body cavity myiasis, 305–6
boosted protease inhibitors, 111
bot fly, 305
breathlessness, 11, 12
  with wheezing, 14
brucellosis, 262
  clinical features, 262–3
  diagnosis, 263–4
  epidemiology, 262
  follow-up, 265
  public health aspects, 265
  treatment, 264–5
brugian filariasis, 135–6
bullae, 32
Buruli ulcer, 301
  clinical features, 301–2
  differential diagnosis, 302
  epidemiology, 301
  investigations, 302

management, 302–3
microbiology, 301
prevention and public health aspects, 303

C

Calabar swelling, 138
cataracts, 364–5
causes, 243
cell mediated immunity (CMI), 163
central nervous system (CNS) infections
    CSF findings, 22, 23
cephalosporins, third-generation, 271
cerebral malaria, 57
cerebrospinal fluid (CSF)
    findings in CNS infections, 22, 23
Chagas' disease, 3
  clinical features
    acute diease, 148
    chronic disease, 148–9
    immunocompromise, 149
  diagnosis
    other techniques, 149
    parasitological techniques, 149
  epidemiology and control, 149
  parasite, life-cycle and pathogenesis, 148
  treatment, 149
chemoprophylaxis, 67, 109
chest pain, 12
Cheyne–Stokes breathing, 21
chiggers, 305
chikungunya, 273
children
  acute breathless and fever in small
      child, 13–14
  HIV infection, 115
    acute cough and fever, 105
    immunization, 109
    management, 115–16
  leprosy, 173
  malnutrition, 358
    aetiology, 358
    clinical features, 358–9
    community-based therapeutic care, 361–2
    definition, 358
    effect of HIV and tuberculosis, 362
    investigations, 360
    management, 360–61
Chinese paralytic syndrome, 249–50
chloramphenicol, 271
chloroquine (CQ), 61–2, 181
  pregnancy, 65
cholera, 186
  control and prevention, 188–9
  diagnosis, 187
  epidemiology, 186–7
  microbiology and pathogenesis, 186
  treatment
    antimicrobial agents, 188

initial rehydration, 187–8
    maintenance rehydration, 188
chromoblastomycosis, 320
  diagnosis, 320
  treatment, 320
chronic obstructive pulmonary disease
    (COPD), 11
chronic papular onchodermatitis
    (CPOD), 127–8
chyluria, 135
ciprofloxacin, 106
clofazimine, 170
Clostridium difficile, 7
cobalamin (vitamin B12) deficiency, 328
  clinical features, 328
  investigations, 328–9
  management, 329
colitis, 3
Colorado tick fever, 274
coma
  further investigation, 21
  rapid assessment, 18–21
corneal xerosis, 367
co-trimoxazole, 9, 106, 271
  prophylaxis, 109
cough, 11
  chronic, 14
C-reactive protein (CRP), 25
Crimean–Congo haemorrhagic fever, 277, 281
croup, 12
cryptococcal meningitis, 241
  clinical features, 241
  investigation, 241–2
  organisms and epidemiology, 241
  prevention, 242
  treatment, 242
cryptosporidiosis, 106
  clinical features, 192
  investigations, 193
  management, 193
  parasite and life-cycle, 192
cutaneous larva migrans, 307
  clinical features, 307
  parasitology, 307
  prevention, 308
  treatment, 307–8
cutaneous leishmaniasis (CL), 77
  clinical features
    cutaneous leishmaniasis (CL), 77
    diffuse cutaneous leishmaniasis
        (DCL), 77–8
    HIV co-infection, 78
    leishmaniasis recidivans (LR), 78
    mucosal leishmaniasis (ML), 78
  investigations, 79
  management, 79–80
  prevention, 81
  treatment selection, 80
cyanosis, 12
cyclosporiasis, 106, 192
cysticercosis, 196–7

cystoisosporiasis, 106, 192
cytomegalovirus chorioretinitis, 108

D

dapsone, 63, 170
darunavir (DVR), 111
decorticate posturing, 21
dehydration, clinical classification, 6
dengue virus, 274, 277, 283
  classification, 284–5
  clinical features, 283
    dengue fever (DF), 283, 284
    dengue haemorrhagic fever (DHF),
      283, 284
  epidemiology, 283
  investigations, 285
  management
    dengue fever (DF), 286
    dengue haemorrhagic fever (DHF),
      286
    other severe manifestations, 286
  pathogenesis, 286
  prevention, 286–7
depression, 348
dermatological presentations, 29
  creeping eruptions, 30
  papules, 31
  petechial rashes, 32
  pigmentation changes
    hyperpigmentation, 31
    hypopigmented macules, 31
  skin itching, 30
  skin nodules, 31
  skin ulcers, 29–30
  urticaria, 31
  vesicles and bullae, 32
diabetes mellitus
  atypical ketosis-prone type 2 diabetes,
    336
  care organization, 338–9
    algorithm, 339
  causes, 336–7
  complications
    acute complications, 337
    chronic complications, 337
    infection, 337
  diagnosis, 335–6
  epidemiology, 335
  management
    diet, 337
    education, 338
    insulin, 337
    ketoacidosis (DKA) treatment, 337–8
    monitoring, 338
    oral agents, 337
  prevalence, 336
diarrhoea, 4
  clinical features, 7
  clinical syndromes, 6–7
  dehydration, clinical classification, 6

  examination, 6
  history, 4–5
  host factors, 6
  investigations, 7–8
  management, 8–9
  management algorithm, 8
  non-infectious causes, 5
  other illnesses, 5
  pathogens, 7
  pathophysiology and definitions, 4
didanosine (ddI), 111
diethylcarbamazine (DEC), 133, 136
diffuse cutaneous leishmaniasis (DCL),
  77–8
  investigations, 79
dihydrofolate reductase (DHFR), 63
dihydropteroate synthase (DHPS), 63
diloxanide furoate, 181
diphyllobothriasis, 197
dipylidiasis, 197
direct agglutination test (DAT), 72
direct observation of therapy (DOTS)
  strategy, 92–4
doll's eye reflex, 21
doxycycline
  cholera, 188
  filariasis, 136–7
  pregnancy, 66
dracunculiasis 315–16
dysphagia, 3

E

Ebola virus, 277, 280
Echinococcus granulosus
  clinical features, 218–19
  investigations, 219
  life-cycle, 218
  prevention and control, 220
  treatment, 219–20
Echinococcus multilocularis
  clinical features, 220
  investigations, 220
  life-cycle, 220
  treatment, 220–21
efavirenz (EFV), 111
eflornithine, 144–5
elephantiasis, 135
emtricitabine (FTC), 110
encephalitis, 17, 243
  arboviral encephalitis, 243
  causes, 243
  equine encephalitis viruses, 246
  Japanese encephalitis, 243
    clinical features, 243–4
    epidemiology, 243
    investigations, 244
    prevention and public health
      aspects, 244
  La Crosse virus, 246
  management, 246

  Murray Valley virus, 246
  St Louis encephalitis virus, 245
  tick-borne encephalitis virus, 245
  West Nile virus, 245
encephalopathy, 16
eneterovirus, 71, pathophysiology and
  presentation, 249
Entamoeba histolytica, 7
enzyme-linked immunoabsorbent assay
  (ELISA), 72
enzymopathies
  glucose-6-phosphate dehydrogenase
    (G6PD) deficiency
    clinical features, 324
    diagnosis, 324–5
    epidemiology, 324
    management, 325
epilepsy
  care organization
    drug treatment, 346
    education, 346
  causes, 345–6
  complications, 346
  diagnosis, 345
  epidemiology, 345
  management
    drug treatment, 346
    status epilepticus, 346
  prevalence, 345
equine encephalitis viruses, 246
eruptions on skin, 30
erythema nodosum leprosum reaction,
  170–71
ethambutol (E), 87
etravirine (ETR), 111
eye disease, 364
  examination of eye, 364
    red eye, 364
  leprosy, 370–71
  pathways to blindness, 364
    cataracts, 364–5
    microbial keratitis, 365–6
    trachoma, 368–9
    management, 369–70
    vitamin A deficiency, 366–8
eye, pupil reaction to light, 20

F

fast agglutination-screening test (FAST), 72
febrile presentations
  acute fever with negative malarial
    blood film, 26
  clinical approach
    examination, 24–5
    history, 24
    initial investigation, 25–6
  common clinical problems, 27–8
    autoimmune and connective tissue
      disorders, 26–7
    malignancy, 27

febrile presentations, *(cont'd)*
  pathogenesis and symptomatic
    treatment, 24
  treatment for common causes
    (<2 weeks), 26
  treatment for common causes
    (>2 weeks), 27
fever–arthralgia–rash arboviruses (FAR)
  chikungunya, 273
  Colorado tick fever, 274
  dengue virus, 274
  O'nyong nyong, 274
  Ross River virus, 274
filarial fever, 135
filarial lymph node enlargement, 135
filariasis, 126
  bancroftian filariasis
    clinical effects, 134–5
    life-cycle, 134
  brugian filariasis, 135–6
  control, 137–8
    vector control, 138
  diagnosis and monitoring, 136
  lymphatic filariasis (LF), 134
  management, 136–7
    individual patients, 137
  prevention of morbidity, 137
fluconazole, 80
fluoroquinolones, 9, 270–71
folate deficiency, 327
  clinical features, 328
  investigations, 328
  management, 328
formol gel test (FGT), 72
furazolidone, 188

G

gastrointestinal presentations, 3
  abdominal pain, 3–4
  diarrhoea, 4
    clinical features, 7
    clinical syndromes, 6–7
    dehydration, clinical classification,
      6
    examination, 6
    history, 4–5
    host factors, 6
    investigations, 7–8
    management, 8–9
    management algorithm, 8
    non-infectious causes, 5
    other illnesses, 5
    pathogens, 7
    pathophysiology and definitions, 4
  dysphagia/odynophagia, 3
  haematemesis, 3
  malabsorption, 4
    tropical sprue, 4
genital ulcer flowchart, 43
Giardia lamblia, 4

giardiasis, 106
  clinical features, 190–91
  differential diagnosis, 191
  epidemiology, 190
  investigations, 191
  management, 191
  parasite and life-cycle, 190
  prevention and public health aspects,
    192
Glasgow coma scale, 19
Global Alliance for the Elimination of
    Lymphatic Filariasis (GAELF), 137
Global Programme to Eliminate
    Lymphatic Filariasis (GPELF), 134
glucose-6-phosphate dehydrogenase
    (G6PD) deficiency
  clinical features, 324
  diagnosis, 324–5
  epidemiology, 324
  management, 325
Guillain–Barré syndrome
  pathophysiology and presentation, 249
guinea worm infection, 315
  clinical features, 315
  control, 316
  diagnosis, 315
  life-cycle, 315
  treatment, 315–16

H

haematemesis, 3
haematinic deficiencies, 326
  cobalamin (vitamin B12) deficiency,
    328
    clinical features, 328
    investigations, 328–9
    management, 329
  folate deficiency, 327
    clinical features, 328
    investigations, 328
    management, 328
  iron deficiency, 326
    clinical features, 326
    investigations, 326–7
    management, 327
haemoglobinopathies
  sickle cell anaemia, 321
    clinical features, 322
    diagnosis, 322–3
    epidemiology, 322
    management, 323
    protection against malaria, 322
  β thalassaemia, 323
    clinical features, 323
    diagnosis, 323
    epidemiology, 323
    management, 323–4
haemolytic uraemic syndrome (HUS), 183
haemoptysis, 11
halofantrine, 62

Hansen's disease, 163
hantaan, 277
headache, 16
helminths, soil-transmitted, 199–200
  ascariasis, 200–201
hemiparesis, 21
hepatitis, viral, 205
  clinicoepidemiological features, 205
  hepatitis A (HAV), 205–6
  hepatitis B (HBV), 206–9
    immunization, 209
    prevalence, 208
  hepatitis C (HCV), 210–11
  hepatitis D (HDV), 210
  hepatitis E (HEV), 211–12
hepatocellular carcinoma (HCC), 206,
    207, 212
histoplasmosis, 317
  African histoplasmosis, 318
  classical histoplasmosis
    clinical features, 317
    diagnosis, 317
    treatment, 317–8
HIV infection, 96
  antiretroviral therapy (ART)
    4-S guide, 112–14
    adult prescription flowchart, 125
    boosted protease inhibitors, 111
    common drugs and regimens, 110
    delivery, 115
    follow-up visit format, 113
    Immune Reconstitution Inflammatory
      Syndrome (IRIS), 114–15
    non-nucleoside reverse
      transcriptase inhibitors (NNRTIs),
      111
    nucleoside reverse transcriptase
      inhibitors (NRTIs), 110–11
    post-exposure prophylaxis (PEP),
      109–10
    public health approach, 110–11
    screening tests, 112
    special population regimens, 112
  children, 115
    management, 115–16
  clinical problems in adults, 102
    acute cough and fever, 103–4
    central nervous system disease, 107–8
    chronic cough and fever, 104–5
    chronic diarrhoea, 105–6
    eye disease, 108
    high fever without focus, 105
    jaundice, 108
    Kaposi's sarcoma, 107
    oral and oesophageal candidiasis,
      106–7
    skin conditions, 102–3
  clinical problems in children
    acute cough and fever, 105
  control strategies, 116–17
    Prevention of Mother-to-Child
      Transmission (PMTCT), 117

cutaneous leishmaniasis (CL)
co-infection, 78
epidemiology, 98
global seroprevalence, 98–9
flowcharts
ART prescription in adults, 125
cough, 119
diarrhoea, 121
fever, 120
headache, 123
painful feet, 124
sore mouth/difficulty swallowing,
122
incidence in tropics, 16
myelopathy, 252–3
natural history, 101
acute seroconversion illness, 101–2
early disease, 102
immune activation phase, 102
late disease (AIDS), 102
pathogenesis, 99–100
progressive immunosuppression,
100–101
prophylaxis
childhood immunization, 109
co-trimoxazole, 109
other infections, 109
preventing pneumococcal disease,
109
TB chemoprophylaxis, 109
respiratory disease, 14–15
schistosomiasis, 162
staging, 101
testing and counselling, 97
test selection, 97–8
testing at STI clinics, 45
transmission
infected blood, 99
risk factors, 99
sexual transmission, 99
vertical transmission, 99
tuberculosis (TB), effect upon, 85, 93–4
clinical features, 86
viruses, 96
differences between, 96–7
visceral leishmaniasis (VL) coinfection, 71–2
hookworm, 201
clinical features, 202
investigations, 202
management, 202
parasites and life-cycle, 201
prevention and public health aspects,
202
humanitarian emergencies, 351
emergency phase, 351
control of communicable diseases
and epidemics, 354
coordination, 354
food and nutrition, 352–3
health care, 354
human resources and training, 354

initial assessment, 351–2
measles immunization, 352
public health surveillance, 354
shelter and site planning, 353
water and sanitation, 352
post-emergency phase, 355
hydatid disease, 218–21
hymenolepiasis, 197
hyperreactive malarial splenomegaly,
48–9
hyperpigmentation, 31
hypertension
care organization, 341–2
algorithm, 342
causes and risk factors, 340
complications, 340
diagnosis, 339–40
epidemiology, 339
hypertensive crisis, 341
management
drug therapy, 341
treatment principles,
340–41
prevalence, 340
special situations, 341
hyperventilation, 21
hypochlorhydria, 6
hypopigmented macules, 31

Immune Reconstitution Inflammatory
Syndrome (IRIS), 114–15, 163
indirect fluorescent antibody test (IFAT),
72
indoor residual spraying (IRS), 66–7
insecticide-treated bednets (ITNs),
66–7
Integrated Management of Adult Illness
(IMAI), 102
Integrated Management of Childhood
Illness (IMCI), 13–14
integrated vector management (IVM),
374
intermittent presumptive therapy (IPT),
65
intestinal flukes, 216
intestinal tuberculosis (TB), 4
intraconazole, 79
intravenous drug use (IVDU), 72
iodoquinol, 181
iron deficiency, 326
clinical features, 326
investigations, 326–7
management, 327
irritable bowel syndrome (IBS), 3
isoniazid (H), 87
preventive therapy, 92
itching, 30
ivermectin, 131–2, 133, 136
strongyloidiasis, 313

J
Japanese encephalitis, 243
clinical features, 243–4
epidemiology, 243
investigations, 244
management, 246
pathophysiology and presentation, 249
prevention and public health aspects,
244
Jarisch–Herxheimer reaction (JHR), 290
jaundice in HIV infections, 108
jiggers, 305

K
kala-azar, 70
Kaposi's sarcoma, 107
Kato–Katz technique, 200
Kérandel's sign, 143
Kernig's sign, 20
ketoacidosis, diabetic (DKA), 337–8
ketoconazole, 79
Koplick's spots, 25
kwashiokor, 359
Kyasanur Forest disease, 281

L
La Crosse virus, 246
lamivudine (3TC), 110
laryngotracheobronchitis, 12
Lassa fever, 277, 280
leishmaniasis
cutaneous leishmaniasis (CL), 77
clinical features 77–8
investigations, 79
management, 79–80
prevention, 81
treatment selection, 80
leishmaniasis recidivans (LR), 78
investigations, 79
leishmanin test (Montenegro test), 79
mucosal leishmaniasis (ML), 78
investigations, 79
visceral leishmaniasis (VL), 70
clinical features, 71
epidemiology, 70
HIV co-infection, 71–2
investigations 72–3
management, 73–4
parasite life-cycle, 70–71
post-kala-azar dermal leishmaniasis
(PKDL), 74–5
prevention, 75–6
viscerotropic leishmaniasis, 71
leprosy, 163
classification, 166–7
borderline lepromatous leprosy, 168
borderline leprosy, 168

leprosy, *(cont'd)*
  borderline tuberculoid leprosy, 168
  eye involvement, 168, 169
  lepromatous leprosy, 168
  other forms, 168
  tuberculoid leprosy, 167–8
clinical features, 165
  nerve damage, 165
  skin lesions, 165
control and prevention
  general health services, 173
  vaccination, 173
diagnosis, 168
  differential diagnosis, 169
  peripheral nerve examination, 169
  skin, 168
  slit skin smears, 169
epidemiology, 163
eye disease, 370–71
immune response, 163–5
management, 169
  chemotherapy, 169–70
  infectivity and screening, 171–2
  multidrug therapy, 170
  new nerve damage and neuritis, 171
  reactions and nerve damage,
    170–71
microbiology, 163
prevention of disability, 172
  childhood, 173
  reconstructive surgery, 172
  women, 172–3
leptospirosis, 294
  clinical features, 294–5
  diagnosis, 295
  epidemiology, 294
  microbiology, 294
  pathogenesis, 294
  prevention, 295–6
  treatment, 295
levamisole, 201, 202
lice, 309–10
lichenified onchodermatitis (LOD), 128
liposomal amphotericin B, 74
liver flukes
  clinical features, 214
  epidemiology, 214
  investigations, 214–15
  management, 215
  parasites and life-cycles, 214
  prevention and public health aspects,
    215
liver flukes, oriental
  clinical features, 215
  epidemiology, 215
  investigations, 215–16
  management, 216
  parasites and life-cycles, 215
  prevention and public health aspects,
    216
Löffler's syndrome, 200
log–normal distribution, 153–4

loiasis, 126, 138
  diagnosis and treatment, 138–9
lopinavir (LPV), 111
louse-borne relapsing fever (LBRF), 289
louse-borne typhus, 292
  clinical features, 292
  treatment, 292
lower abdominal pain in women
    flowchart, 42
lower respiratory tract infection (LRTI),
    13–14
Lujo virus, 277, 281
lumbar puncture, 22–3
  cerebrospinal fluid (CSF) findings,
    22, 23
  guidelines, 22
lumefantrine, 62
lung flukes, 229
  clinical features, 229
    ectopic disease, 229
    lung disease, 229
  diagnosis, 229
  life-cycle, 229
  treatment, 230
lung function testing, 13
lymphatic filariasis (LF), 134

M

macrocytic anaemia, 35–6
malabsorption, 4, 7
  tropical sprue, 4
malaria, 53
  clinical features, 56–7
    complications, 58
    severe disease, 57–8
  control and eradication, 66–7
  diagnosis, 58–60
  drug treatment
    antibiotics, 63
    antifolate drugs, 63
    artemisinin derivatives, 60–61
    atovaquone, 63
    interactions, 66
    quinoline derivatives, 61–3
    resistance to, 63–4
  epidemiology, 53
  hyperreactive splenomegaly, 48–9
  immunity, 56
  life-cycle, 53–5
    targeting, 68
  pregnancy, 58
  prevention for travellers, 67
  sickle cell anaemia protection from,
    322
  treatment, 60
  treatment recommendations
    imported malaria in travellers, 65
    pregnancy, 65–6
    relapse and recrudescence, 66
    severe malaria, 64–5

  uncomplicated malaria, 64
malnutrition
  adults, 362
    nicotinic acid/niacin (B group), 362–3
    vitamin A, 363
    vitamin B1 (thiamine), 363
    vitamin C, 363
    vitamin D, 363
  children, 358
    aetiology, 358
    clinical features, 358–9
    community-based therapeutic care,
      361–2
    definition, 358
    effect of HIV and tuberculosis, 362
    investigations, 360
    management, 360–61
malnutrition-related diabetes mellitus
    (MRDM), 336
Marburg virus, 277, 280
marine envenoming
  fish, 333
  jellyfish, 333
mass drug administration (MDA), 126,
    137–8
Mazzotti test, 131
mebendazole
  ascariasis, 201
  hookworm, 202
mefloquine, 62
meglumine antimonate, 73
melarsoprol, 144–5
melioidosis
  clinical features, 297
  diagnosis, 297
  epidemiology, 297
  pathogenesis, 297
  prognosis, 298
  treatment, 297–8
menigitis, 12, 17
meningism, 16
mental illness, 347
  assessment, 347–8
  bipolar affective disorder, 348–9
  care organization, 350
  depression, 348
  post-traumatic stress disorder (PTSD),
    349–50
  schizophrenia, 348
  treatment, 348
  suicidal patients, 349
metrifonate, 159
metronidazole, 9, 106
  amoebiasis, 181
microbial keratitis, 365–6
microcytic anaemia, 34–5
microsporida, 192–3
miltefosine, 74, 80
mononeuritis multiplex, 18
Montenegro test (leishmanin test), 79
moxidectin, 132
moxifloxacin, 94

mucosal leishmaniasis (ML), 78
  investigations, 79
Murray Valley virus, 246
mycetoma, 319
  clinical features, 319
  diagnosis, 319
  epidemiology, 319
  treatment, 319–20
mycobacteria other than tuberculosis
    (MOTT), 82
Mycobacterium tuberculosis (MTB)
    complex, 82
myelitis, 17
myiasis, 305
  body cavity myiasis, 305–6
  bot fly, 305
  chiggers, 305
  Tumbu fly, 305

N

neck stiffness, 20
Neglected Tropical Diseases (NTDs), 372
  common features
    costs and benefits, 374–5
    drug donation programmes, 375
    examples of success, 375
    impact and burden, 374
    policy considerations, 376
    research needs, 375–6
    wider social dimensions, 375
  health systems and partnerships, 377–9
  strategic approaches, 372
  successes in controlling NTDs, 376–7
  'tool-deficient' diseases, 373
  'tool-ready' diseases, 372–3
  vector control, 374
  zoonotic NTDs, 373
neurological presentations, 16
  disease causes, chronic, 18
  disease causes (VIMTO), 17
  further investigation of coma, 21
  increased incidence in tropics, 16
  lumbar puncture, 22–3
    cerebrospinal fluid (CSF) findings,
        22, 23
    guidelines, 22
  pathological processes, 17–18
  rapid assessment of coma, 18–21
  syndromes, 16
neuropathy, 17
nevirapine (NVP), 111
nifurtimox, 145
nitazoxanide, 9, 106
  amoebiasis, 182
  ascariasis, 201
nodules on skin, 31
non-communicable diseases (NCDs)
  disease spectrum, 334
  epidemiological transition, 334–5
  mortality patterns, 334

non-nucleoside reverse transcriptase
    inhibitors (NNRTIs), 111
normocytic anaemia, 36
nucleoside reverse transcriptase
    inhibitors (NRTIs), 110–11
nystagmus, 21

O

ocular larva migrans (OLM), 203–4
oculocephalic reflex (OCR), 21
oculovestibular reflex (OVR), 21
odynophagia, 3
oedematous malnutrition, 359, 360
oesophageal candidiasis, 3
onchocerciasis (river blindness), 126
  clinical features, 127
    eye disease, 129–30
    general health, 130
    skin, 127–8
    subcutaneous nodules, 129
  control, 132–3
  diagnosis, 130
    microfilariae, 130–31
    other evidence, 131
  epidemiology, 127
  life-cycle, 126–7
  treatment, 131–2
    individual patients, 132
    recommended strategies, 133
Onchocerciasis Control Programme
    (OCP), 132
Onchocerciasis Elimination Programme
    for the Americas (OEPA), 132–3
O'nyong nyong, 274
oriental liver flukes
  clinical features, 215
  epidemiology, 215
  investigations, 215–16
  management, 216
  parasites and life-cycles, 215
  prevention and public health aspects,
      216
oxamniquine, 159

P

packed cell volume (PCV), 34
papular pruritic dermatosis (PPD), 103
papules, 31
paralysis, 16
parasite reduction ratio (PRR), 60
paratyphoid fever, *see* typhoid and
    parathyroid fevers
paromomycin (aminosidine), 74, 106, 181
pentamidine, 74
petechial rashes, 32
piperaquine, 62
piperazine, 201
pleural effusion, 12–13, 14

pneumonia, 222
  clinical features
    differential diagnosis, 223
    signs of acute disease, 223
    symptoms of acute disease, 223
  epidemiology, 222
  future developments
    antibiotic resistance, 227–8
    pneumococcal vaccines, 228
  investigations, 224
    HIV testing, 225
    other investigations, 225
    other microbiological tests, 225
    pleural aspiration, 225
    pulse oximetry, 225
    radiology, 224
    sputum Gram stain, 225
    sputum Ziehl–Neelsen stain, 225
    trans-thoracic lung aspirate, 225
  management, 225
    complications, 227
    flowchart, 226
    inpatient therapy, 225–7
    outpatient therapy, 225
  microbiology, 222
  prevention
    active vaccination, 227
    chemoprophylaxis, 227
  risk factors, 222–3
polio pathophysiology and presentation,
    248
polyradiculopathy, 18
post-exposure prophylaxis (PEP),
    109–10
post-kala-azar dermal leishmaniasis
    (PKDL), 71, 74–5
post-traumatic stress disorder (PTSD),
    349–50
praziquantel, 159, 160
  cestode infections, 197
pregnancy and malaria, 58
  treatment, 65–6
Preventative Chemotherapy and
    Transmission Control (PCT), 137
Prevention of Mother-to-Child
    Transmission (PMTCT), 117
primaquine in pregnancy, 66
productive coughs, 11
pupil reaction to light, 20
Putzi fly, 305
pyrantel pamoate, 201, 202
pyrazinamide (Z), 87
pyrexia, *see* febrile presentations
pyrimethamine, 63
pyrogenic meningitis, 233
  clinical features, 235
  diagnosis, 235–6
  endemic control, 238–9
  epidemiology, 233
    Haemophilus influenzae type b
        epidemiology, 234
    meningococcal epidemiology, 233–4

pyrogenic meningitis, *(cont'd)*
    pneumococcal epidemiology, 234
    vaccines, 234
  management, 236
    empirical therapy, 237
    Haemophilus influenzae disease, 237
    meningococcal disease, 236-7
    pneumococcal disease, 237
    steroid use, 237-8

Q

quinfamide, 181
quinine, 61
  in pregnancy, 65
quinoline derivatives, 61
  amodiaquine (AQ), 62
  chloroquine (CQ), 61-2
  halofantrine, 62
  lumefantrine, 62
  mefloquine, 62
  piperaquine, 62
  quinine, 61
  tafenoquine, 63

R

rabies, 254
  clinical features, 254-5
  diagnosis
    during life, 255
    postmortem, 255
  dogs as reservoirs, 254
  other animals as reservoirs, 254
  post-exposure treatment, 255
    first aid, 255-6
    immediate treatment, 256
    immunization, 256
  post-exposure vaccine regimens, 256-7
    flexibility, need for, 257
    nerve tissue vaccines, 257
    WHO recommendations, 257
  pre-exposure immunization, 257
  prevention, 257
  treatment, 255
    precautions, 255
refugee health
  asylum seekers, 355
    health assessment, 355-6
    infectious diseases, 356
    torture and traumatic experiences,
      356
  humanitarian emergencies, 351
    emergency phase, 351-4
    post-emergency phase, 355
  Sphere Project, 355
relapsing fevers, 289
  clinical features, 290
  diagnosis, 290
  differential diagnosis, 290

epidemiology, 289
  pathology, 289
  prevention and control, 290
  treatment, 290
renal syndrome, 281
respiratory presentations, 11
  assessment
    breathlessness, 11, 12
    chest pain, 12
    cough, 11
    history, 11
    non-respiratory illness, 12
    respiratory history, 12
  common presentations, 13
    acute breathless and fever in adults,
      14
    acute breathless and fever in small
      child, 13-14
    breathlessness and wheeze, 14
    chronic cough and malaise, 14
    pleural effusion, 14
  examination, 12-13
  HIV and respiratory disease, 14-15
  investigations
    blood cultures, 13
    chest X-ray, 13
    lung function testing, 13
    pleural fluid, 13
    sputum/respiratory secretions, 13
rickettsial infections, 292
  African tick typhus, 293
    clinical features, 293
    treatment, 293
  louse-borne typhus, 292
    clinical features, 292
    treatment, 292
  scrub typhus, 292
    clinical features, 292-3
    treatment, 293
Ridley–Jopling classification, 167
rifampicin (R), 87
  leprosy, 169-70
rifaximin, 106
Rift Valley fever, 277, 281
ritonavir (RIT), 111
river blindness, *see* onchocerciasis
Roll Back Malaria (RBM) partnership, 66
Romaña's sign, 148
Ross River virus, 274

S

saquinavir (SQV), 111
scabies, 309
schistosomiasis, 151
  clinicopathological features
    acute disease, 154-5
    cercarial penetration, 154
    egg release, 155
    egg retention, 155-6
    initial illness, 154

neuroschistosomiasis, 156-7
  pathology at unusual sites, 157
epidemiology
  exposure and immunity, 153-4
  patterns, 153
  prevalence, 152
  progression to disease, 154
  reservoir hosts, 152-3
  transmission requirements, 152
future developments
  interactions with HIV, 162
  new diagnostics, 161
  new interventions, 161-2
investigation
  clinical syndromes, 158-9
  direct diagnosis, 157-8
  indirect diagnosis, 158
management, 159
  drug treatment, 159
  specific presentations, 160
parasitology, 151
  life-cycle, 151-2
prevention and public health aspects,
  160
  attack on snails, 160
  mass chemotherapy, 161
  reducing contact with infection,
    160-61
  reducing water contamination, 160
schizophrenia, 348
  treatment, 348
scorpion stings, 332
  management, 332
scrub typhus, 292
  clinical features, 292-3
  treatment, 293
sexually transmitted infections (STIs), 38
  flowchart use, 44
  flowcharts
    genital ulcer, 43
    lower abdominal pain in women,
      42
    urethral discharge in men, 40
    vaginal discharge, 41
  HIV testing, 45
  local adaptations, 39-40
  public health approach, need for, 38
  syndromic management, 38-9, 44
    advantages, 44-5
    disadvantages, 45
shigellosis, 183
sickle cell anaemia, 321
  clinical features, 322
  diagnosis, 322-3
  epidemiology, 322
  management, 323
  protection against malaria, 322
skin atrophy, 128
skin depigmentation, 128
skin itching, 30
skin nodules, 31
skin ulcers, 29-30

snakebite
    clinical features, 330
    diagnosis and initial assessment,
        330–31
    epidemiology and prevention, 332
    first aid, 330
    management, 331
        antivenom, 331
        other therapy, 331–2
sodium stibogluconate, 73
soil-transmitted helminths, 199–200
    ascariasis, 200–201
South American trypanosomiasis
    clinical features
        acute disease, 148
        chronic disease, 148–9
        immunocompromise, 149
    diagnosis
        other techniques, 149
        parasitological techniques, 149
    epidemiology and control, 149
    parasite, life-cycle and pathogenesis, 148
    treatment, 149
space-occupying lesions, 18
spastic paralysis, 251
    cause and anatomy, 251
    importance causes
        tuberculosis (TB), 251–2
    patient assessment, 251
    spinal epidural abscess, 252
        HIV myelopathy, 252–3
        subacute combined degeneration of
            the spinal cord (SACD), 253
        transverse myelitis, 252
        tropical spastic paraparesis, 253
Sphere Project, 355
spider bites, 332
    banana spiders, 333
    funnel-web spiders, 333
    recluse spiders, 332
    widow spiders, 332
spirometry, 13
splenic aspirate, 73
splenomegaly, 47
    causes, 47
    diagnostic clues, 48
    differential diagnosis, 71
    hyperreactive malarial splenomegaly,
        48–9
    massive tropical splenomegaly, 47
    splenectomy, 49
sporotrichosis, 320
    clinical features, 320
    treatment, 320
St Louis encephalitis virus, 245
stavudine (d4T), 110
steroids, 271
streptomycin (S), 87
Strongyloides stercoralis, 4
strongyloidiasis, 311
    autoinfection life-cycle, 311
    clinical features, 311–12

acute infection, 312
chronic disease, 312
hyperinfection, 312–13
diagnosis, 313
epidemiology and control, 313–14
treatment, 313
usual life-cycle, 311
subacute combined degeneration of the
    spinal cord (SACD), 253
suicidal patients, 349
sulfadoxine, 63
sulfalene, 63
suramin, 144

T

tachycardia, 12
tachypnoea, 12
tafenoquine, 63
tapeworms, 195
    clinical features, 196
    investigations, 196
    parasites and life-cycle, 195–6
    prevention and public health aspects,
        197–8
tenofovir (TDF), 111
tetanus
    bacteriology and pathogenesis, 259
    clinical manifestations, 259
        cephalic tetanus, 260
        generalized tetanus, 259
        localized tetanus, 260
        neonatal tetanus, 259
    diagnosis, 260
    epidemiology and prevention, 260
    treatment, 260
tetracycline, 181
    cholera, 188
β thalassaemia, 323
    clinical features, 323
    diagnosis, 323
    epidemiology, 323
    management, 323–4
tiabendazole, 313
tick-borne encephalitis virus, 245
tick-borne relapsing fever (TBRF), 289
tinidazole, 181
‹tool-deficient› diseases, 373
‹tool-ready› diseases, 372–3
torture and traumatic experiences, 356
toxocariasis
    clinical features, investigations and
        management, 203–4
    epidemiology, 203
    parasite and life-cycle, 203
    prevention and public health aspects,
        204
trachoma, 368–9
    management, 369–70
transverse myelitis, 252
triclabendazole, 215

trichuriasis
    clinical features, 203
    epidemiology, 202
    investigations, 203
    management, 203
    parasite and life-cycle, 202–3
    prevention, 203
Trichuris trichiura, 7
tropical pulmonary eosinophilia (TPE),
    231
    clinical features, 231
    diagnosis, 231
    epidemiology, 231
    investigation, 231
    prevention, 232
    treatment, 232
tropical spastic paraparesis, 253
tropical sprue, 4
tropical ulcer, 299
    clinical features, 299
    complications, 300
    epidemiology, 299
    microbiology, 299
    prevention, 300
    treatment, 300
trypanosomiasis, African, 141
    clinical picture
        early stage, 142–3
        late stage symptoms and signs, 143
    control and surveillance, 146
    diagnosis
        early stage, 143–4
        immunological diagnostic methods,
            144
        late stage (CNS involvement),
            144
    disease
        immune response and pathogenesis,
            142
        local effects, 141
        systemic effects, 141–2
    epidemiology, 145–6
    life-cycle, 141
    parasites, 141
    treatment, 144
        early stage, 144
        late stage, 144–5
        relapse, 145
trypanosomiasis, South American
    clinical features
        acute disease, 148
        chronic disease, 148–9
        immunocompromise, 149
    diagnosis
        other techniques, 149
        parasitological techniques, 149
    epidemiology and control, 149
    parasite, life-cycle and pathogenesis,
        148
    treatment, 149
tsetse flies, 141
tuberculoid leprosy, 167–8

tuberculosis (TB), 82
  clinical features
    extrapulmonary TB symptoms, 86
    HIV infection, effect of, 86
    pulmonary TB signs, 86
    pulmonary TB symptoms, 85
    pulmonary vs. extrapulmonary, 85
    systemic symptoms, 85
  epidemiology
    HIV infection, effect on TB, 85
    infection and immunity, 83–4
    prevalence, 82–3
    progression to disease, 84
    risk factors, 84
    transmission, 83
  future developments
    new diagnostics, 94
    new interventions, 94
  investigations, 86–7
  management
    adjunctive corticosteroid therapy, 92
    chemotherapy principles, 87–8
    isolation, 91–2
    multidrug-resistant (MDR) and
      extremely drug-resistant (XDR)
      TB, 90
    patients, new, 89–90
    patients, previously treated, 90
    regimen selection, 89, 91
    treatment monitoring, 90–91
  pleural effusion, 14
  prevention, 92
    BCG vaccination, 92
    DOTS strategy, 92–4
    HIV infection, 93–4
    isoniazid preventive therapy, 92
    Stop TB Strategy, 94
  spastic paralysis, 251–2
tuberculosis (TB), intestinal, 4
Tumbu fly, 305
typhoid and paratyphoid fevers, 267
  carrier state, 271
    treament of chronic carriers, 271
  diagnosis
    culture, 269
    other laboratory findings, 269
    serodiagnosis, 269
  infection mode, 267
  organisms, 267
  paratyphoid A and B, 272
  paratyphoid C, 272
  treatment, 269
    amoxicillin, 271
    azithromycin, 271
    cephalosporins, third-generation, 271

chemotherapy, 269–70
    chloramphenicol, 271
    co-trimoxazole, 271
    fluoroquinolones, 270–71
    steroids, 271
  typhoid fever, 267–8
    clinical fever, 268
    complications, 268–9
    physical signs, 268
  typhoid vaccine, 271–2

U

ulcerated skin, 29–30
urethral discharge in men flowchart, 40
urticaria, 31

V

vaginal discharge flowchart, 41
vesicles, 32
viral haemorhhagic fevers (VHFs), 276
  Crimean–Congo haemorrhagic fever,
    281
  diagnosis, 279
    differential diagnosis, 279
  Ebola and Marburg haemorrhagic
    fevers, 280
  ecological overview, 277
  emerging viruses, 281
  epidemiology, 276
  identification in febrile patients, 276
    algorithm, 278
  Lassa fever, 280
  management, 276, 279–80
  pathogenesis, 276
  renal syndrome, 281
  Rift Valley fever, 281
  South American haemorrhagic fevers,
    280
viral hepatitis, 205
  clinicoepidemiological features, 205
  hepatitis A (HAV), 205–6
  hepatitis B (HBV), 206–9
    immunization, 209
    prevalence, 208
  hepatitis C (HCV), 210–11
  hepatitis D (HDV), 210
  hepatitis E (HEV), 211–12
visceral larva migrans (VLM), 203
visceral leishmaniasis (VL), 70
  clinical features, 71
  epidemiology, 70

HIV co-infection, 71–2
  investigations
    circumstantial evidence, 72
    parasitological evidence, 72–3
    serological tests, 72
    splenic aspirate, 73
  management, 73
    aminosidine (paromomycin), 74
    amphotericin B, 73–4
    amphotericin B, liposomal, 74
    combination treatment, 74
    miltefosine, 74
    pentamidine, 74
    pentavalent antimonials (SbV), 73
  parasite life-cycle, 70–71
  post-kala-azar dermal leishmaniasis
    (PKDL), 74–5
  prevention, 75
    prospects for Indian subcontinent,
      76
    targeting reservoir host, 75
    targeting vector, 75–6
  viscerotropic leishmaniasis, 71
vitamin A, 363
  deficiency leading to eye disease,
    366–8
vitamin B1 (thiamine), 363
vitamin B12 deficiency, 328
  clinical features, 328
  investigations, 328–9
  management, 329
vitamin C, 363
vitamin D, 363

W

West Nile virus, 245
wheezing, 14
whitewater Arroyo virus, 280
whooping cough, 11–12
Winterbottom's sign, 142

Y

yellow fever, 277
  clinical features, 287
  control, 287
  epidemiology, 287

Z

zidovudine (AZT; ZDV), 110